CARDIOVASCULAR
TOXICOLOGY

TARGET ORGAN TOXICOLOGY SERIES

Series Editors

A. Wallace Hayes, John A. Thomas, and Donald E. Gardner

Cardiovascular Toxicology, Fourth Edition. *Daniel Acosta, Jr., editor, 712 pp., 2008*

Toxicology of the Gastrointestinal Tract. *Shayne C. Gad, editor, 384 pp., 2007*

Immunotoxicology and Immunopharmacology, Third Edition. *Robert Luebke, Robert House, and Ian Kimber, editors, 676 pp., 2007*

Toxicology of the Lung, Fourth Edition. *Donald E. Gardner, editor, 696 pp., 2006*

Toxicology of the Pancreas. *Parviz M. Pour, editor, 720 pp., 2005*

Toxicology of the Kidney, Third Edition. *Joan B. Tarloff and Lawrence H. Lash, editors, 1200 pp., 2004*

Ovarian Toxicology. *Patricia B. Hoyer, editor, 248 pp., 2004*

Cardiovascular Toxicology, Third Edition. *Daniel Acosta, Jr., editor, 616 pp., 2001*

Nutritional Toxicology, Second Edition. *Frank N. Kotsonis and Maureen A. Mackey, editors, 480 pp., 2001*

Toxicology of Skin. *Howard I. Maibach, editor, 558 pp., 2000*

Neurotoxicology, Second Edition. *Hugh A. Tilson and G. Jean Harry, editors, 386 pp., 1999*

Toxicant–Receptor Interactions: Modulation of Signal Transductions and Gene Expression. *Michael S. Denison and William G. Helferich, editors, 256 pp., 1998*

Toxicology of the Liver, Second Edition. *Gabriel L. Plaa and William R. Hewitt, editors, 444 pp., 1997*

Free Radical Toxicology. *Kendall B. Wallace, editor, 454 pp., 1997*

Endocrine Toxicology, Second Edition. *Raphael J. Witorsch, editor, 336 pp., 1995*

Carcinogenesis. *Michael P. Waalkes and Jerrold M. Ward, editors, 496 pp., 1994*

Developmental Toxicology, Second Edition. *Carole A. Kimmel and Judy Buelke-Sam, editors, 496 pp., 1994*

Nutritional Toxicology. *Frank N. Kotsonis, Maureen A. Mackey, and Jerry J. Hjelle, editors, 336 pp., 1994*

Ophthalmic Toxicology. *George C. Y. Chiou, editor, 352 pp., 1992*

Toxicology of the Blood and Bone Marrow. *Richard D. Irons, editor, 192 pp., 1985*

Toxicology of the Eye, Ear, and Other Special Senses. *A. Wallace Hayes, editor, 264 pp., 1985*

Cutaneous Toxicity. *Victor A. Drill and Paul Lazar, editors, 288 pp., 1984*

CARDIOVASCULAR TOXICOLOGY

FOURTH EDITION

Edited by
Daniel Acosta, Jr.
University of Cincinnati
Cincinnati, Ohio, USA

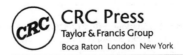

CRC Press
Taylor & Francis Group
Boca Raton London New York

CRC Press is an imprint of the
Taylor & Francis Group, an **informa** business

CRC Press
Taylor & Francis Group
6000 Broken Sound Parkway NW, Suite 300
Boca Raton, FL 33487-2742

First issued in paperback 2019

© 2008 by Taylor & Francis Group, LLC
CRC Press is an imprint of Taylor & Francis Group, an Informa business

No claim to original U.S. Government works

ISBN-13: 978-1-4200-4473-7 (hbk)
ISBN-13: 978-0-367-38695-5 (hbk)

Library of Congress Cataloging-in-Publication Data

Cardiovascular toxicology / edited by Daniel Acosta Jr. — 4th ed.
    p. ; cm. — (Target organ toxicology series ; 25)
    Includes bibliographical references and index.
    ISBN-13: 978-1-4200-4473-7 (hb : alk. paper)
    ISBN-10: 1-4200-4473-7 (hb : alk. paper) 1. Cardiovascular toxicology. I. Acosta, Daniel, 1945- II. Series.
    [DNLM: 1. Cardiovascular Diseases–chemically induced.
  2. Cardiovascular System—drug effects. WG 100 C267 2008]
    RC677.C37 2008
    616.1'07—dc22

                                      2008015485

For Corporate Sales and Reprint Permissions call 212-520-2700 or write to: Sales Department, 52 Vanderbilt Avenue, 7th floor, New York, NY 10017.

Visit the Informa Web site at
www.informa.com

and the Informa Healthcare Web site at
www.informahealthcare.com

Preface

The first three editions of *Cardiovascular Toxicology* provide the foundation for the latest, fourth edition of this monograph. The first edition, edited by Ethard Van Stee, was published in 1982, and the next two editions, edited by Daniel Acosta, Jr., were published in 1992 and 2001, respectively. The central theme of this book is to provide an in-depth overview of myocardial and vascular toxicity of chemical agents.

It is one of the few toxicology texts that focus entirely on toxicity of chemicals to the cardiovascular system. In addition, the monograph separates the discussion of the cardiovascular system into the heart and vascular system, which is not commonly found in other texts.

The latest edition continues to focus on mechanistic and molecular aspects of chemical injury to the heart and the vasculature. Furthermore, it comprises several key sections beyond general cardiovascular toxicology, such as a major review on advances in the field, an up-to-date review of ischemic cell injury, and advances in methodology for measuring and evaluating cardiovascular function and toxicity. An attempt has been made to provide pertinent information on key, well-known cardiovascular toxicants. Thus, many of the chapters are categorized as to the cardiovascular toxic effects of major chemical and therapeutic classes of drugs, industrial agents, and pollutants. The authors have revised and updated all of the previous chapters with the latest findings in their respective areas of interest; several of the chapters have new authors, which brings a new perspective to the topic.

We believe that the fourth edition will serve as a useful reference to clinicians, public health officials, industrial and experimental toxicologists, and other interested professionals. This monograph may also serve as a recommended or supplementary text for advanced graduate courses in target organ toxicology and may assist students and health professionals pursuing a career in academia, industry, or government.

Daniel Acosta, Jr.
September, 2008

Contributors

Peter G. Anderson Department of Pathology, University of Alabama at Birmingham, Birmingham, Alabama, U.S.A.

Amarjit S. Arneja Institute of Cardiovascular Sciences, St. Boniface General Hospital Research Centre, and Departments of Physiology and Internal Medicine, Faculty of Medicine, University of Manitoba, Winnipeg, Canada

Scott M. Belcher Department of Pharmacology and Cell Biophysics, University of Cincinnati College of Medicine, Cincinnati, Ohio, U.S.A.

Paul J. Boor Department of Pathology, University of Texas Medical Branch, Galveston, Texas, U.S.A.

Nachman Brautbar Keck School of Medicine, University of Southern California, Los Angeles, California, U.S.A.

Brigitta C. Brott Interventional Cardiology, University of Alabama at Birmingham, Birmingham, Alabama, U.S.A.

L. Maximilian Buja Department of Pathology and Laboratory Medicine, The University of Texas Health Science Center, and Department of Cardiovascular Pathology, Texas Heart Institute, St. Luke's Episcopal Hospital, Houston, Texas, U.S.A.

Cynthia A. Carnes College of Pharmacy, and Davis Heart and Lung Research Institute, The Ohio State University, Columbus, Ohio, U.S.A.

Enrique Chacon Organ Transport Systems, Inc., Frisco, Texas, U.S.A.

Daniel J. Conklin Department of Medicine, Division of Cardiology, University of Louisville, Louisville, Kentucky, U.S.A.

Melissa R. Dent   Institute of Cardiovascular Sciences, St. Boniface General Hospital Research Centre, and Departments of Physiology and Internal Medicine, Faculty of Medicine, University of Manitoba, Winnipeg, Canada

Naranjan S. Dhalla   Institute of Cardiovascular Sciences, St. Boniface General Hospital Research Centre, and Departments of Physiology and Internal Medicine, Faculty of Medicine, University of Manitoba, Winnipeg, Canada

Colleen Doherty   Millennium Pharmaceuticals, Inc., Cambridge, Massachusetts, U.S.A.

Mitchell S. Finkel   Departments of Medicine; Behavioral Medicine and Psychiatry; Physiology and Pharmacology; Robert C. Byrd Health Sciences Center, West Virginia University School of Medicine, Morgantown, West Virginia and Louis A. Johnson VA Medical Center, Clarksburg, West Virginia, U.S.A.

Shayne C. Gad   Gad Consulting Services, Cary, North Carolina, U.S.A.

Gary Gintant   Department of Integrative Pharmacology, Global Pharmaceutical Research and Development, Volwiler Society, Abbott Laboratories, Abbott Park, Illinois, U.S.A.

Stanton A. Glantz   Division of Cardiology, Department of Medicine, Center for Tobacco Control Research and Education, Cardiovascular Research Institute, University of California, San Francisco, California, U.S.A.

Robert Hamlin   Veterinary Biosciences, Davis Heart and Lung Research Institute, The Ohio State University, Columbus, Ohio, U.S.A.

Daniel P. Healy   James L. Winkle College of Pharmacy, University of Cincinnati Health Science Center, Cincinnati, Ohio, U.S.A.

Vivek Kadambi   Millennium Pharmaceuticals, Inc., Cambridge, Massachusetts, U.S.A.

Y. James Kang   Department of Medicine, University of Louisville School of Medicine, Louisville, Kentucky, U.S.A.

Richard H. Kennedy   Department of Physiology, Loyola University Medical Center, Stritch School of Medicine, Maywood, Illinois, U.S.A.

John J. Lemasters   Departments of Pharmaceutical & Biomedical Sciences and Biochemistry & Molecular Biology, Medical University of South Carolina, Charleston, South Carolina, U.S.A.

Russell B. Melchert   Department of Pharmaceutical Sciences, University of Arkansas for Medical Sciences, College of Pharmacy, Little Rock, Arkansas, U.S.A.

Donald Mishra Departments of Medicine; Behavioral Medicine and Psychiatry; Physiology and Pharmacology; Robert C. Byrd Health Sciences Center, West Virginia University School of Medicine, Morgantown, West Virginia and Louis A. Johnson VA Medical Center, Clarksburg, West Virginia, U.S.A.

William F. Pettit Department of Behavioral Medicine and Psychiatry; West Virginia Initiative for Innate Health and Robert C. Byrd Health Sciences Center, West Virginia University School of Medicine, Morgantown, West Virginia, U.S.A.

Jane Pruemer University of Cincinnati College of Pharmacy, Cincinnati, Ohio, U.S.A.

Kenneth S. Ramos Department of Biochemistry and Molecular Biology, University of Louisville School of Medicine, Louisville, Kentucky, U.S.A.

Franco Rossi Cardiovascular Research Institute, Department of Cell Biology and Molecular Medicine, University of Medicine and Dentistry of New Jersey, New Jersey Medical School, Newark, New Jersey, U.S.A.

Zadok Ruben Patoximed Consultants, Westfield, New Jersey, U.S.A.

You-Tang Shen Cardiovascular Research Institute, Department of Cell Biology and Molecular Medicine, University of Medicine and Dentistry of New Jersey, New Jersey Medical School, Newark, New Jersey, U.S.A.

Joseph W. Starnes Department of Kinesiology, University of Texas at Austin, Austin, Texas, U.S.A.

Stephen F. Vatner Cardiovascular Research Institute, Department of Cell Biology and Molecular Medicine, University of Medicine and Dentistry of New Jersey, New Jersey Medical School, Newark, New Jersey, U.S.A.

E. Spencer Williams Chemrisk, Inc., Houston, Texas, U.S.A.

John A. Williams, II Nachman Brautbar, M.D., Inc., Los Angeles, California, U.S.A.

Michael P. Wu Nachman Brautbar, M.D., Inc., Los Angeles, California, U.S.A.

Advances in Cardiovascular Toxicology

Y. James Kang

*Department of Medicine, University of Louisville School of Medicine,
Louisville, Kentucky, U.S.A.*

INTRODUCTION

Cardiovascular toxicity is virtually associated, directly or indirectly, with all chemicals and drugs that cause deteriorating effects in mammalian system. However, cardiovascular toxicology has not been fully developed until recently. The significance of cardiovascular toxicity in environmental health, clinical practice, and drug discovery and development had been underestimated. There were not enough clinical and environmental studies that addressed the issue of cardiovascular toxicity, and drug discovery and development had largely ignored the concern of cardiovascular toxicity. However, over the past decade, cardiovascular toxicity has become a growing concern of clinical practice, environmental health, and drug discovery and development. There are several review articles that have provided some current knowledge of cardiovascular toxicology (1–4). In this book, advances in different aspects of cardiovascular toxicology are presented in respective chapters. In this chapter, a general view of new understanding of cardiovascular toxicology will be discussed with a focus on basic concepts and critical areas that significantly affect the advances in cardiovascular toxicology.

The most significant advance in cardiovascular toxicology over the past decade is the realization of cardiovascular toxicology as an important subdiscipline of toxicology, of which we previously only had a superficial understanding. The advances in cardiovascular toxicology have been benefited from two important areas of development in cardiovascular medicine; the first is the application of the most advanced approaches and technology in the cardiovascular system, and the second is new knowledge of molecular biology of the cardiovascular system. Advanced approaches include more sophisticated animal models such as gene knock-in and knock-out rodent models of cardiovascular diseases. Recent exploration of genomics and proteomics in cardiovascular system has greatly helped generate new knowledge of cardiovascular signaling pathways, which also becomes an invaluable asset in understanding cardiovascular toxicology. The application of metabolomics is another new technological advance in cardiovascular toxicology, which in combination with genomics and proteomics would provide a multiple dimensional view of cardiovascular toxicity and greatly assist the development and validation of biomarkers for cardiovascular toxicity.

Several areas of cardiovascular studies have provided new insights into cardiovascular toxicity. Toxic effects on or toxic interference with signaling pathways in cardiovascular system have been extensively explored. Cardiovascular adaptive versus maladaptive responses to toxic substances under environmental exposure or clinical setting have drawn more attention to the field. We now appreciate much more than before the crucial role of mitochondrial damage in the development of cardiovascular toxicity as well as the contribution of the persistence of mitochondrial damage to irreversible cardiovascular injury. Among the most important advances in this field is the toxic effect of chemicals and drugs on myocardial regeneration and the subsequent effect on myocardial recovery from injuries.

The most intensive and devoted area of studies in cardiovascular medicine over the past decade, perhaps, is apoptosis. The role of apoptosis in the initiation and progression of cardiovascular diseases has been repeatedly studied in both animal models and human patients. Apoptosis is also the central topic in cardiovascular toxicology. The emergence of some new areas of cardiovascular medicine has called for the expertise in cardiovascular toxicology. The link between air pollution and cardiovascular diseases has been recognized and has drawn attention from both clinical practice and environmental health action. This gives rise to an opportunity as well as a challenge in the field of cardiovascular toxicology to provide a comprehensive understanding of the link between air pollution and cardiovascular diseases. The treatment of AIDS by a highly active antiretroviral therapy (HAART) has proven to be highly effective. However, this treatment is associated with cardiovascular toxicity, to which clinical monitoring or treatment has to be implemented. The cardiovascular toxicity of the HAART has thus become another area of studies in the field. The most explored area in drug discovery and development in both the pharmaceutical industry and regulatory sectors is the cardiovascular toxicity test. Several of the tests such as QT prolongation that had been ignored in the past have now become mandatory for drug development. These new challenges in environmental health, clinical practice, and drug development thus demand reliable biomarkers to predict as well as diagnose cardiovascular toxicity. The development and validation of biomarkers for cardiovascular toxicity has been an important undertaking over the past decade.

Cardiovascular toxicology is at an exponential phase of growth. Looking to the future, the demand for a comprehensive understanding of cardiovascular toxicology is very high. The mechanisms of action of drugs that have been known to cause cardiovascular toxicity have not been fully understood. New areas of cardiovascular toxicity of drugs or therapeutics are emerging. For instance, cardiotoxicity of cellular therapy for cardiac diseases and side effects of mechanical assist device for heart failure on cardiovascular system are new challenges in the field. The adaptation of more advanced approaches and techniques to formulate more integrated assessment of cardiovascular toxicity will greatly help the creation of new knowledge of cardiovascular toxicology.

ADVANCED APPROACHES TO THE UNDERSTANDING OF CARDIOVASCULAR TOXICOLOGY

Over the past decade, new techniques and novel animal models for cardiovascular diseases have greatly assisted the understanding of cardiovascular toxicology. The ultimate functional effect of cardiac toxic manifestations is the decreased cardiac output and reduced peripheral tissue perfusion, resulting from alterations in signaling pathways, energy metabolism, cellular structure and function, electrophysiology, and contractility of the heart. The studies of the effects of xenobiotics on these cellular and molecular events in the cardiovascular system have been greatly benefited from the advanced approaches and techniques.

Genetic Manipulation Animal Models

Manipulation of genes responsible for cardiac function began in the mid 1990s (5). The most important conclusion of these studies is that a sustained expression of any single mutated functional gene, either in the form of gain-of-function or loss-of-function, can lead to a significant phenotype, often in the form of cardiac hypertrophy and heart failure (5,6). Although there are not many genetic manipulation animal models that were specifically generated as a surrogate for cardiovascular toxicity screening, the studies of cardiovascular toxicity have employed many fully characterized genetic manipulation animal models for the understanding of mechanisms of cardiovascular toxicity. Studies using these genetic manipulation animal models have concluded that it is difficult to apply the knowledge generated from these animal models to human patients. First, the acquired cardiac disease such as heart failure is the result of interaction between environmental factors and genetic susceptibility, indicating the role of polymorphisms. Second, extrinsic and intrinsic stresses produce lesions that cannot be explained by a single gene or a single pathway, suggesting complexity between deleterious factors and the cardiovascular system. A comprehensive understanding of the consequence of the interaction between the exposure to environmental stressors and genetic susceptibility is required to pave the road of translation of the knowledge generated from these animal models to human patients.

Genomics and Proteomics

Many more mechanistic insights into cardiovascular diseases have been obtained from the studies of cardiovascular genomics and proteomics. Although there are fundamental differences between genomics and proteomics, from the subjective area to the technology platform, they are complementary. The knowledge of DNA sequence and expression control through genomic studies is essential, but not sufficient. A more meaningful understanding of gene expression can be achieved through characterization of the products expressed from the genes. A comprehensive understanding of cardiovascular diseases thus requires an integrated approach employing both genomics and proteomics techniques. The application of genomics and proteomics in cardiovascular toxicology started only very recently. Multiple genes that were affected by exposure to environmental toxic substances or therapeutic drugs have been analyzed under different experimental settings (7–9). These studies focused on expressional genomics, i.e., the profile of changes in gene expression under toxic exposure conditions. It is, however, important to understand the sequential aspect of these changes through the study of functional genomics. Proteomic analysis of toxic exposure to cardiovascular system has paralleled the progression of genomics studies. Further exploration of genomics and proteomics in cardiovascular toxicology for more meaningful understanding of cardiovascular toxicity is required and can be predicted to be fruitful.

Metabolomics in Cardiovascular Toxicology

The application of metabolomics has just begun in cardiovascular biology and medicine. The significance of metabolomics in cardiovascular toxicology has not been fully appreciated, but the impact of metabolomics on the understanding of cardiovascular toxicity would be unprecedentedly vast. Metabolomics is a recently developed technology to evaluate the metabolic status of a subject under different conditions, or a patient under disease conditions. This technology is based on the principle that homeostatic alterations during disease processes or toxic exposure can be reflected directly or indirectly in the blood, and many ultimately leave biomolecular traces in urine. Therefore, the metabolic profile of a subject under different conditions provides diagnostic indication of the disease progression or the extent of toxicosis. Traditional biomarkers of diseases or toxic exposure are a panel of metabolic indicators, and each biomarker has been measured individually. However, the application of metabolomics is to evaluate the disease condition or the status of toxic exposure through recognition of patterns of changes of many metabolic molecules, providing a comprehensive diagnosis and prediction. In addition, metabolomics will greatly assist the identification, development, and validation of new biomarkers for cardiovascular toxicology.

TOXIC EFFECTS ON SIGNALING PATHWAYS IN CARDIOVASCULAR SYSTEM

The most dramatic exploration of the knowledge in the cardiovascular system is the signal transduction pathways over the past decade. This knowledge greatly benefits the growth of cardiovascular toxicology. It is, however, important to distinguish the toxic effect on signaling pathways from toxic signaling pathways in the cardiovascular system. Most of the cardiovascular toxicology studies, if not all, have addressed the effect of toxic exposure on signal transduction pathways in the system. Although some toxic signaling pathways have been identified, such as the high-affinity binding of 2,3,7,8-tetrachlorodibenzo-p-dioxin (TCDD) to the aryl hydrocarbon receptor (AhR), the significance of these toxic signaling pathways in the cardiovascular system has not been fully understood. However, it has been shown that the AhR-null mice develop cardiac hypertrophy (10).

Cardiac Responses to Toxic Exposure

In the heart, a dynamic change takes place in response to toxic or pathological insults. At the cellular level, these changes express in the form of cell death, cell growth in size or hypertrophy, and renewal of lost myocardial cells—regeneration. Cell death in the mode of apoptosis is controlled by specified signaling pathways, which will be discussed in the section of apoptosis and cardiovascular toxicity. It had been viewed that after birth, the myocytes in the heart, i.e., a terminally differentiated organ can undergo hypertrophy growth—an increase in the size of individual myocytes, but not hyperplasia—an increase in the number of myocytes. This view has been challenged recently because of the identification of cardiac progenitor cells that are capable of differentiating to cardiac myocytes and forming vascular structures (11). Myocardial regeneration is a new area of cardiac biology and medicine. The signaling pathways leading to myocardial regeneration remain elusive. In contrast, the signaling pathways leading to cardiac hypertrophy have been extensively studied. Many studies addressing toxic effects on signaling pathways in the heart have focused on cardiac hypertrophy signal transduction pathways.

Signaling Pathways That Lead to Cardiac Hypertrophy

The stimuli for cardiac hypertrophy can be simply categorized into mechanical and neurohumoral. We now have a much better understanding of the neurohumoral factors and their signal transduction pathways that lead to cardiac hypertrophy, but little understanding of the mechanical signal transduction pathways. Ligands, including hormones, cytokines, chemokines, and peptide growth factors, trigger the signal transduction pathways by interaction with a

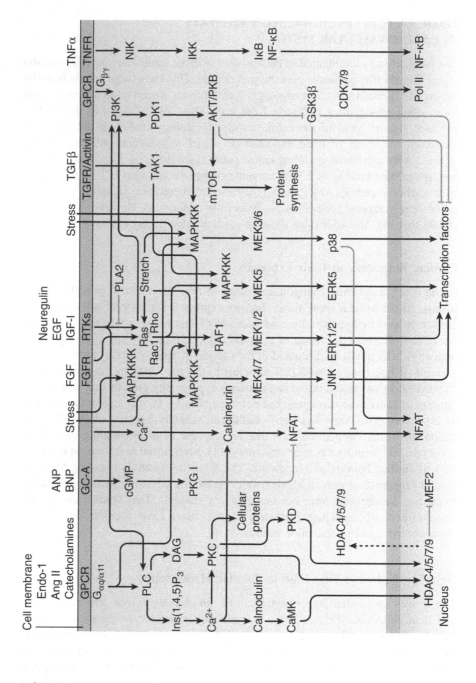

Scheme 1

(*Continued*)

diversity of membrane-bound G-protein-coupled receptors, receptors that have intracellular serine/threonine, or tyrosine kinase domains, and gp130-linked receptors. The signal transduction pathways mediating the action of these ligands are multitude and complex. The major pathways that have been demonstrated in the heart of animal models include mitogen-activated protein kinase (MAPK) pathways, calcineurin-nuclear factor of activated T cells (NFAT) pathway, insulin-like growth factor-I-phosphatidylinositol-3-kinase (PI3K)-AKT/protein kinase B (PKB) pathway, and guanosine $3',5'$-cyclic monophosphate (cGMP)/protein kinase G (PKG) pathway (a negative regulatory pathway). Scheme 1 summarizes these signal transduction pathways and their interactions.

Toxic Effects on the Signal Transduction Pathways

The toxic effect on signaling pathways can be simply viewed as a process that switches the adaptive responses to the deteriorating signaling pathways. This process can be expressed by switching the cell survival to the cell death (both apoptosis and necrosis) program, the adaptive to the maladaptive or pathological hypertrophy, and the reversible to the irreversible injury through inhibition of regeneration. In the following sections, each of these aspects will be discussed. It is, however, important to note that in response to toxic insults, several signaling

←——————————————————————————————

Scheme 1 Overview of signaling transduction pathways involved in cardiac hypertrophic growth and their cross-talk interactions. The signalling that occurs at the sarcolemmal membrane is shown at the top, and the intermediate transduction of signals by various kinases and phosphatases is shown in the middle. The nucleus is shown at the bottom. *Abbreviations*: ANP, atrial natriuretic peptide; Ang II, angiotensin II; BNP, B-type natriuretic peptide; CaMK, calmodulin-dependent kinase; CDK, cyclin-dependent kinase; DAG, diacylglycerol; EGF, epidermal growth factor; Endo-1, endothelin-1; ERK, extracellular signal-regulated kinase; FGF, fibroblast growth factor; FGFR, FGF receptor; GC-A, guanyl cyclase-A; GPCR, G-protein-coupled receptors; GSK3β, glycogen synthase kinase-3β; HDAC, histone deacetylases; IκB, inhibitor of NF-κB; IGF-I, insulin-like growth factor-I; IKK, inhibitor of NF-κB kinase; Ins(1,4,5)P₃, inositol-1,4,5-trisphosphate; JNK, c-Jun N-terminal kinase; MAPKKK, mitogen-activated protein kinase kinase kinase; MAPKKKK, MAPKKK kinase; MEF, myocyte enhancer factor; MEK, mitogen-activated protein kinase kinase; mTOR, mammalian target of rapamycin; NFAT, nuclear factor of activated T cells; NF-κB, nuclear factor-κB; NIK, NF-κB-inducing kinase; PDK, phosphoinositide-dependent kinase; PI3K, phosphatidylinositol 3-kinase; PKB, protein kinase B; PKC, protein kinase C; PKD, protein kinase D; PLA2, phospholipase A2; PLC, phospholipase C; Pol II, RNA polymerase II; RTK, receptor tyrosine kinase; TAK, TGFβ-activated kinase; TGFb, transforming growth factor-b; TGFR, TGF receptor; TNFα, tumor necrosis factor-α; TNFR, TNFα receptor. *Source*: From Ref. 51.

pathways involved in the stress response in the heart are activated, leading to adaptive responses. Although these responses can be referred to as an indication of toxic insults, these adaptive responses cannot be considered as toxicosis. Only the adaptive process is switched to the deteriorating consequence should cardiac toxicity express. In this context, activation of MAPK pathways in the heart in response to toxic exposure is a stress response that may lead to adaptation in the form of cardiac hypertrophy. However, if myocardial cell death, cardiac dysfunction, cardiomyopathy, and eventual heart failure result from the toxic exposure, the heart is considered to undergo toxicosis.

APOPTOSIS AND CARDIOVASCULAR TOXICITY

The recognition of the role of apoptosis in the development of heart failure over the past decade has significantly enhanced our knowledge of cardiovascular diseases (12–14). The attention to the role of apoptosis in cardiomyopathy has been far more intense than any other topics in the investigation of cardiovascular toxicity over the past decade. Virtually, all drugs and chemicals whose cardiovascular toxicity is of concern can cause apoptosis (1). There are two major pathways that have been identified to function extensively in the cardiovascular system to regulate apoptosis: the mitochondrion-controlled pathway (15) and the death receptor-mediated pathway (16).

Mitochondrial Factors in Cardiovascular Cell Death

Cytochrome c and pro-caspase-3 are factors that are preexisting and activated by toxic insults. The early event of mitochondrion-controlled apoptotic pathway is the mitochondrial permeability transition (MPT) pore opening and cytochrome c release (17). There are several potential mechanisms that control the MPT pore opening. The first is related to defective oxidative phosphorylation (18). Such a change may cause the loss of mitochondrial homeostasis and high-amplitude mitochondrial swelling. Since the inner membrane has a larger surface area than the outer membrane, mitochondrial swelling can cause the rupture of the outer membrane, releasing intermembrane proteins such as cytochrome c into the cytosol. Another possible mechanism that leads to mitochondrial cytochrome c release is the action of Bax, a proapoptotic protein of the Bcl-2 family (19). Overexpression of Bax under oxidative stress conditions has been observed in a number of studies on the heart. It has been shown that Bax is translocated from cytosol to mitochondria and forms pores in mitochondrial outer membranes, leaving the inner membranes intact. A newly identified mechanism is that cardiac mitochondria initiate slow waves of depolarization and Ca^{2+} release, which propagate through the cell to form a traveling wave that involves MPT pore opening and cytochrome c-mediated apoptosis (20).

Death Receptor-Mediated Apoptotic Signaling Pathway

Cytokines that trigger the death receptor signaling pathways have been studied in cardiovascular system. Among these cytokines is tumor necrosis factor α (TNF-α) (21), the most studied cytokine in myocardial cell death signaling pathways. Cardiomyocytes are both the source and the target of this cytokine. The pathway leading to TNF-α-induced myocardial apoptosis is mediated by TNF receptors, TNFR1 and TNFR2. TNF-α binding to these receptors leads to activation of caspase-8, which in turn cleaves BID, a BH3 domain-containing proapoptotic Bcl-2 family member. The truncated BID is translocated from cytosol to mitochondria, inducing first the clustering of mitochondria around the nuclei and release of cytochrome c, and then the loss of mitochondrial membrane potential and activation of the apoptotic program. Caspase-8 also directly activates caspase-3, leading to apoptosis. Besides TNF-α, Fas ligand is also able to induce apoptosis of cardiomyocytes through the death receptor-mediated signaling pathway (22).

Interactions Between Cell Death Pathways

These multiple pathways mediated by mitochondrial factors and death receptors suggest that there is a bewildering diversity of programmed cell death paradigms, eventually leading to caspase-3 activation and apoptosis. Under chronic toxic insults, the relative importance of mitochondrial electron transport defects, MPT, cytochrome c leakage, and nonmitochondrial factors needs to be carefully examined. There are two important questions that need to be carefully addressed. First, how important is apoptosis in the overall pathogenesis of the cardiovascular system under different conditions? It is essentially a universal observation that apoptosis is involved in the cardiovascular toxicity of drugs and chemicals; however, there is very limited information regarding its significance in quantitative contributions to cardiovascular diseases. This concern is followed by the second important question: Can caspase inhibitors offer long-term protection against cell death leading to prevention of cardiovascular toxicity? It is important to note that apoptosis and necrosis are linked phenomena. For instance, some studies have shown that caspase inhibitors effectively inhibited apoptosis, but cell death still occurs by necrosis (23). It is thus important to define the most efficient approach in blocking cell death in the cardiovascular system rather than in inhibiting a particular cell death program (1). Such studies would greatly benefit from the application of genomics, proteomics, and metabonomics in the cardiovascular system.

ADAPTIVE AND MALADAPTIVE RESPONSES TO TOXIC EXPOSURE

Myocardial adaptation refers to the general process by which the ventricular myocardium changes in structure and function in response to endogenous and exogenous stressors. This process is often referred to as "remodeling." During maturation, myocardial remodeling is a normal feature for adaptation to increased demands. However, in response to pathological stimuli, such as exposure to environmental toxicants, myocardial remodeling is adaptive in the short term, but is maladaptive in the long term, and often results in cardiac dysfunction. The central feature of myocardial remodeling is an increase in myocardial mass associated with a change in the shape of the ventricle (24).

At the cellular level, the increase in myocardial mass is reflected by cardiac myocyte hypertrophy, which is characterized by enhanced protein synthesis, heightened organization of the sarcomere, and the eventual increase in cell size. At the molecular level, the phenotype changes in cardiac myocytes are associated with reintroduction of the so-called fetal gene program, characterized by the patterns of gene expression mimicking those seen during embryonic development. These cellular and molecular changes are observed in both adaptive and maladaptive responses, thus distinguishing adaptive from maladaptive responses is difficult.

Adaptive Response

In response to physiological stimulation or pathological or toxic insults, the heart undergoes molecular, anatomical, and physiological changes to maintain its function. This process is an adaptive response. Thus, physiological hypertrophy is considered as an adaptive response, which is an adjustment of cardiac function for an increased demand of cardiac output. Such an adaptive hypertrophy is the increase in cardiac mass after birth and in response to exercise. A biochemical distinction of the adaptive hypertrophy is that myocardial accumulation of collagen does not accompany the hypertrophy. Functionally, the increased mass is associated with enhanced contractility and cardiac output. In response to toxicologic stresses, the heart also often increases its mass, which has been viewed as an adaptive response as well. However, most recent evidence suggests that cardiac hypertrophy along with decreased contractility is a maladaptive process of the heart in response to intrinsic and extrinsic stresses.

Maladaptive Response

Although toxic stress–induced hypertrophy can normalize wall tension, it is a risk factor for sudden cardiac death and has a high potential to progress to overt heart failure. A distinction between adaptive and maladaptive hypertrophy is whether or not the hypertrophy is necessary for the compensatory function of the heart under stress conditions. Many studies using genetically manipulated mouse models, either in the form of gain-of-function or loss-of-function, have supported the hypothesis that cardiac hypertrophy is neither required nor necessarily compensatory. For instance, a forced expression of a dominant negative calcineurin mutant confers protection against hypertrophy and fibrosis after abdominal aortic construction (25). But, the elimination of hypertrophy by calcineurin suppression does not cause compromised hemodynamic changes over a period of several weeks (26). Therefore, in these experimental approaches, hypertrophic growth could be abolished in the presence of continuous pressure overload, but the compensatory response could not be compromised. An interesting observation is that an almost complete lack of cardiac hypertrophy in response to aortic banding in a transgenic mouse model was accompanied with a significant slower pace of deterioration of systolic function (27). These observations indicate that cardiac hypertrophy in response to extrinsic and intrinsic stress is not a compensatory response. However, cardiac hypertrophy under pathological or toxic exposure conditions increases the risk for malignant arrhythmia and heart failure, and thus is now viewed as a maladaptive response.

MYOCARDIAL REGENERATION AND RECOVERY FROM TOXIC INJURY

Cardiac injury is reversible if the injury can be recovered after the etiology is removed. Some toxic exposures lead to a long-term, persistent damage, which is irreversible. Myocardial regeneration is an area that is now extensively explored, but the effect of xenobiotics on myocardial regeneration has not been studied in parallel.

Myocardial Degeneration

The ultimate response of the heart to toxic exposure is myocardial degeneration, which can be measured by both morphological and functional changes. However, myocardial degeneration should not be considered an irreversible toxic response. In the past, the heart has been considered incapable of regenerating, so that cardiac injury in the form of cell loss or scar tissue formation was considered permanent damage to the heart. However, evidence now indicates that heart is capable of regeneration and recovery from injuries. Cardiac toxic responses or damage can also be divided into reversible and irreversible.

Myocardial cell death, fibrosis (scar tissue formation), and contractile dysfunction are considered as degenerative responses, which can result in cardiac arrhythmia, hypertrophy, and heart failure. If acute cardiac toxicity does not affect the capacity of myocardial regeneration, the degenerative phenotype is reversible, otherwise irreversible. Both acute and chronic toxic stresses can lead to irreversible degeneration, depending on whether or not the cardiac repair mechanisms are damaged. Cell death is the most common phenotype of myocardial degeneration. Both apoptosis and necrosis occur along with hypertrophy of the remaining cardiac myocytes so that in the hypertrophic heart, the total number of cardiac myocytes is often reduced but the size or volume of individual cells is increased.

Myocardial remodeling

After cell death, not only is there an increase in the size of existing cardiac myocytes, but also cardiac fibrosis takes place. Myocardial fibrosis results from excess accumulation of extracellular matrix (ECM), which is mainly composed of collagens. The net accumulation of ECM connective tissue results from enhanced synthesis or diminished breakdown of the matrix, or both. Collagen contents, predominately type I and III, are the major fibrous proteins in ECM, and their synthesis may increase in response to toxic insults. The degradation of ECM is dependent on the activity of matrix metalloproteinases (MMPs). According to their substrate specificity, MMPs fall into five categories: colla-genases (MMP-1, -8, -13), gelatinases (MMP-2, -9), stromelysins (MMP-3, -7, -10, -11), membrane type MMPs (MMP-14, -15, -16, -17, -24, -25), and metal-loelastase (MMP-12). These MMPs are organ specific so that not all are present in the heart. The activities of these enzymes are altered during the processes of fibrogenesis and fibrinolysis. Under toxic exposure conditions, the imbalance between fibrogenesis and fibrinolysis leads to enhanced fibrogenesis and excess collagen accumulation—fibrosis.

Myocardial Regeneration

The mainstay of cardiac medicine had centered on the concept that the heart is a terminally differentiated organ and that cardiac myocytes are incapable of pro-liferating. Thus, cell death would lead to a permanent loss of the total number of cardiac myocytes. However, this view has been challenged recently because of the identification of cardiac progenitor cells (11). These cells are characterized and proposed to be responsible for cardiac repair because these cells can make myocytes and vascular structures. These cells possess the fundamental properties of stem cells; therefore, they are also called cardiac stem cells. They are self-renewing, clonogenic, and multipotent, as demonstrated by reconstitution of infarcted heart by intramyocardial injection of cardiac progenitor cells or the local activation of these cells by growth factors. It is important to note that toxicological studies of the cardiac progenitor cells have not been done. One speculation is that when cardiac progenitor cells are severely damaged, the potential for recovery from severe cardiac injury would be limited.

The removal of scar tissue or fibrosis in the myocardium in the past has been considered impossible. Although there are no studies that have shown whether or not the scar tissue is removable, there are observations in animal models of hypertensive heart disease that myocardial fibrosis is recoverable (28). It appears that if toxic exposure affects the capacity of collagen removal in the heart, such as inhibition of collagenases, the recovery from cardiac injury would be impaired and the injury would become irreversible.

Myocardial vascularization is required for myocardial regeneration. Many toxic insults affect the capacity of angiogenesis in the myocardium, so that cardiac ischemia occurs. The combination of cardiac ischemia and the direct toxic insults to cardiomyocytes constitute a synergistic damage to the heart. During regeneration, coronary arterioles and capillary structures are formed to bridge the dead tissue (scar tissue) and supply nutrients for the survival of the regenerated cardiomyocytes. There is an orderly organization of myocytes within the myocardium and a well-defined relationship between the myocytes and the capillary network. This proportion is altered under cardiac toxic conditions; either toxicologic hypertrophy or diminished capillary formation can lead to hypoperfusion to myocytes in the myocardium. Unfortunately, our understanding of toxic effects on myocardial angiogenesis is limited.

MITOCHONDRIAL DAMAGE AND CARDIOVASCULAR TOXICITY

The role of mitochondria in cardiovascular response to toxicants as well as therapeutic drugs has long been a focus of investigation. However, most of the studies in this field had remained descriptive. Over the past decade, a sharp increase in the number of studies on mitochondrial pathogenesis and its contribution to cardiomyopathy was observed. There are some new insights into mitochondrion-mediated cardiovascular toxicity. These studies appeared to confirm the essential role of mitochondria in triggering as well as propagating cardiovascular toxic response; however, the molecular mechanisms leading to mitochondrial involvement in the pathogenesis remain elusive. There are several aspects of mitochondrion-mediated cardiovascular toxicity that are worthy to be highlighted, including the role of mitochondria in controlling myocardial cell death, defective mitochondrial oxidative phosphorylation, abnormal mitochondrial biosynthesis, and generation of reactive oxygen species (ROS).

Mitochondrial Control of Cell Death

There are many studies that have focused on the role of mitochondria in controlling myocardial cell death in response to different toxic insults and under different disease conditions. There are a few studies that have provided notable insights into the mitochondrial control of myocardial cell death. It has been shown that in response to apoptotic agents, cardiac mitochondria initiate slow waves of depolarization and Ca^{2+} release, which propagate through the cell. The traveling waves trigger MPT pore opening, leading to cytochrome c release, caspase activation, and apoptosis (20). Mitochondrial Ca^{2+} uptake is critical for the wave propagation, and at the origin of waves, mitochondria take up Ca^{2+} more effectively. Thus, in response to apoptotic agents, mitochondria are transformed to an exciting state, and expansion of the local excitation by mitochondrial waves may play an important role in the activation of the apoptotic machinery in cardiomyocytes.

Defective Mitochondrial Oxidative Phosphorylation

This is a topic that has been studied extensively ever since the identification of mitochondrial function of oxidative phosphorylation. Current studies, however, have been focused more on the link between defective oxidative phosphorylation and pathogenesis of cardiomyopathy (29). There are some new aspects related to the impact of defective oxidative phosphorylation of mitochondria on myocardial cellular dynamics. Of note is that the early phase of defects in oxidative phosphorylation increases mitochondrial outer membrane permeability, leading to cytochrome c release, thus resulting in cytochrome c-mediated caspase-9 activation and thereby caspase-3 activation, leading to apoptosis. The defected oxidative phosphorylation also leads to depletion of cellular adenosine 5'-triphosphate (ATP) levels, resulting in necrosis. These new understandings thus shift the attention to the role of defective oxidative phosphorylation in mitochondrion-controlled cell death. Detection of mutated or otherwise defective components in the oxidative phosphorylation thus becomes a new direction for understanding and development of ultimate suppression of myocardial cell death by toxicants.

Abnormal Mitochondrial Biosynthesis

Recent studies have identified that abnormal mitochondrial biosynthesis plays a crucial role in myocardial pathogenesis and reversibility of cardiomyopathy. Nuclear DNA encodes mitochondrial proteins, thus nuclear DNA damage can lead to mutated products and abnormal mitochondrial biosynthesis. On the other hand, mitochondrial DNA encodes essential elements for mitochondrial function and is subjected to far more oxidative injury than nuclear DNA because of the lack of histones and much higher chances to expose to ROS generated by the electron transport chain. It has also been augured that mitochondria do not have DNA repair mechanism, but recent data showed that mitochondrial DNA repair exists although the repair is not as efficient as that of nuclear DNA repair. Because of these unique characteristics of mitochondrial DNA, cumulative mitochondrial DNA damage under oxidative stress conditions such as Adriamycin treatment, leading to irreversible mitochondrial dysfunction in the heart (30). This cumulative and irreversible oxidative mitochondrial dysfunction concept has an important impact on our understanding of the chronic as well as the late-onset cardiomyopathy of anthracyclines. These drugs cause cardiomyopathy sometimes months to years after cessation of the drug therapy. During the delayed development period, subtle pathological changes that may not be detectable but may continue to accumulate and lead to an overt toxic event. The cumulative and irreversible mitochondrial dysfunction might significantly contribute to the delayed myocardial pathogenesis.

Mitochondrial ROS Generation

Generation of ROS has long been ascribed to the "unwanted" function of mitochondria. Xenobiotics leading to ROS production and accumulation have been studied extensively regarding the mechanism leading to ROS generation; however, debate has continued regarding the significance of each identified pathway or the site of ROS generation in mitochondria. In general, it is accepted that changes in mitochondrial membrane potential are critically involved in ROS generation in mitochondria. There are two important advances in the studies of mitochondrial membrane potential. The first is the importance of mitochondrial ATP-sensitive potassium channels (31) and the second is the contribution of Ca^{2+}-activated potassium channels in the cardiac inner mitochondrial membrane (32). It has been shown that diazoxide opens mitochondrial ATP-sensitive potassium channels and preserved mitochondrial integrity and suppressed hydrogen peroxide–induced apoptosis in cardiomyocytes (31). The Ca^{2+}-activated potassium channels, on the other hand, significantly contribute to mitochondrial potassium uptake of myocytes, and the opening of these channels protects the heart from infarction (32). The link between these channels and the generation of ROS in mitochondria has not been established; however, the involvement of these channels in the mito-chondrial membrane integrity would implicate their relation to ROS production.

CARDIOVASCULAR TOXICITY OF AIR POLLUTION

It has long been known that fine particulate matter of air pollution leads to pathogenesis of respiratory system as well as carcinogenesis (33). The link of air pollution to cardiovascular toxicity, however, has been recognized only over the past decade (33). Both epidemiological and experimental animal studies have provided evidence to support the hypothesis that increased exposure to partic-ulate matter in air pollution contributes to cardiovascular morbidity, hospital-ization, and mortality (33,34).

There are several obstacles in the systemic study of cardiovascular toxicity by particulate air pollution. One of the major challenges is the complexity of the particulate components of air pollution. Current consensus in the field is to divide the airborne particulates into classes according to aerodynamic diameters. There are three major classes: coarse (PM_{10}, 2.5–10 μm), fine ($PM_{2.5}$, <2.5 μm), and ultrafine ($PM_{0.1}$, <0.1 μm). However, ambient air particulate matter consists of a mixture of combustive by-products and resuspended crustal materials, of which the contents are highly related to geographical region, leaving an extreme challenge for studying mechanisms by which particulate air pollution causes cardiotoxicity.

There are three major new additions to our current understanding of car-diovascular toxicity of particulate matter. First, Pope and colleagues (33) have studied mortality data on 500,000 individuals throughout the United States between 1979 and 2000 and found that for every 10-μg/m^3 increase in fine particles ($PM_{2.5}$), all-cause mortality increased by 6% annually and car-diopulmonary mortality by 9%, whereas for every 10-μg/m^3 increase in coarse particles (PM_{10}), the increase in all-cause mortality was by 0.51% and in car-diopulmonary mortality by 0.68%. Thus, the study comes to a conclusion that long-term exposure to fine particulate air pollution is an important environ-mental risk factor for cardiopulmonary mortality.

Second, attempts have been made to provide insights into the mechanistic link between particulate air pollution and cardiovascular toxicity, although it has a long way to go. The documented cardiac toxic effects of particulate air pollution in the past have been limited to changes in the electrocardiograph, including arrhythmia, decreased heart rate variability, and exacerbation of ST-segment changes in experimental models of myocardial infarction (33,35). Some studies also reported the association of particulate air pollution with myocardial infarction (34). In a study examining air pollution and C-reactive protein (CRP) levels from 631 men aged 45 to 64 years conducted in Augsburg, Germany, the association between elevated CRP and increased concentrations of particulate and sulphur oxide air pollution has been identified. Thus it concludes that ambient air pollution elicits an acute phase response, leading to an increased cardiac risk (36). Another study has followed a cohort of patients with established coronary heart disease with biweekly submaximal exercise tests over a six-month period (37). The result showed that the risk of developing ischemia during exercise was significantly elevated at two days after exposure to increased environmental levels of fine particulate air pollution, thus indicating that myocardial ischemia is a potential mechanism responsible for the adverse cardiac effects of air pollution. Other studies have explored that alterations in endothelial function serves as a candidate mechanism for the cardiovascular toxicity induced by particulate air pollution (38). Studies using a rat model have shown that animals with acute myocardial infarction were significantly more sensitive to the cardiac toxic effect of $PM_{2.5}$ (39). The fine particulate matter caused an elevation of serum endothelins and acute myocardial infarction resulted in an upregulation of endothelin receptors in the heart. The result thus suggests that upregulation of the endothelin system is likely involved in the particulate air pollution-induced cardiotoxicity.

Third, studies using animal models have provided evidence for the epidemiological observation that patients with compromised cardiovascular system are more sensitive to the cardiotoxicity of fine particulate air pollution (40). In addition, new data have shown that patients with diabetes were more susceptible to the cardiovascular damage by airborne particles than those without (41). In this study, the effect of coarse particulate (PM_{10}) instead of fine particulate ($PM_{2.5}$) was examined and diabetes had doubled the risk of the PM_{10}-associated cardiovascular admission compared with the absence of diabetes. It is interesting to know whether or not $PM_{2.5}$ would cause more severe cardiovascular damage in patients with diabetes.

There are, of course, many other studies that either confirmed or provided additional evidence to support previous epidemiological observation and experimental results. Overall, cardiotoxicity of air pollution has been significantly explored. The mechanistic link between air pollution and cardiotoxicity is expected from the continued effort in this emerging field.

CARDIOVASCULAR TOXICITY OF HAART

Cardiotoxicity induced by antiviral drugs was known as early as 1992 (42). It was reported that zidovudine (AZT), a widely used antiviral drug, caused dilated cardiomyopathy in a small number of adult patients. The report also noticed that the discontinuation of the treatment with AZT resulted in an improved left ventricular function (42). However, until recently the prognosis for people with AIDS was so low that concerns about adverse effects of drug treatment were relatively ignorable. The advent of HAART has significantly improved survival of patients with AIDS, thus making the issue of the adverse effects of the drugs an important concern. The standard HAART treatment is a combination of two nucleoside reverse transcriptase inhibitors (NRTIs) and one protease inhibitor (PI) or one nonnucleoside reverse transcriptase inhibitor (NNRTI). Besides the known cardiac toxic effect of AZT (42), the enhanced cardiotoxicity of the HAART treatment has been reported (43). The currently existing evidence shows that cardiotoxicity of HAART is convincing. Questions yet to be addressed are what are the mechanisms of cardiotoxicity of these drugs and what are the intervention measures that can prevent cardiotoxicity of HAART.

There are a significantly increased number of studies that have addressed the cardiotoxicity of HAART as well as AIDS per se. However, most of these studies have extended current literature information rather than provided novel insights into the problem that needs to be addressed in the field. Of note, there are a few studies that have reported some interesting results. A study performed by Twu et al. has examined cardiomyopathy of HIV infection (44). In this study, 18 AIDS hearts were studied. Among the AIDS hearts there are 5 with and 13 without cardiomyopathy. It was revealed that in the HIV cardiomyopathy (HIVCM) hearts, cardiomyocytes underwent apoptosis, which corresponds to positive immunohistochemical detection of active caspase-9, a component of mitochondrion-mediated apoptotic pathway, tumor necrosis factor-α and Fas ligand, the major components of death receptor-controlled pathway. The results thus demonstrate that in patients with HIVCM, apoptotic pathways are activated through both mitochondrion-mediated and death receptor-controlled mechanisms, leading to myocardial cell death. This study thus provides new insights into the cellular event of the HIVCM. However, in this study, whether or not these patients were treated with HAART was not identified, leaving an ambiguous wonder whether HIV or HAART or their combination caused myocardial apoptosis.

Studies using animal models would help dissect the distinct cardiotoxic effect of HIV infection from that of HAART treatment. A study using a murine AIDS model generated by infecting mice with LP-BM5 murine leukemia retrovirus has shown that the animals with AIDS had a larger infarct size in the left ventricle compared with controls after a 30 minute of left anterior descending coronary artery occlusion followed by 120-minute reperfusion (45). This study thus demonstrates that AIDS itself is associated with adverse effects on the heart. Another study using a different animal AIDS model has demonstrated the effect of HAART on the heart (46). In this study, eight-week-old hemizygous transgenic AIDS mice (NL4-3Δ *gag/pol*) were used. The HAART including ATZ, lamivudine, and indinavir were used to treat the animals for 10 or 35 days. At the end of each dosing period, echocardiography, molecular markers, and biochemical parameters of cardiomyopathy were determined in these mice. The results showed that after 35 days treatment, the transgenic AIDS mice displayed increased left ventricular mass. The level of mRNA for atrial natriuretic factor was increased (250%), and the mRNA level for sarcoplasmic calcium ATPase was decreased (57%). Plasma lactate concentration was also significantly increased, and pathological and ultrastructural examination revealed granular cytoplasmic changes and enlarged mitochondria in cardiomyocytes. The same HAART treatment for 10 days only caused the increase in the atrial natriuretic factor mRNA levels in the transgenic AIDS mice. However, neither 10-days nor 35-days treatment with the same HAART caused any of these pathological, biochemical, molecular, and morphological changes in the wild type control mice. This study thus demonstrates that cumulative HAART treatment caused cardiomyopathy in the transgenic AIDS mice. That the same treatment did not cause cardiomyopathy in the wild type control mice suggests that the combination of AIDS and HAART treatment is essential for cardiac pathogenesis.

Most of the studies on cardiotoxicity of HAART have reported mitochondrial damage, thus contributing to a popular hypothesis that the mechanism of HAART cardiotoxicity is related to the toxic effect of the drugs on mitochondria. Biochemical evidence has provided support for this hypothesis because AZT acts as a competitive as well as a noncompetitive inhibitor of mitochondrial DNA polymerase (47). However, other mechanisms other than mitochondrial damage would also make significant contributions to cardiotoxicity of HAART, among these is the generation of ROS and thereby ROS-mediated signaling transduction pathways. These hypotheses need to be experimentally tested and have been the focus of most recent studies. Novel insights would be expected in the near future.

CARDIOVASCULAR TOXICITY OF NEW DRUGS

Research on cardiovascular toxicity of new drugs has been a major focus in drug discovery and development over the past decade. New regulation has been implemented by regulatory agencies such as that the U.S. Food and Drug Administration has now required cardiac toxicity tests, including QT prolongation for drug development. There are some new drugs that have been identified to be associated with cardiac toxicity; some of them, such as Vioxx, have been withdrawn from the market.

Arsenic trioxide has been shown to be highly effective in the treatment of relapsed and refractory acute promyelocytic leukemia (APL). A Trisenox brand of arsenic trioxide was approved for clinical use in the United States in 2000. Recent clinical reports have shown a serious ventricular tachycardia by arsenic trioxide in APL patients (48). To understand the cardiotoxic effect of arsenic trioxide and to investigate possible mechanisms of the cardiotoxicity, an animal study was undertaken (49). In this study, mice were treated with arsenic trioxide in a dose regiment that has been shown to produce plasma concentrations of arsenic within the range of those present in arsenic-treated APL patients. After a daily administration of 5 mg/kg arsenic trioxide for 30 days, arsenic-induced myocardial functional changes were found, including a significant decrease in the maximum rate of rise in intraventricular pressure during ventricular contraction (MAX dP/dt), and significant increases in the end diastolic pressure and ventricle minimum diastolic pressure. In response to β-adrenergic stimulation by isoproterenol the arsenic-treated heart did not show increase in MAX dP/dt, which was observed as a stress response in the saline-treated controls. Cardiomyopathy was revealed by histopathological and ultrastructural examination, along with myocardial apoptosis, determined by a terminal deoxynucleotidyl transferase-mediated dUTP nick-end labeling assay and confirmed by caspase-3 activation detected by an enzymatic assay. This study thus demonstrates that arsenic trioxide, in a dose regiment that could produce clinically comparable serum concentrations to those observed in humans, causes cardiotoxicity.

Nonsteroidal anti-inflammatory drugs (NSAIDs) include aspirin, Motrin, and Naprosyn, which are classified as nonselective NSAIDs because they are inhibitors for both cyclooxygenase-1 (COX-1) and COX-2. Inhibition of COX-1 is associated with gastrointestinal toxicity because COX-1 exerts a protective effect on the lining of the stomach. A newer class of NSAIDs has been developed, including rofecoxib (Vioxx), celecoxib (Celebrex), and valdecoxib (Bextra), which are selective inhibitors of COX-2. In September 2004, Vioxx was voluntarily withdrawn from the market on the basis of the data from a clinical trial that showed that after 18 months of use, Vioxx increased the relative risk for cardiovascular events, such as heart attack and stroke. In April 2005, Bextra was removed from the market on the basis of the potential increased risk for serious cardiovascular adverse events and increased risk of serious skin reactions (e.g., toxic epidermal necrolysis, Stevens-Johnson syndrome, erythema multiforme). Emerging information indicates the risk of cardiovascular events may be increased in patients receiving Celebrex. The cardiovascular events induced by COX-2 inhibitors are presumably related to thrombotic events. Studies have also indicated the link of Vioxx to long QT syndrome and the increased risk for torsade de pointes (TdP) and sudden cardiac death.

Recognition of QT prolongation and its associated adverse effects on the heart has been a major focus in drug discovery and development over the past decade. A number of drugs have been found to cause QT prolongation and TdP, and thus were removed from the market or relabeled for restricted use. It has been known for a long time that quinidine causes sudden cardiac death; however, the severe and lethal side effect of QT prolongation had not drawn sufficient attention until the last decade, because of the lack of knowledge and experimental approaches to obtain a comprehensive understanding of QT prolongation. Knowledge on QT prolongation has accumulated and regulatory guidelines for a battery of preclinical tests to assess QT liability of a potential drug are recommended.

DEVELOPMENT AND VALIDATION OF BIOMARKERS

Cardiovascular injury can be divided into two major classes: structural and nonstructural injuries. The structural damage of the cardiovascular system includes cell death and the associated histopathological changes. Functional deficits often accompany the structural injury. Nonstructural damage represents functional deficits without apparent structural alterations. In clinical practice and experimental approach, biomarkers are referred to as indexes of cardiovascular injury measured from blood samples. The fundamental principle of the biomarkers is that molecules that are released from the cardiovascular system under various injury conditions are readily detectable from blood samples.

Validation of Biomarkers

For a biomarker to be indicative of tissue damage, an important question that needs to be addressed is what characteristics are required for a valid biomarker. In year 2000, an Expert Working Group (EWG) on biomarkers of drug-induced cardiac toxicity was established under the Advisory Committee for Pharmaceutical Sciences of the Center for Drug Evaluation and Research of the U.S. Food and Drug Administration. The report from this EWG has summarized the characteristics of ideal cardiac toxic injury biomarkers (50). These characteristics include cardiac specificity, sensitivity, predictive value, robust, bridge preclinical to clinical, and noninvasive procedure/accessibility. These characteristics are adapted as a standard for development and validation of a biomarker of cardiovascular injury.

Availability of Biomarkers

Currently validated biomarkers that are included in clinical diagnostic testing guidelines for cardiac disease are all related to myocardial structural injury. Developing biomarkers for nonstructural injury is the most challenging and demands implantation of more advanced technologies such as genomics, proteomics, and metabolomics. In addition, currently available biomarkers have limitations, although they are useful.

Creatine Kinase

There are three major creatine kinase (CK) isoenzymes identified: CK-MM is the principal form in skeletal muscle, CK-MB presents in myocardium in which CK-MM is also found, and CK-BB is the predominant form in brain and kidney.

Elevation of serum CK-MB is considered a reasonably specific marker of acute myocardial infarction.

Myoglobin

Myoglobin is found in all muscle types and its value as a biomarker of myocardial injury is based on the fact that serum concentrations of myoglobin increase rapidly following myocardial tissue injury, with peak values observed one to four hours after acute myocardial infarction. Elevation of serum myoglobin is likely reflective of the extent of myocardial damage.

B-Type Natriuretic Peptide

B-type natriuretic peptide (BNP) is a cardiac neurohormone secreted by the ventricular myocardium in response to volume and pressure overload, and the release of BNP appears to be directly correlated with the degree of ventricular wall tension. BNP is now accepted as a biomarker for congestive heart failure and is included in the European guideline for the diagnosis of chronic heart failure.

C-Reactive Protein

The acute-phase reactant C-reactive protein (CRP) is a marker of systemic and vascular inflammation, which appears to predict future cardiac events in asymptomic individuals. In particular, inflammation has been shown to play a pivotal role in the inception, progression, and destabilization of atheromas. A predictive value of CRP for the prognosis of coronary heart disease is thus proposed.

Cardiac Troponins

Cardiac troponin T (cTnT) and cardiac troponin I (cTnI) are constituents of the myofilaments and expressed exclusively in cardiomyocytes. It is thus of absolute myocardial tissue specificity. In healthy persons, serum cTnT or cTnI is rarely detectable. Therefore, any measurable concentrations of serum cTnT or cTnI reflect myocardial injury such as myocardial infarction. The clinical experience has arrived at a recommendation that cTn measurement becomes the "Gold Standard" for diagnosis of acute myocardial infarction.

Biomarker Applications and Limitations

All of the biomarkers described above have been used as indexes of myocardial injury in clinical practice and experimental studies and the same use continues. The major concern of most of the biomarkers is their specificity. CK-MB is present in small quantities in skeletal muscle and other tissues, thus elevations of CK-MB occur in some diseases involving skeletal muscle injury. Myoglobin is found in all muscle types, and the concentrations of myoglobin vary significantly between species and even within species. BNP has been proposed to be used as a prognostic indicator of disease progression and outcome of congestive heart failure. However, the actual utility of this biomarker is untested. BNP is also included in the counterregulation of heart hypertrophy, thus the changes in serum BNP concentrations as function of time in the transition from cardiac hypertrophy to heart failure need to be understood comprehensively. Higher levels of BNP may not necessarily indicate more severity of the heart disease, indicating that more scrutiny analysis is needed. CRP is a biomarker of inflammation, and its use in myocardial injury is more supplementary to other tests than having independently predictive value. A significant advance in the development and validation of biomarkers for myocardial injury is the promising clinical experience with cTn, which has absolute myocardial tissue specificity and high sensitivity. It is now accepted by clinical community that cardiac troponins are used as the biomarker of choice for assessing myocardial damage in humans. Its preclinical value for monitoring drug cardiac toxicity and in drug development needs to be evaluated.

LOOKING TO THE FUTURE

Over the past decade, there have been exciting progresses in our understanding of cardiovascular toxicity. The foremost is that cardiovascular toxicity has been recognized as a critical issue in clinical practice, environmental health, and drug development. Many studies have provided novel insights into mechanisms of cardiovascular toxicity, and the same studies will continue in the future. Further investigation of cardiovascular toxicity induced by well-studied drugs and chemicals will generate more critical insights into mechanistic link between exposure to xenobiotics and toxicologic cardiomyopathy. The identification and characterization of emerging drugs and chemicals that cause cardiovascular toxicity will enrich our current knowledge of cardiovascular toxicology. Novel therapeutics for cardiac diseases such as stem cell therapy for ischemic cardiac disease and gene therapy for cardiovascular disease are new areas that have generated the concerns of cardiovascular toxicity. The application of nanotechnology in cardiovascular system greatly enhances drug delivery efficiency and therapeutic efficacy, but the issue of cardiovascular toxicity is also accompanied with this new technology. The left ventricle assist device designation therapy for heart failure will greatly improve the health care for cardiovascular patients, but cardiovascular toxicity will become a new challenge. All of these new exploring areas of cardiovascular medicine and therapy will definitely call for attention from the cardiovascular toxicology field. Further exploration of the state-of-the-art approaches such as genomics, proteomics, and metabonomics will ensure further advances in our knowledge of cardiovascular toxicology. An integrated approach that combines the advanced technologies will greatly assist the development and validation of biomarkers in cardiovascular toxicology. It is highly predictable that more comprehensive understanding and new knowledge of cardiovascular toxicology will be created in the future at a much faster pace than ever before.

REFERENCES

1. Kang YJ. Molecular and cellular mechanisms of cardiotoxicity. Environ Health Perspect 2001; 109 (suppl. 1):27–34.
2. Kang YJ. New understanding in cardiotoxicity. Curr Opin Drug Discov Devel 2003; 6:110–116.
3. Melchert RB, Joseph J, Kennedy RH. Interaction of xenobiotics with myocardial signal transduction pathways. Cardiovasc Toxicol 2002; 2:1–23.
4. Chen QM, Tu VC, Purdon S, et al. Molecular mechanisms of cardiac hypertrophy induced by toxicants. Cardiovasc Toxicol 2001; 1:267–283.
5. Robbins J. Genetic modification of the heart: exploring necessity and sufficiency in the past 10 years. J Mol Cell Cardiol 2004; 36:643–652.
6. Olson EN. A decade of discoveries in cardiac biology. Nat Med 2004; 10:467–474.
7. Imumorin IG, Dong Y, Zhu H, et al. A gene-environment interaction model of stress-induced hypertension. Cardiovasc Toxicol 2005; 5:109–132.
8. Jones WK, Brown M, Wilhide M, et al. NF-kappaB in cardiovascular disease: diverse and specific effects of a "general" transcription factor? Cardiovasc Toxicol 2005; 5:183–202.
9. Heideman W, Antkiewicz DS, Carney SA, et al. Zebrafish and cardiac toxicology. Cardiovasc Toxicol 2005; 5:203–214.
10. Thackaberry EA, Gabaldon DM, Walker MK, et al. Aryl hydrocarbon receptor null mice develop cardiac hypertrophy and increased hypoxia-inducible factor-1alpha in the absence of cardiac hypoxia. Cardiovasc Toxicol 2002; 2:263–274.
11. Anversa P, Leri A, Kajstura J. Cardiac regeneration. J Am Coll Cardiol 2006; 47:1769–1776.
12. Haunstetter A, Izumo S. Apoptosis: basic mechanisms and implications for cardiovascular disease. Circ Res 1998; 82:1111–1129.
13. James TN. Normal and abnormal consequences of apoptosis in the human heart. From postnatal morphogenesis to paroxysmal arrhythmias. Circulation 1994; 90:556–573.
14. Sabbah HN, Sharov VG. Apoptosis in heart failure. Prog Cardiovasc Dis 1998; 40:549–562.
15. Bishopric NH, Andreka P, Slepak T, et al. Molecular mechanisms of apoptosis in the cardiac myocyte. Curr Opin Pharmacol 2001; 1:141–150.
16. Bergmann MW, Loser P, Dietz R, et al. Effect of NF-kappa B Inhibition on TNF-alpha-induced apoptosis and downstream pathways in cardiomyocytes. J Mol Cell Cardiol 2001; 33:1223–1232.
17. Green PS, Leeuwenburgh C. Mitochondrial dysfunction is an early indicator of doxorubicin-induced apoptosis. Biochim Biophys Acta 2002; 1588:94–101.
18. Fosslien E. Mitochondrial medicine—molecular pathology of defective oxidative phosphorylation. Ann Clin Lab Sci 2001; 31:25–67.
19. Jung F, Weiland U, Johns RA, et al. Chronic hypoxia induces apoptosis in cardiac myocytes: a possible role for Bcl-2-like proteins. Biochem Biophys Res Commun 2001; 286:419–425.

20. Pacher P, Hajnoczky G. Propagation of the apoptotic signal by mitochondrial waves. EMBO J 2001; 20:4107–4121.
21. Kubota T, Miyagishima M, Frye CS, et al. Overexpression of tumor necrosis factor-alpha activates both anti- and pro-apoptotic pathways in the myocardium. J Mol Cell Cardiol 2001; 33:1331–1344.
22. Hayakawa K, Takemura G, Koda M, et al. Sensitivity to apoptosis signal, clearance rate, and ultrastructure of fas ligand-induced apoptosis in in vivo adult cardiac cells. Circulation 2002; 105:3039–3045.
23. Suzuki K, Kostin S, Person V, et al. Time course of the apoptotic cascade and effects of caspase inhibitors in adult rat ventricular cardiomyocytes. J Mol Cell Cardiol 2001; 33:983–994.
24. Frey N, Olson EN. Cardiac hypertrophy: the good, the bad, and the ugly. Annu Rev Physiol 2003; 65:45–79.
25. Zou Y, Hiroi Y, Uozumi H, et al. Calcineurin plays a critical role in the development of pressure overload-induced cardiac hypertrophy. Circulation 2001; 104:97–101.
26. Hill JA, Karimi M, Kutschke W, et al. Cardiac hypertrophy is not a required compensatory response to short-term pressure overload. Circulation 2000; 101: 2863–2869.
27. Esposito G, Rapacciuolo A, Naga Prasad SV, et al. Genetic alterations that inhibit in vivo pressure-overload hypertrophy prevent cardiac dysfunction despite increased wall stress. Circulation 2002; 105:85–92.
28. Weber KT. Are myocardial fibrosis and diastolic dysfunction reversible in hypertensive heart disease? Congest Heart Fail 2005; 11:322–324.
29. Fosslien E. Mitochondrial Medicine—Cardiomyopathy caused by defective oxidative phosphorylation. Ann Clin Lab Sci 2003; 33:371–395.
30. Zhou S, Starkov A, Froberg MK, et al. Cumulative and irreversible cardiac mitochondrial dysfunction induced by doxorubicin. Cancer Res 2001; 61:771–777.
31. Akao M, Ohler A, O'Rourke B, et al. Mitochondrial ATP-sensitive potassium channels inhibit apoptosis induced by oxidative stress in cardiac cells. Circ Res 2001; 88:1267–1275.
32. Xu W, Liu Y, Wang S, et al. Cytoprotective role of Ca2+- activated K+ channels in the cardiac inner mitochondrial membrane. Science 2002; 298:1029–1033.
33. Pope CA III, Burnett RT, Thun MJ, et al. Lung cancer, cardiopulmonary mortality, and long-term exposure to fine particulate air pollution. JAMA 2002; 287: 1132–1141.
34. Peters A, Dockery DW, Muller JE, et al. Increased particulate air pollution and the triggering of myocardial infarction. Circulation 2001; 103:2810–2815.
35. Magari SR, Hauser R, Schwartz J, et al. Association of heart rate variability with occupational and environmental exposure to particulate air pollution. Circulation 2001; 104:986–991.
36. Peters A, Fröhlich M, Döring A, et al. Particulate air pollution is associated with an acute phase response in men; results from the MONICA-Augsburg Study. Eur Heart J 2001; 22:1198–1204.
37. Pekkanen J, Peters A, Hoek G, et al. Particulate air pollution and risk of ST-segment depression during repeated submaximal exercise tests among subjects with coronary heart disease: the exposure and risk assessment for fine and ultrafine particles in ambient air (ULTRA) study. Circulation 2002; 106:933–938.

38. Brook RD, Brook JR, Urch B, et al. Inhalation of fine particulate air pollution and ozone causes acute arterial vasoconstriction in healthy adults. Circulation 2002; 105: 1534–1536.
39. Kang YJ, Li Y, Zhou Z, et al. Elevation of serum endothelins and cardiotoxicity induced by particulate matter (PM2.5) in rats with acute myocardial infarction. Cardiovasc Toxicol 2002; 2:253–261.
40. Wellenius GA, Saldiva PH, Batalha JR, et al. Electrocardiographic changes during exposure to residual oil fly ash (ROFA) particles in a rat model of myocardial infarction. Toxicol Sci 2002; 66:327–335.
41. Zanobetti A, Schwartz J. Cardiovascular damage by airborne particles: are diabetics more susceptible? Epidemiology 2002; 13:588–592.
42. Herskowitz A, Willoughby SB, Baughman KL, et al. Cardiomyopathy associated with antiretroviral therapy in patients with HIV infection: a report of six cases. Ann Intern Med 1992; 116:311–313.
43. Fantoni M, Autore C, Del Borgo C. Drugs and cardiotoxicity in HIV and AIDS. Ann N Y Acad Sci 2001; 946:179–199.
44. Twu C, Liu NQ, Popik W, et al. Cardiomyocytes undergo apoptosis in human immunodeficiency virus cardiomyopathy through mitochondrion- and death receptor-controlled pathways. Proc Natl Acad Sci U S A 2002; 99:14386–14391.
45. Chen Y, Davis-Gorman G, Watson RR, et al. Vitamin E attenuates myocardial ischemia-reperfusion injury in murine AIDS. Cardiovasc Toxicol 2002; 2:119–127.
46. Lewis W, Haase CP, Raidel SM, et al. Combined antiretroviral therapy causes cardiomyopathy and elevates plasma lactate in transgenic AIDS mice. Lab Invest 2001; 81:1527–1536.
47. Lee H, Hanes J, Johnson KA. Toxicity of nucleoside analogues used to treat AIDS and the selectivity of the mitochondrial DNA polymerase. Biochemistry 2003; 42: 14711–14719.
48. Unnikrishnan D, Dutcher JP, Varshneya N, et al. Torsades de pointes in 3 patients with leukemia treated with arsenic trioxide. Blood 2001; 97:1514–1516.
49. Li Y, Sun X, Wang L, et al. Myocardial toxicity of arsenic trioxide in a mouse model. Cardiovasc Toxicol 2002; 2:63–73.
50. Wallace KB, Hausner E, Herman E, et al. Serum troponins as biomarkers of drug-induced cardiac toxicity. Toxicol Pathol 2004; 32:106–121.
51. Heineke J, Molkentin JD. Regulation of cardiac hypertrophy by intracellular signalling pathways. Nat Rev Mol Cell Biol 2006; 7:589–600.

2

Pathobiology of Myocardial Ischemic Injury—Implications for Pharmacology and Toxicology

L. Maximilian Buja

Department of Pathology and Laboratory Medicine, The University of Texas Health Science Center, and Department of Cardiovascular Pathology, Texas Heart Institute, St. Luke's Episcopal Hospital, Houston, Texas, U.S.A.

INTRODUCTION

Myocardial ischemia is a condition of myocardial impairment, which results from inadequate delivery of oxygenated blood through the coronary arteries relative to the metabolic demands of the myocardium (1–6). Thus, ischemic heart disease, also known as coronary heart disease, involves an imbalance in the normal integrated function of the coronary vasculature and the myocardium. The major consequences of acute myocardial ischemia are depressed myocardial contractile function, arrhythmias, and myocardial necrosis (infarction). The multiple clinical manifestations of acute myocardial ischemia are referred to as acute coronary syndrome (ACS), which includes unstable angina pectoris, acute myocardial infarction (AMI), and sudden cardiac death. Ischemic heart disease also encompasses stable angina pectoris and chronic ischemic heart disease. The myocardial response to ischemic injury can be modulated by a number of biological processes, particularly preconditioning and reperfusion (Table 1).

Table 1 Myocardial Responses to Alterations in Coronary Perfusion

Dysfunction during transient ischemia (angina pectoris)
Stunning following acute ischemia
Hibernation during chronic ischemia
Ischemic preconditioning
Second window of protection
    Against stunning
    Against infarction
Acute myocardial infarction
    Subendocardial, transmural
    Extension, expansion
    Complications
Reperfusion effects
    On myocardial function
    On myocardial injury
Preconditioning
Postconditioning
Remodeling
Chronic ischemic heart disease
Ischemic cardiomyopathy

Source: From Ref. 4.

Therapeutic approaches to ameliorate the natural progression of myocardial ischemic injury include catheter-based interventions and surgical approaches as well as pharmacological treatments, which may have toxicological complications.

ROLE OF CORONARY ALTERATIONS IN MYOCARDIAL ISCHEMIA

Observations in Humans

The inflammatory process is critically important in atherogenesis, so that atherosclerosis is now considered to be an inflammatory disease (7–12). Atherosclerosis develops as a response of the arterial wall to chronic repetitive injury produced by risk factors, including hyperlipidemia, hypertension, cigarette smoking, and diabetes mellitus, and progresses particularly fast in individuals with familial hypercholesterolemia (13). Atherosclerosis leads to progressive narrowing of the coronary arteries and predisposes to the development of ischemic heart disease (7–12). However, the pathogenesis of acute ischemic heart disease involves the occurrence of acute pathophysiological alterations in the coronary arteries superimposed on coronary atherosclerosis of variable severity (14–31). The acute pathophysiological event may involve a stress-induced increase in myocardial oxygen demand or an impairment in the oxygen-carrying capacity of the blood. However, most cases of ACS result from a primary alteration in the coronary vasculature, leading to decreased delivery of

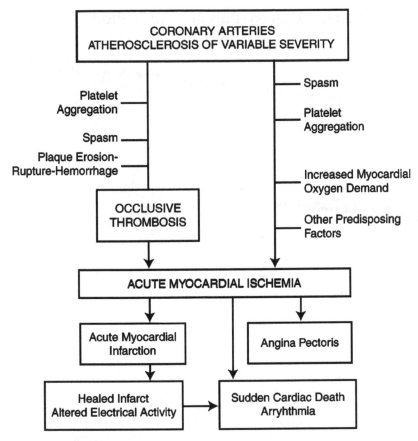

Figure 1 Pathogenetic mechanisms of acute ischemic heart disease and potential clinical outcomes. *Source*: Adapted from Ref. 14.

blood to the myocardium (Fig. 1). These alterations involve platelet aggregation, vasoconstriction (coronary spasm), and thrombosis superimposed on atherosclerotic plaques (Fig. 2).

An acute alteration of an atherosclerotic plaque often initiates acute narrowing or occlusion of the coronary artery. Acute changes in plaques consist of erosion, fissure, ulceration, and rupture, with injury to the endothelium and surface cap of the plaque as the initiating event (18–21,27–31). Vulnerable plaques are plaques that are predisposed to develop these acute complications (18–21,27–36). These vulnerable plaques have been characterized as thin fibrous cap atheromas, which are prone to rupture; thick fibrous cap atheromas, which are prone to erosion; and calcified nodular lesions, in descending order of frequency (Figs. 3,4) (30,31). Precipitation of the acute changes likely requires chronic or recurrent local injury to the atherosclerotic vessel, which involves toxic effects of products produced by degeneration of the plaque constituents,

Platelet Aggregation and Activation

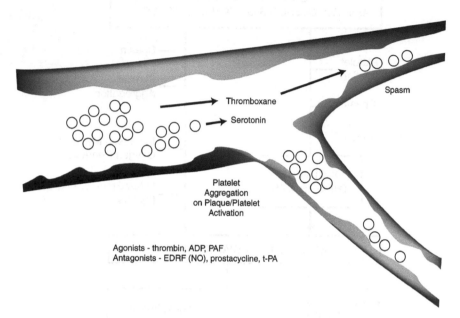

Figure 2 A schematic diagram indicating the role of platelet-mediated mechanisms of induction of acute myocardial ischemia. Platelet aggregation develops in atherosclerotic coronary arteries at sites of endothelial injury. Aggregating platelets release mediators, including thromboxane A2 (TxA2) and serotonin (5HT), which cause further platelet aggregation downstream and vasoconstriction. Factors favoring platelet aggregation include thrombin, ADP, and PAF. Factors inhibiting platelet aggregation include endothelium-derived relaxing factor (NO), prostacycline, and t-PA. *Abbreviations*: ADP, adenosine diphosphate; PAF, platelet activating factor; NO, nitric oxide; t-PA, tissue plasminogen activator. *Source*: Adapted from Ref. 15,22.

inflammation, and hemodynamic trauma (32–36). Vulnerable plaques exhibit increased numbers of T lymphocytes and macrophages adjacent to the surface, and the latter cells release stromolysin, collagenases, metallomatrix proteinases, and other degradative enzymes, which contribute to destabilization of the plaque capsule. Occlusive coronary thrombi overlying eroded, fissured, ulcerated, or ruptured plaques are found in over 90% of cases of acute transmural myocardial infarction (18–21). In ACSs of ischemic heart disease other than AMI, including unstable angina pectoris and sudden cardiac death, acute alterations of the coronary arteries also are frequently observed (18–21,37–44). These include endothelial disruption, plaque fissuring, platelet aggregation, and nonocclusive or occlusive thrombi. These findings form the basis for the successful application of thrombolytic therapy to produce coronary reperfusion for the treatment of AMI (45–49). Intensive efforts also are underway for the development and

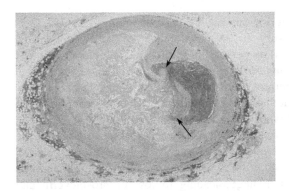

Figure 3 Coronary occlusion with plaque rupture and thrombosis. The ruptured plaque has a large lipid-laden core and a thin fibrous capsule. Note the separation of the capsule (*arrowheads*), outward displacement of plaque contents across the rupture site, and communication with the overlying thrombus. Plaque hemorrhage was present in other sections of the lesion. (Hematoxylin and eosin: × 10). *Source*: From Ref. 18.

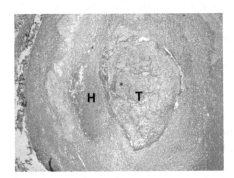 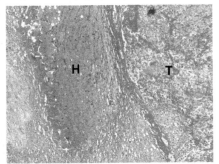

Figure 4 Coronary occlusion with thrombosis of the lumen and plaque erosion and hemorrhage. (**A**) Low-power photomicrograph of the coronary artery shows the thrombus (T) adjacent to a focus of plaque erosion and hemorrhage (H). (**B**) High-magnification photomicrograph shows the erosion of the plaque surface with plaque hemorrhage (H) and adjacent thrombus in the lumen. [Hematoxylin and eosin: (**A**) × 11, (**B**) × 108]. *Source*: From Ref. 3.

application of various imaging and other techniques for the clinical detection of vulnerable coronary lesions (50–53).

Observations in Experimental Models

Insights into the role of coronary factors in the pathogenesis of acute myocardial ischemia have been provided by a canine model in which coronary stenosis with endothelial injury has been produced by placement of a plastic constrictor on a roughened area of the left anterior descending coronary artery (22–25). Coronary injury in the model results in the development of cyclic blood flow alterations that are characterized by periods of progressive reduction to a nadir of blood flow, followed by abrupt restoration of blood flow. These cyclic blood flow alterations are due to recurrent platelet aggregation at the site of coronary stenosis. There is evidence that the process is driven by several platelet-derived mediators, including thromboxane A_2 (TxA_2) and serotonin (22–25). The cyclic blood flow alterations are mediated both by anatomic obstruction of the coronary artery by aggregated platelets as well as by excessive vasoconstriction produced by TxA_2, serotonin, and possibly by other products released from the platelets (Fig. 2). Endothelial damage, leading to loss of prostacyclin and endothelium-derived relaxing factor [nitric oxide (NO)], also contributes to the process. The cyclic blood flow alterations can be inhibited by treatment with TxA_2 synthesis inhibitors, TxA_2 receptor antagonists, ADP receptor antagonists, serotonin receptor antagonists, and glycoprotein IIb/IIIa receptor antagonists (22–25). In a chronic model with cyclic blood flow alterations for several days, the animals develop intimal proliferation at the site of coronary stenosis, with further narrowing of the lumen (22–25). This process is likely mediated by multiple growth factors, including platelet-derived growth factor (PDGF) released from platelets. The intimal proliferation can be attenuated by treatment with inhibitors of leukocyte and platelet receptors and chemical mediators (22–25).

Clinical Correlates

The observations derived from the canine cyclic blood flow model have implications for the pathogenesis of acute ischemic heart disease (14–27,36). Endothelial injury developing at a site of coronary stenosis can initiate changes leading to impaired coronary perfusion and myocardial ischemia. Endothelial injury predisposes to recurrent platelet aggregation, which produces anatomic obstruction compounded by vasoconstriction. TxA_2 and serotonin are important mediators of the process (15,16,22–27). Recurrent episodes of platelet aggregation may lead to further coronary stenosis as a result of intimal proliferation (14–27,36). A clinical counterpart of the latter phenomena may be the intimal proliferation that frequently occurs following percutaneous transluminal coronary angioplasty (PTCA) in man. The process of recurrent platelet aggregation may result at any stage in the development of occlusive coronary thrombosis, although spontaneous resolution is also possible. Studies in man have also provided evidence of platelet aggregation as well as release of TxA2 and serotonin in patients with unstable angina pectoris (15,16,21,27,36). Antiplatelet therapies, including ADP receptor and glycoprotein IIb/IIIa receptor antagonists, are clinically effective in patients with ACSs (15,16,21,26,27,36,45–49). Thus, there is strong evidence that endothelial injury and platelet aggregation are key factors in the mediation of acute ischemic heart disease.

ACSs are divided clinically into those presenting with the electrocardiographic pattern of ST segment elevation myocardial ischemia or infarction (STEMI) and non-ST segment elevation myocardial ischemia or infarction (NSTEMI) (45–49). ACS patients are commonly treated with thrombolytic therapy, percutaneous coronary intervention (PCI), or both, depending on presentation (54,55). Relevant pharmacological agents include (*i*) anticoagulant therapy, including low molecular weight heparin; (*ii*) thrombolytic therapy, including tissue plasminogen activating factor; and (*iii*) antiplatelet agents, including ADP receptor and glycoprotein IIb and IIIa receptor antagonists (26,27,45–49). PCIs include PTCA and placement of coronary stents. Coronary stents were developed in an attempt to reduce the 30% to 40% incidence of coronary restenosis within 6 to 12 months of PTCA (54–59). This restenosis is due to a combination of thrombosis and intimal proliferation, as shown in the experimental work described above. Stent technology led to the development of stents coated with antiproliferative agents, including sirolimus and paclitaxel (60,61). Results with these coated stents initially showed better results than bare metal stents. However, recent studies have revealed a problem of late thrombosis of the coated stents (62–64). Optimal therapy of the complications of PTCA will continue to require ongoing investigation. A recent study has found no differences in morbidity and mortality in patients with chronic stable angina pectoris treated with angioplasty compared with medication without PCI (65). However, there remains an important role for emergent PCI for patients with impending AMI.

MECHANISMS OF MYOCARDIAL ISCHEMIC INJURY

Metabolic Alterations

Regulation of myocardial metabolism has important clinical relevance (66–71). The major metabolic alterations induced by myocardial ischemia involve impaired energy and substrate metabolism (1–6). These metabolic alterations initiate alterations leading to reversible and, subsequently, irreversible injury of cardiomyocytes (Fig. 5). Oxygen deprivation results in a rapid inhibition of mitochondrial oxidative phosphorylation, the major source of cellular ATP synthesis. Initially, there is compensatory stimulation of anaerobic glycolysis for ATP production from glucose. However, glycolysis leads to the accumulation of hydrogen ions and lactate with resultant intracellular acidosis and inhibition of glycolysis (1–6,66,67). There is a shift from glucose to fatty acid as a fuel source. However, energy metabolism from fatty acids is less efficient than from glucose (68). Furthermore, fatty acid metabolism as well as glucose metabolism is impaired (1–6,66–71). Free fatty acids in the ischemic myocardium are derived from endogenous as well as exogenous sources, namely circulating free fatty acids mobilized from lipid stores, with the magnitude of fatty acid influx depending on the degree of collateral perfusion. Inhibition of mitochondrial β-oxidation leads to the accumulation of long-chain acylcarnitine, long-chain

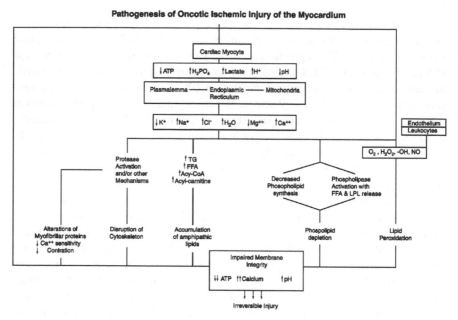

Pathogenesis of Oncotic Ischemic Injury of the Myocardium

Figure 5 Postulated sequence of alterations involved in the pathogenesis of oncotic ischemic injury of the myocardium. Oxygen deficiency induces metabolic changes, including decreased ATP, decreased pH, and lactate accumulation, in ischemic myocytes. The altered metabolic milieu leads to impaired membrane transport with resultant derangements in intracellular electrolytes. An increase in cytosolic Ca^{2+} triggers the activation of proteases and phospholipases with resultant cytoskeletal damage and impaired membrane phospholipid balance. Alterations of myofibrillar contractile proteins lead to decreased Ca^{2+} sensitivity and decreased contraction despite the increased cytosolic Ca^{2+}. Lipid alterations include increased PL degradation with release of free fatty acids and LPL and decreased phospholipid synthesis. The accumulation of amphipathic lipids alters membrane fluidity. Lipid peroxidation occurs as a result of attack by free radicals produced, at least in part, by the generation of excess electrons (e-) in oxygen-deprived mitochondria. Free radicals may also be derived from the metabolism of arachidonic acid and catecholamines, the metabolism of adenine nucleotides by xanthine oxidase in endothelium (species dependent), and the activation of neutrophils and macrophages. The irreversible phase of injury is mediated by severe membrane damage caused by phospholipid loss, lipid peroxidation, and cytoskeletal damage. *Abbreviations*: ATP, adenosine triphosphate; PL, phospholipid; LPL, lysophospholipids. *Source*: Adapted from Ref. 4.

acyl CoA, and free fatty acids (72–74). Initially, the free fatty acids are esterified into triglycerides, giving rise to fatty change in the myocardium. However, as esterification becomes blunted, free fatty acids increase.

Myocardial ischemia is initially manifested by impaired excitation contraction coupling with resultant reduction in contractile activity of the ischemic myocardium (1–6). The sudden regional loss of intravascular pressure appears to be the primary cause of the immediate decline in contractile function following coronary occlusion (75). Subsequent progression of contractile failure is related to the associated early metabolic changes that include a declining ATP level, leakage of potassium from myocytes, intracellular acidosis, and accumulation of inorganic phosphate (1–6). The loss of contractile activity probably has a beneficial secondary effect by prolonging myocardial viability as a result of a major reduction in the demand for ATP.

Altered Ionic Homeostasis

The metabolic derangements discussed above lead to dysfunction of membrane pumps and channels, with resultant derangements in intracellular electrolyte homeostasis. The earliest manifestation of membrane dysfunction is a net loss of potassium due to accelerated efflux of the ion from ischemic myocardial cells (1–6,76–78). Although the potassium efflux occurs before a severe reduction in ATP, more rapid depletion of a localized component or compartment of ATP may lead to activation of ATP-dependent K^+ efflux channels (77). Once ATP reduction is of sufficient magnitude, impaired function of the sodium, potassium ATPase occurs. This is accompanied by an accumulation of sodium, chloride, and water in the cells; further loss of potassium; loss of cell volume regulation; and cell swelling (79,80). Another early change involves an initial increase in free intracellular magnesium level, followed by progressive loss of magnesium (78). This is related in part to release of magnesium ATP complexes as ATP depletion occurs. Finally, progressive changes in intracellular calcium homeostasis occur, which may be of particular importance in the development of lethal cell injury.

Role of Calcium

The intracellular calcium level regulates normal cardiac function, and deranged calcium balance contributes significantly to the pathogenesis of myocardial cell injury (81–83). The intracellular calcium level is regulated by several processes (81–87). At the level of the sarcolemma, the voltage-dependent calcium channel is responsible for the slow inward current of the normal action potential; the sodium-calcium exchanger modulates intracellular calcium levels; and the calcium ATPase mediates a calcium efflux pathway. At the level of the sarcoplasmic reticulum, the calcium magnesium ATPase and phospholamban mediate calcium uptake and release on a beat-to-beat basis. Intracellular calcium levels also are modulated by uptake and storage of calcium in the mitochondria and binding of calcium to calcium-binding proteins.

The total intracellular calcium concentration is on the order of 1 to 2 mmol/L, with most of this calcium bound to cellular proteins (81–83). The free cytosolic ionized calcium (Ca^{2+}) concentration is approximately 100 to 300 nmol/L during diastole and approximately 1 µmol/L during systole. Beat-to-beat regulation of the cell calcium level involves voltage-dependent calcium influx across the sarcolemma, followed by calcium-induced calcium release from the sarcoplasmic reticulum, with the latter providing the major source of the calcium that binds to the myofilaments and activates cardiac contraction. Diastole is mediated by a reuptake of calcium into the sarcoplasmic reticulum, thereby lowering the cytosolic-free calcium level.

At an early stage of myocardial hypoxic and ischemic injury, normal calcium transients are lost and the cytosolic-free calcium concentration increases into the μmol/L range (88–91). Multiple mechanisms may be involved, including a net influx of calcium across the sarcolemma as well as loss of calcium from intracellular storage sites in the sarcoplasmic reticulum and mitochondria (88–91). These changes reflect membrane dysfunction, which is induced by ATP depletion and intracellular acidosis. The postulated consequences of an increase in cytosolic calcium include activation of phospholipases, proteinases, and calcium-dependent ATPases. Contractile depression persists in spite of the increase in cytosolic calcium as a result of damage to the myofibrillar proteins, thereby decreasing their sensitivity to calcium (4–6).

Progressive Membrane Damage

The conversion from reversible to irreversible ischemic myocardial injury is mediated by progressive membrane damage (Fig. 5). A number of factors may contribute to the more advanced stages of membrane injury. Cellular and organellar membranes consist of a phospholipid bilayer containing cholesterol and glycoproteins. The phospholipid bilayer is maintained by a balance between phospholipid degradation and synthesis. In myocardial ischemia, progressive phospholipid degradation occurs, probably as a result of the activation of one or more phospholipases secondary to an increase of cytosolic calcium or possibly other metabolic derangements (4–6). Phospholipase A– and phospholipase C–mediated pathways may be involved. Phospholipid degradation results in a transient increase in lysophospholipids, which are subsequently degraded by other lipases as well as the release of free fatty acids. Thus, phospholipid degradation contributes to the accumulation of various lipid species in ischemic myocardium. These lipids include free fatty acids, lysophospholipids, long-chain acyl CoA, and long-chain acylcarnitines (1–6,72–74,92–95). These molecules are amphiphiles (molecules with hydrophilic and hydrophobic portions). As a result of their amphiphatic property, these molecules accumulate in the phospholipid bilayer, thereby altering the fluidity and permeability of the membranes (72–74,96).

Initially, phospholipid degradation appears to be balanced by energy-dependent phospholipid synthesis. However, degradation eventually becomes predominant, with the result that net phospholipid depletion on the order of approximately 10% of total phospholipid content occurs after three hours of coronary occlusion (92). Although this net change in total phospholipid content is relatively small, it is associated with the development of significant permeability and structural defects, which are inhibited by agents that inhibit phospholipid degradation (93–95).

Myocardial ischemia also induces the generation of free radicals and toxic oxygen species derived from several sources (97–100). As a result of impaired oxidative metabolism, ischemic mitochondria generate an excess number of reducing equivalents that may initiate the generation of free radicals. Free radicals also can be produced by the enzymatic and nonenzymatic metabolism of arachidonic acid derived from phospholipid degradation and of catecholamines released from nerve terminals (see below). Endothelium of several species contains xanthine dehydrogenase, which may be converted to xanthine oxidase during ischemia. The xanthine oxidase can then metabolize adenine nucleotides derived from the metabolism of ATP. Neutrophils and macrophages invading ischemic tissue represent another source of free radicals. One major free radical cascade involves a generation of superoxide anions, followed by the production of toxic oxygen species, including the hydroxyl radical. Another major free radical cascade involves the production of excessive amounts of NO (101,102). A major target of free radicals is cell membranes where the free radicals act on unsaturated fatty acids in membrane phospholipids, leading to their peroxidation. Thus, free radicals can be generated during myocardial ischemia, and this process can be accelerated by reoxygenation.

Another factor in membrane injury involves disruption of the cytoskeleton, thereby, affecting the anchoring of the sarcolemma to the interior of the myocyte (103–105). Dystrophin and vinculin have been identified as cytoskeletal proteins involved in this process. It is postulated that ischemia leads to disruption of cytoskeletal filaments connecting the sarcolemma to the myofibrils, as a result of activation of proteases by increased cytosolic calcium or other mechanisms. Loss of immunostaining for dystrophin is characteristic of this process (106,107). After such disruption, the ischemic myocyte becomes more susceptible to the effects of cell swelling following accumulation of sodium and water. This process leads to the formation of subsarcolemmal blebs, followed by rupture of the membrane.

Such injury culminating with cell swelling (oncosis) and rupture is accelerated by the effects of reperfusion, which allows for increased sodium, chloride, water, and calcium accumulation in the injured cells. Marked reactivation of contraction occurs as a result of marked calcium influx coupled with transient regeneration of ATP by mitochondria resupplied with oxygen. The resultant hypercontracture will accelerate membrane rupture following cytoskeletal disruption. Reperfusion also leads to an oxidative burst, which generates free radicals. The processes just described are important mechanisms of reperfusion injury (4–6,108–114).

Thus, the transition from reversible to irreversible myocardial damage appears to be mediated by membrane injury secondary to progressive phospholipid degradation, free radical effects, and damage to the cytoskeletal anchoring of the sarcolemma. The consequences of this vicious cycle are loss of membrane integrity and further calcium accumulation with secondary ATP depletion (Fig. 5).

Apoptosis, Oncosis, Autophagy, and Necrosis

The above description presents the well-documented pathophysiology of cell injury and cell death in cardiac myocytes subjected to a major ischemic or hypoxic insult. However, it is now known that other pathophysiological mechanisms may contribute to myocardial cell injury and death. Apoptosis has now been recognized as a major and distinctive mode of cell death (115–121). Multiple reports have implicated apoptosis in myocardial infarction, reperfusion injury, and other forms of cardiovascular pathology (4–6,122–127). Apoptosis (programmed cell death I) is characterized by a series of molecular and biochemical events, including (*i*) gene activation (programmed cell death); (*ii*) perturbations of mitochondria, including membrane permeability transition and cytochrome C release; (*iii*) activation of a cascade of cytosolic aspartate-specific cysteine proteases (caspases); (*iv*) endonuclease activation leading to double-stranded DNA fragmentation; and (*v*) altered phospholipid distribution of cell membranes and other surface properties with preservation of selective membrane permeability (Fig. 6) (118–121). Apoptosis may be produced by activation of an extrinsic pathway initiated by activation of the TNF/Fas receptor and then caspase-8 or by activation of an intrinsic pathway involving perturbation of the mitochondria, leading to leakage of cytochrome C into the cytoplasm and activation of caspase-9. A third pathway involves Ca^{2+} release from the endoplasmic reticulum and activation of caspase-12. The final effector pathway involves activation of caspase-3. Apoptosis is also characterized by distinctive morphological alterations featuring cell and nuclear shrinkage and fragmentation. In contrast, numerous studies have reported ischemic myocardial damage to be characterized by cell swelling and altered cellular ionic composition as a result of altered membrane permeability. This pattern of cell injury and death with cell swelling has been termed "oncosis."

Oncosis represents a common form of cell injury and death that can result from multiple causes, including toxic and chemical injury, as well as hypoxia and ischemia (115–117). The pathogenesis of oncotic cell death leading to necrosis involves progressive damage to the cell membrane or sarcolemma, which has been characterized as having three stages: (*i*) potentially reversible discrete alterations in membrane ionic transport protein systems; (*ii*) a transitional state of progressive loss of the selective permeability barrier function of the phospholipid bilayer and increased nonspecific permeability; and (*iii*) irreversible physical disruption of the membrane of the swollen cell (Table 2) (115). The pathogenesis of the membrane damage can be initiated by at least four mechanisms: (*i*) direct damage to the cell membrane by certain toxic chemicals, products of activated leukocytes, the complement attack complex (C5b-9), and osmotic fluctuations, such as the calcium paradox, thereby permitting an uncontrolled influx of ions, especially Ca^{2+}, into the cell; (*ii*) damage to the respiratory apparatus of the mitochondria, with inhibition of oxidative phosphorylation, leading to decreased ATP production and increase in hydrogen ions

Mechanisms of Apoptosis

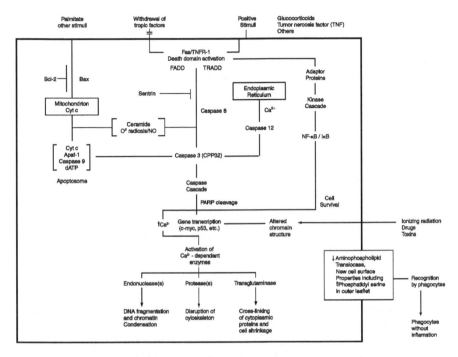

Figure 6 Mechanisms of cell death by apoptosis. Apoptosis may be initiated by activation of extrinsic or intrinsic pathways. The extrinsic pathway involves activation of the death domain of the TNFR/Fas with subsequent activation of caspase-8. The major intrinsic pathway involves perturbation of mitochondria, leading to activation of the membrane permeability transition, release of cytochrome C, and formation of the apoptosome with cytochrome C, Apaf-1, caspase-9, and d-ATP. The mitochondrial response is regulated by the Bcl-2 family of proteins involving the antiapoptotic Bcl-2 and the proapoptotic Bax and other proteins. Another intrinsic pathway involves Ca^{2+} release from the endoplasmic reticulum and activation of caspase-12. Activation of certain adaptor proteins can trigger a kinase cascade, leading to activation of NFκB and a cell survival outcome. However, if the pro-apoptotic pathways predominate, then a final common pathway to apoptosis is initiated by activation of caspase-3. Various substrates are cleaved, including PARP, and an apoptotic gene profile is activated. Outcomes include double-stranded DNA fragmentation and shrinkage necrosis. *Abbreviations*: TNFR, tumor necrosis factor receptor; NFκB, nuclear factor κB; Apaf-1, apoptotic protease activating factor-1; PARP, poly-ADP ribose polymerase. *Source*: Adapted from Ref. 4.

(drop in pH, intracellular acidosis) and initiation of free radical production; (*iii*) proteolysis of membrane-associated cytoskeletal proteins, including dystrophin and the dystrophin-associated protein complex, the vinculin-integrin link, and the spectrin-based submembranous cytoskeleton; and (*iv*) unregulated membrane phospholipid degradation due to activation of phospholipases and membrane

Table 2 Three Stages of Cell Membrane Injury and Associated Cellular Ionic Alterations

Discrete alterations in ionic transport systems
  K^+ efflux
  Mg^{2+} increase followed by Mg^{2+} loss
  Ca^{2+} increase
  Na^+, Cl^-, and H_2O increases and further K^+ decrease
Increased permeability of the phospholipid bilayer
  Increased permeability to Ca^{2+} with potential for Ca^{2+} loading and increase in
    total cell Ca^{2+}
  Further changes in Na^+, Cl^-, K^+, Mg^{2+}, and H_2O
  Leakage of smaller macromolecules
Physical disruption of the membrane
  Holes in the membrane
  Leakage of larger macromolecules
Equilibrium between the constituents of cell interior and exterior

Abbreviations: K^+, potassium ion; Mg^{2+}, magnesium ion; Ca^{2+}, calcium ion; Na^+, sodium ion;
Cl^-, chloride ion; H_2O, water.
Source: From Ref. 115.

lipid peroxidation due to the generation of oxygen-based free radicals and toxic oxygen species (1–6,106,107,115). The initial alterations of energy metabolism and ionic fluxes, especially the rise in intracellular free Ca^{2+}, are important in initiating the pathways leading to membrane damage (Fig. 5).

Although some reports have proposed a predominant role for apoptosis in myocardial ischemic injury and infarction, such a role for apoptosis may be overstated because of overinterpretation of evidence of DNA fragmentation, which is not specific for apoptosis (4,5,106,107,117). Other assays, including hairpin 1 and 2 polymerases, have been proposed to be more reliable for detection of patterns of DNA fragmentation characteristic of apoptosis and oncosis (4,5,106,107,117). However, the occurrence and extent of apoptosis needs to be confirmed by multiple assays, optimally including an assay for activated caspase, and with serial measurements over time. Variable results have been obtained using various caspase inhibitors to reduce the extent of myocardial ischemic damage. However, mutant mouse models have provided proof of principle that apoptosis does contribute significantly to myocardial infarction through activation of both the extrinsic and intrinsic pathways. The data suggest that apoptosis and oncosis each contribute about 50% to the evolution of myocardial infarction after coronary occlusion and reperfusion (122–126). The rate and magnitude of ATP reduction appears to be a critical determinant of whether an injured myocyte progresses to death by apoptosis or oncosis, since an ATP analog, d-ATP, is a key component of a molecular complex that mediates cytochrome C release with activation of the caspase cascade and apoptotic death (128–130). It is likely then that severely ischemic myocytes progress rapidly to cell death with swelling (oncosis), whereas less severely ischemic myocytes may progress to cell death by apoptosis. A hybrid form of injury may involve activation of apoptotic and oncotic pathways in the same cardiomyocytes. Necrosis, strictly defined, is the sum of degradative changes following irreversible cell injury by any of the known mechanisms. Thus, myocardial ischemic injury can be considered a generic term encompassing the multiple mechanisms leading to irreversible injury of cardiomyocytes and nonmyocytic cells as a result of a major ischemic insult.

Recently, autophagy (programmed cell death II) has been recognized as a third mode of cell death. Autophagic cell death involves unregulated catabolism and lysosomal degradation of cell proteins and organelles (131,132). Autophagic cell death has been implicated along with apoptosis and oncosis in negative remodeling, leading to fatal heart failure in patients with chronic ischemic heart disease and cardiomyopathies (106,107).

Autonomic Alterations and Arrhythmogenesis

Myocardial ischemia is accompanied by significant alterations in the autonomic nervous system. A major acute ischemic episode generates a stress reaction leading to elevation of circulating catecholamines as well as free fatty acids. Within the ischemic myocardium, norepinephrine is released from injured nerve terminals resulting, initially, in a redistribution of catecholamines, followed by their eventual depletion (133). Alterations in adrenergic receptors develop, including increases in the numbers of β- and α-adrenergic receptors expressed on the sarcolemmal membrane (134,135). Initially, excess catecholamine stimulation is coupled with increased intracellular metabolism mediated in part through the adenylate cyclase system. Eventually, uncoupling occurs between intracellular metabolism and receptor stimulation. However, this coupling can be restored and heightened upon reperfusion. Excess catecholamine stimulation can have a number of untoward consequences, including enhanced intracellular calcium influx as well as arrhythmogenesis.

Arrhythmias and conduction disturbances occur commonly in association with myocardial ischemia and may range from mild alterations to ventricular fibrillation. Arrhythmias are particularly common during the early phase of an ischemic episode as well as at the onset of reperfusion (2,42–44). It is likely that different mechanisms operate in different phases of ischemic arrhythmias. The arrhythmias may be mediated by (*i*) metabolic alterations, including a high concentration of potassium in the extracellular space adjacent to cardiac myocytes and nerve terminals (2); (*ii*) accumulation of lysophospholipids, long-chain acyl compounds, and free fatty acids in myocardial membranes (72–74); (*iii*) the alterations in the adrenergic system described above (133–135); and (*iv*) intracellular electrolyte alterations, including accumulation of intracellular calcium (136).

EVOLUTION OF MYOCARDIAL INFARCTION

Progression of Myocardial Ischemic Injury

In humans, the left ventricular subendocardium is the region most susceptible to myocardial ischemic injury. This is also true for the dog, which is a common species used for experimental studies of myocardial ischemia, whereas other species, such as the pig, have few native collaterals (1–6). The susceptibility of the subendocardium relates to a more tenuous oxygen supply-demand balance in this region versus the subepicardium. This in turn is related to the pattern of distribution of the collateral circulation as well as local metabolic differences in subendocardial versus subepicardial myocytes.

Following coronary occlusion, the myocardium can withstand up to about 20 minutes of severe ischemia without developing irreversible injury. However, after about 20 to 30 minutes of severe ischemia, irreversible myocardial injury develops. The subsequent degradative changes give rise to recognizable myocardial necrosis. In the human and dog, myocardial necrosis first appears in the ischemic subendocardium, because this area generally has a more severe reduction in perfusion compared with the subepicardium. Over the ensuing three to four hours, irreversible myocardial injury progresses in a wavefront pattern from the subendocardium into the subepicardium (2,137). In the experimental animal and probably in humans as well, most myocardial infarcts are completed within approximately three to four hours after the onset of coronary occlusion. A slower pattern of evolution of myocardial infarction, however, can occur when the coronary collateral circulation is particularly prominent and/or when the stimulus for myocardial ischemia is intermittent, e.g., in the case of episodes of intermittent platelet aggregation before occlusive thrombosis.

Histological and Ultrastructural Changes

Established myocardial infarcts have distinct central and peripheral regions (Fig. 7-11) (2,82,83,137–139). In the central zone of severe ischemia, the necrotic myocytes exhibit clumped nuclear chromatin; stretched myofibrils with widened I bands; mitochondria containing amorphous matrix (flocculent) densities composed of denatured lipid and protein and linear densities representing fused cristae; and defects (holes) in the sarcolemma. In the peripheral region of an infarct, which has some degree of collateral perfusion, many necrotic myocytes exhibit disruption of the myofibrils with the formation of dense transverse (contraction) bands; mitochondria containing calcium phosphate deposits as well as the amorphous matrix densities; variable amounts of lipid droplets; and clumped nuclear chromatin. A third population of cells at the outermost periphery of infarcts contain excess numbers of lipid droplets but do not exhibit the features of irreversible injury just described. The three patterns of myocardial necrosis have been characterized as typical coagulation necrosis, coagulative myocytolysis (contraction band

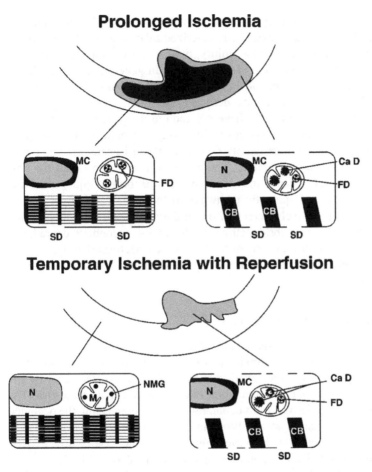

Figure 7 A schematic diagram comparing the pathobiological features of a transmural infarct produced by permanent coronary occlusion (*top*) and a subendocardial infarct produced by temporary coronary occlusion, followed by reperfusion (*bottom*). With prolonged coronary occlusion, myocardial necrosis is established in the subendocardium within 40 to 60 minutes, progresses in a wavefront pattern into the subepicardium of the region at risk (risk zone), and is completed in three to four hours. With prolonged coronary occlusion, the myofibrils of myocytes in the central infarct region are hyper-relaxed as compared with those in the normal tissue, depicted in the lower panel, and the mitochondria contain flocculent densities composed of denatured lipid and protein. The myofibrils of myocytes in the peripheral infarct region are formed into contraction bands, and the mitochondria show calcium deposits as well as flocculent densities. With temporary ischemia and reperfusion, injury is limited to the subendocardium and is characterized by myofibrillar contraction bands and early mitochondrial calcification. *Abbreviations*: N, nucleus; MC, marginated chromatin; SD, sarcolemmal defect; FD, flocculent (amorphous) density; NMG, normal matrix granule; CB, contraction band; CaD, calcium deposit. *Source*: From Ref. 83.

necrosis), and colliquative myocytolysis (myocytolysis) (140,141). The pattern of injury seen in the infarcted periphery characterized by contraction band necrosis is also characteristic of myocardial injury produced by temporary coronary occlusion, followed by reperfusion (1–6,108–114). In general, the most reliable ultrastructural features of irreversible injury are the amorphous matrix densities in the mitochondria and the sarcolemmal defects (Figs. 7–11).

Takemura and Fujiwara (127) have pointed out the paucity of histological and ultrastructural features of apoptosis involving ischemic cardiomyocytes, whereas such features are more readily demonstrable in ischemic nonmyocytic cells in evolving myocardial infarcts. These observations have raised the possibility that myocardial ischemia may involve a hybrid form of injury involving activation of oncotic and apoptotic pathways in the same cardiomyocytes, as discussed above. Alternatively, retention of cardiomyocytes irreversibly injured by oncotic, apoptotic, or hybrid pathways allows for secondary degradative changes manifest as myocardial necrosis. Myocardial necrosis then leads to an exudative inflammatory reaction with subsequent organization and healing with scar formation.

Determinants of Myocardial Infarct Size

The myocardial bed-at-risk, or risk zone, refers to the mass of myocardium that receives its blood supply from a major coronary artery that develops occlusion (137). Following occlusion, the severity of the ischemia is determined by the amount of preexisting collateral circulation into the myocardial bed-at-risk. The collateral blood flow is derived from collateral channels connecting the occluded and nonoccluded coronary systems. With time, there is progressive increase in coronary collateral blood flow. However, much of this increase in flow may be too late to salvage significant amounts of myocardium (2–6,137,142).

The size of the infarct is determined by the mass of necrotic myocardium within the bed-at-risk (2–6,137,142). The bed-at-risk will also contain viable but injured myocardium. The border zones refer to the nonnecrotic but dysfunctional myocardium within the ischemic bed-at-risk. The size of the border zone varies inversely with the relative amount of necrotic myocardium, which increases with time as the wavefront of necrosis progresses. The border zone exists primarily in the subepicardial half of the bed-at-risk and has very little lateral dimension, owing to a sharp demarcation between vascular beds supplied by the occluded and patent major coronary arteries.

Thus, the major determinants of ultimate infarct size are the duration and severity of ischemia, the size of the myocardial bed-at-risk, and the amount of collateral blood flow available shortly after coronary occlusion (2–6, 137–139,142). Infarct size also can be influenced by the major determinants of myocardial metabolic demand, which are heart rate, wall tension (determined by blood pressure), and myocardial contractility. Myocardial infarct size is a major determinant of prognosis, since the development of highly lethal cardiogenic shock correlates with loss of 40% or more of functioning left ventricular myocardium (143,144).

Measurement of Myocardial Infarct Size

Pathological analysis of infarct size has provided a "goal standard" in accessing the accuracy of various noninvasive diagnostic tests for myocardial infarction and the efficacy of various interventions and treatment. Application of a strict criterion for proof of a direct positive effect of a therapeutic intervention involves measurement of a reduction in infarct size without a change in collateral coronary blood flow (2–6,145,146). Although extensive investigation in this area has been conducted, noninvasive determination of infarct size remains a challenge. Techniques that have been used to image coronary arteries and myocardium have included various electrocardiographic methods, quantitation of serum enzyme release, and various imaging approaches, including intravascular ultrasound, echocardiography, radionuclide scintigraphy, positon emission tomography, computed tomography, and magnetic resonance imaging (147–150). In the early phase of development of myocardial imaging, our group extensively evaluated the use of technetium stannous pyrophosphate scintigraphy for detection and sizing of myocardial infarcts, while other groups evaluated other

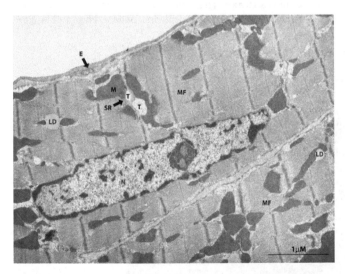

Figure 8 Normal left ventricular canine myocardium. The myocardium is compact and exhibits normal ultrastructure. The cardiomyocytes show myofibrils with sarcomeric units comprising two bands, narrow I bands, and wide A bands; they contain abundant glycogen (G), a few small lipid droplets (LD), sarcoplasmic reticulum (SR), T tubules (T), normal mitochondria (M), and a central nucleus (N). The capillary is expanded and is lined by a thin endothelium (E). The interstitial space is very narrow. (Electron micrograph: ×6800). *Source*: From Ref. 79.

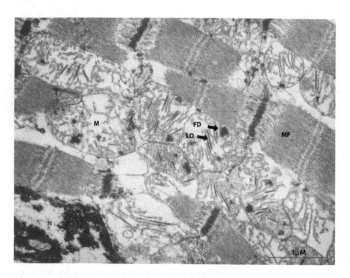

Figure 9 Cardiomyocyte showing ultrastructural features of irreversible ischemic injury in the severely ischemic central region of an evolving canine myocardial infarct. Note the separation of the organelles, indicative of mild intracellular edema and cell swelling. The myofibrils are relaxed. The mitochondria (M) are swollen and contain flocculent densities (FD) (amorphous matrix densities), and linear densities [fused cristae (LD)]. The nucleus (N) is shrunken and has clumped chromatin (×16900). This is the typical pattern of severe ischemic myocardial injury resulting from rapid and severe ATP depletion. *Source*: From Ref. 6.

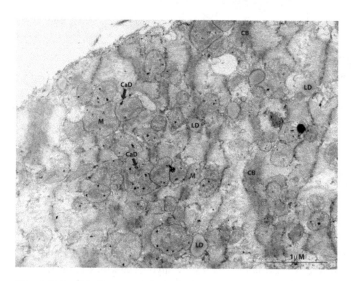

Figure 10 Cardiomyocyte with ultrastructural features of contraction band injury and calcium overloading as seen in the peripheral zone of an evolving canine myocardial infarct with collateral blood flow. Note the foci of myofibrils condensed into bands (CB), the lipid droplets (LD), and granular calcium deposits (calcium phosphate, CaD ×6500). *Source*: From Ref. 6.

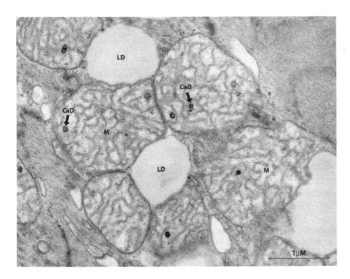

Figure 11 Ultrastructural detail of ischemic cardiomyocyte with lipid deposits (LD) and swollen mitochondria containing very electron dense, annular-granular calcium phosphate deposits (CaD ×26,000). As ATP is reduced, mitochondrial oxidative capacity is decreased, leading to an accumulation of re-esterified fatty acids as liquid droplets, and the sarcolemmal function becomes impaired, leading to increased calcium influx, which becomes excessive with a ready supply of extracellular fluid. The excess calcium triggers hypercontraction of the myofibrils manifest as contraction bands. The mitochondria accumulate the excess calcium at the expense of further ATP production; the calcium binds with inorganic phosphate to form calcium phosphate deposits. *Source*: From Ref. 6.

scintigraphic approaches (138,139). Now the multiple other imaging approaches have been developed. However, ongoing work is needed to perfect methods for noninvasive detection and quantification of the myocardial bed-at-risk and the extent of reversible and irreversible damage. This then will allow an analysis of absolute infarct size as well as infarct size as a percentage of the bed-at-risk.

MODULATION OF MYOCARDIAL ISCHEMIC INJURY

Modulating Influences of Preconditioning, Stunning, Postconditioning, Reperfusion, and Remodeling

A number of factors can significantly modulate the myocardial response and subsequent outcome following an ischemic episode (4–6). The progression of myocardial ischemia can be profoundly influenced by reperfusion (Fig. 12). However, the effects of reperfusion are complex (108–114). Reperfusion can clearly limit the extent of myocardial necrosis if instituted early enough after the onset of coronary occlusion. However, reperfusion also changes the pattern of

Reperfusion Within Thirty Minutes of Coronary Occlusion

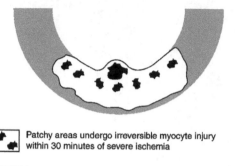

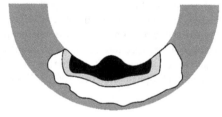 Patchy areas undergo irreversible myocyte injury within 30 minutes of severe ischemia

Large areas of myocardium undergo reversible injury during 30 minutes of coronary occlusion and are salved
A by reperfusion but with transient dysfunction (stunning)

Reperfusion Within Two Hours of Coronary Occlusion

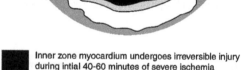

Inner zone myocardium undergoes irreversible injury during intial 40-60 minutes of severe ischemia

Mid zone myocardium becomes severely injured during coronary occlusion and is subject to irreversible injury upon reperfusion (reperfusion-induced cell death)

Outer zone myocardium becomes less severely injured during coronary occlusion and is salvageable upon reperfusion
B but with transient dysfunction (stunning)

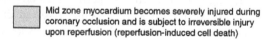
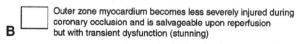

Figure 12 Influences of duration of coronary occlusion and timing of reperfusion on the response of the ischemic myocardium. (**A**) When reperfusion is achieved within 30 minutes of coronary occlusion, minimal irreversible injury occurs and most of the ischemic myocardium is salvaged but with transient dysfunction (stunning). (**B**) When reperfusion occurs within two hours of coronary occlusion, a significant amount of subendocardial myocardium develops irreversible injury, including some myocytes that become irreversibly injured at the time of reperfusion (reperfusion-induced cell death); however, reperfusion also results in significant salvage of subepicardial myocardium that would have developed irreversible injury with permanent coronary occlusion. *Source*: From Ref. 4.

myocardial injury by causing reduced reflow ("no-reflow phenomenon") and hemorrhage within the severely damaged myocardium and by producing a pattern of myocardial injury characterized by contraction bonds and calcification. Reperfusion also accelerates the release of intracellular enzymes from damaged myocardium. This may lead to a marked elevation of serum levels of these enzymes without necessarily implying further myocardial necrosis. The timing of reperfusion is critical to the outcome, with the potential for myocardial salvage being greater with earlier intervention. Although reperfusion can clearly salvage myocardium, it may also induce additional injury. The concept of reperfusion injury implies the development of further damage, as a result of the reperfusion, to myocytes that were injured but that remained viable during a previous ischemic episode. Such injury may involve functional impairment, arrhythmia, and/or progression to cell death (108–114). Reperfusion injury is mediated by bursts of Ca^{2+} influx and oxygen radical generation, with the oxygen radicals generated in the reperfused myocardial cells and neutrophils, which accumulate in the microvasculature and interstitium and, thereby, contribute to the reduced reflow phenomenon.

The rate of progression of myocardial necrosis can be influenced by prior short intervals of coronary occlusion and reperfusion. Specifically, experimental evidence indicates that the extent of myocardial necrosis after 60 to 90 minutes of coronary occlusion is significantly less in animals that had been pretreated with one or more five-minute intervals of coronary occlusion before the induction of permanent occlusion. However, after 120 minutes of coronary occlusion, the effect on infarct size is lost. This phenomenon is known as preconditioning (151,152). A reduced rate of ATP depletion correlates with the beneficial effects of preconditioning (151,152). Further studies have suggested that activation of adenosine receptors and ATP-dependent potassium channels in the sarcolemma and particularly in the mitochondria may mediate the process of preconditioning (Fig. 13) (4–6,114,153–155). After a refractory period, a second late phase of myocardial protection during a subsequent ischemic event develops (155,156). This phenomenon, known as the second window of protection (SWOP), is related to ischemia-induced gene activation with production of various gene products, including stress (heat shock) proteins and NO synthase (4–6,155,156).

Controlled reperfusion with several very brief temporary periods of coronary occlusion before sustained reperfusion can reduce the extent of reperfusion injury. This phenomenon is known as postconditioning (157,158). Coupling timely postconditioning with pharmacological agents has the potential of greatly reducing ischemic injury and reperfusion injury.

Prolonged functional depression, requiring up to 24 hours or longer for recovery, develops on reperfusion even after relatively brief periods of coronary occlusion, on the order of 15 minutes, which is insufficient to cause myocardial necrosis. This phenomenon has been referred to as myocardial stunning (4–6). A related condition, termed hibernation, refers to chronic depression of myocardial

Postulated Mechanisms of Early Ischemic Myocardial Preconditiong and Second Window of Protection

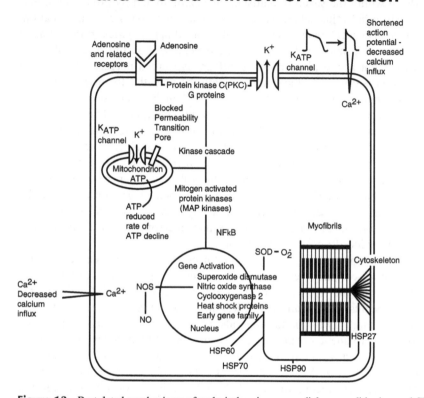

Figure 13 Postulated mechanisms of early ischemic myocardial preconditioning and SWOP. Brief periods of coronary occlusion lead to an initially slower rate of ATP decline and reduced rate of progression to irreversible injury and necrosis during subsequent prolonged coronary occlusion; this phenomenon is ischemic preconditioning. Experimental evidence indicates that key events in ischemic preconditioning are activation of adenosine and related receptors, activation of PKC, and opening of ATP-dependent K^+ channels in the sarcolemma and mitochondria. The activated receptors couple to G protein, which stimulates a phospholipase that leads to degradation of phospholipids and formation of DAG. DAGs then activate PKC through a process that apparently involves translocation of certain PKC isoforms from the cytosol to the cell membrane. PKC then phosphorylates various molecules, including K_{ATP} channels. One hypothesis is that sarcolemmal K^+ efflux leads to shortening of the action potential duration, decreased Ca^{2+} influx, and subsequent blunting of injury induced by Ca^{2+} overload. However, the current leading hypothesis is that opening of mitochondrial K_{ATP} channels leads to mitochondrial swelling, blockade of opening of the permeability transition pore, ROS generation, and preservation of ATP. Brief episodes of coronary occlusion lead to early ischemic preconditioning, followed by a refractory period and the subsequent onset of a SWOP. The SWOP is related to gene activation mediated by a kinase cascade, including MAP kinases, and NFκB. Gene products implicated in the SWOP include superoxide dismutase, NO synthase and its product, NO, and heat shock proteins, including HSP27, which interacts with the cytoskeleton. *Abbreviations*: SWOP, second window of protection; PKC, protein kinase C; DAG, diacyglycerides; ROS, reactive oxygen species; MAP, mitogen-activated protein; NFκB, nuclear factor κB. *Source*: From Ref. 4.

function owing to a chronic moderate reduction of perfusion (4–6). Pre-conditioning and stunning are independent phenomena, since the preconditioning effect is short term, transient, and not mediated through stunning. Free radical effects and calcium loading have been implicated in the pathogenesis of stun-ning, as well as other components of reperfusion injury (159,160). After longer intervals of coronary occlusion, on the order of two to four hours, necrosis of the subendocardium develops and even more severe and persistent functional depression occurs (161). In experimental studies, after two hours of coronary occlusion LV regional sites of moderate dysfunction during ischemia recovered normal or near-normal regional contractile function after one to four weeks of reperfusion, whereas after four hours of coronary occlusion, contractile dys-function persisted after four weeks of reperfusion (161).

Therefore, depending on the interval of coronary occlusion before reper-fusion, various degrees of contractile dysfunction, necrosis, or both are seen with reperfusion. These observations emphasize the need for early intervention to salvage myocardium (1–6,137). On balance, early reperfusion results in a major net positive effect making early reperfusion an important goal in the treatment of acute ischemic heart disease (45–49).

Following myocardial infarction, progressive changes occur in viable myocardium in response to increased stress on the ventricular wall. This process, known as myocardial remodeling, involves hypertrophy of cardiomyocytes; vascular and connective tissue proliferation; loss of cardiomyocytes by oncosis, apoptosis, and autophagy; and apparent formation of new cardiomyocytes from stem cells (4,106,107,162). Effective remodeling in response to a moderate insult can result in normalization of wall stress. However, ineffective or inadequate remodeling in response to a major insult can lead to fixed structural dilatation of the ventricle, heart failure, and ischemic cardiomyopathy (163,164).

Therapeutic Interventions

Continuing efforts have been made to develop therapeutic approaches to limiting infarct size since the extent of myocardial necrosis is a major determinant of prognosis following myocardial infarction. Experimental studies have shown that evaluation of a therapeutic agent should take into account both the influence of the size of the myocardial bed-at-risk and the amount of collateral perfusion over a given time interval of coronary occlusion (Fig. 14) (142,145,146). If an intervention produces a smaller infarct as a percentage of the bed-at-risk at any given level of residual perfusion, then it can be concluded that the intervention has an independent effect on myocardial ischemic cell injury. Various phar-macological approaches have been aimed at improving myocardial metabolism, increasing myocardial blood flow, reducing cellular calcium overload, and preventing free radical-mediated effects (Table 3) (142,145,146,165–167). In spite of the promise of experimental studies, demonstration of major reduction of infarct size by pharmacological means has not been forthcoming in man. However, some pharmacological approaches, such as treatment with propranolol,

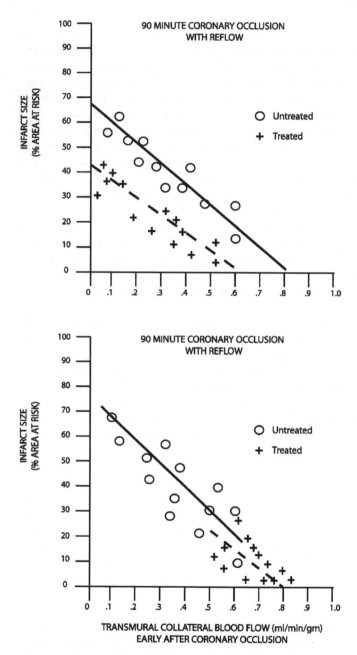

Figure 14 Theoretical outcomes of experiments performed to determine the potential effect of an intervention on limiting infarct size after 90 minutes of temporary coronary occlusion and reperfusion in the dog. Infarct size, expressed as a percentage of the area at risk, is plotted against transmural collateral blood flow measured shortly after coronary occlusion. Smaller infarct size at any level of residual collateral blood flow is shown in the

Table 3 Interventions Demonstrated to Reduce the Extent of Myocardial Infarction in Experimental Animals

---

Interventions that increase coronary blood flow
  Isosorbide dinitrate and nitroglycerin infusion
  Calcium antagonists, including nifedipine
  Mechanical circulatory assistance, including intraaortic balloon counterpulsation and
    external compression of the lower extremities
  Reperfusion after temporary coronary artery occlusion
Interventions that reduce myocardial oxygen demand
  β-Adrenergic blocking agents, including propranolol
  Selected calcium antagonists, including verapamil and diltiazem
Interventions that increase substrate availability
  Glucose, potassium, and insulin
  Carnitine
  Certain amino acids, including the L-isomers of glutamate, arginine, ornithine, and
    aspartate
Interventions that protect the myocardial cell directly and/or decrease inflammation
  Hyaluronidase
  Hypertonic agents, including mannitol (protection may last only 40–60 min)
  Ibuprofen or flurbiprofen
  Single doses of steroids
  Specific phospholipase inhibitors
  Free radical scavengers

Source: From Ref. 142.

have been shown to have a positive effect on morbidity and mortality (45–49). This is reflected by the difficulties in establishing efficacy for an experimentally proven intervention, glucose-insulin-potassium infusion, in patients, while conventional therapy is in constant evolution (168–172).

The most important advance in recent years has been the advent of PCIs, including thrombolytic therapy and stent placement, to provide reperfusion of the ischemic myocardium. This approach is the hallmark of the current era of treatment of AMI (54,55). Ongoing investigations are aimed at developing pharmacological interventions, which can be coupled with thrombolytic therapy

←——————————————————————————

treated versus untreated group (*top*). This result supports the conclusion that the intervention reduced infarct size by a direct effect on the ischemic myocytes without affecting coronary blood flow. As another potential result, the treated group has smaller infarcts associated with greater collateral blood flow compared with the untreated group (*bottom*). This result supports the conclusion that the intervention reduced infarct size by increasing collateral blood flow and decreasing the severity of ischemia rather than by a direct effect on the ischemic myocytes. Alternatively, this result could have occurred by bias in selecting animals with greater native collaterals for the treated group. *Source*: From Ref. 146.

to provide optimal protection and salvage of the ischemic myocardium. Control and treatment of arrhythmias and conduction disturbances include both pharmacological approaches, pacemakers and defibrillators.

Pathology of Interventionally Treated Coronary Artery Disease

PTCA can produce a variety of acute effects, including dilatation of the vessel caused by stretching of the intima and media, damage to the endothelial surface, multiple fissures in the plaque, and dissection of the media (56–59,173,174). The acute injury initiates a reparative response that leads to intimal proliferation (22–26,56–59,173,174). Similar effects occur after atherectomy and laser angioplasty (174,176). The resultant fibrocellular tissue is composed of modified smooth muscle cells (myofibroblasts) and connective tissue matrix without lipid deposits. A similar lesion is seen in animal models of arterial injury (22–26). Experimental evidence supports a role for platelet activation in the pathogenesis of the lesion (22–26). This process of intimal proliferation leads to restenosis of lesions in 30% to 40% of cases within six months. The use of vascular stents in conjunction with angioplasty has significantly improved the long-term patency rates, although the stents do invoke some intimal reaction (57–61). The introduction of drug-eluting stents coated with antiproliferative agents has further improved the short-term patency rates (62–64). However, late thrombosis is a cause of concern. Conventional therapy has recently been found to be equally effectual as PCI and stent placement in patients with stable angina pectoris.

Saphenous vein coronary artery bypass grafts (SVCABG) develop diffuse fibrocellular intimal thickening, medial degeneration and atrophy, and vascular dilatation within several months after implantation (174,177–179). Subsequently, the grafts are prone to development of eccentric intimal plaques with lipid deposition (atherosclerosis). Plaque fissuring and thrombosis may also develop. Therefore, all of the changes seen in naturally occurring atherosclerosis may also develop in the saphenous veins, thereby creating a finite limit to the beneficial effects of these grafts. With improvements in surgical technique, the use of internal mammary arteries for coronary bypass has taken on more widespread application. The internal mammary arteries are more resistant to the intimal injury and intimal proliferation observed in saphenous veins, and, therefore, the arterial bypass grafts have prolonged potency (180–182).

New Approaches to Myocardial Modulation

A new era in the treatment of ischemic heart disease is developing on the basis of the therapeutic application of new insights regarding the pathogenesis of myocardial ischemic disease. New pharmacological interventions are being tested on the basis of the possible contribution of apoptosis as well as oncosis in myocardial infarction (4–6,123–126). Ongoing work is being conducted to successfully achieve genetic manipulation (gene therapy) of the processes responsible for the response of the arterial wall to injury, with the goals of retarding or preventing intimal proliferation and thrombosis at sites of coronary injury (183–186). Alternative approaches are also being explored for the treatment of intractable angina pectoris (173,174,187,188). One surgical approach is the use of transmyocardial laser treatment to create new myocardial microvasculature (189–191). An alternate approach is the intravascular delivery of genetically engineered growth factors, including VEGF and FGF (186,192–195).

The debate regarding whether or not cardiac myocytes are terminally differentiated has been revived (196,197). Molecular mechanisms responsible for the mitotic block of mature myocytes are under investigation with the potential for genetic manipulation of myocyte proliferation (198,199). The myocardium has been found to have a population of endogenous cardiac stem cells as well as circulating stem cells that are home to the myocardium (162,200–203). However, naturally occurring myocardial regeneration in response to injury in the mammalian heart is biologically limited (204). Other approaches are being explored, including microinjection of genetically engineered myocytes and allogenic stem cells for repopulation of damaged myocardium (205–207). Strategies are being explored to reduce the extent of myocardial damage and repair the myocardium by activating and enhancing and promoting myocytic differentiation of stem cells. The considerable promise of these approaches for the treatment of ischemic myocardial disease is the focus of ongoing basic research and clinical investigation and application.

REFERENCES

1. Hillis LD, Braunwald E. Myocardial ischemia. N Engl J Med 1977; 296:971; 1034; 1093.
2. Reimer KA, Ideker RE. Myocardial ischemia and infarction: anatomic and biochemical substrates for ischemic cell death and ventricular arrhythmias. Hum Pathol 1987; 18:462.
3. Willerson JT, Hillis LD, Buja LM. Ischemic Heart Disease: Clinical and Pathophysiological Aspects. New York: Raven Press, 1982.
4. Buja LM. Modulation of the myocardial response to ischemia. Lab Invest 1998; 78:1345.
5. Buja LM. Myocardial ischemia and reperfusion injury. Cardiovasc Pathol 2005; 14:170.
6. Willerson JT, Buja LM. Myocardial reperfusion: biology, benefits and consequences. Dialogues Cardiovasc Med 2006; 11:267.
7. Ross R. The pathogenesis of atherosclerosis: a perspective for the 1990s. Nature 1993; 362:801.
8. Ross R. Atherosclerosis: an inflammatory disease. N Engl J Med 1999; 340:115.
9. Libby P. Inflammation in atherosclerosis. Nature 2002; 420:868.
10. Libby P, Ridker PM, Maseri A. Inflammation and atherosclerosis. Circulation 2002; 105:1135.

11. Hansson GD, Libby P, Schönbeck U, et al. Innate and adaptive immunity in the pathogenesis of atherosclerosis. Circ Res 2002; 91:281.

12. Hansson GK. Inflammation, atherosclerosis, and coronary artery disease. N Engl J Med 2005; 352:1685.

13. Buja LM, Clubb FJ Jr., Bilhelmer DW, et al. Pathobiology of human familial hypercholesterolemia and a related animal model, the Watanabe heritable hyperlipidemic rabbit. Eur Heart J 1990; 11(suppl E):41.

14. Buja LM, Hillis LD, Petty CS, et al. The role of coronary arterial spasm in ischemic heart disease. Arch Pathol Lab Med 1981; 105:221.

15. Hirsh PD, Campbell WB, Willerson JT, et al. Prostaglandins and ischemic heart disease. Am J Med 1981; 71:1009.

16. Fitzgerald DJ, Roy L, Catella F, et al. Platelet activation in unstable coronary disease. N Engl J Med 1986; 315:983.

17. Davies MJ, Thomas AC, Knapman PA, et al. Intramyocardial platelet aggregation in patients with unstable angina pectoris suffering sudden ischemic cardiac death. Circulation 1986; 73:418.

18. Buja LM, Willerson JT. Clinicopathological correlates of acute ischemic heart disease syndromes. Am J Cardiol 1981; 47:343.

19. Buja LM, Willerson JT. The role of coronary artery lesions in ischemic heart disease: insights from recent clinicopathologic, coronary arteriographic, and experimental studies. Hum Pathol 1987; 18:451.

20. Buja LM, Willerson JT. Relationship of ischemic heart disease to sudden cardiac death. J Forensic Sci 1991; 36:25.

21. Fuster V, Badimon L, Badimon JJ, et al. The pathogenesis of coronary artery disease and the acute coronary syndromes. N Engl J Med 1992; 326:242; 310.

22. Willerson JT, Golino P, Eidt J, et al. Specific platelet mediators and unstable coronary artery lesions. Experimental evidence and potential clinical implications. Circulation 1989; 80:198.

23. Willerson JT, Yao S-K, McNatt J, et al. Frequency and severity of cyclic flow alternations and platelet aggregation predict the severity of neointimal proliferation following experimental coronary stenosis and endothelial injury. Proc Natl Acad Sci U S A 1991; 88:10624.

24. Golino P, Ambrosio G, Ragni M, et al. Inhibition of leukocyte and platelet adhesion reduces neointimal hyperplasia after arterial injury. Thromb Haemost 1997; 77:783.

25. Anderson HV, McNatt J, Clubb FJ, et al. Platelet inhibition reduces cyclic flow variations and neointimal proliferation in normal and hypercholesterolemic-atherosclerotic canine coronary arteries. Circulation 2001; 104:2331.

26. Schulman SP, Goldschmidt-Clermont PJ, Topol EJ, et al. Effects of integrelin, a platelet glycoprotein IIb/IIIa receptor antagonist, in unstable angina. A randomized multicenter trial. Circulation 1996; 94:2083.

27. Theroux P, Fuster V. Acute coronary syndromes: unstable angina and non-Q-wave myocardial infarction. Circulation 1998; 97:1195.

28. Virmani R, Kolodgie FD, Burke AP, et al. Lessons from sudden coronary death: a comprehensive morphological classification scheme for atherosclerotic lesions. Arterioscler Thromb Vasc Biol 2000; 20:1262.

29. Kolodgie FD, Gold HK, Burke AP, et al. Intraplaque hemorrhage and progression of coronary atheroma. N Engl J Med 2003; 349:2316.

30. Schaar JA, Muller JE, Falk E, et al. Terminology for high-risk and vulnerable coronary artery plaques. Eur Heart J 2004; 25:1077.
31. Virmani R, Burke AP, Farb A, et al. Pathology of the vulnerable plaque. J Am Coll Cardiol 2006; 47(suppl C):C13.
32. van der Wal AC, Becker AE, van der Loos CM, et al. Site of intimal rupture or erosion of thrombosed coronary atherosclerotic plaques is characterized by an inflammatory process irrespective of the dominant plaque morphology. Circulation 1994; 89:36.
33. Buja LM, Willerson JT. Role of inflammation in coronary plaque disruption. Circulation 1994; 89:503.
34. Burke AP, Farb A, Malcomb GT, et al. Plaque rupture and sudden death related to exertion in men with coronary artery disease. JAMA 1999; 281:921.
35. Burke AP, Farb A, Malcomb GT, et al. Effect of risk factors on the mechanism of acute thrombosis and sudden coronary death in women. Circulation 1998; 97:2110.
36. Fuster V, Moreno PR, Fayad ZA, et al. Atherothrombosis and high-risk plaque. Part I: evolving concepts. J Am Coll Cardiol 2005; 46:937.
37. Virmani R, Burke AP, Farb A. Sudden cardiac death. Cardiovasc Pathol 2001; 10:275.
38. Farb A, Burke AP, Tang A, et al. Coronary plaque erosion without rupture into a lipid core. A frequent cause of coronary thrombosis in sudden coronary death. Circulation 1996; 93:1354.
39. Burke AP, Farb A, Malcomb GT, et al. Coronary risk factors and plaque morphology in men with coronary disease who die suddenly. N Engl J Med 1997; 336:1276.
40. Burke AP, Farb A, Malcomb GT, et al. Effect of risk factors on the mechanism of acute thrombosis and sudden coronary death in women. Circulation 1998; 97:2110.
41. Burke AP, Farb A, Malcomb GT, et al. Plaque rupture and sudden death related to exertion in men with coronary artery disease. JAMA 1999; 281:921.
42. Zipes DP, Wellens HJ. Sudden cardiac death. Circulation 1998; 98:2334.
43. Huikuri HV, Castellanos A, Myerburg RJ. Sudden death due to cardiac arrhythmias. N Engl J Med 2001; 345:1473.
44. Winslow RD, Mehta D, Fuster V. Sudden cardiac death: mechanisms, therapies and challenges. Nat Clin Pract Cardiovasc Med 2005; 2:352.
45. Van de Werf F, Ardissino D, Betriu A, et al. Management of acute myocardial infarction in patients with ST-segment elevation. Eur Heart J 2003; 24:28.
46. Bertrand ME, Simoons ML, Fox KA, et al. Management of acute coronary syndromes in patients presenting without persistent ST-segment elevation. Eur Heart J 2002; 23:1809.
47. Antman EM, Anbe DT, Armstrong PW, et al. ACC/AHA guidelines for management of patients with ST-elevation myocardial infarction. Circulation 2004; 110(5):588.
48. Braunwald E, Antman EM, Beasley JW, et al. ACC/AHA guideline update for the management of patients with unstable angina and non-ST-segment elevation myocardial infarction—2002. Circulation 2002; 106:1893.
49. Gibbons RJ, Fuster V. Therapy for patients with acute coronary syndromes—new opportunities. N Engl J Med 2006; 354:1524.
50. Madjid M, Zarrabi A, Litovsky S, et al. Finding vulnerable atherosclerotic plaques: is it worth the effort? Arterioscler Thromb Vasc Biol 2004; 24:1775.

51. Hamilton AJ, Huang SL, Warnick D, et al. Intravascular ultrasound molecular imaging of atheroma components in vivo. J Am Coll Cardiol 2004; 43:453.

52. Fuster V, Fayad ZA, Moreno PR, et al. Atherothrombosis and high-risk plaque. Part II: approaches by noninvasive computed tomographic/magnetic resonance imaging. J Am Coll Cardiol 2005; 46:1209.

53. Sanz J, Moreno PR, Fuster V. Update on advances in atherothrombosis. Nat Clin Pract Cardiovasc Med 2007; 4:78.

54. Smith SC Jr., Feldman TE, Hirshfeld JW Jr., et al. ACC/AHA/SCAI 2005 guideline update for percutaneous coronary intervention. Circulation 2006; 113:156.

55. Silber S, Albertsson P, Avilés FF, et al. Guidelines for percutaneous coronary interventions. Eur Heart J 2005; 26:804.

56. Buja LM, Willerson JT, Murphree SS. Pathobiology of arterial wall injury, atherosclerosis, and coronary angioplasty. In: Black AJR, Anderson HV, Ellis SG, eds. Complications of Coronary Angioplasty. New York, NY: Marcel Dekker, 1991:11.

57. Farb A, Lindsay J Jr., Virmani R. Pathology of bailout coronary stenting in human beings. Am Heart J 1999; 137:621.

58. Farb A, Sangiorgi G, Carter AJ, et al. Pathology of acute and chronic coronary stenting in humans. Circulation 1999; 99:44.

59. Farb A, Kolodgie FD, Hwang JY, et al. Extracellular matrix changes in stented human coronary arteries, Circulation 2004; 110:940.

60. Virmani R, Farb A, Guagliumi G, et al. Drug-eluting stents: caution and concerns for long-term outcome, Coron Artery Dis 2004; 15:313.

61. Schwartz RS, Chronos NA, Virmani R. Preclinical restenosis models and drug eluting stents: still important, still much to learn. J Am Coll Cardiol 2004; 44:1373.

62. Curfman GD, Morrissey S, Jar Cho JA, et al. Drug-eluting coronary stents – promise and uncertainty. N Engl J Med 2007; 356:1059.

63. Serruys PW, Daemen J. Are drug-eluting stents associated with a higher rate of late thrombosis than bare metal stents? Late stent thrombosis: a nuisance in both bare metal and drug-eluting stents. Circulation 2007; 115:1433.

64. Camenzind E, Steg G, Wijns W. Stent thrombosis late after implantation of first-generation drug-eluting stents: a cause for concern. Circulation 2007; 115:1440.

65. Boden WE, O'Rourke RA, Jeo KK, et al. Optimal medical therapy with or without PCI for stable coronary disease. N Engl J Med 2007; 356:1503.

66. Neely JR, Grotyohann LW. Role of glycolytic products in damage to ischemic myocardium. Dissociation of adenosine triphosphate levels and recovery of function of reperfusion ischemic hearts. Circ Res 1984; 55:816.

67. Morgan HE. Fueling the heart. Circ Res 2003; 92:1276.

68. Gibala MJ, Young ME, Taegtmeyer H. Anaplerosis of the citric acid cycle: role in energy metabolism of heart and skeletal muscle. Acta Physiol Scand 2000; 168:657.

69. Moore ML, Park EA, McMillin JB. Upstream stimulatory factor represses the induction of carnitine palmitoyltransferase-Iβ expression by PCG-1. J Biol Chem 2003; 278:17263.

70. Taegtmeyer H, Golfman L, Sharma S, et al. Linking gene expression to function: metabolic flexibility in normal and diseased heart. Ann N Y Acad Sci 2004; 1015:202.

71. Taegtmeyer H, Wilson CR, Razeghi P, et al. Metabolic energetics and genetics of the heart. Ann N Y Acad Sci 2005; 10147:208.

72. Katz AM, Messineo FC. Lipid-membrane interactions and the pathogenesis of ischemic damage in the myocardium. Circ Res 1981; 48:1.
73. Corr PB, Gross RW, Sobel BE. Amphipathic metabolites and membrane dysfunction in ischemic myocardium. Circ Res 1984; 55:135.
74. Buja LM. Lipid abnormalities in myocardial cell injury. Trends Cardiovasc Med 1991; 1:40.
75. Koretsune Y, Corretti MC, Kusuoka H, et al. Mechanism of early ischemic contractile failure. Inexcitability, metabolite accumulation or vascular collapse? Circ Res 1991; 68:255.
76. Carmeliet E. Myocardial ischemia: reversible and irreversible changes. Circulation 1984; 70:149.
77. Venkatesh N, Lamp ST, Weiss JN. Sulfonylureas, ATP-sensitive K + channels, and cellular K+ loss during hypoxia, ischemia, and metabolic inhibition in mammalian ventricle. Circ Res 1991; 69:623.
78. Thandroyen FT, Bellotto D, Katayama A, et al. Subcellular electrolyte alterations during hypoxia and following reoxygenation in isolated rat ventricular myocytes. Circ Res 1992; 71:106.
79. Willerson JT, Scales F, Mukherjee A, et al. Abnormal myocardial fluid retention as an early manifestation of ischemic injury. Am J Pathol 1977; 87:159.
80. Buja LM, Willerson JT. Abnormalities of volume regulation and membrane integrity in myocardial tissue slices after early ischemic injury in the dog: effects of mannitol, polyethylene glycol, and propranolol. Am J Pathol 1981; 103:79.
81. Braunwald E. Mechanism of action of calcium-channel-blocking agents. N Engl J Med 1982; 307:1618.
82. Buja LM, Hagler HK, Willerson JT. Altered calcium homeostasis in the pathogenesis of myocardial ischemic and hypoxic injury. Cell Calcium 1988; 9:205.
83. Hagler HK, Buja LM. Subcellular calcium shifts in ischemia and reperfusion. In: Piper HM, ed. Pathophysiology of Severe Ischemic Myocardial Injury. Dordrecht/ Boston/London: Kluwer Academic Publishers, 1990:283.
84. Yamamoto T, Su Z, Moseley AE, et al. Relative abundance of alpha 2 Na^+ pump isoform influences Na^+-Ca^{2+} exchanger currents and Ca^{2+} transients in mouse ventricular myocytes. J Mol Cell Cardiol 2005; 39:113.
85. Seguchi H, Ritter M, Shizukuishi M, et al. Propagation of Ca^{2+} release in cardiac myocytes: role of mitochondria. Cell Calcium 2005; 38:1.
86. Kadono T, Zhang XQ, Srinivasan S, et al. CRYAB and HSPB2 deficiency increases myocyte mitochondrial permeability transition and mitochondrial calcium uptake. J Mol Cell Cardiol 2006; 40:783.
87. Barry WH. Na^+ "Fuzzy space": does it exist, and is it important in ischemic injury? J Cardiovasc Electrophysiol 2006; 17(suppl 1):S43.
88. Morris AC, Hagler HK, Willerson JT, et al. Relationship between calcium loading and impaired energy metabolism during Na+, K+ pump inhibition and metabolic inhibition in cultured neonatal rat cardiac myocytes. J Clin Invest 1989; 83:1876.
89. Lee HC, Smith N, Mohabir R, et al. Cytosolic calcium transients from the beating mammalian heart. Proc Natl Acad Sci U S A 1987; 84:7793.
90. Marban E, Kitakaze M, Kusuoke H, et al. Intracellular free calcium concentrations measured with 19F NMR spectroscopy in intact ferret hearts. Proc Natl Acad Sci USA 1987; 84:6005.

91. Steenbergen C, Murphy E, Levy L, et al. Elevation in cytosolic free calcium concentration early in myocardial ischemia in perfused rat heart. Circ Res 1987; 60:700.

92. Chien KR, Han A, Sen A, et al. Accumulation of unesterified arachidonic acid in ischemic canine myocardium. Relationship to a phosphatidylcholine deacylation-reacylation cycle and the depletion of membrane phospholipids. Circ Res 1984; 54:313.

93. Jones RL, Miller JC, Hagler HK, et al. Association between inhibition of arachidonic acid release and prevention of calcium loading during ATP depletion in cultured neonatal rat cardiac myocytes. Am J Pathol 1989; 135:541.

94. Buja LM, Fattor RA, Miller JC, et al. Effects of calcium loading and impaired energy production on metabolic and ultrastructural features of cell injury in cultured neonatal rat cardiac myocytes. Lab Invest 1990; 63:320.

95. Sen A, Miller JC, Reynolds R, et al. Inhibition of the release of arachidonic acid prevents the development of sarcolemmal membrane defects in cultured rat myocardial cells during adenosine triphosphate depletion. J Clin Invest 1988; 82:1333.

96. Buja LM, Miller JC, Krueger GRF. Altered membrane fluidity occurs during metabolic impairment of cardiac myocytes. In Vivo 1991; 5:239.

97. Burton KP. Superoxide dismutase enhances recovery following myocardial ischemia. Am J Physiol 1985; 248:H637.

98. Burton KP. Evidence of direct toxic effects of free radicals on the myocardium. Free Radic Biol Med 1988; 4:15.

99. McCord JM. Oxygen-derived free radicals in postischemic tissue injury. N Engl J Med 1985; 312:159.

100. Burton KP, Morris AC, Massey KD, et al. Free radicals alter ionic calcium levels and membrane phospholipids in cultured rat ventricular myocytes. J Mol Cell Cardiol 1990; 22:1035.

101. Ferdinandy P, Appelbaum Y, Csonka C, et al. The role of nitric oxide and TPEN, a potent metal chelator, in ischeamic and reperfused rat hearts. Clin Exp Pharmacol Physiol 1998; 25:496.

102. Zhang X, Xie YW, Nasjletti A, et al. ACE inhibitors promote nitric oxide accumulation to modulate myocardial oxygen consumption. Circulation 1997; 95:176.

103. Steenbergen C, Hill ML, Jennings RB. Volume regulation and plasma membrane injury in aerobic, anaerobic, and ischemic myocardium in vitro. Effects of osmotic cell swelling on plasma membrane integrity. Circ Res 1985; 57:864.

104. Steenbergen C, Hill ML, Jennings RB. Cytoskeletal damage during myocardial ischemia changes in vinculin immunofluorescence staining during total in vitro ischemia in canine heart. Circ Res 1987; 60:478.

105. Ganote CE, Vander Heide RS. Cytoskeletal lesions in anoxic myocardial injury. A conventional and high-voltage electronmicroscopic and immunofluorescence study. Am J Pathol 1987; 129:327.

106. Kostin S, Pool L, Elsässer A, et al. Myocytes die by multiple mechanisms in failing human hearts. Circ Res 2003; 92:715.

107. Kostin S. Pathways of myocyte death: implications for development of clinical laboratory biomarkers. Adv Clin Chem 2005; 40:37.

108. Hearse DJ, Bolli R. Reperfusion-induced injury: manifestations, mechanisms and clinical relevance. Cardiovasc Res 1992; 26:101.

109. Maxwell SRJ, Lip GYH. Reperfusion injury: a review of the pathophysiology, clinical manifestations and therapeutic options. Int J Cardiol 1997; 58:95.
110. Park JL, Lucchesi BR. Mechanisms of myocardial reperfusion injury. Ann Thorac Surg 1998; 68:1905.
111. Ambrosio G, Tritto I. Reperfusion injury: experimental evidence and clinical implications. Am Heart J 1999; 138:S69.
112. Virmani R, Kolodgie FD, Forman MB, et al. Reperfusion injury in the ischemic myocardium. Cardiovasc Pathol 1992; 1:117.
113. Gross GJ, Auchampach JA. Reperfusion injury: does it exist? J Mol Cell Cardiol 2007; 42:12.
114. Yellon DM, Hausenloy DJ. Myocardial reperfusion injury. N Engl J Med 2007; 357:1121.
115. Buja LM, Eigenbrodt ML, Eigenbrodt EH. Apoptosis and necrosis. Basic types and mechanisms of cell death. Arch Pathol Lab Med 1993; 117:1208.
116. Majno G, Joris I. Apoptosis, oncosis and necrosis. An overview of cell death. Am J Pathol 1995; 146:3.
117. Buja LM, Entman ML. Modes of myocardial cell injury and cell death in ischemic heart disease. Circulation 1998; 98:1355.
118. Reed JC. Mechanisms of apoptosis. Am J Pathol 2000; 157:1415.
119. Scorrano L, Oakes SA, Opferman JJ, et al. BAX and BAK regulation of endoplasmic reticulum Ca^{2+}: a control point for apoptosis. Science 2003; 300:135.
120. Demaurex N. Distelhorst C. Cell biology. Apoptosis—the calcium connection. Science 2003; 300:65.
121. Danial NN, Korsmeyer SJ. Cell death: critical control points. Cell 2004; 116:205.
122. Takashi E, Ashraf M. Pathologic assessment of myocardial cell necrosis and apoptosis after ischemia and reperfusion with molecular and morphological markers. J Mol Cell Cardiol 2000; 32:209.
123. Foo RS, Mani K, Kitsis RN. Death begets failure in the heart. J Clin Invest 2005; 115:565.
124. Jugdutt BI, Idikio HA. Apoptosis and oncosis in acute coronary syndromes: assessment and implications. Mol Cell Biochem 2005; 270:177.
125. Kunapuli S, Rosanio S, Schwarz ER. "How do cardiomyocytes die?" Apoptosis and autophagic cell death in cardiac myocytes. J Card Fail 2006; 12:381.
126. Kajstura J, Bolli R, Sonnenblick EH, et al. Cause of death: suicide. J Mol Cell Cardiol 2006; 40:425.
127. Takemura G, Fujiwara H. Morphological aspects of apoptosis in heart diseases. J Cell Mol Med 2006; 10:56.
128. Leist M, Single B, Castoldi AF, et al. Intracellular adenosine triphosphate (ATP) concentration: a switch in the decision between apoptosis and necrosis. J Exp Med 1997; 185:1481.
129. Tatsumi T, Shiraishi J, Keira N, et al. Intracellular ATP is required for mitochondrial apoptotic pathways in isolated hypoxic rat cardiac myocytes. Cardiovasc Res 2003; 59:428.
130. Schaper J, Kostin S. Cell death and adenosine triphosphate: the paradox. Circulation 2005; 112:6.
131. Shintani T, Klionsky DJ. Autophagy in health and disease: a double-edged sword. Science 2004; 306:990.
132. Gonzalez-Polo RA, Boya P, Pauleau AL, et al. The apoptosis/autophagy paradox: autophagic vacuolization before apoptotic death. J Cell Sci 2005; 118:3091.

133. Muntz KH, Hagler HK, Boulas JH, et al. Redistribution of catecholamines in the ischemic zone of dog heart. Am J Pathol 1984; 114:64.

134. Sharma AD, Saffitz JF, Lee BI, et al. Alpha adrenergic-mediated accumulation of calcium in reperfused myocardium. J Clin Invest 1983; 72:802.

135. Thandroyen FT, Muntz KH, Buja LM, et al. Alterations in beta-adrenergic receptors, adenylate cyclase, and cyclic AMP concentrations during acute myocardial ischemia and reperfusion. Circulation 1990; 82(suppl 2):30.

136. Thandroyen FT, Morris AC, Hagler HK, et al. Intracellular calcium transients and arrhythmia in isolated heart cells. Circ Res 1991; 69:810.

137. Reimer KA, Jennings RB. The "wavefront phenomenon" of myocardial ischemic cell death. II. Transmural progression of necrosis within the framework of ischemic bed size (myocardium at risk) and collateral flow. Lab Invest 1979; 40:633.

138. Buja LM, Parkey RW, Stokely EM, et al. Pathophysiology of technetium-99m stannous pyrophosphate and thallium-201 scintigraphy of acute anterior myocardial infarcts in dogs. J Clin Invest 1976; 57:1508.

139. Buja LM, Tofe AJ, Kulkarni PV, et al. Sites and mechanisms of localization of technetium-99m phosphorus radiopharmaceuticals in acute myocardial infarcts and other tissues. J Clin Invest 1977; 60:724.

140. Baroldi G. Different types of myocardial necrosis in coronary heart disease: a pathophysiological review of their functional significance. Am Heart J 1975; 89:742.

141. Baroldi G, Falzi G, Mariani F. Sudden coronary death. A postmortem study in 208 selected cases compared to 97 "control" subjects. Am Heart J 1979; 98:20.

142. Buja LM, Willerson JT. Infarct size-can it be measured or modified in humans? Prog Cardiovasc Dis 1987; 29:271.

143. Page DL, Caulfield JB, Kastor JA, et al. Myocardial changes associated with cardiogenic shock. N Engl J Med 1971; 285:133.

144. Alonso DR, Scheidt S, Post M, et al. Pathophysiology of cardiogenic shock. Quantification of myocardial necrosis, clinical and electrocardiographic correlations. Circulation 1973; 48:588.

145. Reimer KA, Jennings RB, Cobb FR, et al. Animal models for protecting ischemic myocardium (AMPIM): results of the NHLBI Cooperative Study. Comparison of unconscious and conscious dog models. Circ Res 1985; 56:651.

146. Buja LM, Willerson JT. Experimental analysis of myocardial ischemia. In: Silver MD, ed. Cardiovascular Pathology. 2nd ed. New York, NY: Churchill Livingstone, 1991:621.

147. Orn S, Manhenke C, Squire IB, et al. Effect of left ventricular scar size, location, and transmurality on left ventricular remodeling with healed myocardial infarction. Am J Cardiol 2007; 99:1109.

148. Brodoefel H, Reimann A, Klumpp B, et al. Assessment of myocardial viability in a reperfused porcine model: evaluation of different MSCT contrast protocols in acute and subacute stages in comparison with MRI. J Comput Assist Tomogr 2007; 31:290.

149. Trindade ML, Caldas MA, Tsutsui JM, et al. Determination of size and transmural extent of acute myocardial infarction by real-time myocardial perfusion echocardiography: a comparison with magnetic resonance imaging. J Am Soc Echocardiogr 2007; 20:126.

150. Gibbons RJ, Valeti US, Araoz PA, et al. The quantification of infarct size. J Am Coll Cardiol 2004; 44:1533.

151. Murry CE, Jennings RB, Reimer KA. Preconditioning with ischemia: a delay of lethal cell injury in ischemic myocardium. Circulation 1986; 74:1124.
152. Murry CE, Richard VJ, Reimer KA, et al. Ischemic preconditioning slows energy metabolism and delays ultrastructural damage during a sustained ischemic episode. Circ Res 1990; 66:913.
153. Liu GS, Thornton J, Van Winkle DM, et al. Protection against infarction afforded by preconditioning is mediated by A_1 adenosine receptors in rabbit heart. Circulation 1991; 84:350.
154. Cleveland JC Jr., Meldrum DR, Rowland RT, et al. Adenosine preconditioning of human myocardium is dependent upon the ATP-sensitive K^+ channel. J Mol Cell Cardiol 1997; 29:175.
155. Yellon DM, Downey JM. Preconditioning the myocardium: from cellular physiology to clinical cardiology. Physiol Rev 2003; 83:1113.
156. Kuzuya T, Hoshida S, Yamashita N, et al. Delayed effects of sublethal ischemia on the acquisition of tolerance to ischemia. Circ Res 1993; 72:1293.
157. Vinten-Johansen J, Zhao ZQ, Jiang R, et al. Myocardial protection in reperfusion with postconditioning. Expert Rev Cardiiovasc Ther 2005; 3:1035.
158. Zhao ZQ, Vinten-Johansen J. Postconditioning: reduction of reperfusion-induced injury. Cardiovasc Res 2006; 70:200.
159. Kusuoka H, Porterfield JK, Weisman HF, et al. Pathophysiology and pathogenesis of stunned myocardium. Depressed Ca^{2+} activation of contraction as a consequence of reperfusion-induced cellular calcium overload in ferret hearts. J Clin Invest 1987; 79:950.
160. Bolli R, Patel BS, Jeroudi MO, et al. Demonstration of free radical generation in "stunned"' myocardium of intact dogs with the use of the spin trap alpha-phenyl N-tert-butyl nitrone. J Clin Invest 1988; 82:476.
161. Bush LR, Buja LM, Tilton G, et al. Effects of propranolol and diltiazem alone and in combination on the recovery of left ventricular segmental function after temporary coronary occlusion and long term reperfusion in conscious dogs. Circulation 1985; 72:413.
162. Nadal-Ginard B, Kajstura J, Leri A, et al. Myocyte death, growth, and regeneration in cardiac hypertrophy and failure. Circ Res 2003; 92:139.
163. Mann DL, Bristow MR. Mechanisms and models of heart failure: the biochemical model and beyond. Circulation 2005; 111:2837.
164. Fedak PW, Verma S, Weisel RD, et al. Cardiac remodeling and failure: From molecules to man (Parts I, II and III). Cardiovasc Pathol 2005; 14:1; 49; 109.
165. Willerson JT, Buja LM. Protection of the myocardium during myocardial infarction: pharmacologic protection during thrombolytic therapy. Am J Cardiol 1990; 65:35I.
166. Hearse DJ. Myocardial protection during ischemia and reperfusion. Mol Cell Biochem 1998; 186:177.
167. Braunwald E. Personal reflections on efforts to reduce ischemic myocardial damage. Cardiovasc Res 2002; 56:332.
168. Bucciarelli-Ducci C, Bianchi M, De Luca L, et al. Effects of glucose-insulin-potassium infusion on myocardial perfusion and left ventricular remodeling in patients treated with primary angioplasty for ST-elevation acute myocardial infarction. Am J Cardiol 2006; 98:1349.

169. Rasoul S, Ottervanger JP, Timmer JR, et al. One year outcomes after glucose-insulin-potassium in ST elevation myocardial infarction. The glucose-insulin-potassium study II. Int J Cardiol 2007; 122:52.

170. Díaz R, Goyal A, Mehta SR, et al. Glucose-insulin-potassium therapy in patients with ST-segment elevation myocardial infarction. JAMA 2007; 298:2399.

171. Deedwania P, Kosiborod M, Barrett E, et al. Hyperglycemia and acute coronary syndrome. A scientific statement from the American Heart Association Diabetes Committee of the Council on Nutrition, Physical Activity, and Metabolism. Circulation. 2008; 117:1610.

172. Opie LH. Metabolic management of acute myocardial infarction comes to the fore and extends beyond control of hyperglycemia. Circulation. 2008; 117:2172.

173. Waller BF. "Crackers, breakers, stretchers, drillers, scrapers, shavers, burners, welders and melters"—the future treatment of atherosclerotic coronary artery disease? A clinical-morphologic assessment. J Am Coll Cardiol 1989; 13:969.

174. Schoen FJ, Edwards WD. Pathology of cardiovascular interventions, including endovascular therapies, revascularization, vascular replacement, cardiac assist/replacement, arrhythmia control, and repaired congenital heart disease. In: Silver MD, Gotlieb AI, Schoen FF, eds. Cardiovascular Pathology. 3rd ed. New York, NY: Churchill Livingstone, 2001, chap. 22.

175. Farb, Roberts DK, Pichard AD, et al. Coronary artery morphologic features after coronary rotational atherectomy: insights into mechanisms of lumen enlargement and embolization. Am Heart J 1995; 129:1058.

176. Topaz O, McIvor M, Stone GW, et al. Acute results, complications, and effect of lesion characteristics on outcome with the solid-state, pulsed-wave, mid-infrared laser angioplasty system: final multicenter registry report. Lasers Surg Med 1998; 22:228.

177. Lie JT, Lawrie GM, Morris GC Jr. Aortocoronary bypass saphenous vein graft atherosclerosis. Anatomic study of 99 vein grafts from normal and hyper-lipoproteinemic patients up to 75 months postoperatively. Am J Cardiol 1977; 40:906.

178. Bulkley BH, Hutchins GM. Pathology of coronary artery bypass graft surgery. Arch Pathol Lab Med 1978; 102:273.

179. Grondin CM, Campeau L, Lesperance J, et al. Atherosclerotic changes in coronary vein grafts six years after operation. Angiographic aspects in 110 patients. J Thorac Cardiovasc Surg 1979; 77:24.

180. Loop FD, Lytle BW, Cosgrove DM, et al. Influence of the internal-mammary-artery graft on 10-year survival and other cardiac events. N Engl J Med 1986; 314:1.

181. Shelton ME, Forman MB, Virmani R, et al. A comparison of morphologic and angiographic findings in long-term internal mammary artery and saphenous vein bypass grafts. J Am Coll Cardiol 1988; 11:297.

182. Tatoulis J, Buxton BF, Fuller JA. Patencies of 2127 arterial to coronary conduits over 15 years. Ann Thorac Surg 2004; 77:93.

183. Nabel EG. Gene therapy for cardiovascular diseases. Circulation 1995; 91:541.

184. Simari RD, Sam H, Rekhter M, et al. Regulation of cellular proliferation and intimal formation following balloon injury in atherosclerotic rabbit arteries. J Clin Invest 1996; 98:225.

185. Zoldhelyi P, McNatt J, Xu XM, et al. Prevention of arterial thrombosis by adenovirus-mediated transfer of cyclooxygenase gene. Circulation 1996; 93:10.

186. Kishore R, Losordo DW. Gene therapy for restenosis: biological solution to a biological problem. J Mol Cell Cardiol 2007; 42:461.
187. Mulcahy D, Knight C, Stables R, et al. Lasers, burns, cuts, tingles and pumps: a consideration of alternative treatments for intractable angina. Br Heart J 1994; 71:406.
188. Schoebel FC, Frazier OH, Jessurun GAJ, et al. Refractory angina pectoris in end-stage coronary artery disease: evolving therapeutic concepts. Am Heart J 1997; 134:587.
189. Sundt TM III, Rogers JG. Transmyocardial laser revascularization for inoperable coronary artery disease. Curr Opin Cardiol 1997; 12:441.
190. Kwong KF, Kanellopoulos GK, Nickols JC, et al. Transmyocardial laser treatment denervates canine myocardium. J Thorac Cardiovasc Surg 1997; 114:883.
191. Schumacher B, Pecker P, von Specht BU, et al. Induction of neoangiogenesis in ischemic myocardium by human growth factors: first clinical results of a new treatment of coronary heart disease. Circulation 1998; 97:645.
192. Losordo DW, Vale PR, Symes JF, et al. Gene therapy for myocardial angiogenesis: initial clinical results with direct myocardial injection of phVEGF165 as sole therapy for myocardial ischemia. Circulation 1998; 98:2800.
193. Folkman J. Angiogenic therapy of the human heart. Circulation 1998; 97:628.
194. Folkman J, D'Amore PA. Blood vessel formation: what is its molecular basis? Cell 1996; 87:1153.
195. Nabel EG. Delivering genes to the heart—right where it counts! Nat Med 1999; 5:141.
196. Anversa P, Kajstura J. Ventricular myocytes are not terminally differentiated in the adult mammalian heart. Circ Res 1998; 83:1.
197. Soonpaa MH, Field LJ. Survey of studies examining mammalian cardiomyocyte DNA synthesis. Circ Res 1998; 83:15.
198. Rubart M, Field LJ. Cardiac regeneration: repopulating the heart. Ann Rev Physiol 2006; 68:29.
199. Pasumarthi KB, Nakajima H, Nakajima HO, et al. Targeted expression of cyclin D2 results in cardiomyocyte DNA synthesis and infarct regression in transgenic mice. Circ Res 2005; 96:110.
200. Leri A, Kajstura J, Anversa P. Cardiac stem cells and mechanisms of myocardial regeneration. Physiol Rev 2005; 85:1373.
201. Anversa P, Kajstura J, Leri A, et al. Life and death of cardiac stem cells: a paradigm shift in cardiac biology. Circulation 2006; 113:1451.
202. Urbanek K, Cesselli D, Rota M, et al. Stem cell niches in the adult mouse heart. Proc Natl Acad Sci U S A 2006; 103:9226.
203. Chen X, Wilson RM, Kubo H, et al. Adolescent feline heart contains a population of small, proliferative ventricular myocytes with immature physiological properties. Circ Res 2007; 100:536.
204. Vela D, Buja LM. Quest for the cardiovascular holy grail: mammalian myocardial regeneration. Cardiovasc Pathol 2008; 17:1.
205. Rubart M, Field LJ. Cell-based approaches for cardiac repair. Ann N Y Acad Sci 2006; 1080:34.
206. Evans SM, Zbinden S, Epstein SE. Progenitor cells for cardiac repair. Semin Cell Dev Biol 2007; 18:153.
207. Laflamme MA, Zbinden S, Epstein SE, et al. Cell-based therapy for myocardial ischemia and infarction: pathophysiological mechanisms. Annu Rev Pathol Mech Dis 2007; 2:307.

3

Nonclinical Safety Assessment of the Cardiovascular Toxicity of Drugs and Combination Medical Devices

Shayne C. Gad

Gad Consulting Services, Cary, North Carolina, U.S.A.

INTRODUCTION

Toxicologists in the pharmaceutical and medical device industries have as their prime responsibility the identification of any potential risks associated with therapeutics that their employers intend to take to market and into potential clinical use. In almost all cases, toxicologists in industry (although they may possess an individual expertise in one or more target organ systems) must perform as generalists, evaluating a compound for a broad range of adverse effects. Many of the standardized experimental designs that serve for detecting whether such effects are present (so-called regulatory toxicology studies) are subject to regulatory mandate and review. This fact and the usual restraints of timing and cost has historically limited and guided what is done to identify cardiotoxic agents, including the determination that an effect exists, at what dose levels, and occasionally to determine whether the effect is reversible. Since the early 2000s, experience with postmarket identification of cardiovascular adverse effects of drugs (not limited to those for cardiovascular indications) and medical devices in patients using these products has dictated a series of changes to the preclinical evolution of potential products prior to late-stage clinical development. While changes have been made in the collection or analysis of data to address specific concerns that arise, such as the exposure of the potential for induction of valvular heart disease by fenfluramine (Table 1), such changes are limited in nature to either conducting additional studies or adding measures or means of analysis to existing study designs. More importantly, such concerns have lead to additional test requirements as well as modifications to existing study designs. Tests now required or recommended are both in vitro and in vivo, and will be considered in these contexts (Table 2).

Compounds with therapeutic potential are the particular domain of interest of the pharmaceutical toxicologist (1). In this arena, the task becomes considerably more challenging. The challenge occurs because pharmaceutical agents are intended to be administered to a target species (usually humans, except for veterinary drugs) and are intended to have biologic effects. Occasionally, the commercial objective is to produce a therapeutic agent, which alters the function of the cardiovascular system. To the pharmaceutical toxicologists, the task of evaluating cardiotoxicity frequently is expanded to identifying and understanding

Table 1 Noncardiac Drugs Known to Induce or Worsen Heart Failure According to the Suggested Mechanism(s) Implicated

Drug class	Drug
Cardiomyopathy	
Cytotoxic drugs	Doxorubicin, epitubicin, and other anthracyclines, mitoxantrone, cyclophosphamide, 5-fluorouracil, capecitabine
Immunomodulating drugs/antibodies	Trastuzumab, interferon-a-2, interleurkin-2, infliximav, etanercept
Antifungal drugs	Itraconasole, amphotericin B
Antipsychotic drugs	Clozapine
Pulmonary hypertension	
Antimigraine drugs	Methysergide, ergotamine
Appetite suppressants	Fenfluramine, fluramine, phentermine
Heart-valve abnormalities	
Antimigraine drugs	Methysergide, ergotamine
Appetite suppressants	Fenfluramine1, dexfenfluramine, phentermine
Antiparkinsonian drugs	Pergolide
Fluid overload	
NSAIDs, including cyclo-oxygenase-2 inhibitors	All
Antidiabetic drugs	Rosigiltaxone, piogiltaxone, trogiltazone
Glucocorticoids	All
Herbal drugs	Herbal drugs containing liquorice or adulterated with NSAIDs

Abbreviation: NSAIDs, nonsteroidal anti-inflammatory drugs.

the mechanism of action, the relevance of findings to the target species, and quantitating the therapeutic dose (i.e., the separation between the dose with a desired effect and the higher dose that has an adverse effect). Indeed, the case of detecting cardiovascular toxicity as a function of the underlying mechanism of other toxicity, particularly if we are talking about individuals with preexisting cardiovascular disease, is a complex one. More careful consideration of clinical experiences with drugs continues to reveal that the scope of possible, therapeutically limiting cardiotoxicities is broad but ill defined, as shown by the recent cases of nonsteroidal anti-inflammatory drugs (NSAIDs), cyclo-oxygenase 2 (COX-2) inhibitors, and monoclonal antibody anticancer agents. Electrocardiograms (EKGs) and histopathology are critical and usually the definitive tools in such assessments.

The basic principles of cardiovascular function and mechanisms of cardiovascular toxicity are presented elsewhere in this book, or in other reviews of cardiovascular toxicity, (9–11) and are not addressed here.

Evaluations of cardiotoxicity, with the exception of one special case, tend to be performed by adding measurements and observations to existing "pivotal" test designs. These measures look at alterations in myocardial and vascular structure (pathology, clinical pathology) and function (EKGs, clinical pathology, and clinical observations) (Table 2). Tests focused on the cardiovascular system are designed and executed only if an indication of an effect is found. The special case exceptions are so-called safety pharmacology studies, which seek to look at exaggerated pharmacologic effects in rather focused target organ functional studies. Additionally, there are currently efforts by the Food and Drug Administration (FDA) and others to develop (or refine existing) tests to detect agents affecting valvular tissue better. Such development is complicated by the fact that preexisting conditions (hypertension) predispose individuals for the adverse effects.

PHARMACOLOGIC PROFILING

The profiling of the pharmacologic effects of a new drug on the cardiovascular system is an essential element in early evaluations and development. Broad assessments of the effects on critical target organ functions (cardiovascular, renal, pulmonary, immune, peripheral, and central nervous systems) for which no action is intended are often called safety pharmacology, although other purposes (such as the serendipitous discovery of additional desirable pharmacologic activities, i.e., new therapeutic opportunities) are also served. These assessments are carried out in the therapeutic to near-therapeutic dosage range, e.g., from the projected human ED_{50} (effective dose therapeutically in 50% of the patient population) to perhaps the projected ED_{90}.

Such evaluations can reveal other actions that were unintended and undesirable (side-effects), or extensions, exaggerations of the intended pharmacology, which are either unacceptable or essential for interpreting results in actual toxicology studies (Table 2) (11). The regulatory guidelines for such

Table 2 Test Systems for Evaluation of Cardiovascular Toxicity of Therapeutics

Description	Comments
In vitro ligand-binding assay	
Fast and sensitive assay that uses HEK 293 cells stably and transfected with the hERG channel and radiolabeled ligand, e.g., dofetilide6 or MK-499. High throughput of >100 compounds per day. Low-cost assay.	Can correlate well with electrophysiology. No functional activity can be inferred. May not detect compounds that act at sites distinct to the ligand-binding site, leading to lack of correlation with electrophysiology.
In vitro electrophysiology hERG assay	
Manual patch clamp electrophysiology used for more detailed work (e.g., temperature dependence of hERG block). Automated electrophysiology in the form of PatchXpress (7). Manual patch clamp has low throughput of <50 data points per wk. PatchXpress has high throughput of up to 1200 data points per wk.	Can detect activity at any binding site and can offer information on state/use dependence of a channel. Reported to correlate well with QT prolongation in vivo. False negatives may arise as a result of hydrophobic interactions between compounds and the apparatus used in the experiment.
Ex vivo—Langendorff-perfused isolated heart preparation	
Records MAPs in isolated Langendorff-perfused rabbit heart and evaluates APD, conduction, instability, triangulation, and reverse-use dependency. High-cost, low-throughput assay.	Offers information on several markers of proarrhythmia liability, which have been violated with drugs known to induce TdP, and those not associated with proarrhythmia in clinical settings.
Ex vivo—Purkinje fibers	
Measures transmembrane action potential. Prolongation of the QT interval and subsequent risk of arrhythmia is related to prolongation of the APD in Purkinje fibers. High cost, low throughput of around 1 compound per wk.	The intensive use of animals (primarily dogs) is unattractive from an ethical perspective. Currents measured cannot be correlated to man, inhibiting a translational approach.

Table 2 Test Systems for Evaluation of Cardiovascular Toxicity of Therapeutics (*Continued*)

Description	Comments
In vivo—animal models	
The methosamine-sensitized rabbit model (15) has been widely used to assess proarrhythmic liability.	Markets of repolarization liability other than APD of QT prolongation may have higher predicative value owing to better correlation with TdP.
The AV dog model (11,14) involves a structural, mechanical, and electrical remodeling process that increases the susceptibility to arrhythmia on exposure to drugs that delay ventricular repolarization.	The reported rabbit and dog models use anesthetized animals and have been mainly used for class III antiarrhythmics.
Other animal models include guinea pig [EKG of conscious restrained guinea pigs (16,104)], pig, and monkey.	Guidelines suggest that safety pharmacology should be studied in *conscious* animals, thereby excluding possible interferences of anesthetics. Guidance is required on appropriate dose selection of nonantiarrhythmic drugs where clinical data on relevant exposures or efficacy are unavailable.
High-cost, low-throughput series of assays.	

Abbreviations: hERG, human ether a-go-go gene; MAP, monophasic action potential; APD, action potential duration; TdP, torsade de pointes; AV, atrioventricular; EKG, electrocardiogram.

"secondary" pharmacologic evaluations currently vary among the United States, the United Kingdom, and Europe (Table 3).

Such interpretations are more difficult, of course, when the agent is intended to have therapeutic cardiovascular effects. Brunner and Gross (13) and Brunton (14) should be reviewed by anyone undertaking such an effort to ensure familiarity with basic cardiovascular pharmacology.

Focusing on cardiovascular effects, the concerns are for both direct (on the heart and vasculature) and indirect (such as on adrenal release) effects in the short term. Accordingly, these studies look at function in the short term (hours to perhaps 3 days). The dog and the rat are generally the model species (although mice and primates may also be used), with parameters being evaluated including the following:

- Physiologic functions: systemic arterial blood pressure, heart rate, EKG, blood gases, and blood flow.
- Biochemistry: enzyme release [lactate dehydrogenase (LDH), creatinine phosphokinase (CPK)], oxygen consumption, calcium transport, and substrate utilization.

Table 3 Safety Pharmacological Evaluation of New Chemical Entities

United Kingdom and Europe	United States
Central nervous system	Neuropharmacology
Autonomic system	Cardiovascular/respiratory
Cardiovascular system	Gastrointestinal
Respiratory system	Genitourinary
Gastrointestinal system	Endocrine
Other systems where relevant	Anti-inflammatory
	Immunoactive
	Chemotherapeutic
	Enzyme effects
	Other

Note: These lists and terminologies are derived from the recommendations of the respective regulatory authorities, as laid out in the *EEC Notice of Applicants,* ISBN 92-825-9503-X, and in the *Guideline for the Format and Content of the Nonclinical Pharmacology, Toxicology Section of an Application,* Center for Drug Evaluation and Research, FDA, Washington, DC; 1987.

Several of these (EKG, LDH, and CPK) are also evaluated in traditional pivotal safety/toxicology studies at higher doses (up to 100 times the intended human dose) and are discussed in further detail later. Such studies also depend on evaluation of clinical signs to indicate problems. By definition, the functional cardiovascular system is very dynamic. Accordingly, the times of measurement (sampling) must be carefully considered.

All these could also be of concern for nondrug chemical entities but are generally only evaluated to the extent described later under pivotal studies (if at all).

IN VITRO EVALUATION OF CARDIOVASCULAR TOXICITY

In vitro models, at least as screening tests, have been with us in toxicology since the 1980s. The last 10 to 15 years have brought a great upsurge of interest in such models. This increased interest is due to economic and animal welfare pressures as well as technologic improvements. This is particularly true in industry, and cardiotoxicity is one area where in vitro systems have found particularly attractive applications. Specific requirements for evaluating cardiovascular risk potential are now mandated for all but a few new human pharmaceuticals (17–19).

Since the mid 1990s, several drugs (such as Seldane—terfenadine) had to be or were withdrawn from the market due to inducing fatal arrhythmia, evoking a condition called torsade de pointes (TdP) (7). Those drugs (Table 4) were found to evoke QT interval prolongation and subsequently, TdP (19–21).

Table 4 Drugs Linked to Torsade de Pointes (TdP)

Drugs with risk of TdP		
Amiodarone	Erythromycin	Pentamidine
Arsenic trioxide	Erythromycin E.E.S	Pimozide
Bepridil	Halofantrine	Procainamide
Chloroquine	Haloperidol	Procainamide
Chlorpromazine	Ibutilide	Quinidine
Cisapride	Levomethadyl	Quinidine
Clarithromycin	Mesoridazine	Sotalol
Dofetilide	Methadone	Sparfloxacin
Domperidone	Methadone	Terfenadine
Droperidol	Pentamidine	Thioridazine
Drugs with possible risk of TdP		
Alfuzosin	Granisetron	Roxithromycin
Amantadine	Indapamide	Tacrolimus
Azithromycin	Isradipine	Tamoxifen
Chloral hydrate	Levofloxacin	Telithromycin
Clozapine	Lithium	Tizanidine
Dolasetron	Lithium	Vardenafil
Felbamate	Moexipril/HCTZ	Venlafaxine
Flecainide	Moxifloxacin	Voriconazole
Foscarnet	Nicardipine	Ziprasidone
Fosphenytoin	Octreotide	Quetiapine
Gatifloxacin	Ofloxacin	Ranolazine
Gemifloxacin	Ondansetron	Risperidone

Source: From Refs. 2,22.

Most agents that prolong QTc and/or cause TdP are hERG blockers (human ether-a-go-go related gene—so named because the fruit flies it was first described in appeared to dance). Others agents affect hERG indirectly. Significant progress has been made in characterizing the medicinal chemistry of structures affecting the specific potassium channel (23–26).

The hERG Assay

Patch-Clamp Studies Using Recombinant Cells Expressing hERG Channels

Most pharmaceuticals associated with TdP inhibit rapidly delayed rectifier potassium current, I_{Kr}. Therefore, particular attention to assays for I_{Kr} is prudent for assessing risk of QT interval prolongation.

Using the voltage-clamp technique, outward or inward ionic currents can be measured from single cell preparations. Because of inherent difficulties associated with recording I_{Kr} in native myocytes, much of the available data for this current have been obtained using recombinant cell lines expressing hERG.

Inhibition of other outward (repolarizing) currents (e.g., I_{TO}, I_{KI}, I_{Ks}) or increase in inward (depolarizing) ionic currents (e.g., I_{Na}) could also lead to QT interval prolongation, and therefore should be considered when investigating the mechanisms for QT interval prolongation (27–29).

hERG Protein Expression System

When transfected with hERG alone or hERG in association with genes for potential regulating subunits (e.g., MiRP1), appropriate cell systems express a K^+ channel that displays biophysical and pharmacologic properties similar to hERG. Several expression systems have been used to test the activity of test substances on hERG current.

With the presence of endogenous currents, the presence or absence of subunits (directly associated regulatory proteins) and kinases or phosphatases controlling regulatory phosphorylation sites can affect the pharmacology of the expressed channel protein relative to native cardiac ion channels.

Mammalian [e.g., Chinese hamster ovary (CHO), human embryonic kidney (HEK)-293, COS-7] rather than *Xenopus* oocytes should be selected for expressing hERG because a major limitation of the *Xenopus* model is that test substances can accumulate in the oocyte yolk, resulting in significant variability and error in potency estimates (Fig. 1).

hERG rather than I_{Kr}-present murine atrial tumor AT-1 or HL-1 cells derived from transgenic mice should be preferred. The channels expressed by

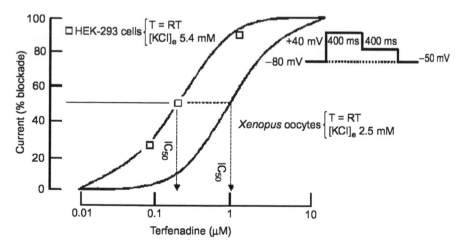

Figure 1 Effects of terfenadine on hERG channels expressed in HEK-293 cells and *Xenopus* oocytes.

Table 5 IC50 of Several Drugs Against hERG Channel (HEK-293)

Drug	IC50 (μM) at 22°C	IC50 (μM) at 35°C
Terfanadine	0.02	0.3
Loratadine	4.7	7.9
Dephenidramine	3.9	2.7
Fexofenadine	11	13.6
Cisapride	0.03	0.04
Sotalol	810	270
Erythromycin	3158	200

Conveyed current determined at 22°C and 35°C. *Abbreviations*: hERG, human ether a-go-go gene.

these cells are similar to neonatal/fetal mouse cardiac myocytes, raising some concerns about dedifferentiation in these tumor-derived cells. Test results obtained are also clearly dependent on culture temperature (Table 5) and must be clearly specified with any provided or published data.

- Objective: Detection potential of blocking the cardiac rapid component of the I_{Kr}).
- Study design:
  - Cells expressing the human gene encoding the major part of the ion channel carrying I_{Kr} (hERG)
  - At least three concentrations up to solubility limit or 30 μM.
- End point:
  - IC50 and IC20 to be calculated (fitting of the concentration-response curve) if an inhibition above 50% is seen at top concentration.
  - Drugs that achieve IC20 are considered to possibly present a clinical safety issue, therefore, cardiac safety index (CSI) approach elicits clinical effects.
- CSI
  - Ratio: hERG conc./efficacious conc.
  - 30 × >> comfortable.
  - 100 × >> OK.

Relevance of hERG to QT Prolongation

Compounds associated with adverse drug reactions (ADRs) of QT prolongation and arrhythmias such as TdP and sudden death predominantly have a secondary pharmacologic interaction with the rapidly activating I_{Kr}. The gene encoding this channel has been identified as hERG. Testing of compounds for interactions with the HERG channel allows the identification of potential risk of QT prolongation in humans and can be used as a screen in development of candidate selection.

HEK-293 cells have been transfected with cDNA for hERG-1 to produce a stable expression system.

The relevance and relative importance of these measurements in conjunction with all of the other components of cardiovascular safety assessment has become cleaner as data on both hERG and clinical effects of drugs have become available. Certainly it is influential in making drug candidate screening and lead designation decisions, but should not be a critical determining factor by itself.

Purkinje Fiber Assays

Isolated Purkinje fibers (usually from the rabbit) provide a useful model for evaluating the potential prearrhythmic potential of drugs and other therapeutic agents. With some drug-induced arrhythmias, e.g., arrhythmias triggered by steps after depolarization, have been described and characterized in cardiac Purkinje fibers, a main conducting tissue. While these afterdepolarization-induced triggered activities have been identified in ventricular cells located in the midmyocardium region (M cells), they are rarely seen in other types of ventricular myocytes (30). Some drug-induced afterdepolarizations that are facilitated by additional β-adrenergic stimulation preferentially occur during low pacing (e.g., 20 pulses/min). These arrhythmic events, termed "early after-depolarizations" (EADs), are defined by a depolarization occurring before full repolarization of the cell membrane. In contrast, other specific Purkinje fiber–related arrhythmic events are dependent on rapid pacing (e.g., 180 pulses/min for a few minutes). These arrhythmias, referred to as "delayed after depolarizations" (DADs), are defined by a depolarization occurring after total repolarization of the cell membrane. Such abnormal spontaneous depolarizations are liable to provoke extrasystoles and triggered activities that are characterized by tachyarrhythmias showing a marked diastolic depolarization slope and triggered by premature extrasystoles. In the clinic and in laboratory animals, these triggered activities are believed to be responsible for the development of TdP, which are life-threatening ventricular tachycardias (31).

There are some excellent sources, which should be referred to for detailed descriptions of rabbit Purkinje fiber responses (30).

As predictive systems of the specific target organ toxicity, and particularly in the case of cardiotoxicity, any in vitro system having the ability to identify those agents with a high potential to cause damage in a specific target organ at physiologic concentrations is extremely valuable.

In Vitro Systems as Screens

The second use of in vitro models is largely specific. This is to serve as tools to investigate, identify, and/or verify the mechanisms of action for selective target organ toxicities. Such mechanistic understandings then allow one to know whether such toxicities are relevant to humans (or to conditions of exposure to humans), to develop means either to predict such responses while they are still reversible or to form the means to intervene in such toxicosis (i.e., first aid or therapy), and finally potentially to modify molecules of interest to avoid unwanted effects while maintaining desired properties (particularly important in drug design). Such uses are not limited to studying chemicals, drugs, and manufactured agents; they can also be used in the study of such diverse things as plant, animal, and microbial toxins, which may have commercial, therapeutic, or military applications or implications because of their cardiotoxicity.

There is currently much controversy over the use of in vitro test systems. Will they find acceptance as "definitive test systems," or will they only be used as preliminary screens for such final tests? Or, in the end, will they not be used at all? Almost certainly, all three of these cases will be true to some extent. Depending on how the data generated are to be used, the division between the first two is ill defined at best.

Before trying to answer these questions definitively in a global sense, each of the end points for which in vitro systems are being considered should be overviewed and considered against the factors outlined up to this point.

Substantial potential advantages exist in using an in vitro system in toxicologic testing. These advantages include isolation of test cells or organ fragments from homeostatic and hormonal control, accurate dosing, and quantitation of results. It should be noted that, in addition to the potential advantages, in vitro systems per se have a number of limitations that can contribute to their not being acceptable models. Findings from an in vitro system, which either limit their use in predicting in vivo events or make them totally unsuitable for the task, include wide differences in the doses needed to produce effects or differences in the effects elicited.

Tissue culture has the immediate potential to be used in two very different ways by industry. First, it has been used to examine a particular aspect of the toxicity of a compound in relation to its toxicity in vivo (i.e., mechanistic or explanatory studies). Second, it has been used as a form of rapid screening to compare the toxicity of a group of compounds to a particular form of response. Indeed, the pharmaceutical industry has used in vitro test systems in these two ways for years in the search for new potential drug entities: as screens and as mechanistic tools.

Mechanistic and explanatory studies are generally called for when a traditional test system gives a result that is either unclear or for which the relevance to the real life human exposure is doubted. In vitro systems are particularly attractive for such cases because they can focus on every defined single aspect of a problem or pathogenic response, free of the confounding influence of the multiple responses of an intact higher-level organism. Note, however, that first one must know the nature (indeed the existence) of the questions to be addressed. It is then important to devise a suitable model system that is related to the mode of toxicity of the compound.

One must consider what forms of markers are to be used to evaluate the effect of interest. Initially, such markers have been exclusively morphologic (in that there is a change in microscopic structure), observational (is the cell/preparation dead or alive or has some gross characteristic changed), or functional (does the model still operate as it did before). Recently, it has become clear that more sensitive models do not just generate a single endpoint type of data, but rather a multiple set of measures that, in aggregate, provide a much more powerful set of answers.

There are several approaches to in vitro cardiotoxicity models. The oldest is that of the isolated organ preparation (32–35). Perfused and superfused tissues and organs have been used in physiology and pharmacology since the late 19th century. There is a vast range of these available, and a number of them have been widely used in toxicology. Almost any end point can be evaluated, and these are the closest to the in vivo situation and therefore generally the easiest from which to extrapolate or conceptualize. Those things that can be measured or evaluated in the intact organism can largely also be evaluated in an isolated tissue or organ preparation. The drawbacks or limitations of this approach are also compelling, however.

An intact animal generally produces one tissue preparation. Such a preparation is viable generally for a day or less before it degrades to the point of being useless. As a result, such preparations are useful as screens only for agents that have rapidly reversible (generally pharmacologic or biochemical) mechanisms of action. They are superb for evaluating mechanisms of action at the organ level for agents that act rapidly—but not generally for cellular effects or for agents that act over the course of more than a day.

The second approach is to use tissue or organ culture. Such cultures are attractive because they maintain the ability for multiple cell types to interact in at least a near physiologic manner. They are generally not as complex as the perfused organs but are stable and useful over a longer period of time, increasing their utility as screens somewhat. They are truly a middle ground between the perfused organs and the cultured cells.

The third and most common approach is that of cultured cell models (32,36,37). These can be either primary or transformed (immortalized) cells, but the former have significant advantages in use as predictive target organ models. Such cell culture systems can be utilized to identify and evaluate interactions at the cellular, subcellular, and molecular level on an organ- and species-specific basis. The advantages of cell culture are that single organisms can generate multiple cultures, the cultures are stable and useful for protracted periods of time, and effects can be studied very precisely at the cellular and molecular level. The disadvantages are that isolated cells cannot mimic the interactive architecture of the intact organ and will respond over time in a manner that becomes decreasingly representative of what happens in vivo. An additional concern is that, with the exception of hepatocyte cultures, the influence of systemic metabolism is not factored in unless extra steps are taken. Any such cellular

Table 6   Representative In Vitro Test Systems for Cardiovascular Toxicity

System	End point	Evaluation	Reference
Coronary artery smooth muscle cells (S)	Morphological evaluation: vacuole formation	Correlates with in vivo results	37
Isolated perfused rabbit or rat heart (M,S)	Functional: operational, electrophysiologic, biochemical, and metabolism	Long history of use in physiology and pharmacology	33
Isolated superfused atrial and heart preparations (S,M)	Functional: operational and biochemical	Correlation with in vivo findings for antioxidants	34,35
Myocytes (S,M)	Functional and morphologic	Correlates well with in vivo results on a local concentration basis	39,40

Abbreviations: S, screening; M, mechanistic.

systems would be more likely to be accurate and sensitive predictors of adverse effects if their function and integrity were evaluated while they were operational.

A wide range of target organ-specific models have already been developed and utilized. Their incorporation into a library-type approach requires that they be evaluated for reproducibility of response, ease of use, and predictive characteristics under the intended conditions of use. These evaluations are probably at least somewhat specific to any individual situation. Table 6 presents an overview of representative systems for cardiovascular toxicity. Not mentioned in this table are any of the new coculture systems in which hepatocytes are "joined up" in culture with a target cell type to produce a metabolically competent cellular system. It should be noted that recently several researchers have advocated the failing rabbit heart as a particularly good model for screening drugs for TdP (38).

IN VIVO PARAMETER EVALUATIONS IN STANDARD STUDIES

For most new chemical entities, the primary screen for cardiotoxicity in industry consists of selected parameters incorporated into the pivotal or systemic toxicity of various lengths. These "shotgun" studies (so called because they attempt to collect as much data as possible to identify and crudely characterize toxicities associated with a drug or chemical) are exemplified by the 13-week study shown in Figure 2. In general, evaluations are performed to determine functional, structural, and biochemical (enzymatic) indicators of toxicity.

As shown, a large number of variables are measured, with only a few of them either acting directly or indirectly as predictors of cardiovascular toxicity.

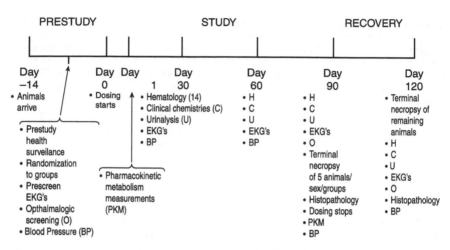

Figure 2 Line chart for a standard or "pivotal" 13-week toxicity study. Four or more groups of 16 (8 male and 8 female) beagle dogs each; daily dosing (5 days/wk for chemicals, 7 days/wk for pharmaceuticals or food additives) at selected dose levels, with one group being controls and receiving only vehicle or sham exposure; mortality and morbidity checks twice per day, detailed clinical observations at least once per week; FOB on days 0, 4, 11, and 87; body weights of every animal on days −7, −1, 0, 4, 7, 11, and weekly thereafter; food consumption weekly. For the sake of illustration what is shown is a dog study. The design is the same (except for the number of animals) for studies conducted in other species (rats, primates, etc.). Dosing is by the appropriate route and frequency (usually, however, once daily in the morning). *Abbreviation*: FOB, functional observational battery.

These measures are taken at multiple time points and in aggregate compose a powerful tool set for identifying the existence of problems. Their sensitivity and value are limited, however, by several design features incorporated into the pivotal studies, i.e., those that use dogs, primates, etc., and the number of times that specific measurements are made. Both are limited by cost and logistics, and these limitations decrease the overall power of the study. The second feature is the complications inherent in dealing with background variability in many of these parameters. Although individual animals are typically screened prior to inclusion in a study to ensure that those with unacceptable baselines for parameters of interest (very typically EKGs, clinical chemistries, and hematologies) are eliminated, clearly some degree of variability must be accepted on grounds of economics or practicality. Proper analysis of the entire data set collected as an integrated whole is the key to minimizing these weaknesses.

Electrocardiograms

Properly used and analyzed, EKGs represent the most sensitive early indicator of cardiac toxicity or malfunction. Long before the other functional measures (blood pressure or clinical signs) or before the invasive measures (clinical chemistries or histopathology), the EKG should generally reveal that a problem exists.

Deceptively simple in form (Fig. 3), EKGs present a great deal of information (41). Much of this information (amplitudes of the various waves, the lengths of intervals, and the frequency of events, i.e., heart rate) is quantitative in nature and can be analyzed by traditional statistical techniques. For this larger portion of the information in EKGs, the problems are that (*i*) baselines vary significantly from species to species (making interpretation of the relevance of changes seen in some models difficult) and (*ii*) the task of actually collecting the EKGs and then extracting quantitative data from them is very labor intensive. There are now some computer-assisted analysis programs, such as that described by Watkinson et al. (42), which perform the quantitative aspects of data extraction and analysis well.

There is also a significant amount of information in EKGs that is not quantitative, but is rather more of a pattern-recognition nature. This requires a learned art and a great deal of experience for the more complex changes.

Interpretation of the underlying causes of changes in EKGs requires knowledge of cardiac pathophysiology. Sodeman and Sodeman (43) present excellent overviews of this area, and Doherty and Cobbe (44) review the special cases of EKG changes in animal models.

Attention to technique is critical in the proper performance and interpretation of EKGs. Each species has different requirements for the placement and even the type of electrodes used (16,44,45). In addition, there are differences in electrocardiographic effects between sedated and nonsedated animals. Additionally, there are rather marked differences in EKGs between species, with the dog having a very labile T wave and the rat ST segment being short to nonexistent (Fig. 3). In recent years, the QT interval (most often evaluated in the dog) has become of particular interest. Increases in QT interval duration by a number of drugs have been associated with ventricular arrhythmias in humans (46).

More elegant techniques, such as positron emission tomography (PET) scanning, can be utilized to identify effects on hERG channel function in intact animals (47,48), but are impractical for use in the broad screening studies conducted to meet regulatory safety assessment requirements.

Blood Pressure and Heart Rate

These two traditional noninvasive measures of cardiovascular function have the advantages of being easy and inexpensive to perform. Their chief disadvantage is that they are subject to significant short-term variability, which significantly degrades their sensitivity and reliability. Techniques do exist for minimizing these disadvantages in various animal model species (49,50), and careful attention to general husbandry and handling helps.

If EKGs are collected, then it is easy to extract the heart rate from the tracings. Most automated systems will, in fact, perform this calculation as a matter of course. Blood pressure, meanwhile, is attractive because it is a

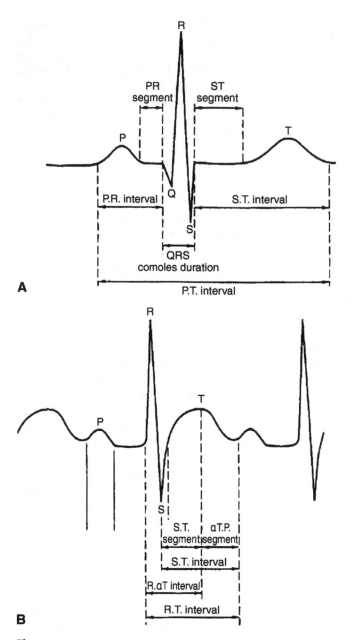

Figure 3 Styled EKGs for (**A**) humans and (**B**) adult rats. Although there are similarities between species, it is important to be aware of differences here and of differences that are dependent on age.

noninvasive measure of vascular function. Techniques for collecting it have improved significantly in recent years.

Neither of these measures is commonly collected in the pivotal or standard safety study, however. If clinical signs, particularly in larger (nonrodent) species, indicate that an effect is present, these should readily be added to a study.

Flow Measurement Techniques

The major techniques (dye dilution, thermal dilution, and microspheres) are available to allow investigation of blood flow down to the capillary level, using the direct Flick technique as a calculation basis. This technique is based on a careful measurement of oxygen consumption of an individual and the determination of the amount of oxygen in the arterial and venous blood. By estimating the metabolic rate of the subject, one can determine the volume of blood that would be required to carry the volume of oxygen consumed in a set interval. This relationship yields the flow volume in milliliters per minute. The equation for calculating flow is as follows:

$$Q = q^2 / [O_2]pv - [O_2]pa$$

where Q is the cardiac output, q^2 is the oxygen consumption of the body, $[O_2]$ is the oxygen concentration, pv is the pulmonary vein, and pa is the pulmonary artery.

The direct Flick technique demands that stringent requirements are met to ensure accuracy of the flow measurements including (*i*) a stable metabolic rate over the sampling period, (*ii*) the accurate determination of oxygen consumption and oxygen content in arterial and venous blood, (*iii*) a representative venous blood sample or venous admixture, and (*iv*) a valid method to determine metabolic rate. A cardinal rule for all of these techniques is that indicator is neither gained nor lost during the measurement period.

Indocyanine green has been used for many years for the determination of cardiac output using the Flick technique. A small amount of indocyanine green at a specific concentration is administered into the left side of the heart. Arterial blood then is sampled, preferably from the aorta, by constant withdrawal through an optical cuvette sensitive to the specific absorption spectrum of indocyanine green. The concentration of indocyanine green in the blood is automatically determined as the sample is withdrawn through the cuvette, plotted graphically, and described by a curve. By integrating the area under the curve and comparing this with a sample standard of known concentration, the average concentration of dye is calculated over the length of the sampling period. The volume of blood pumped per unit time then equals the cardiac output. A stringent requirement for this technique is that the withdrawal rate of blood through the cuvette must be constant and that the rate must be fast enough to obtain a representative sample of blood before recirculation of the dye begins. Also, the sampling catheter between the withdrawal pump and the animal must be kept as short as possible to reduce mixing of blood with dye and blood without dye.

Thermal dilution is a variation on the indicator dilution technique, which uses a bolus of cold, or room temperature, physiologic saline as the indicator and an intravascular thermocouple or thermistor as the detector. The bolus of cool saline is injected into the left side of the heart and the thermocouple is placed in the ascending aorta. The calculations of cardiac output with this technique are almost identical to those used for the indocyanine green determinations. The requirements for this technique are that a constant temperature of cold bolus must be injected and that no heat must be gained or lost by the blood as it circulates between the site of injection and the site of detection. Repetitive sampling is possible using this technique.

Microspheres are the third major indicator used for the determination of blood flow. Microspheres are small, carbonized spheres, usually 15 μm in diameter, that flow evenly distributed within the bloodstream and are trapped in the circulation at the arteriolar level. The microspheres can be used to determine qualitative flow by examining the organ for the presence of microspheres. As microspheres can be labeled with different radioactive tracers, tissue samples can be taken from the site in question to determine the radioactive level using a radioactive counting device (e.g., gamma counter). The total number of microspheres is proportional to the total number of counts recorded per unit time when compared with a standard dilution of such radiolabeled microspheres. To determine the effect of different interventions, different radiolabels can be used for each flow determination. Implantable sensors are also now becoming available to measure these parameters (pressure flow and heart rates) in species sizes down to and including mice (51,52).

Imaging Technologies: Magnetic Resonance Imaging and Echocardiography

As imaging technology has improved (particularly with improved image resolution) and its costs have declined, nonclinical safety evaluation of both drugs and medical device (particularly devices intended for cardiovascular uses) have begun to utilize imaging technologies for the evaluation of safety of new therapeutics.

MRI. Magnetic resonance imaging (MRI) relies mainly on the detection of hydrogen nuclei in water and fat to construct high-resolution images. The contrast in these images results from different T1 and T2 relaxation times for hydrogen nuclei in different tissue environments. MRI is based on the same principles as liquid-state nuclear magnetic resonance (NMR), i.e., the behavior of nuclei in a magnetic field under the influence of radio frequency (RF) pulses, but the hardware, pulse sequences, and data processing are somewhat different. Improvements in electronics and computers since the mid 1990s have given MRI resolution capabilities in intact organisms down to approximately 3 mm, and therefore tremendous potential as a tool for studying mechanisms of toxicology. MRI techniques provide detailed information on the response of specific organs to toxicants and can also be used to monitor xenobiotic metabolism in vivo. In addition, they could reduce the number of animals required for toxicology studies, as a single animal can be followed over an extended period of time to monitor internal changes.

Angiography, using X-rays to image coronary vasculature and blood flow in discrete regions during a study, has become a standard tool for evaluating effects on vascular function (including evaluating blockage, revascularization, and angiogenesis) when such are concerns or desired outcomes of treatment. Performance of such angiography in preclinical studies is usually restricted to use in dogs and swine, where it is a valuable tool for evaluating vascular/flow functional effects (46).

Echocardiography. Echocardiography (ECHO) is the use of ultrasound technology to assess various aspects of cardiac function and morphology. By using different ECHO windows (standard placements of the ECHO probe) and types of ultrasound propagation, qualitative information can be obtained regarding indices of cardiac size, systolic function, diastolic function, and hemodynamics. Furthermore, certain parameters are a reflection of an integrated input of cardiac functions and can be used for a global impression of cardiac function (53).

In the present studies, the parameters measured varied because of differences in heart size, anatomy, species, movement artifacts, and equipment used. However, certain parameters are constant across the studies and these are used for comparative purposes. Two of these parameters (or surrogate) are also those used in the *Common Terminology Criteria for Adverse Events* (CTCAE), version 3 (v3), an adverse event rating, which is used for assessing adverse events during clinical trials. These parameters include an assessment of left ventricular ejection fraction and fractional shortening of the left ventricle.

Table 7 presents a glossary of the terms used, how these reflect indices of cardiac function, and how changes in these parameters reflect decreases in cardiac function.

Clinical studies in oncology tumor vascular disrupting agents have shown indications of cardiac effects, including QTc interval prolongation, measurable plasma troponin-T levels, cardiac hypoxia, and cardiac ischemia. GLP IND-enabling studies of several agents have indicated minimal-slight cardiopathology in the dog and rat. Following such observations, the cardiotoxic potentials have been investigated by means of ECHO, together with histopathology and cardiac biochemistry, in dog, pig, and cynomolgus monkey.

Results with studies suggest that the use of ECHO can demonstrate changes in cardiac function at lower doses that can be predictive of more significant changes at higher doses.

Studies on cardiac function in the dog and monkey have shown neither troponin I nor the cardiac selective isoform of creatine kinase that appeared to be reliable indicators of cardiac pathology or systolic dysfunction.

Histopathologic examination of the heart is necessarily an integral part of the echocardiographic studies performed to investigate effects on cardiac

Table 7 Glossary of Echocardiographic Terms and Changes Associated with a Decreased Cardiac Function

---

Heart size

Decrease in parameters is associated with a decrease in cardiac function, as there is a reduced volume
  - LVIDd: left ventricular inner diameter at diastole (mm)
  - LAD: left atrial diameter (mm)

Systolic function
  - FxS: fractional change in left ventricular diameter (%)

    – A decrease is associated with decreased cardiac function, reflecting reduced systolic contraction

  - FxArea: fractional change in left ventricular area (%)

    – A decrease is associated with decreased cardiac function, reflecting a reduced area of systolic contraction

  - LVIDs: left ventricular inner diameter (mm)

    – An increase is associated with decreased cardiac function, reflecting reduced systolic contraction

  - PEP/LVET: ratio of the preejection period to left ventricular ejection time

    – An increase is associated with deficits in contractility or high afterload, a relatively shortened period of systolic contraction

  - VCFm: mean velocity of circumferential fiber shortening (circ/sec)

    – A decrease is associated with decreased cardiac function, reflecting a reduced rate of systolic contraction or reduced contractility

Diastolic function
  - IVRT: left ventricular isovolumic relaxation time (ms)

    – An increase is often associated with impaired myocardial relaxation

Hemodynamics
  - Heart rate (bpm)
  - VTI: velocity time integral of aortic flow profile (mm)

    – Related to stroke volume
    – Decreased with a decrease in cardiac function

  - VTI × HR: proportional to cardiac output (mm/min)

    – Decreased with a decrease in cardiac function

  - AoVel: peak aortic velocity (mm/sec)

    – Decreased with a decrease in cardiac function

Global function
  - EPSS: separation of the mitral leaflets from the septal wall during the early wave of mitral flow (mm)

    – Increased with a decrease in cardiac function, may be associated with mitral regurgitation.

---

function in the dog and monkey. Properly formulated patterns of histopathologic findings similar to those reported in the safety and toxicology studies, with myocardial necrosis of the papillary muscle, intraventricular septum, and left ventricular wall, are seen.

Minimally, cardiotoxic Cmax values for such agents appear to vary considerably between species and also with the use of different formulations. A further confounding factor to consider is the variability in sampling times between studies, a critical aspect when dealing with an intravenously administered compound with a short half-life (~ 2 hours) as is the case with many protein therapeutic agents.

Results with studies suggest that the use of ECHO can demonstrate changes in cardiac function at lower doses that can be predictive of more significant changes at higher doses.

CLINICAL SIGNS/OBSERVATIONS

Clinical signs represent the oldest noninvasive assessment of general health and provide in animal studies a crude but broad and potentially very valuable screen-identifying adverse responses. Training, experience, and continuity of the observer are vitally important to these signs being both meaningful and reliable. A rigorous, regular, and formatted collection of such signs in an objective manner (54) provides an essential component of any systemic toxicity study.

A number of the observations collected in the standard clinical signs measurements either directly or indirectly address cardiovascular function. These include body temperature, the occurrence of cyanosis, flushing, weakness, pulse, and the results of careful palpitation of the cardiac region.

CLINICAL PATHOLOGY

Traditional systemic or "general" toxicology studies place their greatest reliance for detecting cardiotoxicity on the last two sets of tools presented here—clinical and anatomic pathology. Both of these are invasive, but not necessarily terminal, therefore, entailing either instilling at least some stress in test animals or (for smaller animals) euthanasia of the animals, but these studies are considered to be reasonably unequivocal in their interpretation. Also, both require a significant amount of experience/knowledge as to the normal characteristics of the model species.

Clinical pathology entails both hematology and clinical chemistry. Here, we are interested only in the latter because cardiovascular toxicity is not generally reflected in the hemogram. Urinalysis is likewise not a useful component of the clinical chemistry screen for detecting cardiotoxicity. Rather, serum levels of selected parameters are of primary interest. During actual myocardial infarction (MI), there occurs a leakage of cellular constituents with rapid losses of ions and metabolites, resulting in transient increases in serum concentrations of these parameters. Later, there is a release of specific enzymes and proteins, which are in turn slowly cleared from the plasma. One can broadly classify the measurements made in serum as electrolytes, enzymes, proteins (other than enzymes), and lipids. Analysis of the findings as to their increases and decreases tends to be more powerful when it looks at patterns of changes across several end points, such as increases in CPK, γ-hydroxybutyrate dehydrogenase (γ-HBDH), and LDH, and in serum glutamic-oxaloacetic transaminase (SGOT).

Although the most important parameters are generally considered to be CPK, γ-HBDH, LDH, and SGOT, each of which is primarily a muscle enzyme (and therefore increased levels of which may be indicative of either skeletal or cardiac muscle damage), it is appropriate to consider the entire range of chemistry end points (55).

Electrolytes

Maintenance of the intracellular concentrations of cations (sodium, potassium, calcium, magnesium, and zinc) is essential for proper cardiovascular function. Alterations of the concentration of these cations may result in increased cardiac tissue sensitivity, arrhythmias, or significant adverse changes in vascular permeability. Concentrations of these cations are interrelated, making any significant disturbance of the ionic balance for one cation a consequence for the concentrations of the remaining ions. This interrelationship is observed with cardiac glycosides, which inhibit the sarcolemmal sodium pump Na^+/K^+–adenosine triphosphatase (ATPasc), causing increased intracellular sodium concentration, followed by increases of intracellular calcium and cardiac contractility. Where cardiac output is decreased, disturbances of plasma electrolytes may be the result of consequential alterations of renal function, e.g., reduced glomerular filtration rate (GFR). GFR may be evaluated by plasma creatinine and urea measurements. In addition, hypernatremia or hyponatremia may be observed in cardiac failure, depending on the volemic state of the animal.

When considering the effects of calcium and magnesium on cardiac function, the concentrations not bound to proteins (free) are more important than the total plasma concentration. Depending on the species, approximately 40% of the total plasma calcium and 30% of the plasma magnesium are bound to proteins. The need to consider plasma-free calcium concentration to protein-bound calcium concentration has been demonstrated by doxorubicin-induced cardiotoxicity in rabbits. Hypercalcemia is not apparent when total plasma calcium is measured in doxorubicin-treated rabbits, as there is a concomitant reduction of plasma albumin caused by renal toxicity. Increased plasma ionized levels observed in these rabbits may therefore be partly due to the renal function. Excessive stress and use of restraining procedures during blood collection will markedly affect the potassium, calcium, and magnesium levels. The sites selected for blood collection and anesthetic techniques will also influence these plasma cation measurements.

Although changes of plasma anion concentrations often follow disturbances incationic balance, these changes are of lesser significance for cardiac function. Plasma anions (chloride, bicarbonate, and inorganic phosphate) are poor marker anions as their plasma concentrations may be altered for many reasons other than those associated with cardiac function.

Osmolality and Acid-Base Balance

Plasma osmolality determinations may be meaningful in conditions such as congestive cardiac failure, in which total body sodium concentration and extracellular fluid volume are increased but there is evidence of hyponatremia. Several formulas for the calculation of plasma osmolality from plasma concentrations of sodium, urea, and glucose have been used with humans but have limited applicability with other species, in which the component concentrations vary. Acid-base balance determinations can be used to monitor cardiotoxic effects on respiratory and metabolic functions, but the variability due to collection procedures on these determinations in small laboratory animals limit their regular use in toxicologic studies.

Enzymes

Heart muscle tissue is rich in enzymes but only a few have proved to be useful indicators of myocardial damage and congestive cardiac failure. A major limitation in animal studies is the relatively short half-life of these markers after damage has occurred. This makes the sampling design shown in Figure 2 very much a hit-or-miss proposition, particularly as different doses of the same compound will cause damage (and therefore evoke enzyme release) at different times. Additionally, it must be remembered that these enzymes are released by cells that are dead or dying. Damage that is functionally impairing to the organ or organism may not kill enough cells to be detected by this end point. There are also real limits on how many samples may be drawn from smaller animals, particularly when a large enough volume must be drawn for evaluation of other clinical pathology parameters.

Plasma enzyme activity depends on the enzyme concentrations in different tissues, the mass of damaged tissue, the severity of damage, the molecular size of the enzyme, and the rate of clearance from the plasma. The distribution of enzymes in different tissues varies between species (56,57). Differences in published data for tissue enzyme concentrations in the same species are in part due to the methods used for tissue preparation and sample collection (because of varying levels of physiologic stress), extraction of the enzyme, and enzyme measurement. The rate for enzyme removal from the intravascular space varies greatly for individual enzymes and species, as reflected by the differing relative half-lives of each enzyme.

For both CPK and LDH measurements, it is preferable to use plasma rather than serum, owing to the relatively high concentration of these enzymes in platelets and, hence, their release into serum during blood coagulation. Plasma samples with visible evidence of hemolysis should not be used because of the high enzyme concentrations in erythrocytes. Blood collection procedures may influence plasma enzyme values, particularly in rodents.

Creatine phosphokinase

CPK has two subunits, B and M, which can form three cytosolic isoenzymes: the dimer consisting of two M (muscle) subunits (CPKMM) is the "muscle-type" isoenzyme, the hybrid dimer (CPK-MB) is the "myocardial-type" isoenzyme, and the third dimer (CPK-BB) is the "brain-type" isoenzyme. A fourth iso-enzyme (CPKm) is located in the mitochondria of cardiac and other tissues.

Intramuscular injections cause increased plasma CPK activities. However, if blood samples are collected approximately five minutes after injection of an anesthetic agent sufficient to anesthetize rats fully, no effect on CPK is observed. The age of an animal may affect plasma CPK, with activities generally being higher in younger animals. Values also may be affected by stress and severe exercise.

Myoglobin

Myoglobin, as with creatine kinase (CK), is primarily found in the cytoplasm of both skeletal and cardiac myocytes. In clinical medicine, the primary utility for serum myoglobin analysis is in early detection of acute MI and response to thrombolytic treatment. Although the analyte lacks specificity for cardiac muscle and occurs in higher (though species- and age-variable) proportion in skeletal muscle, it displays a clinically advantageous short circulating half-life for early postinjury monitoring. A circulating half-life of about 20 minutes to 20 hours in humans and less than 10 minutes in dogs has been reported (58). Accordingly, serum myoglobin in humans and laboratory species has generally been found to increase quickly following myocardial injury (with adequate perfusion) and to return rapidly to baseline with resolution of tissue damage (59,60). Peak arterial plasma myoglobin in dogs, as determined with an in-house developed enzyme-linked immunoassay (ELISA), occurred within 20 to 40 minutes after release of a two-hour coronary artery occlusion (59).

Currently, commercial ELISA kits that are marketed for evaluation of myo-globin in several different laboratory species are available. These assays utilize species-specific reference material. Automated clinical assays for human myoglobin incorporate a variety of proprietary reagent antibodies with nonstandardized reference material and manufacturers do not claim cross-reactivity with the nonhuman specimens (61). Notably, despite extensive conservation of myoglobin amino acid sequences across mammalian species, cross-reactivity of antibodies developed against the protein in one species with myoglobin from another has not been in accordance with regional sequence similarity. This is partly due to amino acid substitutions that influence tertiary structure and other antigenic features of the protein (62).

Lactate Dehydrogenase

LDH is a cytosolic tetrameric enzyme with five major isoenzymes consisting of M (muscle) and H (heart) subunits; a sixth isoenzyme of C subunits is found in some tissues. The five isoenzymes are numbered according to relative mobility during electrophoretic separation: LDH, consists of four H subunits; LDH 5 consists of four identical M units; and LDH2', LDH 3', and LDH 4 are hybrid combinations of the two subunits (HHHM, HHMM, and HMMM, respectively). The distribution of LDH in various tissues is often described as ubiquitous, and variations occur between species. For these reasons and because of the broad normal plasma LDH ranges often encountered in laboratory animals, the total plasma LDH values are often difficult to interpret; separation (and quantification) of plasma LDH isoenzymes therefore is helpful in cardiotoxicity studies.

Plasma α-hydroxybutyrate dehydrogenase (HBD) measurements reflect the activities of LDH1 and LDH2 isoenzymes. In 7 of 10 species examined, tissue HBD activities are highest in cardiac tissue. LDH5 is the dominant isoenzyme in normal rat and dog plasma, whereas LDH1 and LDH2 are the dominant isoenzymes in plasma of several primates. Where LDH5 is the major isoenzyme in the plasma, it may require a considerable increase of LDH1 before total LDH values change significantly. Some drugs (such as streptokinase) modify the electrophoretic mobility of some LDH isoenzymes.

Serum Glutamic-Oxaloacetic Transaminase and Serum Glutamic-Pyruvic Transaminase

These two enzymes are commonly used as indicators of hepatotoxicity, but their plasma activities may also be altered following myocardial damage. Neither of these is tissue specific; in many laboratory animal species, cardiac tissue SGOT concentration is higher than in most other major tissues, whereas cardiac tissue serum glutamic-pyruvic transaminase (SGPT) concentrations vary between species. In the rat, dog, and mouse, hepatic tissue SGPT concentrations are generally higher than those in other major tissues, but hepatic and cardiac tissue concentrations are similar in several primate species. The plasma SGOT/SGPT ratio may be useful in detecting cardiac damage, but the ratios vary with species

Table 8 Differentiation Based on Serum Enzyme Findings for Major Classes of Cardiac Damage and Related/Confounding Events

Condition	SGOT	SGPT	CPK	LDH
Myocardial cell death (infarct)	Increased	No change	Increased	Increased
Congestive heart failure (liver congestion)	Increased	Increased	No change	Increased
Muscle necrosis	Increased	No change	Increased	Increased
Lung embolism	No change	No change	Minimal increased	Increased

Abbreviations: SGOT, serum glutamic-oxaloacetic transaminase; SGPT, serum glutamic-pyruvic transaminase; CPK, creatine phosphokinase; LDH, lactate dehydrogenase.

and often cannot be compared with published data because the ratios are dependent on methods.

There are two isoenzymes of SGOT—cytosolic and mitochondrial isoenzymes; SGOT also has cytosolic and mitochondrial isoenzymes, but SGPT often is commonly believed to be entirely cytosolic owing to the higher proportion of cytosolic to mitochondrial isoenzyme.

Table 8 broadly summarizes these patterns of change for the major classes of damage seen in or confused with cardiac toxicity.

Heart Fatty Acid–Binding Protein

Similar to myoglobin, heart fatty acid–binding protein (H-FABP) is an early clinical laboratory marker of myocardial injury and response to thrombolytic treatment. H-FABP is also of comparable size with myoglobin, found in high concentration in myocyte cytoplasm, and rapidly released into blood with cell injury. H-FABP is one of the several structurally diverse long-chain fatty acid–binding proteins that have differential tissue expression. At least nine immunologically and genetically distinct fatty acid–binding proteins have been reported in humans, and at least three distinct FABPs have been found in rodent tissues (63–65). A physiologic role commonly assigned to H-FABP in all species is transport of hydrophobic long-chain fatty acids from the cell membrane to intracellular sites of metabolism in the mitochondria. Other functions of the protein have also been suggested.

In contrast with myoglobin, H-FABP is considered relatively more cardiospecific because the concentration in heart muscle is severalfold greater than that in skeletal muscle. In humans, myogobin has approximately a twofold greater concentration in skeletal muscle than heart (when expressed per gram of tissue wet weight), while H-FABP is approximately 10-fold greater in heart than in most skeletal muscles (66). Similarly in rodents, H-FABP has been found to occur in all striated muscles, but is greatest in proportion in cardiac muscle. The protein or gene expression of H-FABP in rodents has also been found in a few other tissues, including kidney and brain, although generally in much lower levels. The actual concentration of H-FABP in cardiac muscle relative to other tissues in nonhuman species, however, is variable between species, as well as between muscle region and during development.

In humans with MI, circulating H-FABP generally peaks within six hours and returns to reference limits by 24 hours after the onset of the injury (66,67). H-FABP also appears rapidly in urine, and both plasma and urinary H-FABP concentrations have been correlated with severity of myocardial injury and infarct size in humans (67).

Similarly, in vitro and in vivo studies of the rat and dog have indicated that H-FABP is rapidly released into circulation from injured myocytes and quickly cleared intact through the kidneys (68–70). In a rat model of myocardial ischemia, peak plasma H-FABP occurred within 15 minutes and concentrations were generally proportional to the size of affected area (68). Elimination kinetics in dogs-administered exogenous H-FABP indicated a mean plasma half-life of approximately 30 minutes and peak level in urine of seven minutes. In a dog model of coronary artery occlusion, plasma and urinary H-FABP levels showed rapid increase after reperfusion (70). To strengthen the distinction between skeletal and cardiac muscle injury with H-FABP analysis in nonclinical and clinical studies, the ratio of myoglobin to H-FABP must be determined. Use of the ratio has been particularly advocated for nonclinical studies because of common concomitant skeletal muscle injury that occurs in association with animal handling. However, studies on the benefit of this ratio compared to simple analysis of H-FABP absolute values in nonclinical studies have not been published. Notably, because H-FABP renal clearance is different than that of myoglobin, impaired renal excretion can also alter this ratio.

Commercial automated assays for analysis of human H-FABP are available. However, considerable differences in amino acid sequences between the human and rodent protein have been documented, and at least some antibodies to human H-FABP tested with rodent and nonrodent animal samples have shown only 26% to 60% cross-reactivity with the nonhuman protein. Commercial species-specific ELISA kits for H-FABP are available for several laboratory species.

In conclusion, H-FABP levels in circulation and urine has potential value as a bridging biomarker that is more cardiac specific than myoglobin for early detection of myocardial injury. H-FABP may also be useful in estimation of severity or extent of acute myocardial injury in nonhuman species. However, as with myoglobin, H-FABP has only narrow overall utility in nonclinical testing for cardiac injury because of the lack of complete tissue specificity and very short circulating half-life.

Troponins

Troponins are cardiac muscle proteins, which can serve as sensitive markers of heart damage (71,72).

Both cardiac troponin T (cTnT) and cTnI can be measured by immuno-assay systems, which use similar techniques. Levels of cTnT and cTnI in the blood are undetectable by current methods, thus normal values for cTnT and cTnI are effectively zero (73).

Following MI there is death of myocardial tissue and the release into the circulation of intracellular components, including the more familiar cardiac enzyme CK, its MB isoenzyme (CK-MB), and cTnT and cTnI. The latter can be detected at about the same time as CK and CK-MB. All cases of definite MI will have detectable levels of cTnT and cTnI by 12 hours from hospital admission and often much earlier.

Troponin Importance in MI

The cTns have a number of specific features. They are released only following cardiac damage (74).

CK and CK-MB are found in skeletal muscle as well as cardiac muscle. Thus, if there is damage to skeletal muscle, elevations of CK and CK-MB will occur and can make the diagnosis of MI difficult. A good example would be chest pain following a marathon when measurement of CK and CK-MB are unhelpful as both are elevated because of muscle trauma. By contrast, levels of cTnT and/or cTnI will not rise unless MI has occurred.

Unlike CK and CK-MB, cTnT and cTnI are released for much longer duration, with cTnI detectable in the blood for up to five days and cTnT for 7 to 10 days following MI. Thus, MI can be detected if the patient presents late. For example, if a patient comes to the surgery with complain of a chest pain that occurred two to three days ago, measurement of cTnT or cTnI will allow the diagnosis or exclusion of MI as a cause of the chest pain. However, anyone with recent (within the last 12 hours) cardiac sounding chest pain requires rapid hospital assessment.

CK and CK-MB are released from skeletal muscle at a low level all the time so there is always a background value. This does not occur for the cardiac structural proteins such as cTnT and cTnI. Hence, they are very sensitive. One-third of patients admitted with unstable angina, in which MI was apparently excluded by CK and CK-MB measurement, have raised levels of cTnT and cTnI. Follow-up studies show that these patients are at significantly greater risk of death, subsequent MI, or readmission with unstable angina than patients who did not have detectable levels cTnT or cTnI (75,76).

The sensitivity and diagnostic accuracy of cTnT and cTnI have resulted in the European Society of Cardiology and the American College of Cardiology proposing a new set of diagnostic criteria for MI (77). These consider cTnT and cTnI to be the gold standard for biochemical tests. MI is therefore considered to have occurred if any (or all) of the following apply:

- Definitive EKG changes (Q waves or ST segment elevation)
- Ischemic EKG changes
- Possible cardiac symptoms plus a rise (and fall) of cTnT or cTnI

Problems

It must be remembered that failure to show a rise in cTnT or cTnI does not exclude the diagnosis of ischemic heart disease.

A patient who is admitted with a suspected diagnosis of MI, but does not have detectable cTnT or cTnI, still requires further investigation such as an exercise stress test or other cardiac imaging to exclude a flow-limiting stenosis. Clinical studies have shown that for most applications there is little to choose between measurements of cTnT and cTnI.

However, the multiplicity of cTnI methods means that not all give the same result or show equal sensitivity. It is most important that general practitioners are aware of the method their local laboratory uses and its sensitivity and reproducibility (especially at the cutoff for diagnosis of MI). Another problem arises from the exquisite sensitivity and specificity of cTnT and cTnI for the detection of cardiac damage. Elevation of cTnT or TnI is absolutely indicative of cardiac damage, but this can occur as a result of causes other than MI.

Hence myocarditis, cardiac trauma from surgery or road accident, coronary artery spasm from cocaine, severe cardiac failure, and pulmonary embolus can cause cardiac damage with an accompanying elevation of cTn(s).

Finally, both cTnT and cTnI may be elevated in patients with chronic renal failure and indicate a higher long-term risk of death. They can be distinguished from changes because of MI by repeating the tests. MI causes a rise and fall in cTnT or cTnI, but in renal failure the elevated levels are sustained.

The role of cTn measurements can be summarized as follows:

- To confirm or exclude a diagnosis of MI within 12 hours from admission with possible cardiac symptoms.
- To guide treatment decisions in patients admitted with unstable angina.
- To confirm or exclude a diagnosis of MI in patients presenting late, e.g, two to three days, after an episode of possible cardiac symptoms where immediate hospital admission may not be appropriate.
- To confirm or exclude a diagnosis of MI in patients in whom other tests (CK, CK-MB) are not useful because of trauma or extreme exercise.

Other Proteins

Plasma albumin acts as a marker of plasma volume following cardiac damage; changes may simply reflect edema or plasma volume differences following congestive cardiac failure. Plasma albumin can be measured by dye-binding methods or more specific immunoassays. Plasma protein electrophoresis can confirm decreased plasma albumin levels and detect changes of other protein fractions. Serial plasma protein electrophoretic measurements may be useful in monitoring inflammatory processes, but changes are not specific for cardiac damage.

Plasma myoglobin can be used as a marker of myocardial damage, but the changes of plasma myoglobin occur more rapidly than those observed for plasma CPK. The myoglobin structure varies between different vertebrates, and the amino acid sequence imparts varying immunogenic properties, thus preventing the use of some latex agglutination and radioimmunoassay methods with certain species. Again, myoglobinemia may be caused by disease processes other than cardiovascular disorders.

Plasma fibrinogen is a useful measurement, particularly in the assessment of thrombolytic agents and episodic thrombolysis. Chromogenic substrates designed for human plasma fibrinogen assays do not react identically with samples from other species, and some assays for determining fibrin degradation products do not work with all species.

Lipids

As markers of lipid metabolism, plasma lipids are indicators of potential risks for cardiotoxicity in contrast to some of the preceding markers, which directly or indirectly reflect cardiac tissue damage. In rabbits fed cholesterol-enriched vegetable oil, the relationship between hyperlipidemia and the resulting lesions of the aorta and coronary arteries were demonstrated over 70 years ago. Whereas hypolipidemic agents are designed to prevent atherosclerosis, some drugs may inadvertently moderate or modify metabolic pathways for lipid, lipoproteins, or apolipoproteins (through biliary secretion or lipid surface receptors). Adverse effects on lipid metabolism can be monitored by measuring plasma total cholesterol and triglycerides, with additional measurements of plasma lipoproteins, total lipids, phospholipids, apolipoproteins, and nonesterified fatty acids.

Plasma lipid patterns vary with age, sex, diet, and the period of food withdrawal prior to collection of blood samples. There are both qualitative and quantitative differences in the lipid metabolism of different laboratory animal species; these occur because of differences in the rates and routes of absorption, synthesis, metabolism, and excretion. In the rat, ferret, dog, mouse, rabbit, and guinea pig, the major plasma lipoprotein classes are the high-density lipoproteins, contrasting with old-world monkeys and humans, in which the low-density lipoproteins are the major lipoproteins in plasma.

For a more thorough review of the expected ranges for clinical chemistries in model species and their interpretation, one should consult Loeb and Quimby (78), Evans (79), Wallach (80), or Mitruka and Rawnsley (81).

PATHOLOGY

As with plasma chemistries, major considerations in the use of anatomic pathology as a tool for detecting and evaluating cardiotoxicity are associated with sampling (i.e., how many sections are to be taken and from where). Histopathology is generally a terminal measure [the exception being the use of in situ biopsy techniques, such as those proposed by Fenoglio and Wagner (82)], so the time point for study termination governs whether a lesion will have had time to develop and whether its interpretation will not be complicated by subsequent (after the injury of interest) events. Similarly, it is of concern how representative sections will be taken from collected tissues.

The heart shares a primary property with the nervous system, having cells with electrically excitable membranes, a potentially vulnerable target for toxins, i.e., membranes coupled to an intracellular contraction system and two properties, excitation and contraction, having high energy requirements. The heart has the highest energy demands on a weight basis of any organ in the body and requires a continued supply of oxygen to support aerobic metabolism. Oxygen supply and utilization are therefore another area of vulnerability. To clarify the basic principles of cardiac toxicology, the heart can simply be considered as an oxygen-dependent mass of contractile cells driven by excitable membranes that are subject to neuroliumoral control. As a result, cardiotoxicity may be caused because of alterations in oxygen transport or neurohormonal release.

Cardiotoxicity is a relatively infrequent adverse observation in humans because of the "weeding out" of potential cardiotoxic materials during preclinical testing of drugs. However, a large number of compounds of potential therapeutic value in cardiovascular or neurologic disease are administered at high doses to animals in development studies, and cardiotoxicity may frequently be encountered. The vast majority of effects are acute, transient functional responses and are reversible if the animal does not die. These functional responses include bradycardia, tachycardia, and various forms of arrhythmia, and like their equivalents in the nervous system these "cardiotoxicities" are generally considered to be exaggerated pharmacologic effects.

In many of the best-studied cases of functional abnormalities, the mechanism is related to alterations in the ion shifts across the cell membrane (sarcolemma), which are used in the action potential. Digitalis and related cardiotonic chemicals are probably toxic by inhibiting membrane $Na^+/K^+/Ca^{2+}$-ATPase, which maintains the normal transcellular gradients of these ions. Other chemicals disturbing ion transport across the cell membrane are tetrodotoxin, tetraethyl ammonium, and verapamil, which reduce the inflow of Na^+, K^+, and Ca^{2+} respectively. Other toxins are thought to act on intracellular sites. Heavy metals alter mitochondrial function and may depress the energy production vital to excitation-contracting coupling. The depression of cardiac contractility by halothane may be related in part to inhibition of myosin ATPase activity. Thus, there are many potential intracellular mechanisms by which toxins may interfere with excitation-contraction coupling to produce functional abnormalities. Many cardiotoxic agents probably interfere with this process at several sites.

Cardiomyopathy

In contrast to the frequent occurrence of functional effects, relatively few cardiotoxic agents cause structural changes in the heart. When effects are noted, they are usually characterized by degeneration followed by inflammation and repair. These lesions are designated cardiomyopathies. Myocardial (cardiac) necrosis is the most frequently studied cardiomyopathy. In principle, this can result indirectly by disturbance of the blood supply to the myocyte (hypoxic injury) or by direct chemical insult to the myocyte (cytotoxic injury) or by a combination of both effects. The end result, necrosis, is essentially the same, but the location of the lesion may differ. Hypoxic injury tends to affect fairly specific sites, whereas cytotoxic injury may be more widespread.

The classic cardiotoxic drugs that cumulatively cause congestive cardiomyopathy are the anthracycline anticancer/antibiotic drugs, exemplified by doxorubicin and daunomycin. For these, with continued dosing, there is widespread vacuolization of the intracellular membrane-bound compartments and mitochondrial degeneration occurring in a cumulative dose-responsive manner (83).

Bronchodilators and vasodilators are the compounds classically producing site-specific necrosis. One or a few doses of isoproterenol produce acute cardiac necrosis in rat heart with a striking tendency for the subendocardial regions at the apex of the left ventricle. The vasodilator hydralazine acutely produces similar lesions; in beagles, the apex of the left ventricular papillary muscles is the favored site. Continued administration of hydralazine does not increase the incidence or severity of the lesions, and the initial acute lesions heal by fibrosis. Such acute cardiornyopathies could easily be missed in long-term studies, unless specific connective tissue stains [such as aniline black, Masson trichromal, van Gieson, or phosphotungstic acid hematoxylin (PTAH)] (84) are used to highlight the fibrosis.

The pathogenetic mechanism of this site-specific necrosis is not totally understood, but myocardial hypoxia probably plays an important role. Vasodilation may lower coronary perfusion and tachycardia increases oxygen demand. As the capillary pressure is lowest subendocardially, this area is at most risk to oxygen deprivation. The papillary muscles supporting the forces on the valves have the greatest oxygen requirement and are similarly at risk. The sites of injury are thus consistent with the hypothesis of myocardial hypoxia (85). Acute cardiac necrosis produced by vasoactive drugs can be considered to be the result of an exaggerated, pharmacologic effect.

Myocardial hypoxia depletes intracellular high-energy phosphate stores required to maintain membrane ion shifts. Disturbances of Ca^{2+} transport lead to increased cytosolic Ca^{2+}, increasing the adenosine triphosphate (ATP) breakdown already initiated by hypoxia. Calcium overload ultimately leads to cell death. Histologically, the dead myofibers have homogeneous eosinophilic cytoplasm (hyaline necrosis) and shrunken or fragmented nuclei. The subsequent inflammatory infiltrate consists mainly of macrophages, with healing by fibrosis.

Cytotoxic injury is often chronic, in contrast to the acute lesion caused by vasodilators. The lesions resulting from antineoplastic anthracycline antibiotics, such as daunorubicin and doxorubicin, frequently appear several months after the start of therapy. The clinical picture is generally a chronic congestive cardiomyopathy. Morphologically, the two main features are cardiac dilatation and myofiber degeneration. The degeneration consists of myofibrillar loss, producing lightly stained cells, and vacuolation due to massive dilatation of the sarcoplasmicc reticulum. At the ultrastructural level, many cellular components are affected. A similar chronic dose-related cardiomyopathy with congestive failure can be produced in animal models, and in rabbits the lesions tend to be distributed around blood vessels. The pathogenesis of the anthracycline cardiomyopathy is unclear.

Chronic cardiomyopathies can be produced by cobalt and brominated vegetable oils. Cobalt-induced cardiomyopathy was first discovered among heavy beer drinkers in Canada. Vacuolation, swelling, loss of myofibrils, and necrosis occur in experimentally poisoned rats and are found mainly in the left ventricle. Cobalt ions can complex with a variety of biologically important molecules and the potential sites for toxicity are numerous.

The cardiotoxicity of brominated vegetable oils is not characterized by necrosis but by fat accumulation affecting the whole myocardium. Focal necrosis may occur in the more severely affected hearts. The hearts of rats treated with brominated cottonseed oil show a dose-related reduction in the ability to metabolize palmitic acid, probably accounting for the accumulation of lipid globules in the myofibers.

Cardiac Hypertrophy

Cardiac hypertrophy is usually viewed as a compensatory response to hemodynamic stress. It can however also be a risk factor for QT prolongation and cardiac sudden death (86,87). Such increase in the mass of heart muscle is occasionally found in toxicity studies. This is usually a compensatory response to an increase in workload of the heart, and in compound-related cases, this is usually secondary to effects on the peripheral vasculature. Primary cardiac effects are rare, but can be produced by hormones such as growth hormones. A common challenge is distinguishing adaptive from maladaptive changes.

Pigment deposits in the heart are a common feature of aging animals. These aging pigments occur in lysosomes in the perinuclear regions of the sarcoplasm, and in extensive cases the heart appears brown at necropsy. This condition is known as brown atrophy. Food coloring pigment such as Brown

FK may also accumulate in a similar manner and in routine hematoxylin and eosin (H&E) section is impossible to differentiate from the lipofuscin of aging animals.

Vasculature

Drug-induced vascular injury in animals, while uncommon, has been a topic of intense discussion and debate in the toxicology, clinical, and regulatory arena since 1990 (88–91). A lack of understanding of the basic mechanisms by which such vascular injury is caused in animals, the absence of specific and sensitive biomarkers, and low cross-species safety multiples have become significant barriers in the development of many classes of therapeutic agents.

Vascular injury has been reported, with increasing frequency, as an adverse histologic observation in preclinical toxicity studies that are conducted to support the safe introduction of new medicines in humans. Vascular lesions, primarily arterial, can be induced within hours of drug administration; their morphologic and pharmacologic reversabilities are not clear. Animals exhibit no clinical signs, and routine clinical pathology data are normal. While reported and postulated mechanisms are varied, vascular injury in animals is induced by altered hemodynamic forces (shear and/or hoop stress), direct drug-induced toxicity, and/or immune-mediated injury of the endothelium and/or medial smooth muscle. Aside from histologic methods, the detection, noninvasively, of acute drug-induced vascular injury in animals or humans is not currently possible due to the lack of specific and sensitive biomarkers of endothelial and/or vascular smooth muscle injury.

In the past, regulatory authorities and pharmaceutical companies have been able to manage the risk of drug-induced cardiovascular toxicity in animals as sufficient data emerged that appeared to correlate the occurrence of myocardial and vascular toxicity with decreases in blood pressure and reflex tachycardia. Founded on this principle, it became generally accepted that as long as therapeutic doses of candidate drugs in humans did not induce hypotension and reflex tachycardia, safety and regulatory concerns were lessened, resulting in many products finding a clear path to the market place and/or approvable status (Table 9).

Hypotension and marked reflex tachycardia are well established as causing myocardial necrosis. This rule, however, may not apply to drugs that cause vascular lesions that are associated with myocardial lesions, as with minoxidil and the phophodiesterase (PDE) 3 inhibitors. Industry is now developing drugs that cause vascular injury in animals, but without changes in systemic blood pressure or heart rate, e.g., endothelin receptor antagonists, dopamine (DA1) agonists, adenosine agonists, second- and third-generation PDE 4 inhibitors, and others. It appears that the two events, myocardial and vascular toxicities, have different pathogenic mechanisms, the former related to myocardial ischemia and the latter unknown.

Table 9 Marketed Drugs That Cause Arterial Toxicity in Animals

Drug	Mechanism	Preclinical cardiovascular effects
Milrinone	PDE 3 inhibitor	Decreased MABP/reflex tachycardia
Fenoldopam	DA1 agonist	Decreased MABP
Theophylline	PDE 3 inhibitor/adenosine antagonist	Decreased MABP/reflex tachcardia
Minoxidil	Potassium channel opener	Decreased MABP/reflex tachycardia
Adenosine and adenosine receptor agonist	A1 agonist	Vasodilator
Hydralazine	Potassium channel opener (88)[a]	Decreased MABP/reflex tachycardia; alterations in gene expression (92)[a].
Bosentan	Endothelin receptor antagonist	No significant change in MABP or HR
Cilomilast	PDE 4 inhibitor	No significant change in MABP or HR
Nicorandil	Potassium channel opener/ nitrate	Decreased MABP/reflex tachycardia
Indolidan	PDE inhibitor (88)[a]	Decreased MABP/reflex tachycardia

[a]Reference (in parentheses).
Abbreviations: PDE, phophodiesterase; MABP, mean arterial blood pressure; HR, heart rate; DA1, dopamine.

When toxicities in animals, e.g., drug-induced vascular injury, are reported and the therapeutic index and/or safety margins are either low or negative and there are no obvious associations with predictive biomarkers, it is incumbent on industry to provide data to confirm that the new drug will be reasonably safe in humans. In the past, experience with many of the potent vasodilators (minoxidil, PDE III inhibitors, hydralazine) led scientists to conclude that cardiovascular lesions observed in animals were associated with dramatic changes in hemo-dynamics leading to marked reflex tachycardia, which resulted in the induction of cardiovascular lesions. Drug doses that did not cause marked reflex tachy-cardia did not cause lesions. These kinds of drugs progressed to clinical studies where patient safety was monitored by carefully evaluating blood pressure and heart rate and avoiding doses that caused marked decreases in systemic vascular resistance, hypotension, and reflex tachycardia.

Pressures on industry to identify reliable biomarkers have created very high hurdles for drugs that cause vascular injury. Concerns have been heightened by the known association between chronic vascular injury and inflammation (artherosclerosis) and the increased incidence of cardiovascular morbidity in humans. The lack of "safety margins" and biomarkers has hindered development of life-saving therapies in asthma, stroke, cerebral hemorrhage, pulmonary hypertension, chronic obstructive pulmonary disease, and others. However, as noted above, several drugs that cause vascular injury without hypotension and reflex tachycardia have been approved, without evidence of any known increased clinical risk. Although the messages between the regulatory authorities and industry are somewhat confusing, it is clear that industry must strive to develop methods to monitor for endothelial and/or smooth muscle compromise in normal animals and humans to clear the path for effective and efficient drug development in the future.

Adverse vascular toxicity, as described in animals, has not been reported in humans with the compounds listed in Table 1. Some compounds, like fenoldopam, bosentan, and cilomilast did not cause the classical picture of hypotension and reflex tachycardia in animal models, but nevertheless were approved or are approvable. In some of these cases, the animal to human safety multiples are very low or negative. While each drug is approved on the basis of its own merit and safety and risk–benefit analysis, decision making must be based on consistent scientific principles.

The regulatory dilemma of vascular risk management will not be resolved quickly. In the interim, where unique physiology, pharmacology and metabolism, and adequate therapeutic indices and safety margins serve to segregate animal findings from the human, reasonable safety and risk determinations are possible. At this time, while it may not be possible to make generalizations and assumptions of clinical value for humans, decisions regarding clinical safety must continue to be based on weight of evidence and experienced and sound scientific clinical judgment on a case-by-case basis.

Arterial and venular injury is a relatively uncommon hazard identified during preclinical toxicity testing; however, it is commonly observed in over a dozen different pharmacologic classes of drugs, including some that are approved products. The lesions of interest can be induced within hours in selected vascular beds in rats, dogs, pigs, monkeys, and/or mice. Depending on the induction protocol, lesions are usually reversible, although the literature is conflicting on this point. In rat and dog, vascular beds prone to drug-induced vascular injury are also susceptible to development of spontaneous vascular disease.

It is recognized that drugs that induce vascular lesions in animals present a safety assessment dilemma to toxicologists, physicians, and regulators wishing to assess safety of new medicines for humans. This dilemma is confounded by gaps in our knowledge regarding pathogenesis of injury, as well as limited knowledge regarding comparative physiology, pharmacology, and metabolism in various species, and, importantly, the absence of validated preclinical methods for monitoring vascular integrity noninvasively. Contrary to past thinking, preclinical experience with new and novel pharmaceuticals suggests that vascular injury is not associated with systemic changes in blood pressure and heart rate, rendering these parameters of little predictive clinical value. Variation in species responsiveness to vasoactive and nonvasoactive agents and marked differences in reactivity of selected vascular beds, taken together with contributions from numerous reactive cell types (e.g., endothelium, vascular smooth muscle, and inflammatory/immune cells) all add complexity to defining mechanism(s) and identifying robust biomarkers that are sensitive and specific.

There are several ways to produce arteriopathy, but the lesions generally follow a similar course. In acute lesions, the initial change is hyaline or fibrinoid degeneration of the intima and media. The increased eosinophilia seen histologically may be due to insudation of plasma proteins, necrosis of medial smooth muscle cells, or both. An inflammatory response often follows and the lesion may be described as an acute arteritis. Repair of the lesion is by proliferation of medial myofibroblasts extending into the intima. A broad range of compounds have been shown in National Toxicology Program (NTP) rat bioassay studies to cause cardiac thrombosis (93), undetected except at necropsy.

The two best-known pathways of vascular injury are hemodynamic changes and immune complex deposition. Acute arterial injury can result from rapid marked hemodynamic changes produced by the exaggerated pharmacologic effects of high doses of vasoactive agents on mean arterial pressure (MAP) and heart rate (HR) (88). The bronchodilators and vasodilators producing cardiac necrosis may also cause an arteritis in the dog heart, often in the right atrium. Agents producing vasoconstriction or hypertension, such as norepinephrine or angiotensin infusion, also produce lesions in small arteries in various regions of the body. Lesions also follow alternating doses of vasodilators and vaso-constrictors. The evidence suggests that a combination of plasma leakage due to physical effect on endothelial cells and acute functional demands on the smooth muscle cells plays an important role in the pathogenesis of these acute lesions.

Immune complex lesions such as vasculitis or hypersensitivity angitis have similar features to hemodynamic lesions, but tend to favor small vessels; therefore, fibrinoid change may be less conspicuous. In animals, immune complex lesiorki are produced most readily by repeated injection of foreign serum proteins.

Arteriopathies dominated by the proliferative component have been reported in women taking oral contraceptives. The lesions consist mainly of fibromuscular intimal thickenings with little or no necrosis or leukocyte infiltrations. Vascular lesions can also be produced in mice chronically dosed with steroid hormone.

Hemorrhage

Blood may escape from vessels because of defects in clotting factors, platelets, or the vessel wall, either singly or in combination. Clotting factor and platelet defects lead to hemorrhage by preventing effective closure of an injured vessel.

Hemorrhage due to direct injury of the vessel wall by chemicals is infrequent except as a local toxic effect. The most common form of chemically induced hemorrhage (purpura) is the widespread minor leakages that sometimes occur in the skin and mucous membranes in association with allergic vasculitis.

Hemorrhage is also a common artifact in animals that are dying (agonal artifact), or as a consequence of postmortem techniques. Hemorrhages in the germinal centers of the mandibular lymph node and thymic medulla are observed frequently in rats killed by intraperitoneal injection of barbiturates. These hemorrhages appear as red spots on the surface of the organ. Large areas of hemorrhage may occur in the lungs of rats killed by carbon dioxide inhalation, which may confound the interpretation of inhalation toxicity studies. Pulmonary hemorrhage may also occur in animals killed by physical means such as decapitation or cervical dislocation. A much more complete discussion of the histopathology of drug and chemically induced cardiac disease can be found in Balazs and Ferrans (92) or Bristow (93).

Mitochondrial Damage

The cells of the heart are the most intense of all body cells in their constant need for energy. For this, they are dependent on mitochondria, the organelles that are the bodies' energy source. Although many in vivo models of heart failure have been developed, a suitable in vitro model of heart failure has not yet been described. One of the terminal pathophysiologic features in heart failure was shown to be apoptosis, because the number of apoptotic cells in the heart was greatly increased during the progression of heart failure of various etiologies. Furthermore, impaired energy metabolism is reported to occur in the failing heart and to be responsible for the aggravation of heart failure (94). So far, many inducers of apoptosis in cell lines have been reported. However, compared to anticancer drugs such as doxorubicin, there are few reports of an inducer of apoptosis in primary cultured cardiomyocytes. Compared with other organs, the heart tissue possesses more mitochondria; therefore, it may be speculated that the impaired energy metabolism directly affects cardiac function, resulting in apoptosis (95–97). It has been shown that mitochondrial dysfunction induces apoptosis of cardiomyocytes and that these cardiomyocytes express molecular markers implicated in heart failure, such as ET-1 mRNA and atrial natriuretic peptide (ANP) mRNA, during apoptosis.

To adequately evaluate selective/differential mitochondrial damage in a normal regulatory toxicology study, it is necessary to determine if there is specific damage to the mitochondria. This can be evaluated in several manners but is most readily expressed by a decrease in the number or functioning of the mitochondria in the tissue. Such an assessment requires either careful light microscropy (LM) or electron microscropy (EM) evaluation with special staining, looking for things like mitochondrial swelling. Because the heart has a higher density of mitochondria and is more sensitive to destruction of these organelles, it is advisable to determine the mitochondrial count specifically in these tissues if there is any cause for concern (such as a therapeutic class effect or the observation of mineralization in cardiac tissue). Effects on mitochondrial functionality, even if at a level below clinically detectable, can be evaluated by evaluation of 3-[4,5 dimethylthiazol-2,1]-2-5-diphenyltetrazolium bromide (MTT) admits as a measured redox capability (98).

To maximize the chance of seeing any effect on mitochondrial numbers that might be present via LM in tissues that have already been fixed, it should be specially stained (0.5% periodic acid solution, or periodic acid schiff (PAS), being a recommended stain), examined, and compared with control animals from the same study.

If starting from fresh tissue, one may employ appropriate fixation techniques, followed by sectioning and staining for EM examination. This is usually employed in follow-on (rather than primary regulatory) studies, as the tissues are usually already fixed via an LM appropriate methodology before the need for special examination is discovered.

MEDICAL DEVICES

The assessment of cardiovascular toxicity for cardiovascular medical devices [such as bare metal stents (BMS)] or combination products (drug or biologic medical devices in one implantable product) has become a significant area of scientific, clinical, regulatory, and societal concern. The most prominent of such products are drug-coated stents, particularly the current standard of practice versions, which have a drug embedded in a biosorbable polymer matrix coated on the inside of a metal stent. In such cases, the intent is to impede the process of restenosis—the formation of new tissue growth within and along the interior of the stent, leading to renewed occlusion of the vessel and the progression of such cases. There are specific animal models for assessing the potential of such cases (99).

Such evaluations can be made in situ on stents implanted into dogs or pigs (the preferred models for vascular device evaluation) using either ECHO (discussed previously) or intravascular ultrasound (IVUS). Indeed, in 2007, the use of IVUS to insure proper stent placement has been proposed as a means of reducing the incidence of fatal myocardial events associated with devices.

Beyond this specific case of drug-coated bare metal stents, there are extensive efforts underway to develop drug-coated stents, the bodies of which are composed of a biosorbable polymer antiinfective, long-term indwelling catheters (for uses such as hemodialysis), and bone and spinal graft materials with biologic components to aid in bone attachment and regrowth. Each of these has potential cardiovascular risks, which must be assessed—acid dumping and bulk fragmention with the former, vascular, and systemic toxicity for antimicrobial agents for the latter.

ANIMAL MODELS

No review of the approaches used to identify and characterize cardiotoxic agents in industry would be complete without consideration of which animal models are used and what their strengths and weaknesses are.

Table 10 presents a summary of baseline values for the common parameters associated with cardiovascular toxicity in standard toxicity studies. These are presented for the species that see a degree of regular use in systemic toxicity studies (rat, mouse, dog, miniature swine, rabbit, guinea pig, ferrets, and two species of primates).

Major considerations in the use of the standard animal models to study cardiovascular toxicity are summarized as follows (28):

Rat—Very resistant to development of atherosclerosis; classic model for studying hypertension as some strains are easily induced.

Rabbit—Sensitive to microvascular constriction induced by release of epinephrine and norepinephrine (15).

Dog—Resistant to development of atherosclerosis.

Swine—Naturally developing high incidence of atherosclerosis; for this reason, a preferred model for study of the disease.

Primates—The rhesus is sensitive to the development of extensive atherosclerosis, following consumption of high-cholesterol diets.

More details on species, handling characteristics, and experimental techniques can be found in a study by Gad (28). There are also some special considerations when sudden cardiac death is a potential concern (29). It must be noted that there are gender differences in susceptibility to cardiac repolarization potential in most model species and in humans (99–102), perhaps due to sex hormone levels. This should be considered in both experimental design and interpretation

SUMMARY

Presented here is an overview of current issues in and approaches to detecting and characterizing cardiotoxicity in the assessment of safety of pharmaceuticals and medical devices. This is a field that is continuing to rapidly evolve and has become a critical part of the regulatory toxicology of these products. It depends on some very fixed tool sets to deal with both functional and structural toxicities. When the entire suite of methodology as presented here is used, it has performed reasonably well (as judged by cardiotoxicity, being only an idiosyncratic finding for products properly used and/or handled in humans). However, significant incremental improvements continue in the field, utilizing many of the technologies presented elsewhere in this volume.

Table 10 Baseline (Normal) Values for Parameters Potentially Related to Cardiac Toxicity

Species	HR (bpm)	BP (systolic/diastolic)	CPK (±UI-1)	SGOT (±UI-1)	LDH (±UI-1)	SGPT (±UI-1)
Rat	350–400	116/90	5.6 ± 1.3	200 ± 152	106 ± 78	42.2 ± 3.0
Mouse	300–750	113/81	3.7 ± 1.5	350 ± 108		98 ± 22
Dog (beagle)	100–130	148/100	1.2 ± 1.1	31 ± 7	68 ± 37.85	21.7 ± 8.4
Primate	150–300	159/127	2.06–6.3	26.1 ± 9.4	100–446	14.5 ± 8
(Cynomolgus rhesus)			22–53	27 ± 7	43–426	42.1 ± 21.2
Rabbit	120–300	110/80	1.76	44 ± 26	104.843–30	35 ± 16
Ferret	200–255	152/117		95 ± 52	608–45.6	208 ± 217
Guinea pig	260–400	77/47	0.95 ± 0.2	48 ± 9.5		44.6 ± 7.0
Swine	58–86	128/95		8.2 ± 21.6	96–160	9–17

Note: Values are ± one standard deviation.

Abbreviations: HR, heart rate; BP, blood pressure; bpm, beats per minute; CPK, creatine phosphokinase; SGOT, serum glutamic-oxaloacetic transaminase; LDH, lactate dehydrogenase; SGPT, serum glutamic-pyruvic transaminase.

The results of all these evaluations, generally performed before any FIM (first-in-man) clinical studies, provide an assessment of cardiovascular risk, which dictates how cautiously (and even if) a drug or device will proceed into clinical trials (103).

REFERENCES

1. Guth BD. Preclinical cardiovascular risk assessment in modern drug development. Toxicol Sci 2007; 97:4–20.
2. Morganroth J, Gussak, I. Cardiac Safety of Noncardiac Drugs. Totowa, NJ: Humana Press, 2005.
3. Carlsson L, Amos GJ, Andersson B, et al. Electrophysiological characterization of the prokinetic agents cisapride and mosapride in vivo and in vitro: implications for proarrhythmic potential?J Pharmacol Exp Ther 1997; 282(1):220–227.
4. Slordal L, Spigset O. Heart failure induced by non-cardiac drugs. Drug Saf 2006; 29(7): 567–586.
5. Kerkela R, Grazette L, Yacobi R, et al. Cardiotoxicity of the cancer therapeutic agent imatinab mesylate. Nat Med 2006; 12(8):908–916. (Epub 2006 Jul 23).
6. Connolly HM, Crary JL, McGoon MD, et al. Valvular heart disease associated with fenfluramine–phentermine. NEJM 1997; 337: 581–588.
7. Motsko SP, Rascati KL, Busti AJ, et al. Temporal relationship between use of NSAIDs, including selective COX-2 inhibitors, and cardiovascular risk. Drug Saf 2006; 29(7): 621–631.
8. Mann DL. Targeted cancer therapeutics: the heartbreak of success. Nat Med 2006; 12(8):881–882.
9. Melchert RB, Yuan C, Acosta D. Cardiovascular toxicology: Introductory Notes. In: Acosta D, ed. Cardiovascular Toxicology. New York: Taylor & Francis, 2001:1–30.
10. Ramos KS, Melchent RB, Chacon E, et al. Toxic responses of the heart and vascular systems. In: Klassen CD, ed. Casarett and Doull's Toxicology. 6th ed. New York: McGraw-Hill, 2001.
11. Smith TL, Koman LA, Mosberg AT, et al. Cardiovascular physiology and methods for toxicology. In: Hayes AW, ed. Principles and Methods in Toxicology. New York: Taylor & Francis, 2001:917–958.
12. Gad SC. Safety Pharmacology Boca Raton, FL: CRC Press, 2004.
13. Brunner H, Gross F. Cardiovascular pharmacology. In: Zbinden G, Gross F eds. Pharmacologic Methods in Toxicology. Oxford, UK: Pergamon Press, 1979:63–99.
14. Brunton LL, Parker KL. The Pharmaceutical Basis of Therapeutics. 11th ed. New York: McGraw-Hill, 2006:737–966.
15. D'Alonzo AJ, Zhu JL, Darbenzio RB. Effects of class III antiarrhythmic agents in an in vitro rabbit model of spontaneous torsades de pointe. Eur J Pharmacol 1999; 369(1):57–64.
16. Atta, AG, Vanace PW. Electrocardiographic studies in the *Macaca mulatta* monkey. Ann N Y Acad Sci 1960; 85:811–818.
17. ICH. Guideline S7B: The Nonclinical Evaluation of the Potential for Delayed Ventricular Repolarization (QT Interval Prolongation) by Human Pharmaceuticals. Geneva, Switzerland: International Conference for Harmonization, 2004.

18. Morganroth J. Cardiac repolarization and the safety of new drugs defined by electrocardiography. Clin Pharmacol Ther 2007; 81(1):108–113.
19. Hondeghem LM. Estimation of Proarrhythmic Hazards by QT Prolongation/Shortening: QT Obsession Drug Inf J 2006; 40:275–279.
20. Rampe D, Roy ML, Dennis A, et al. A mechanism for the proarrhythmic effects of cisapride (Propulsid): high affinity blockade of the human cardiac potassium channel HERG. FEBS Lett 1997; 417:28–32.
21. Grisanti S, Morganroth J, Shah RR. A Practical Approach to Cardiac Safety. Appl Clin Trials Oct 2, 2005.
22. Redfern WS, Carlsson L, Davis AS, et al. Relationships between preclinical cardiac electrophysiology, clinical QT interval prolongation and Torsade de Pointes for a broad range of drugs: evidence for a provisional safety margin in drug development. Cardiovasc Res 2003; 58(1):32–45.
23. Jamieson C, Moir EM, Rankovic Z, et al. Medicinal chemistry of hERG optimizations: Highlights and hang-ups. J Med Chem 2006; 49(17):5029–5046.
24. Aronov A. Common Pharmacophores for Unchanged Human Ether-a-go-go-Related Gene (hERG) Blockers. J Med Chem 2006; 49:6917–6921.
25. Cavero I, Crumb WJ. Mechanism-designed assessment of cardiac electrophysiology safety of pharmaceuticals using human cardiac ion channels Business Briefing: Pharma. Tech 2001:1–9.
26. Lacerda AE. et al. Comparison of block among cloned cardiac potassium channels by non-antiarrhythmic drugs. Eur Heart J 2001; (suppl K):K23–K30.
27. Calabrese EJ. Principles of Animal Extrapolation. New York: Wiley, 1983.
28. Gad SC. Animal Models in Toxicology, 2nd ed. New York: CRC Press, 2006.
29. Chan PS, Cervoni P. Current concepts and animal models of sudden cardiac death for drug development. Drug Dev Res 1990; 19:199–207.
30. Aubert M, Osterwalder R, Wagner B, et al. Evaluation of the rabbit Purkinje fiber assay as an *in vitro* tool for assessing the risk of drug-induced Torsades de Pointes in humans. Drug Saf 2006; 29:237–254.
31. Joshi A, Dimino T, Vohra Y, et al. Preclinical strategies to assess QT liability and torsadogenic potential of new drugs: The role of experimental models. J Electrocardiol 2004; 37(suppl):7–14.
32. Werdan K, Melnitzki SM, Pilz G, et al. The cultured rat heart cell: a model to study direct cardiotoxic effects of *Pseudomonas* endo- and exotoxins. In: Second Vienna Shock Forum. New York: Alan R Liss, 1989:247–251.
33. Mehendale HM. Application of isolated perfusion organ techniques in toxicology. In: Hayes AW, ed. Principles and Methods of Toxicology. New York: Taylor & Francis, 2001:1529–1584.
34. Gad SC, Leslie SW, Brown RG, et al. Inhibitory effects of dithiothreitol and sodium bisulfite on isolated rat ileum and atrium. Life Sci 1977; 20:657–664.
35. Gad SC, Leslie SW, Acosta D. Inhibitory actions of butylated hydroxytoluene (BHT) on isolated rat ileal, atrial and perfused heart preparations. Toxicol Appl Pharmacol 11979; 48:45–52.
36. Acosta D, Sorensen EMB, Anuforo DC, et al. An in vitro approach to the study of target organ toxicity of drugs and chemicals. In Vitro Cell Dev Biol 1985; 21:495–504.
37. Ruben Z, Fuller GC, Knodle SC. bisobutamide–induced cytoplasmic vacuoles in cultured dog coronary artery muscle cells. Arch Toxicol 1984; 55:206–212.

38. Kijtawornrat A, Nishijima Y, Roche BM, et al. Use of a failing rabbit heart as a model to predict torsadogenicity. Toxicol Sci 2006; 93(1):205–212. (Epub 2006 Jun 1).
39. Leslie SW, Gad SC, Acosta D. Cytotoxicity of butylated hydroxytoluene and butylated hydroxyanisole in cultured heart cells. Toxicology 1978; 10:281–289.
40. Low-Friedrich L, von Bredow F, Schoeppe W. *In vitro* studies on the cardiotoxicity of chernotherapeutics. Chemotherapy 1990; 36:416–421.
41. Walker MJA, Pugsley MK. Methods in Cardiac Electrophysiology. Boca Raton, FL: CRC Press, 1998.
42. Watkinson WP, Brice MA, Robinson KS. A computer–assisted electrocardiographic analysis system: methodology and potential application to cardiovascular toxicology. J Toxicol Environ Health 1985; 15:713–727.
43. Sodeman WA, Sodeman TM. Pathologic Physiology. Philadelphia, PA: W.B. Saunders, 1985.
44. Doherty JD, Cobbe SM. Electrophysiological changes in an animal model of chronic cardiac failure. Cardiovasc Res 1990; 24:309.
45. Hamlin R. Extracting "more" from cardiopulmonary studies on beagle dogs. In: Gilman MR, ed. The Canine as a Biomedical Model. Bethesda, MD: American College of Toxicology and LRE, 1985:9–15.
46. Goodman JS, Peter CT. Proarrhythmia: primum non nocere. In: Mandel WJ, ed. Cardiac Arrhythmias: their Mechanisms, Diagnosis and Management. Philadelphia, PA: J.P. Lippincot Company, 1995:173–179.
47. Kim SW, Yang SD, Ahn BJ, et al. In vivo targeting of ERG potassium channels in mice and dogs by a positron-emitting analogue of fluoroclofilium. Exp Mol Med 2005; 37(4):269–275.
48. Cheng J. Evidence of the gender-related differences in cardiac repolarization and the underlying mechanisms in different animal species and human. Fundam Clin Pharmacol 2006; 20:1–8.
49. Vatner SF, Patrick TA, Kudel AB, et al. Monitoring of cardiovascular dynamics in conscious animals. In: Acosta DA, ed. Cardiovascular Toxicology. Philadelphia, PA: Taylor & Francis, 2001:79–102.
50. Garner D, Laks MM. New implanted chronic catheter device for determining blood pressure and cardiac output in the conscious dog. Physiology 1985; 363:H681–H685.
51. Webster JG. Medical Instrumentation. New York: John Wiley & Sons, 1998.
52. Riccardi MJ, Beohar N, Davidson CJ. Coronary catheterization and coronary angiography. In: Rosendorf C, ed. Essential Cardiology. Philadelphia, PA: W.B. Saunders, 204–226.
53. Kaddoura S. Echo Made Easy. London, UK: Churchill Livingstone, 2002:190.
54. Gad SC. A neuromuscular screen for use in industrial toxicology. J Toxicol Environ Health 1982; 9:691–704.
55. Wahler DB. Serum chemical biomarkers of cardiac injury for nonclinical safety testing. Toxicol Pathol 2006; 34:94–104.
56. Clampitt RB, Hart RJ. The tissue activities of some diagnostic enzymes in ten mammalian species. J Comp Pathol 1978; 88:607–621.
57. Lindena J, Sommerfeld U, Hopfel C, et al. Catalytic enzyme activity concentration in tissues of man, dog, rabbit, guinea pig, rat and mouse. J Clin Chem Clin Biochem 1986; 24:35–47.
58. Klocke FJ, Copley DP, Krawczyk JA, et al. Rapid renal clearance of immunoreactive canine plasma myoglobin. Circulation 1982; 65:1522–1528.

59. Ellis AK, Little T, Zaki Masud AR, et al. Patterns of myoglobin release after reperfusion of injured myocardium. Circulation 1985; 72:639–647.

60. Spangenthal EJ, Ellis AK. Cardiac and skeletal muscle myoglobin release after reperfusion of injured myocardium of dogs with systemic hypotension. Circulation 1995; 91:2635–2641.

61. Panteghini M, Linsinger T, Wu A, et al. Standardization of immunoassays for measurement of myoglobin in serum. Phase I: evaluation of candidate secondary reference materials. Clin Chim Acta 2004; 341:65–72.

62. Twining SS, Lehmann H, Atassi MZ. The antibody response to myoglobin is independent of the immunized species. Analysis in terms of replacements in the antigenic sites and in environmental residues of the cross-reactions of fifteen myoglobins with sperm-whale myoglobin antisera raised in different species. Biochem J 1980; 191(3):681–697.

63. Heuckeroth RO, Birkenmeier EH, Levin MS, et al. Analysis of the tissue-specific expression, developmental regulation, and linkage relationships of a rodent gene encoding heart fatty acid binding protein. J Biol Chem 1987; 262:9709–9717.

64. Glatz JF, van der Vusse GJ. Nomenclature of fatty acid-binding proteins. Mol Cell Biochem 1990; 98:231–235.

65. Veerkamp JH, Paulussen RJ, Peeters RA, et al. Detection, tissue distribution and (sub) cellular localization of fatty acid-binding protein types. Mol Cell Biochem 1990; 98:11–18.

66. Okamoto F, Sohmiya K, Ohkaru Y, et al. Human heart-type cytoplasmic fatty acid-binding protein (H-FABP) for the diagnosis of acute myocardial infarction. Clinical evaluation of H-FABP in comparison with myoglobin and creatine kinase isoenzyme MB. Clin Chem Lab Med 2000; 38:231–238.

67. Tanaka T, Hirota Y, Sohmiya K, et al. Serum and urinary human heart fatty acid-binding protein in acute myocardial infarction. Clin Biochem 1991; 24:195–201.

68. Knowlton AA, Apstein CS, Saouf R, et al. Leakage of heart fatty acid binding protein with ischemia and reperfusion in the rat. J Mol Cell Cardiol 1989; 21:577–583.

69. Vork MM, Glatz JF, Surtel DA, et al. Release of fatty acid binding protein and lactate dehydrogenase from isolated rat heart during normoxia, low-flow ischemia, and reperfusion. Can J Physiol Pharmacol 1993; 71:952–958.

70. Sohmiya K, Tanaka T, Tsuji R, et al. Plasma and urinary heart-type cytoplasmic fatty acid-binding protein in coronary occlusion and reperfusion induced myocardial injury model. J Mol Cell Cardiol 1993; 25:1413–1426.

71. Wallace KB, Hausner E, Herman E, et al. Serum troponins as biomarkers of drug-induced cardiac toxicity. Toxicol Pathol 2004; 32:106–121.

72. Tarducci A, Abate O, Borgarelli M, et al. Serum values of cardiac troponin-T in normal and cardiomyopathic dogs. Vet Res Commun. 2004; 28(suppl 1):385–388.

73. Antman EM, Tanasijevic MJ, Thompson B, et al. Cardiac- specific troponin I levels to predict the risk of mortality in patients with acute coronary syndromes. N Engl J Med 1996; 335:1342–1349.

74. Collinson PO. Troponin T or troponin I or CK-MB (or none?). Eur Heart J 1998; 19 (suppl N):N16–N24.

75. Hamm CW, Ravkilde J, Gerhardt W, et al. The prognostic value of serum troponin T in unstable angina. N Engl J Med 1992; 327:146–150.

76. Stubbs P, Collinson P, Moseley D, et al. Prospective study of the role of cardiac troponin T in patients admitted with unstable angina. BMJ 1996; 313:262–264.

77. Myocardial infarction redefined—a consensus document of The Joint European Society of Cardiology/American College of Cardiology Committee for the redefinition of myocardial infarction. Eur. Heart J. 2000; 21:1502–1513.
78. Loeb WF, Quimby FW. The Clinical Chemistry of Laboratory Animals. 2nd ed. Philadelphia, PA: Taylor & Francis, 1999.
79. Evans GO. Biochemical assessment of cardiac function and damage in animal species. J Appl Toxicol 1991; 11:15–22.
80. Wallach J. Interpretation of Diagnostic Tests. Boston, MA: Little, Brown & Company, 1978.
81. Mitruka BM, Rawnsley HM. Clinical Biochemical and Hematological Reference Values in Normal Experimental Animals. New York: Masson, 1977.
82. Fenoglio JJ, Wagner BM. Endomyocardial biopsy approach to drug–related heart disease. In: Hayes AW, ed. Principles and Methods of Toxicology. New York: Raven Press, 1989:649–658.
83. Scheulen ME, Kappus H. Anthracyclines as model compounds for cardiac toxicity. In: Dehart W, Neumann HG, eds. Tissue–specific Toxicity. New York: Academic Press, 1992.
84. Luna LG. Manual of Histological Staining Methods of the Armed Forces Institute of Pathology. New York: McGraw-Hill, 1968.
85. Daly AM. Metabolism of the failing heart, Cardioscience 1993; 4:199–203.
86. Picard S, Doineau S, Ronel R. The action potential of the Purkinje fiber: an *in vitro* model for the evaluation of the proarrhythmic potential of cardiac and noncardiac drugs. Current Protocols in Pharmacology. New York: John Wiley & Sons, 2006.
87. Kang YJ. Cardiac hypertrophy: a risk factor for QT-Prolongation and cardiac sudden death. Toxicol Pathol 2006; 34:58–66.
88. Louden C, Brott D, Katein A, et al. Biomarkers and mechanisms of drug-induced vascular injury in non-rodents. Toxicol Pathol 2006; 34:19–26.
89. Emerson BE, Lin A, Lu B, et al. Acute drug-induced vascular injury in Beagle dogs: Pathology and correlating genomic expression. Toxicol Pathol 2006; 34:27–32.
90. Yoshiyama K, Kissling GE, Johnson JA, et al. Chemical-induced atrial thrombosis in NTP rodent studies. Toxicol Pathol 2006; 33:517–532.
91. Expert working group on drug-induced vascular injury. Drug-induced vascular injury- a quest for biomarkers. Toxicol Appl Pharmacol 2005; 203:62–87.
92. Balazs T, Ferrans JJ. Cardiac lesions induced by chemicals. Environ Health Perspect 1978; 26:181–191.
93. Bristow MR. Drug–induced Heart–Disease. New York: Elsevier, 1980.
94. Storey KB. Functional Metabolism: Regulation and Adaptation. Hoboken, NJ: Wiley-Liss, 2004.
95. Dunnick J, Johnson J, Horton J, et al. Bis(2-chloroethoxy)methane-Induced Mitochondrial and Myofibrillar Damage: Short-Term Time-Course Study. Toxicol Sci 2004; 81:243–225.
96. Kakinuma Y, Miyauchi T, Yuki K, et al. Mitochondrial dysfunction of cardiomyocytes causing impairment of cellular energy metabolism induces apoptosis, and concomitant increase in cardiac endothelin-1 expression. J Cardiovasc Pharmacol 2000; 36(5 suppl 1):S201–S204.
97. Dunnick J, Lieuallen W, Moyer C, et al. Cardiac damage in rodents after exposure to Bis(2-chloroethoxy)methane. Toxicol Pathol 2004; 32:309–317.

98. Golomb E, Schneider A, Houminer E, et al. Occultcardiotoxicity: subtoxic dosage of Bis(2-Chloroethoxy) methane impairs cardiac response to simulated ischemic injury. Toxicol Pathol 2007; 35:383–387.
99. Touchard AG, Schwartz RA. Preclinical restenosis models: challenges successes. Toxicol Pathol 2006; 34:11–18.
100. Achhorn W, Whitworth AB, Weiss EM, et al. Differences between men and women in side effects of second-generation antipsychotics. Nervenarzt July 28,2006.
101. Liu X-K, Katchman A, Drici M-D, et al. Gender differences in the cycle length-duration QT and potassium currents in rabbits. JPBT 1998; 285:672–679.
102. Drici MD, Burklow TR, Haridasse Y, et al. Sex hormones prolong the QT interval and downregulate potassium channel expression in the rabbit heart. Circulation 1996; 94:1471–1474.
103. ICH. Guideline E14: Clinical Evaluation of QT/QTc Interval Prolongation and Proarrhythmic Potential for Non-Antiarrhythmic Drugs. Geneva, Switzerland: International Conference for Harmonization, 2005.
104. Testai L, Breschi MC, Martinotti E, et al. OT Prolongation in guinea pigs for preliminary screening of torsadogenicity of drugs and drug candidates. II J Appl Toxicol 2007; 27:270–275.

4

Novel Approaches in The Evaluation of Cardiovascular Toxicity

Enrique Chacon

Organ Transport Systems, Inc., Frisco, Texas, U.S.A.

Joseph W. Starnes

Department of Kinesiology, University of Texas at Austin, Austin, Texas, U.S.A.

Vivek Kadambi and Colleen Doherty

Millennium Pharmaceuticals, Inc., Cambridge, Massachusetts, U.S.A.

John J. Lemasters

Departments of Pharmaceutical & Biomedical Sciences and Biochemistry & Molecular Biology, Medical University of South Carolina, Charleston, South Carolina, U.S.A.

INTRODUCTION

The ever-increasing number of chemical compounds synthesized by chemical and pharmaceutical industries has prompted the development of innovative in vitro research methods for optimizing potential drug candidates. Many of these new approaches show promise for effective and inexpensive toxicity assessment. In addition to providing potential toxicity assessments, in vitro methods serve as ideal models to investigate and understand mechanisms of action. In the previous edition (1), we discussed in vitro cytotoxicity modeling and the credence of in vitro models. Three important criteria need to be considered in the selection of an in vitro method are (*i*) the assay must correlate well with the in vivo biological response being modeled; (*ii*) the assay must have a biological basis that links it to the cell injury or pharmacological process; and (*iii*) the assay should be technically reliable and reasonably easy to conduct if used for screening purposes. In this chapter, we present a summary of the use of cardiac myocytes and two newer approaches being used to assess cardiotoxicity. Specifically, the two new models presented are the working heart model to evaluate cardiovascular toxicity and hERG channel assessment to evaluate QT interval prolongation.

PRIMARY HEART CELL CULTURES FOR CYTOTOXICITY SCREENING

Many investigators use cell cultures as in vitro models to evaluate the toxicity of xenobiotics (2,3). The progression of injury in primary cell cultures is usually similar to in vivo models. The onset of irreversible injury in vivo or in cultured cell monolayers is a time-dependent event. In cell culture models, the time dependence of cell injury can be identified after both acute and chronic exposures. Cell culture systems permit assessment of cellular responses that are technically difficult in vivo (4). In particular, cardiac cell culture systems have served to further our understanding of the cellular and molecular basis of myocardial cell injury (2,5).

Several cell culture systems are available. Nearly all systems utilize hearts from the chick, rat, or rabbit as the source of tissue. Hearts are separated mechanically and enzymatically into a heterogeneous suspension of muscle and non-muscle cells.

Separation of muscle from non-muscle cells is usually achieved by rate of attachment to cell culture dishes (6) or by centrifugal elutriation (7). Non-muscle cell cultures are generally a mixture of endothelial cells and fibroblasts. It has been argued that cells in culture rely predominantly on glycolysis for their energy supply, a change from the β-oxidation characteristic of muscle cells in vivo. However, experiences from our laboratories with cultured heart cells indicate that mitochondrial metabolism is preserved in cultured myocytes and serves as a vital source of energy. In addition, cardiac cells in culture will utilize β-oxidation as a major energy source provided that appropriate substrates are present (6,8). These characteristics make myocardial cell cultures appropriate models for cardiotoxicity assessment. Furthermore, myocardial cell cultures provide informative data with minimal investment of time and expense compared with models utilizing whole organs or live animals.

Neonatal Cardiac Myocytes

Newborn rats aged two to five days are typically used as a source of cardiac myocytes. Neonatal cardiac myocytes are relatively easy to isolate and can be maintained for weeks in primary culture. To prevent overgrowth of fibroblasts and other cells, myocytes should be purified before culturing. Two methods are routinely used to obtain relatively pure myocyte preparations. The first method is based on the rapid rate of attachment of non-muscle cells to plastic culture dishes (9). Enzymatic digests of whole hearts are placed in shallow plastic culture dishes.

After two to three hours of plating, more than 90% of non-muscle cells will have adhered to the dishes.

Non-attached myocytes are then decanted into separate culture dishes. A second method of separating myocytes from non-muscle cells utilizes the technique of centrifugal elutriation (7). Centrifugal elutriation separates cells based on size. Heart digests are infused into a rotating chamber in a direction against the centrifugal field. Cells remain trapped in the chamber until flow is increased or rotor speed decreased. As the force of flow begins to exceed the force of gravity, cells are eluted from the chamber, with the smallest cells being released first. Purified neonatal cardiac myocytes are plated at 75,000 cells per well in 96-well plates or 106 cells per 35-mm culture dish. After three to four days in culture, a nearly confluent monolayer of spontaneously contracting cells is obtained. Cells isolated by rate of attachment show significant contamination with fibroblasts after five to six days in culture. Cells isolated by elutriation show minimal contaminant cell growth, even after 30 days in culture. As metabolism of cultured cells may change over time, we typically use five- to eight-day cultures of myocytes purified by centrifugal elutriation for cytotoxicity screening.

Adult Cardiac Myocytes

In 1972, Chang and Cummings (10) described the cultivation of myocytes from human heart. Since larger and older animal hearts provide a terminally differentiated myocyte that more closely resembles adult human myocytes, much attention has been given to the development of adult cardiac myocyte cultures. Adult cell isolations frequently demonstrate a "calcium intolerance" that causes isolated rod-shaped cells to hypercontract and lose viability when exposed to physiologic concentrations of calcium. Success in isolating adult cardiac myocytes is dependent on a number of variables. The quality of dissociative enzymes used in the cell isolation process is a major determinant for obtaining viable cells. Variations of digestive enzyme from one lot to another seem particularly important and give rise to great variations of yield and viability. Other important variables include perfusion pressure, digestion time, temperature, electrolyte balance, and method of physical dispersion after perfusion. The difficulty of reliably obtaining large numbers of cardiac myocytes from adult sources has limited their use in cytotoxicity screening.

As in neonatal cell preparations, special attention must be given to the purity of myocardial cell cultures. Overgrowth of fibroblasts and other non-muscle cells can occur within three to five days in culture. Mitotic inhibitors, such as cytosine arabinoside, are frequently used to restrict contamination by fibroblasts and endothelial cells. Unlike neonatal cardiac myocytes, cultured adult cardiac myocytes do not spontaneously contract. However, the cells can be electrically stimulated to duplicate in vivo contractile activity. With the continued development of adult cardiac cell isolation techniques, investigators should be able to exploit the strengths of this model to evaluate the potential cardiotoxic effects of xenobiotics.

ISOLATED PERFUSED HEART FOR THE ASSESSMENT OF CARDIOVASCULAR TOXICITY

A cardiovascular model that stands between cultured cardiac myocytes and the in vivo heart is the isolated perfused heart. The isolated perfused heart is one of the most widely used experimental models in cardiovascular and pharmacological research. Whole-organ perfusion outside of the organism offers certain advantages over most other preparations: (*i*) compounds can be carried directly to the cardiac myocytes through the normal physiological channels by the coronary circulation; (*ii*) the viability of the muscle can be determined in a physiologically meaningful way based on functional parameters such as heart rate, pressure development, cardiac output, and coronary flow; and (*iii*) the model allows for precise control over key variables such as ventricular afterload and preload, rate of coronary flow, blood composition, and temperature. Importantly, almost any compound or stress can be precisely administered to the isolated perfused heart resulting in tightly controlled dose-response studies. There are vast options for biochemical analyses using the cardiac tissue or the coronary effluent. At any-time during perfusion the heart can be easily freeze-clamped to stop metabolic activity and preserve macromolecular integrity for analysis at a later time. By adding glutaraldehyde to the perfusate, the heart can be perfusion fixed for subsequent immunohistochemical techniques. Furthermore, methods and instrumentation are now available for noninvasive monitoring of many key intracellular events, such as high-energy phosphates, substrate use, ion movement, while the perfused organ is performing physiological levels of work.

Primary Methods of the Isolated Perfused Heart

The two primary methods of perfusing the isolated mammalian heart are the classical retrograde preparation described over 100 years ago by Langendorff in 1895 (11) and the more recent working heart preparation credited to Bob Neely (12). Most studies have been carried out on the rat, but larger animals have also been used and the mouse is increasing in popularity. The Langendorff heart preparation is the more widely used and simpler of the two methods as it involves cannulation of only the aorta. The coronary vessels are perfused as perfusion solution is delivered in the retrograde direction down the aorta, either at a constant hydrostatic pressure or at a constant flow rate (Fig. 1). In the working heart preparation, both the aorta and the pulmonary vein are cannulated so that the perfusate can enter the left atrium and flow into the left ventricle to be pumped out through the aorta as occurs in vivo (Fig. 2). Some excellent and detailed descriptions of the isolated perfused heart technique are available (13–19). In this chapter we will summarize some of the basic aspects of the two models.

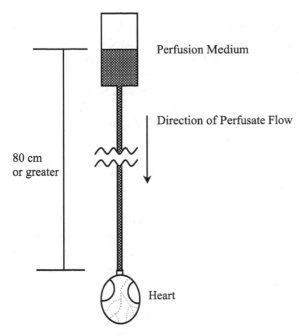

Figure 1 The basic Langendorff preparation. Coronary perfusion pressure is determined by height of perfusion medium above the heart.

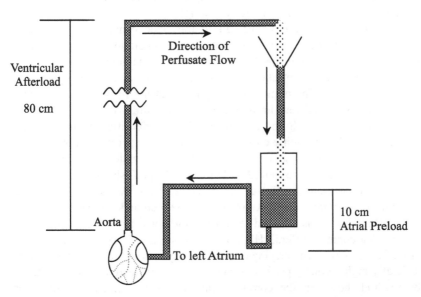

Figure 2 Hemodynamics of working heart preparation. Adjusting the heights of the aortic column and atrial buffer reservoir, respectively, can control afterload and preload. The heights displayed represent typical values.

The first step in the perfusion procedure is the same for both Langendorff and working preparations and involves getting oxygenated perfusion buffer flowing through the coronary arteries before ischemic artifacts occur. The chest cavity of a deeply anesthetized animal is opened to expose the heart, which is then excised with a single cut that retains the appropriate length of aorta for cannulation. In most studies, heparin or another anticoagulant is administered to the animal prior to heart excision in order to prevent thrombi formation. The excised beating heart is immediately dropped into a beaker containing cold (4°C) 0.9% sodium chloride to stop contractions and prevent ischemic injury. With practice an investigator can slip the aortic root over the cannula and begin flow through the coronary arteries within 30 seconds after excising a rat heart; while it may take longer for a mouse heart, which is approximately one-tenth the size of a rat heart. Sutherland et al. (18) suggest that a transition time up to 120 seconds for mouse hearts should be adequate to prevent subsequent ischemic injury, stunning (20), or preconditioning (21). Some investigators cannulate the heart in situ to eliminate any possibility of ischemic effects; however, this is not necessary as long as the transition is carried out quickly and the heart is cooled. Gross heart weight can be quickly obtained during the transition period by placing the beaker on a tared balance and gently squeezing the heart with a gauze to remove blood from the ventricles before dropping the heart into the beaker. Once perfusion has begun extraneous tissue can be cut from the heart, weighted, and subtracted from the gross weight to obtain preperfusion wet weight. Edema occurs during the perfusion process, so weighing before perfusion begins is a convenient way to obtain an accurate wet weight.

Once the aortic root is connected to the fixed cannula and retrograde perfusion begun, the Langendorf preparation is in operation. The perfusate is delivered either at a constant perfusion pressure by maintaining the perfusate reservoir at a constant height above the aortic valve or at a constant flow rate controlled by a pump. The minimum perfusion pressure for adequate coronary perfusion and oxygen delivery in the rat heart is 50 mmHg (13), and it is set in the range of 65 to 80 mmHg in most studies. The composition of the perfusion buffer varies greatly depending on the purpose of the experiment; however, the vast majority of studies use a variation of the physiological salt solution developed by Krebs and Henseleit (22). Typically the perfusion solution contains glucose (with or without insulin) as the exogenous energy providing substrate and is equilibrated with a gas mixture of 95% oxygen and 5% carbon dioxide. The 5% carbon dioxide is required to achieve the correct pH at 37°C in Krebs-Henseleit bicarbonate buffers. High concentrations of oxygen are needed because of the low-oxygen-carrying capacity of crystalloid buffers, which results in artificially high coronary perfusion rates. This is considered to be a limitation of the method; however, the coronary vasculature is still capable of autoregulation and responds appropriately to vasoactive compounds. Some have modified the method by supplementing the Krebs-Henseleit buffer with red blood cells, resulting in the normalization of coronary flow rates (15,23).

Langendorff Preparation

In the Langendorff preparation, the force of the retrograde flow shuts the leaflets of the aortic valve and pushes the perfusion solution into the coronary arteries via the ostia. Thus, when connecting the heart to the perfusion apparatus it is important that the bottom of the aortic cannula is distal to the ostia or the heart will rapidly fail (Fig. 3). After perfusing the entire ventricular mass, the perfusate exits the coronary venous circulation via the coronary sinus and then leaves the heart through the open right atrium and the pulmonary artery. The left ventricle has been described as essentially empty during Langendorff perfusion because no specific provision is made to provide ventricular inflow. However, this is not the case. The left ventricle fills with fluid via thebesian veins and possibly leakage through the aortic valves. Over 40 years ago, Neely and colleagues demonstrated that ventricular filling occurs in the Langendorff preparation during diastole and that some fluid is ejected against the retrograde flow during systole (12). Diastolic aortic pressure never drops below preset perfusion pressure, but diastolic intraventricular pressure is near zero in a normal (non-injured) heart. Peak systolic pressures (both aortic and intraventricular) are slightly above perfusion pressure because the force of the ejected fluid adds to the preset perfusion pressure. The experiments by Neely and colleagues were carried out by inserting a 20-gauge needle into the left ventricle, which could be opened to measure amount of fluid ejected or connected to a pressure transducer to

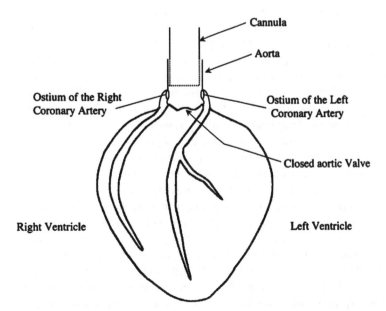

Figure 3 Proper connection of aorta to cannula. The cannula should not block entry into the coronary ostia.

measure intraventricular pressures. Today, most investigators using the Langendorff preparation measure intraventricular pressures with the aid of a fluid-filled balloon inserted into the left ventricle via the mitral valve and connected to a pressure transducer.

The Langendorff heart is commonly referred to as a nonworking heart because no net aortic flow occurs, thus no external mechanical work is performed. However, it is important to point out that it is doing considerable mechanical and metabolic work. As perfusion pressure is raised, corresponding increases also occur for indices of mechanical and metabolic work such as heart rate times developed pressure (intraventricular systolic-diastolic), the pressure-time integral, and oxygen consumption (12). Coronary flow also increases linearly at a slightly steeper slope than oxygen consumption, which assures that the heart remains well oxygenated at the higher work intensities (12).

The Working Heart Preparation

In the working heart preparation, the left side of the heart functions in a manner similar to the in vivo situation. Fluid enters the left ventricle via the left atrium and the ventricle pumps that fluid through the aorta and up the aortic tubing in an anterograde direction (Fig. 2). As mentioned above, the first step is to quickly put the heart in the Langendorff mode for the purpose of getting oxygenated perfusion buffer flowing through the coronary arteries. The left atrium is then cannulated, the atrial inflow line opened, and the aortic line switched from the Langendorff reservoir to allow the stroke volume to travel up the aortic line and be ejected into the air, that is, hydrolic work is accomplished. In this preparation, atrial inflow pressure (preload), peripheral resistance to ventricular pumping (afterload), and heart rate can be controlled. They can be easily manipulated to produce workloads matching any that can occur in vivo. The working heart preparation is considerably more sensitive in the ability to detect functional differences than the Langendorff. This is partially due to the fact that the working heart is entirely responsible for maintaining its perfusion pressure, whereas the Langendorff gets a great deal of assistance in this matter. However, the working heart's responsibility for maintaining its own perfusion pressure is a drawback regarding the amount of dysfunction that it can tolerate. The Langendorff heart can tolerate much more injury or dysfunction before going into total failure because it can be assured of adequate perfusion pressure to maintain tissue oxygenation even if the ventricle cannot pump. In some experiments employing the working heart it may be necessary to temporarily switch to the Langendorff mode. For example, in most studies investigating ischemia-reperfusion injury, the left ventricle is unable to generate enough force immediately after the ischemic bout to keep the coronary arteries adequately perfused. Therefore, if an investigator wants to measure post-ischemic function using the working heart, he/she may need to allow some post-ischemic "recovery time" in the Langendorff mode until the heart can generate enough force to adequately perfuse its coronary arteries without assistance.

Implicit in the attempt to evaluate the effect of a pharmacological intervention on a myocardial response is the assumption that the isolated heart is functionally stable under normal perfusion conditions. In our experience, the isolated working rat heart perfused with well-oxygenated buffer at 37°C is stable for about three hours. The Langendorff preparation can be perfused longer without noticing a drop in function because it is typically performing less mechanical work. The length of time that the isolated heart can remain viable can be extended greatly if quiescent periods are included. For example, studies investigating organ preservation for transplant may keep an isolated heart in a cold, quiescent state for six hours or more before beginning to evaluate its function. Unfortunately, there are a large number of studies in the literature that report significant functional declines after only 30 to 60 minutes of perfusion. Such short viability is almost always due to technical errors, contamination of the perfusate, or a dirty apparatus. Isolated hearts lack the normal intrinsic filtration and scavenging systems associated with the kidney, liver, and blood components. Without these the impact of minute impurities in the form of metal ions, microscopic debris, bacteria, denatured protein, or chemical contamination by buffer reagents is greatly magnified. This is particularly the case for the working heart because of its sensitivity. Filtering the buffer before perfusion and including an in-line filter in the working heart and whenever buffer is to be recirculated helps minimize many, but not all, of the problems. For example, during a stability check before beginning an experiment using the Langendorff preparation, we observed that baseline coronary flow gradually declined to the extent that flow rate was reduced 50% within 60 minutes, followed shortly by increased end-diastolic pressure. We eventually traced the problem to the last thing we expected. The insulin we were using to aid in glucose uptake was from a vial approved for use by humans. It contained the preservative cresol, which while fine for humans, we determined it as highly toxic in the isolated perfused rat heart at a buffer concentration of about 1 ppm. Thus, it is advisable to undertake periodic stability checks and to include control perfusion groups in studies investigating drugs or stresses, that is, ischemia-reperfusion, that can influence some measure of myocardial function. Sutherland et al. recommends a maximum acceptable decline in left ventricular–developed pressure of 15% per hour for isolated perfused mouse hearts (18).

The increased sensitivity of the working heart model over the Langendorff method makes the working heart an ideal method to evaluate the effects of any compound or stress in a tightly controlled dose-response fashion. With practice, a vigilant perfusionist should be able to achieve considerably better stability.

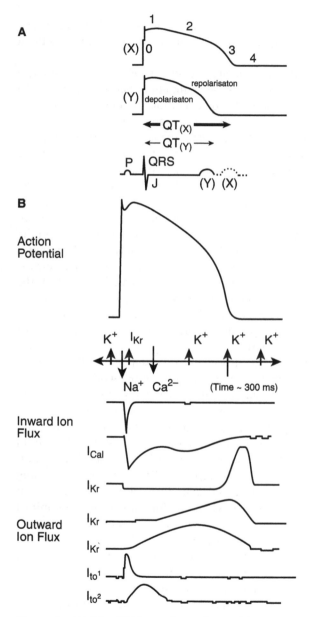

Figure 4 (**A**) The QT interval correlates with the cardiac ventricular action potential duration. The QRS interval plus the JT interval represents the absolute QT interval. In the schematic representation (curves X and Y), the ventricular action potential of (X) is prolonged compared with (Y). The upper action potential is labeled with its phases, including rapid upstroke (0), early repolarization (1), plateau phase (2), late repolarization (3), and postrepolarization. The representation of the ECG shows the timing of QT(X) and QT(Y). (**B**) The profile of a ventricular action potential in association with ion flux across the myocyte membrane and the major currents contributing to the action potential over

USE OF hERG CHANNEL ASSESSMENT TO EVALUATE QT INTERVAL PROLONGATION

Overview of QT Interval Prolongation

As a consequence of the withdrawal of several compounds from the commercial market [Seldane® (terfenadine; Hoechst Marion Roussel, Kansas City, Missouri), Propulsid® (cisapride; Janssen Pharmaceutica, Titusville, New Jersey), Hismanal® (astemizole; Janssen Pharmaceutica, Titusville, New Jersey)], and as evidenced by the release of the International Conference on Harmonisation (ICH) S7A (24), S7B (25), and E14 guidances (26), drug-induced QT interval prolongation has become an issue of significant concern in cardiovascular toxicology.

Proper cardiac function relies on the precise movement of sodium, calcium, and potassium ions through a concert of ion channels for the accurate generation of the action potential in cardiac myocytes. One such ion channel, the hERG channel has gained infamy as the molecular entity at the root of QT interval prolongation. The hERG gene encodes the α-subunit of the voltage-gated potassium channel responsible for the current (I_{Kr}) that produces the rapid phase of ventricular repolarization.

In ventricular myocytes, the I_{Kr} current is active throughout the entire action potential and contributes most significantly to phases 2 and 3 (Fig. 4) (27,28). Inhibition of the I_{Kr} current leads to prolongation of the action potential duration and prolongation, as seen on a surface electrocardiogram, of the QT interval, which represents the time required for ventricular depolarization and repolarization. Delayed repolarization, a functional consequence of hERG channel blockade, leaves the ventricular myocytes vulnerable to early after-depolarizations (EADs). It is these EADs that can trigger episodes of torsade de pointes (TdP), a ventricular tachyarrhythmia that can spontaneously revert, returning the heart to normal sinus rhythm, or can degenerate into ventricular fibrillation (29,30). Because the incidence of TdP following administration of pharmaceutical agents known to prolong the QT interval is low, estimated to range from 1 in 2000 to 1 in over 20,000 (31), the likelihood of identifying a torsadogenic agent in clinical trials is also low. Therefore, surrogate methods for predicting the potential of a pharmaceutical agent to cause TdP are of great importance in pharmaceutical discovery and development. As QT interval prolongation generally precedes episodes of TdP and can be easily measured with electrocardiography, QT interval prolongation has been used as a biomarker for TdP. Correspondingly, interaction between a pharmaceutical agent and the hERG

←

time (300 milliseconds). (For simplicity, not all currents contributing to the action potential are included.) As shown in panel A, inward (downward) currents contribute to depolarization, and outward (upward) currents contribute to repolarization. *Abbreviation*: QRS, on a surface electrocardiogram, the interval from the beginning of the Q wave to the end of the S wave, corresponds to depolarization of the ventricles.

channel has become an indicator of the potential of a pharmaceutical agent to prolong the QT interval [known as acquired long QT syndrome (LQTS)].

Acquired LQTS has been shown to occur with a wide variety of drugs, from a range of pharmacological and structural classes, as a consequence of the interaction of the drug with the hERG channel and the resultant alteration of the I_{Kr} current. Because the ICH S7B guidance emphasized the need for preclinical assessment of the potential of clinical drug candidates to prolong the QT interval, a variety of in vivo and in vitro methods for investigating both QT interval prolongation and hERG channel interactions have been developed and validated. Within the pharmaceutical industry, there has been a continuous movement toward less expensive, higher-throughput in vitro methods for investigating hERG channel interactions to allow evaluation of this potential liability at the earliest possible stage of drug discovery and development.

Functional Assays

The ICH S7B guidance outlines a battery of safety pharmacology studies to be completed to investigate the potential of a pharmaceutical agent to prolong the QT interval. Included in this battery of studies are several functional in vitro electrophysiology assays, which are most commonly performed in an isolated tissue preparation (i.e., ventricular wedge, Purkinje fiber), cardiac myocytes, or a cell line heterologously expressing the hERG channel (32). The aim of these studies is to elucidate alterations in ionic current(s) in the cell or tissue under study by using the voltage clamp technique, which has been used for many years to study ionic currents in several cell types, including neurons, muscle cells, and cardiac myocytes.

Electrophysiology assays performed in cardiac myocytes, Purkinje fibers, or ventricular wedge preparations most closely mimic the in vivo expression of and interplay between sodium, calcium, and potassium ion channels in the generation of an action potential. Because this variety of ion channels is present along with the appropriate auxiliary subunits required for their proper function in vivo, results from these types of in vitro studies may be more predictive of clinical findings. However, because the hERG current in cardiac myocytes is relatively low in comparison to other currents, it may be difficult to measure the hERG current in tissue preparations (33). These studies also present technical challenges, including the need to isolate the tissue or cell of interest fresh for each experiment. Additionally, the presence of multiple ion channels and functional currents may mask individual ion channel effects through compensatory effects on other channels (34).

Patch-clamp electrophysiology is a refinement of the voltage clamp technique and allows the investigation of individual ion channels. Patch-clamp electrophysiology studies are commonly performed in mammalian cells stably transfected with hERG cDNA, which eliminates the need for fresh cell or tissue isolations, thereby decreasing the time and cost associated with these studies. As QT interval prolongation, and hERG channel interaction as a surrogate, has become an issue of increasing regulatory concern and scrutiny, measurement of the hERG channel current, I_{Kr}, by using patch-clamp electrophysiology has become the gold standard in hERG channel assessment. The ability to investigate whether xenobiotics alter the function of the hERG channel has also been invaluable in elucidating the role of the hERG channel in QT interval prolongation.

Numerous experiments have been conducted to demonstrate the validity of hERG channel patch-clamp electrophysiology studies. These experiments illustrate that the vast majority of compounds known to prolong the QT interval and cause TdP in the clinical setting do, in fact, block the I_{Kr} current through direct interaction with the hERG channel. Despite the fact that potential interaction with other ion channels is not accounted for in hERG channel patch-clamp electrophysiology studies, these studies accurately predict whether a compound is likely to cause QT interval prolongation and TdP. Redfern et al. used safety ratios (ratios of IC_{50} values obtained in hERG electrophysiology studies and unbound therapeutic plasma concentrations observed clinically) to categorize marketed compounds by their torsadogenic propensity and correlated the safety ratios with clinical occurrence of TdP (29). This analysis concluded that a safety ratio of less than 30 was associated with clinical occurrence of TdP, demonstrating the predictive ability of the hERG patch-clamp electrophysiology assay (Fig. 5).

Despite the clear utility of this assay, interpretation of the data generated is confounded by the fact that results can vary between studies using different protocols (e.g., performing the assay at room temperature vs. physiological temperature), between laboratories using the same protocol, or even between technicians in the same laboratory (34). Additionally, traditional patch-clamp electrophysiology is a labor-intensive undertaking, requiring highly trained and skilled technicians. Recently, however, automated patch-clamp machinery, such as that marketed by Molecular Devices, has held out the promise of high-throughput generation of reliable functional data.

Nonfunctional Assays

Although the ICH S7B guideline makes no mention of nonfunctional in vitro assays for the assessment of hERG channel interaction, a myriad of such assays has been developed. The primary goal for these assays, which only measure ion channel properties indirectly, should be the concordance of the data with the results of the gold standard, the patch-clamp assay (32). Because assessment of the potential for small molecules to prolong the QT interval via interactions with the hERG channel has become important to the pharmaceutical industry, significant effort has been expended to develop higher throughput methods of nonfunctional in vitro hERG channel assessment.

One of the most widely used nonfunctional in vitro screening assays is the radioligand-binding assay. This assay takes advantage of well-characterized potent hERG binders (e.g., astemizole, dofetilide, and MK-499) and uses membranes isolated from the same heterologous expression system commonly

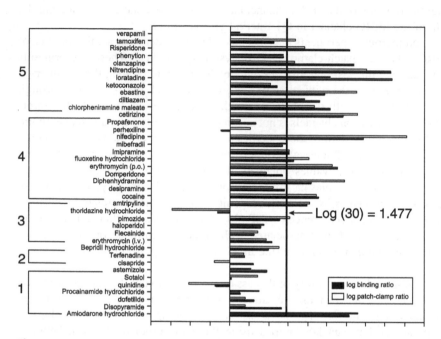

Figure 5 Redfern et al. (29) used safety ratios of electrophysiology IC_{50} values and unbound therapeutic plasma concentrations to categorize marketed compounds according to their torsadogenic propensity and correlated these safety ratios with clinical occurrence of QT interval prolongation and tosade de pointes (TdP). Calculation of safety ratios using radioligand-binding assay K_i values was used to categorize compounds in a similar manner. The hERG binding and electrophysiological methods identified false-positive and false-negative compounds, such as verapamil and amiodarone, respectively with similar efficiencies.

Categories as assigned by Redfern et al. (29). Category 1: Repolarization-prolonging (classes Ia and III) antiarrhythmics. Category 2: Drugs that have been withdrawn or suspended from the market in at least one major regulatory territory due to an unacceptable risk of TdP for the condition being treated. Category 3: Drugs that have a measurable incidence of TdP in humans, or for which numerous case reports exist in the published literature. Category 4: Drugs for which there have been isolated reports of TdP in humans. Category 5: Drugs for which there have been no published reports of TdP in humans.

used in patch-clamp studies to measure the ability of a test article to displace a potent radiolabeled hERG binder (26).

Despite the fact that measurement of radioligand displacement cannot discriminate between agonists and antagonists, several investigators have published excellent correlations between the results of radioligand-binding assays and patch-clamp assays (Fig. 6) (32,35–37). In a manner similar to that used by Redfern et al. to analyze patch-clamp data (29), data generated in radioligand-

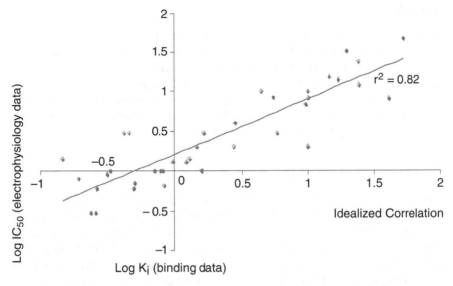

Figure 6 Inhibition curves, determined by test compound inhibition of ^{3}H-dofetilide binding, were used to determine IC_{50} values and calculate K_i values. K_i results from this binding assay showed a good correlation with published electrophysiology values ($r^2 = 0.82$, $n = 36$ marketed compounds).

binding assays have been used to generate safety ratios that can be used to classify compounds according to clinical occurrence of TdP (Fig. 5). In that analysis, data from the radioligand-binding assay were as predictive as those from hERG patch-clamp assays. To capitalize on the higher throughput afforded by radioligand-binding assays, attempts have been made to convert filtration-based hERG channel assays to scintillation proximity assay (SPA) formats amenable to 384-well platforms (38).

Another method for measuring alterations in the hERG channel current is the ion flux assay (33). The permeability of potassium channels to rubidium has been leveraged in the development of this assay, which measures the effect of xenobiotic treatment on the flow of either nonradioactive Rb^+ or radioactive $^{86}Rb^+$ (34). A similar measurement of ionic flux can be accomplished by using voltage-sensitive fluorescent dyes (39). Both platforms have proven to be less sensitive than patch-clamp electrophysiology assays (35).

Fluorescent polarization assays offer an intriguing option for a high-throughput nonfunctional assay. An assay based on this platform would not require the use of radioactivity, but instead would rely on a fluorescently labeled ligand for detection of interactions with the hERG channel. However, Deacon et al., report that high levels of hERG protein expression are required to establish an acceptable signal-to-noise ratio, a potential barrier to the widespread adoption of this assay format (38).

SUMMARY

In the 3rd edition of *Cardiovascular Toxicology*, we discussed the more classical in vitro methods (1). Namely, isolated cardiac myocytes were discussed as in vitro models to evaluate potential cardiac cytotoxicity. Considering that new approaches are constantly being identified to evaluate potential cardiac toxicity, our goal for the present edition was to present two powerful technologies that show significant promise in the investigation of cardiovascular toxicity. We discuss the working heart model and hERG channel assessment.

The Working Heart Model

The working heart model allows for precise control over key variables such as ventricular afterload and preload, rate of coronary flow, blood composition, and temperature. The working heart preparation is considerably more sensitive in the ability to detect functional differences than the Langendorff. Because of this increased sensitivity, the working heart is an ideal method to evaluate the effects of any compound or stress in a tightly controlled dose-response fashion.

QT Interval Prolongation and hERG Channel Assessment

Incidences in which a variety of pharmaceuticals have been shown to cause QT interval prolongation and subsequent ventricular tachyarrhythmias (TdP: torsade de pointes) resulting in sudden cardiac death has caused the emergence of regulatory guidelines to address this potentially lethal effect of new drug candidates. The guidelines require testing the potential of pharmaceutical candidates to interact with the hERG channel and prolong the QT interval. These guidelines have precipitated the development of a variety of in vitro techniques for investigating this potential. Because the incidence of TdP following the administration of pharmaceutical agents known to prolong the QT interval is quite low, the likelihood of an increased incidence of TdP being noted in clinical trials is also low. Preclinical assays that assess the potential of a clinical drug candidate to interact with the hERG channel and prolong the QT interval have become critical in eliminating those drug candidates that exhibit this potential. Although only few of these assays are accepted by regulatory agencies (functional assays such as the action potential duration and hERG patch-clamp assays), others, primarily nonfunctional assays, have been validated as higher throughput, lower-cost alternatives and have been implemented as screening assays early in the drug discovery process.

ACKNOWLEDGMENTS

The authors would like to thank Alexis Khalil at Millennium Pharmaceuticals for her editorial assistance.

REFERENCES

1. Chacon E, Bond JM, Lemasters JJ. Evaluation of in vitro cytotoxicity modeling. In: Acosta D, ed. Cardiovascular Toxicology, 3rd ed. New York, NY: Taylor and Francis, 2001:59–78.
2. McQueen CA. In Vitro Toxicology: Model Systems and Methods. New Jersey: Telford Press, 1989.
3. Acosta D, Sorensen EM, Anuforo DC, et al. An in vitro approach to the study of target organ toxicity of drugs and chemicals. In Vitro Cell Dev Biol 1985;21:495–504.
4. Lemasters JJ, Chacon E, Zahrebelski G, et al. Laser scanning confocal microscopy in living cells. In: Herman B, Lemasters JJ, eds. Optical Microscopy: New Technologies and Applications. San Diego: Academic Press, 1992.
5. Bond JM, Herman B, Lemasters JJ. Recovery of cultured rat neonatal myocytes from hypercontracture after chemical hypoxia. Res Commun Chem Pathol Pharmacol 1991; 71:195–208.
6. Probst I, Spahr R, Schweickhardt C, et al. Carbohydrate and fatty acid metabolism of cultured adult cardiac myocytes. Am J Physiol 1986; 250:H853–H860.
7. Ulrich RG, Elliget KA, Rosnick DK. Purification of neonatal rat cardiac cells by centrifugal elutriation. J Tissue Cult Methods 1989; 11:217–223.
8. Spahr R, Jacobson SL, Siegmund B, et al. Substrate oxidation by adult cardiomyocytes in long-term primary culture. J Mol Cell Cardiol 1989; 21:175–185.
9. Wenzel DG, Wheatley JW, Byrd GD. Effects of nicotine in cultured heart cells. Toxicol Appl Pharmacol 1970; 17: 774–785.
10. Chang TD, Cummings GR. Chronotropic responses of human heart tissue cultures. Circ Res 1972; 30: 628–633.
11. Langendorff O. Untersuchungen am uberlebenden Sagethierherzen. Arch Ges Physiol 1895; 61:291–332.
12. Neely JR, Liebermeister H, Battersby EJ, et al. Effect of pressure development on oxygen consumption by isolated rat heart. Am J Physiol 1967; 212: 804–814.
13. Neely JR, Rovetto MJ. Techniques for perfusing isolated rat hearts. Methods Enzymol 1975; 39:43–60.
14. Larsen TS, Belke DD, Sas R, et al. The isolated working mouse heart: methodological considerations. Pflugers Arch 1999; 437:979–985.
15. Sutherland FA, Hearse DJ. The isolated blood and perfusion fluid perfused heart. Pharmacol Res 2000; 41:613–627.
16. Barr RL, Lopaschuk GD. Methodology for measuring in vitro/ex vivo cardiac energy metabolism. J Pharmacol Toxicol Methods 2000; 43:141–152.
17. Ytrehus K. The ischemic heart—experimental models. Pharmacol Res 2000; 42: 193–203.
18. Sutherland FJ, Shattock MJ, Baker KE, et al. Mouse isolated perfused heart: characteristics and cautions. Clin Exp Pharmacol Physiol 2003; 30:867–878.
19. Skrzypiec-Spring M, Grotthus B, Szelag A, et al. Isolated heart perfusion according to Langendorff—still viable in the new millennium. J Pharmacol Toxicol Methods 2007; 55: 113–126.
20. Bolli R, Marban E. Molecular and cellular mechanisms of myocardial stunning. Physiol Rev 1999; 79:609–634.
21. Murry CE, Jennings RB, Reimer KA. Preconditioning with ischemia: a delay of lethal cell injury in ischemic myocardium. Circulation 1986; 74:1124–1136.

22. Krebs HA, Henseleit K. Untersuchungen über die Harnstoffbildung im Tierkorper. Z Physiol Chem 1932; 210:33–66.

23. Podesser BK, Hallström S, Schima H, et al. The erythrocyte-perfused "working heart" model: hemodynamic and metabolic performance in comparison to crystalloid perfused hearts. J Pharmacol Toxicol 1999; 41:9–15.

24. ICH, ICH Harmonized Tripartite Guidelines (S7A): Safety Pharmacology Studies for Human Pharmaceuticals. http://www.ich.org/LOB/media/MEDIA504.pdf

25. ICH, ICH Harmonized Tripartite Guidelines (S7B): The Non-Clinical Evaluation of the Potential for Delayed Ventricular Repolarization (QT Interval Prolongation) by Human Pharmaceuticals. http://www.ich.org/LOB/media/MEDIA2192.pdf

26. ICH, ICH Harmonized Tripartite Guidelines (E14): The Clinical Evaluation of QT/ QTc Interval Prolongation and Proarrhythmic Potential for Non-Antiarrhythmic Drugs. http://www.ich.org/LOB/media/MEDIA1476.pdf

27. Zhou Z, Gong Q, Ye B, et al. Properties of HERG channels stably expressed in HEK293 cells studies at physiological temperature. Biophys J 1998; 74:230–241.

28. Netzer R, Ebneth A, Bischoff U, et al. Screening lead compounds for QT interval prolongation. Drug Discov Today 2001; 6(2):78–84.

29. Redfern WS, Carlsson L, Davis AS, et al. Relationships between preclinical cardiac electrophysiology, clinical QT interval prolongation and torsade de pointes for a broad range drugs: evidence for a provisional safety margin in drug development. Cardiovasc Res 2003; 58(1):32–45.

30. Sanguinetti MC, Tristani-Firouzi M. hERG potassium channels and cardiac arrhythmia. Nature 2006; 440:463–469.

31. Gad Shayne C. Safety Pharmacology in Pharmaceutical Development and Approval. New York: CRC Press. 2004.

32. Finlayson K, Witchel HJ, McCulloch J, et al. Acquired QT interval prolongation and HERG: implications for drug discovery and development. Eur J Pharmacol 2004; 500:129–142.

33. Gintant GA, Su Z, Martin RL, et al. Utility of hERG assays as surrogate markers of delayed cardiac repolarization and QT safety. Toxicol Pathol 2006; 34:81–90.

34. Fenichel RR, Malik M, Antelevitch C, et al. Drug-induced *torsade de pointes* and implications for drug development. J Cardiovasc Electrophysiol 2004; 15(4):475–495.

35. Chiu PJS, Marcoa KF, Bounds SE, et al. Validation of a [^{3}H]Astemizole binding assay in HEK293 cells expressing HERG K+ channels. J Pharmacol Sci 2004; 95: 311–319.

36. Recanatini M, Poluzzi E, Masetti M, et al. QT prolongation through hERG K+ channel blockade: current knowledge and strategies for the early prediction during drug development. Med Res Rev 2005; 25(2):133–166.

37. Murphy SM, Palmer M, Poole MF, et al. Evaluation of functional and binding assays in cells expressing either recombinant or endogenous hERG channel. J Pharmacol Toxicol Methods 2006; 54(1):42–55.

38. Deacon M, Singleton D, Szalkai N, et al. Early evaluation of compound QT pro-longation effects: a predictive 384-well fluorescence polarization binding assay for measuring hERG blockade. J Pharmacol Toxicol Methods 2007; 55(3):238–247.

39. Xu J, Wang X, Ensign B, et al. Ion-channel assay technologies: quo vadis? Drug Discov Today 2001; 6(24):1278–1287.

5

Nonhuman Primate Models for Cardiovascular Research

You-Tang Shen, Franco Rossi, and Stephen F. Vatner

Cardiovascular Research Institute, Department of Cell Biology and Molecular Medicine, University of Medicine and Dentistry of New Jersey, New Jersey Medical School, Newark, New Jersey, U.S.A.

INTRODUCTION

Most medical advances have been the product of both basic and applied research and are based mainly on research in animal models. However, there have been cases where efficacy and toxicity studies in animals failed to predict clinical outcomes. These differences could be due, in part, to major species differences between the animal models used and humans. Rodents are the most commonly used species for cardiovascular research, whereas nonhuman primates, which have the greatest genetic and physiological similarity to humans, account for less than 0.3% of animal research in the United States.

There are several major cardiovascular differences between rodents and large mammals; only a few will be noted here. One is the myosin isoform change as an adaptation during ventricular hypertrophy. The myosin isoform switch, from V_1 α-myosin heavy chain (α-MHC) to V_3 β-MHC, has been demonstrated in rodent species (1) but not in large mammals (2–4). An additional significant difference between rodents and large mammals is intracellular Ca^{2+} handling. In the rat, approximately 90% of the Ca^{2+} for contraction comes from intracellular stores in the sarcoplasmic reticulum, while most other large animals derive more of their activator Ca^{2+} from extracellular Ca^{2+}, which enters the cell via L-type Ca^{2+}

channels (5,6). With respect to responses to ischemia, we have shown differences in the mechanism of myocardial stunning among rodents and large mammalian models (7). For example, studies in rodent models suggest that the mechanism of reversible, postischemic contractile dysfunction is a reduced sensitivity of myofilaments to Ca^{2+} because of the degradation of Troponin I with no change in Ca^{2+} handling (8,9). In addition to species differences between rodents and large mammals, some major differences also exist between large mammals and nonhuman primates. We have previously demonstrated significant species differences among conscious pigs, dogs, and baboons in their responses to myocardial infarction (10) and myocardial stunning (11). We have also shown major differences in β_3-adrenergic receptor (β_3-AR) regulation between dogs and nonhuman primates (12). Regarding the mechanism of regulation of lipids and hormonal changes, particularly those related to the menstrual cycle, only nonhuman primates are analogous to humans (13). Accordingly, the primate model is particularly useful for the purpose of extrapolating pharmacological efficacy and toxicity data to humans, and it follows that the development of new, more suitable animal model of disease, specifically nonhuman primates, would create an abundance of new and exciting research strategies for the assessment of cardiovascular efficacy and toxicity. Although cardiovascular studies have been conducted in nonhuman primate models, only a few have focused on heart failure (14), which is the final pathway for many cardiovascular diseases.

In the current chapter, we will describe our novel primate model of heart failure that closely mimics the process of congestive heart failure observed in patients. One unique feature of this nonhuman model is that, unlike existing heart failure models, it allows for physiological and biochemical measurements during progressive stages of heart failure, i.e., initial myocardial ischemia, compensated left ventricular (LV) hypertrophy and end-stage congestive heart failure. Therefore, this model has the potential to provide excellent opportunities for evaluating novel therapeutic targets, in terms of efficacy and toxicity, and facilitate the elucidation of the mechanisms involved in the progression to heart failure.

The ability to obtain reliable measurements in the examination of cardiovascular function is vital for the interpretation of experimental results. Technology has been consistently advancing and so have our techniques, which are based on four decades of prior experience in cardiovascular research. We discuss these updated techniques in this chapter. Since nonhuman primates are extremely valuable and also expensive, we emphasize studies that utilize multiple measurements in the same animal model and combine simultaneous and repetitive recordings of several cardiovascular parameters. This feature provides a comprehensive profile of each animal's cardiac function and also provides a link among responses in physiology, pharmacology, toxicology, and other research areas.

Over the past four decades, our laboratory has successfully performed several studies in conscious, chronically instrumented nonhuman primates, i.e., baboons and monkeys (11,12,15–26). Implanted instrumentation include aortic and left and right atrial catheters, a miniature high-frequency LV pressure gauge, an ascending aortic blood flow (ABF) probe, LV wall thickness, short axis, and coronary and aortic ultrasound crystals, right ventricular and atrial pacing leads, a coronary flow probe, and an inferior vena cava occluder. This instrumentation, along with either an implanted hydraulic coronary artery occluder or ligation of a coronary artery, allow us to directly and continuously measure LV systolic and diastolic function, as well as systemic hemodynamics at baseline and following several interventions, e.g., coronary artery occlusion and reperfusion, leading to chronic myocardial remodeling and then to end-stage congestive heart failure.

TECHNIQUES FOR MEASUREMENT OF CARDIOVASCULAR PARAMETERS

Vascular and Ventricular Pressures

Miniature solid-state pressure transducers are used for chronic measurements of arterial pressure, as well as left and right ventricular pressure. These transducers, which were originally developed by Van Citters and Franklin (27), have been used in our laboratory for more than four decades in studies in unrestrained, conscious woodchucks (28), rabbits (29), dogs (30,31), pigs (11,32), sheep (33), cows (19,34), and nonhuman primates (10,17,18,24,35). For chronic implantation, solid-state pressure transducers offer a number of advantages over commonly used, fluid-filled catheter-strain gauge manometer systems. The most important of these advantages are (*i*) a wide frequency range, (*ii*) high sensitivity, which facilitates their use with radiotelemetry systems, and (*iii*) relative freedom from signal distortion, which occurs in fluid-filled systems from catheter clotting or kinking or acceleration effects upon the fluid system. A pressure transducer must have a high-frequency response to accurately reproduce the rapidly changing phases of a pressure signal, such as the leading edge of systole in ventricular pressure. Furthermore, the time derivative of ventricular pressure (*dP/dt*) is often used as an index of cardiac contractility, and to obtain this parameter by analog differentiation, the higher-frequency components of the pressure signal must be preserved. Figure 1 shows a representative recording of the effects of isoproterenol on LV pressure, LV *dP/dt*, phasic and mean arterial pressure, phasic and mean ascending ABF, and heart rate in young and old conscious monkeys.

The pressure transducers used in our laboratory are small (4–7 mm diameter, 1 mm thick) hermetically sealed cylindrical chambers with a titanium diaphragm. Bonded on the back are four silicon-strain gauge elements arranged in a Wheatstone bridge configuration (models P4–P7, Konigsberg Instruments Inc., Pasadena, California, U.S.). The transducer senses pressure changes as a deformation of the diaphragm, which in turn unbalances the bridge and generates an offset signal proportional to the applied pressure. This signal is subsequently amplified and recorded as an analog reproduction of the pressure wave. During

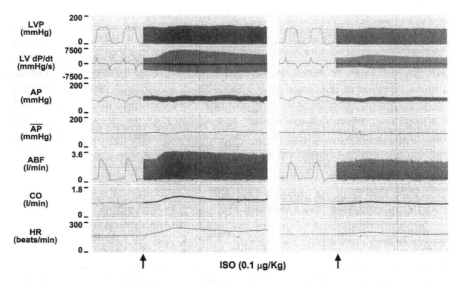

Figure 1 Representative phasic waveform recordings of LV pressure (LVP), LV *dP/dt*, phasic and mean arterial pressure (AP), phasic and mean ascending aortic blood flow (ABF) and mean aortic blood flow, and heart rate in young (A) and old (B) monkeys. Note that responses to (ISO 0.1 µg/kg, IV.) are blunted (desensitized) in the older monkey. *Abbreviations*: ABF, aortic blood flow; AP, arterial pressure; CO, cardiac output. LV, left ventricular; *Source*: From Ref. 18.

each study, the solid-state transducer undergoes an initial *in vitro* calibration before surgical implantation. In addition, transducers are cross-calibrated during experiments, *in vivo,* against a strain gauge transducer connected to fluid-filled, chronically implanted catheters positioned in the aorta and left atrium. Arterial pressure is measured after implanting the solid-state transducer in the thoracic or abdominal aorta through a 1- to 2-cm longitudinal incision closed by interrupted sutures. The right ventricular transducer is inserted through a stab wound in the mid-anterior free wall of the right ventricle, and the LV transducer is most often inserted through a stab wound in the apex of the LV. The ventricular transducers are secured by purse string sutures. As with all implants of this type, the transducer leads are exteriorized through the chest wall and routed subcutaneously to the interscapular area of the animal. The externalized transducer leads are protected by shrink tubing and larger animals are fitted with a tear-resistant nylon vest. In intractable animals (e.g., nonhuman primates), the wires are usually not externalized but are buried subcutaneously until the time of experiments.

The major disadvantages of implantable solid-state pressure transducers, for use chronically, are drifts in zero offset and sensitivity. These problems become critical because, at the time of experiments, it is impossible to calibrate the implanted transducer in terms of absolute pressure. It becomes necessary, therefore, to cross-calibrate these transducers with a calibrated system when experiments are conducted. An electronic calibration of the overall pressure measuring system, exclusive of the transducer, is made at the start and at the end of experiments. The output of the implanted solid-state pressure transducer is then compared with a directly calibrated catheter-strain gauge manometer. This procedure overcomes the problem of changes that may have occurred in the solid-state transducer's transfer function since the last *in vitro* calibration. In our experience, this procedure is repeated approximately weekly for arterial implants, but daily cross-calibration is necessary for experiments in which small variations in zero pressure level are critical (e.g., measurements of LV end-diastolic pressure). Although there are many problems associated with the measurement of pressures in animals with long-term chronic implants, it is clear that there are inherent advantages of the solid-state transducer.

Instead of the implantable solid-state pressure transducer, external, fluid-filled catheter pressure transducers are often used to measure intravascular and atrial pressures. Several types of tubings, such as Tygon, polyethylene, and silicon materials, can be used and connected to the transducers. The fluid-filled catheter pressure transducer allows pressure measurements to be obtained in vessels smaller than 1 mm in diameter. Unlike the miniature solid-state pressure transducers, the fluid-filled catheter pressure transducer can readily be checked for drifts in baseline and sensitivity. The major disadvantage is that the transducers are larger in size and also susceptible to distortion artifacts in the pressure signal. Because of the limitation of frequency response, compared with the miniature solid-state pressure gauge, this type of transducer is less desirable for measurement of LV dP/dt.

Blood Flow Measurements

Doppler and Transonic Flow Techniques

The Doppler technique, i.e., the continuous wave (CW), nondirectional flowmeter, developed by Franklin et al. (36), has been used in our laboratory for the measurement of coronary (22,37–40), cerebral, renal, mesenteric, and iliac blood flows (21,31,41–43). The development of the ultrasonic Doppler flowmeter has proceeded from the original, nondirectional CW implementation to directional CW and, more recently, to a pulsed, directional design, which is the most commonly used device today. All of these devices use the common principle that ultrasound reflected from a target (e.g., the moving blood cells) exhibits a shift in frequency proportional to the velocity of the target. Ultrasound is directed diagonally to the bloodstream and a part of this energy is reflected from moving blood cells. The shift in frequency that is caused by this process provides an average of the instantaneous velocity profile across the vessel lumen and is determined by extracting the frequency difference between transmitted and reflected sonic waves.

Since the early 1960s, transit-time ultrasonic flowmeters have been used in this country. Furthermore, this technique has been improved upon over the past 20 years and is now used in almost all laboratory animals, including mice, for the measurement of blood flow. The basic principle for this technology is to use wide-beam illumination to pass signals back and forth. The speed of the ultra-sound, affected by the flow of liquid, passes through the "acoustic window" of the flow probe and the Transonic meter (Transonic Systems Inc., Ithaca, New York, U.S.) reads the "transit-time." The difference between the upstream- and downstream-integrated transit-times is a measure of volume flow.

Microsphere Technique

Microspheres are used for measurement of blood flow, but require several assumptions as follows: (*i*) Microspheres are thoroughly mixed within the blood stream and uniformly distributed throughout the body according to distribution of blood flow. (*ii*) Microspheres are introduced into the blood stream and then are trapped by different organs, and this does not affect the function in these organs. (*iii*) Microspheres are trapped on the first circulation through an organ and once localized in that organ, do not recirculate. (*iv*) Microspheres have properties similar to those of the formed elements within the blood flow and are distributed throughout the tissues in a similar manner to whole blood. Thus, the major advantage of this technique is that the regional blood flow in almost all vascular beds, including skin, fat, and brain, can be measured. However, the major limitation is that only up to eight time points, referring to the numbers of radioactive labels or colors, can be measured.

The size of microspheres is critical for the measurement of regional blood flow, as microspheres are intended to be trapped in the precapillary coronary circulation during the first circulation, and to do so they cannot pass through arteriole venous shunts and be recirculated. It has also been reported that less than 1% of 8 to 10 μm of microspheres were observed to pass through organs and recirculate in dogs and sheep (44,45), whereas the amount of nonentrapment of 15 μm microspheres was shown to be insignificant in rhesus monkeys (46). Thus, microspheres of about 15 μm have been accepted as both meeting the conditions of distribution similar to red cells as well as demonstrating the absence of nonentrapment.

Microspheres can be either radioactive or colored. For larger animal models, about 1 to 2 million microspheres labeled with ^{95}Nb, ^{85}Sr, ^{141}Ce, ^{46}Sc, ^{51}Cr, ^{113}Sn, ^{114}In, and ^{103}Ru are suspended in 0.01% Tween 80 solution (10% dextran) and placed in an ultrasonic bath for 30 to 60 minutes. Before injection, 1 to 2 mL of Tween 80 solution should first be injected to test for potential adverse cardiovascular effects. Microspheres are usually injected and flushed with saline over a 10- to 20-second period, via a left atrial catheter. Alternatively, microspheres can also be injected via an LV catheter. Arterial blood reference samples are withdrawn at a rate of 7.75 mL/min for a total of

120 seconds, beginning at 30 second before microsphere injection. At the end of the study, tissue samples from different solid-state organs are taken and weighed. All tissue samples, along with the collected blood samples, are counted in a gamma counter with an appropriately selected energy window. After correction of counts for background and crossover, regional blood flow is obtained and expressed as milliliters per minute per gram of tissue.

A similar procedure is used for measurement of blood flow with colored microspheres, with up to 11 different colored microspheres available, i.e., gold, samarium, lutetium, lanthanum, ytterbium, europium, terbium, holmium, rhenium, iridium, and scandium. Since the sensitivity to detect colored microspheres is relatively low, compared with radioactive microspheres, the number of microspheres used should be 4 to 6 million per injection. At the end of experiments, tissue samples from different areas are collected and weighed. These samples, along with blood samples, are then transferred into sodium-free polypropylene vials and dried overnight at a temperature of 70°C in an oven. After spectroscopic analysis, i.e., neutron activation technology, blood flow can be calculated and expressed as milliliters per minute per gram of tissue.

Ventricular and Vascular Dimensions

Ventricular Dimensions

The ultrasonic transit-time dimension gauge, as originally described by Rushmer et al. (47) and improved by Patrick and co-workers (48,49), is routinely used for the measurement of LV internal diameter, right and LV wall thickness, and right and LV regional segment length (50–55). One of the commercially available dimension devices is the "Triton System 6" (Triton Technology Inc., San Diego, California, U.S.). This technique uses pairs of small piezoelectric transducers operating in the frequency range of 3 to 7 MHz, depending on the application. In operation, a burst of sound from one transducer propagates to the second transducer. If the speed of sound is known in the intervening medium (1.58×10^6 mm s^{-1} for blood), then the separation of the transducers can be determined by measuring the transit-time of this sound. This one-way, two-transducer technique contrasts with the ultrasonic echo technique used clinically in cardiac diagnosis. The echo technique uses a single transducer to emit ultrasound, which is then reflected from the internal structures of the body. Although the two-transducer technique is invasive and is limited to a discrete straight line measurement, the capability for enhanced and more discrete reception of the ultrasonic signal can radically improve the accuracy and resolution of dimension measurements. This permits the detection of more subtle changes in regional function than is capable with the pulsed echo technique.

In operation, the dimension gauge measures the acoustic transit-time of bursts of ultrasound propagated between two piezoelectric crystals placed on opposing surfaces of the LV cavity (internal diameter), placed on opposing surfaces of the right or LV free walls (wall thickness), or propagated among pairs of piezoelectric crystals inserted into the free walls of the right or left ventricles (~1–2 cm apart; segmental length). The transit-time dimension gauge can be synchronized to measure up to 12 simultaneous dimensions, thus allowing a multiple assessment of regional myocardial function. The signals can also be differentiated to obtain the rate of myocardial fiber shortening, an index of regional cardiac function. In addition, the intramyocardial electrogram, from each of the transducers, can be assessed using the standard limb, lead arrangements as an indifferent reference. This technique is particularly useful for detecting the graded dysfunction that occurs with regional myocardial ischemia. Both measurements of regional wall thickness and regional segment length are used for these types of studies.

The theoretical resolution of the ultrasonic dimension technique is one-quarter of the wavelength, with the wavelength being determined by the thickness of the crystal. To achieve improved resolution, it is necessary to use thin, high-frequency piezoelectric crystals. We are currently using 7-MHz crystals (0.3 mm thick and 2.0 mm in diameter) for myocardial segment length determination, because transducer separation is typically 1 cm and the signal strength is not adversely affected by this distance. At the other extreme, transducers used for the measurement of ventricular diameter are 3-MHz crystals (0.7 mm thick and 3–4 mm in diameter), because the distance measured is in the 3- to 4-cm range and attenuation of the sound is greater, being proportional to both distance and frequency. Transducers for wall-thickness determination are intermediate, with a 2-mm-diameter, 5-MHz crystal used for the endocardial surface. A similar transducer with a small, Dacron patch is sutured to the epicardium to complete the implant. To measure regional subendocardial and subepicardial wall thickness, an additional crystal is implanted in the mid-wall (51).

Vascular Dimensions

The study of the elastic properties of the aortic wall is fundamental for the understanding of the coupling between the heart and peripheral circulation, the characteristics of vascular mechanoreceptors, and the pathogenesis of important disease states, such as atherosclerosis and hypertension. Moreover, the concept of large coronary artery vasoconstriction as a possible mechanism for Prinzmetal's variant angina (56), as well as typical angina pectoris and myocardial infarction (57,58), underlines the importance of making direct continuous measurements of coronary vascular dimensions (59,60).

The design of the transit-time dimension gauge has recently been modified to permit the measurement of both large (48) and small (59,60) vessel dimensions. These modifications involve refinement of the electronics as well as construction of smaller transducers. The transducers (1 mm × 3 mm) are constructed from 7-MHz piezoelectric materials, with stainless steel wiring and a thin coat of epoxy. To minimize mass loading of the vessel and to facilitate alignment at

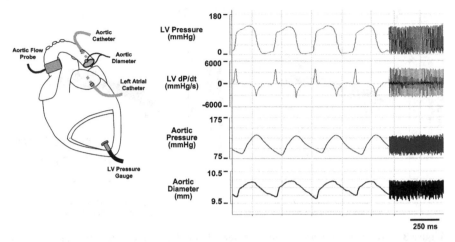

Figure 2 Schematic illustration of instrumentation and representative waveforms of LV pressure, LV *dP/dt*, aortic pressure, and aortic diameter in a young monkey. *Abbreviation*: LV, left ventricular. *Source*: (for left portion of the figure) From Ref. 35.

surgery, these transducers have been constructed without lenses, although a small Dacron patch is attached to the back of the transducer with epoxy for stabilization purposes. The transducers are implanted on opposing sides of the vessel and secured with 5-0 suture. Resistive loading is used to minimize the instrument-ringing artifact. The inhibit pulse is shortened to be adjustable over the range of 0.5 to 10 μs and the sensitivity of postdetection amplifiers is increased to compensate for the smaller signal developed by the shorter transit-time. These modifications result in an instrument that is stable enough to resolve 0.05-mm changes in the diameter of a 3-mm vessel. The measurements are repeatable and constitute a sensitive and accurate method of assessing changes in coronary artery diameter under a variety of interventions in the conscious animal (59,60). Figure 2 shows a schematic illustration of implanted instrumentation for measurements of aortic pressure and diameter, as well as waveforms of aortic pressure and diameter, along with LV pressure and LV *dP/dt*. Figure 3 shows the difference in the aortic pressure-diameter relationships observed among male and female, young versus old conscious monkeys.

BIOMEDICAL TELEMETRY AND DATA ACQUISITION SYSTEMS

Telemetry Systems and Digital Recordings

As an extension of the measurement techniques described above, the radio-telemetry of biological signals has obvious utility in situations where the experimental design precludes the use of cables, tethers, and the laboratory

A

B

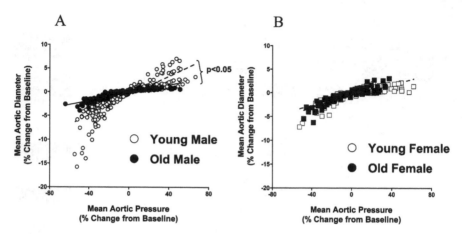

Figure 3 Aortic pressure and aortic diameter relationships, in response to bolus injection of sodium nitroprusside and phenylephrine, are plotted as percent change from baseline in young male (*panel a*) and female (*panel b*) monkeys (*open circles*) and in old male and female monkeys (*closed circles*). The slope of the relationship between mean aortic pressure and aortic diameter in old male monkeys (*dashed line*) is significantly less ($p < 0.05$) than that in young male monkeys (*solid line*), suggesting a stiffer aorta in the old male monkeys. This difference was not observed in female monkeys. *Source*: From Ref. 17.

environment. Examples include activities such as free-ranging exercise and the recording of data from intractable animals such as large nonhuman primates (26), as well as studies of animals in their natural habitat (21,22,41–43,49,61–67). The telemetry systems we use fall into two categories: flow pressure systems and pressure dimension systems. Examples are shown in Figures 4 and 5.

Tether System

Particular care needs to be taken in handling nonhuman primates, as they can be aggressive and dangerous. For an experimental design where telemetry is not practical, a tether system can be used when working with nonhuman primates (17,18,20,35,68,69) (Fig. 6). Tethering also allows for the use of catheters chronically implanted in blood vessels, by extending them away from the caged animal, and also allows for fluid injection (e.g., pharmacological agents) and blood withdrawal to be conducted from a distance. When not in use, catheters must be maintained by a slow infusion of heparin, through the tether system, to avoid blood clots. Another benefit of the tether system is that it allows for simultaneous fluid injection or blood withdrawal and recording of electrical signals from the different transducers chronically implanted in the animal. This is made possible by using gold-plated wire brushes to maintain the electrical continuity as the animal moves freely inside the cage. What differentiates the tether system from other implantable or jacket-mounted telemetry devices is the very small weight the animal carries during the time it is

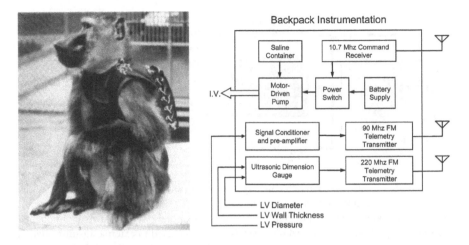

Backpack Instrumentation

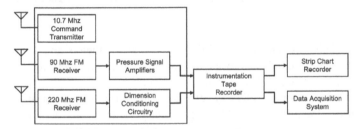

Data Station Instrumentation

Figure 4 Schematic illustration of telemetry system for sending and receiving physiological signals of LV pressure and dimension in conscious, nonhuman primate models. *Abbreviation*: LV, left ventricular.

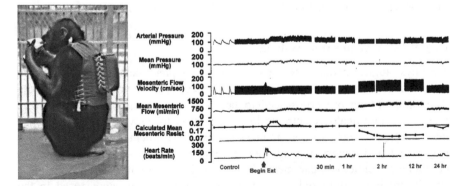

Figure 5 This illustration shows recordings from a chimpanzee in response to feeding at different intervals, up to 24 hours (*Bottom*). *Source*: (for right portion of the figure) From Ref 24.

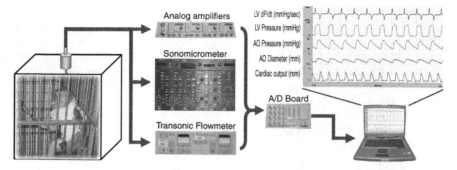

Figure 6 Schematic diagram of a tether system. Dual fluid swivels mounted on top of the cage allow the connection of extracorporeal pressure transducers and allow the withdrawal of blood and infusion of fluids; wire brush electrical swivel allows the implanted transducers, probes, and piezoelectric crystals to be connected to external instrumentation for signal conditioning and amplification; preconditioned and filtered electrical signals are subsequently digitized and recorded via software, as shown to the right of the diagram.

restrained. Tether systems act as a bridge to connect catheters and transducers to the actual monitoring devices located in an adjacent room where the acquisition, conditioning, and recording of the signals take place.

In our laboratories, tether systems containing two fluid couplings (Instech Laboratories, Inc., Plymouth Meeting, Pennsylvania, U.S.) and an electrical swivel, with as many as 10 electrical circuits (Airflyte Electronics Co., Bayonne, New Jersey, U.S.) allow chronic, continuous measurements from conscious animals that are instrumented with an in-dwelling catheter for infusion of fluids, catheters for the measurement of arterial pressure or LV pressure, and a flow probe for the measurement of blood flow. Figure 6 shows the tether system connected with the instrumentation for direct measurements of pressure, diameter, and blood flow, which is converted to a digital signal for computer analysis.

Digital Data Acquisition Systems

The physiological parameters discussed in this chapter, such as pressures, blood flows, dimensions and temperature, are, intrinsically, a function of time. As such, their time-varying properties need to be taken into consideration when using transducers and analog electronic instrumentation to convert these parameters into electronic signals. The transducer and instrumentation characteristics may affect and change the information content of the signal representing a particular physiological parameter (70–72). This is particularly true when these signals are being digitized by digital acquisition systems and stored in the form of numeric data on a computer for further processing or storage. These systems generally consist of a hardware portion for the conversion of the electrical analog signal into a stream of binary digits, and software to derive real time parameters of interest and, at the same time, to allow for control of the hardware.

In the design of such systems and devices, multiple factors need be taken into consideration to ensure the integrity of the information. These factors, which are the major features of a digital data acquisition system, include resolution, linearity, accuracy, sampling rate, aliasing, and oversampling (73–75). In the past decade, hardware and software specifically designed for biomedical research data acquisition has been introduced on the market by different manufacturers: NOTOCORD-hem™ (Notocord Systems SAS, Croissy Sur Seine, France), PowerLab with Chart software (ADInstruments, Inc., Colorado Springs, Colorado, U.S.), and Ponemah Physiology Platform (Data Sciences International, St. Paul, Minnesota, U.S.). Usually, manufacturers also make proprietary A/D hardware systems that can only be controlled and operated by their own software. Besides the individual user interfaces, all the manufacturers mentioned above design software in modules so that only specific functions can be performed on the physiological parameters of interest. Each module analyzes signals in real time and provides beat-to-beat analysis. All the data and results can also be exported to multiple applications to generate graphs, charts, or tables.

CARDIOVASCULAR DISEASE MODELS IN NONHUMAN PRIMATES

Myocardial Ischemia and Reperfusion

Myocardial ischemia and reperfusion in nonhuman primates is achieved by either chronically implanted hydraulic occluders or via ligature during surgery. We have used both procedures in baboons (10,11,76) and monkeys (77).

Heart Failure Models

Heart failure is the final pathway of several cardiovascular diseases, such as coronary artery disease, hypertension, and valvular disease and cardiomyopathy. Although many transgenic murine models of heart failure have been developed and characterized, one of the disadvantages of using murine species is that these models may mimic a specific change or pathway that occurs at the cellular and molecular level. Most importantly, there are major species differences between mice and other larger mammals, which were noted earlier.

The most commonly used experimental models of heart failure in nonhuman primates are either myocardial infarction or rapid ventricular pacing (14). Myocardial infarction has the advantage of mimicking the most common pathogenesis of chronic heart failure seen in humans. However, heart failure in larger animal models cannot generally be induced by myocardial infarction alone, since infarcts large enough to induce heart failure chronically almost uniformly induce fatal arrhythmias or cardiogenic shock. We found that cardiac function and hemodynamics are well maintained even after several months of moderate-sized myocardial infarction in nonhuman primates. Although increases in infarct size could result in cardiac failure, most often we find that either acute heart failure is induced or sudden death occurs before chronic heart failure develops. One disadvantage of the pacing model to induce heart failure is that the biochemical and hemodynamic alterations revert to almost normal values soon after pacing is stopped (78,79). This suggests that the mechanisms of pacing are similar to those of reversible dilated cardiomyopathy (80–82), rather than those of the irreversible failing heart in humans.

We previously developed a heart failure model induced by coronary artery occlusion followed by rapid ventricular pacing in porcine (83) and canine models (84). Unlike the model of heart failure induced by rapid ventricular pacing alone, the severe LV dysfunction and abnormal systemic hemodynamics did not reverse after cessation of pacing, suggesting that the underlying mechanism following combined myocardial infarction and rapid ventricular pacing may be different from pacing-induced heart failure alone. It is conceivable that the nonischemic myocardium can compensate for the loss of regional function after coronary artery occlusion and maintain global LV performance. In the presence of myocardial infarction, rapid pacing increases the energy demand of the non-ischemic myocardium possibly beyond the range of compensation, leading to decompensated cardiac failure.

During the past few years, we have characterized a monkey model of heart failure induced by combined myocardial infarction with rapid ventricular pacing. The protocol to develop the model is shown in Figure 7. Pacing leads are attached to the right ventricular free wall and left atrial appendage for controlled rapid ventricular pacing. Following implantation of this instrumentation, the left anterior descending coronary artery is occluded via permanent ligation at the half distance from its origin, and all branches are also ligated. During surgery, the success of coronary occlusion is confirmed by color change in the myocardium, absence of wall motion, and changes in electrocardiogram (ECG). After all these procedures are completed, the incision is closed and monkeys are allowed to recover from surgery. Approximately two months after coronary artery ligation, baseline hemodynamic measurements are made via the tether system, as shown in Figure 7. The rapid ventricular pacing rate is initiated at 220 bpm for the first three days, and then the rate is increased to 280 to 290 bpm for two to three weeks, when both LV dysfunction and clinical symptoms are obviously present.

In summary, the chronically instrumented, conscious animal model, particularly the nonhuman primate model, is an important tool for exploring the mechanisms of cardiovascular disease and performing high-fidelity assessments of pharmacological and physiological interventions on efficacy and, potentially, toxicity. Nonhuman primates, the closest species to humans, are therefore useful models to allow identification of novel pathways and targets linked with cardiovascular diseases in humans. The nonhuman primate model will be an

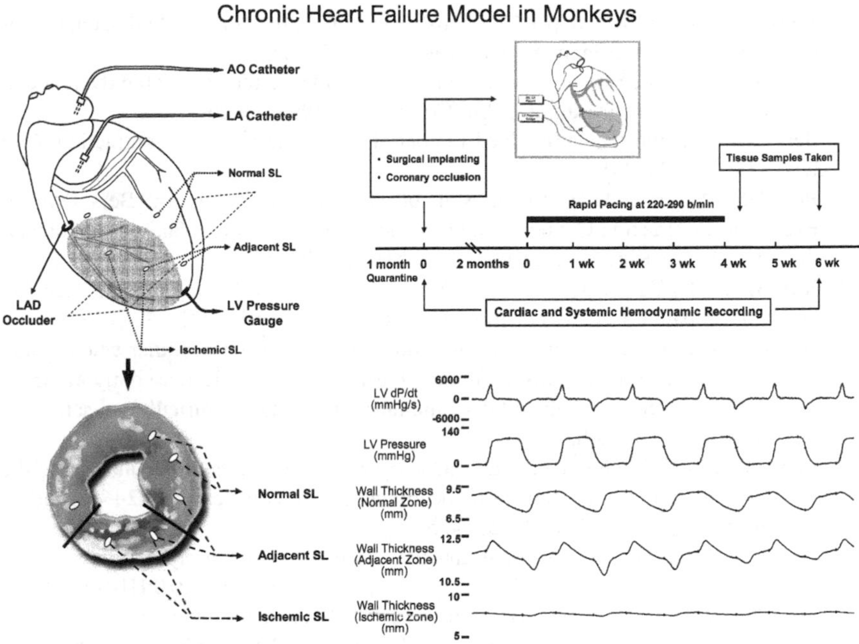

Chronic Heart Failure Model in Monkeys

Figure 7 At time of surgery, the instrumentation is implanted and a branch of the coronary artery is occluded. After recovery, hemodynamics are recorded. Two months after coronary occlusion rapid pacing starts at about 200 to 220 bpm and the pacing rate is progressively increased over a two- to three-week period to reach a steady rate of 290 bpm that will lead to heart failure within a week or two. *Abbreviation*: bpm, beats per minute.

effective and important preclinical step that can reduce the costs associated with drug development and also facilitate new targeted research and development. For example, this model will be useful for the simultaneous study of pharmacodynamics, i.e., time profile of the efficacy of tested substances, and pharmacokinetics, i.e., time course of tested substances in plasma and their metabolite levels. Equally important, as a model for safety assessment, nonhuman primates should also be ideal predictors of potential problems that cannot be detected from studies in other species, but those that would occur in humans. An important feature of conscious, unrestrained nonhuman primate models is the ability to avoid the confounding influence of anesthesia and acute surgical trauma, which would significantly affect the results of any study.

REFERENCES

1. Opie L. The Heart: Physiology and Metabolism. 2nd ed. New York, NY: Raven Press; 1991.
2. Tagawa H, Rozich JD, Tsutsui H, et al. Basis for increased microtubules in pressure-hypertrophied cardiocytes. Circulation 1996; 93:1230–1243.

3. Tsutsui H, Ishihara K, Cooper Gt. Cytoskeletal role in the contractile dysfunction of hypertrophied myocardium. Science 1993; 260:682–687.
4. Zile MR, Koide M, Sato H, et al. Role of microtubules in the contractile dysfunction of hypertrophied myocardium. J Am Coll Cardiol 1999; 33:250–260.
5. Bers DM. Calcium fluxes involved in control of cardiac myocyte contraction. Circ Res 2000; 87:275–281.
6. Bers DM. Major cellular structures involved in E-C coupling. In: Bers DM ed. Excitation-Contraction Coupling and Cardiac Contractile Force. 2nd ed. Dordrecht, the Netherlands: Kluwer Academic Publishers, 2000:1–16.
7. Kim SJ, Kudej RK, Yatani A, et al. A novel mechanism for myocardial stunning involving impaired Ca(2+) handling. Circ Res 2001; 89:831–837.
8. Gao WD, Atar D, Backx PH, et al. Relationship between intracellular calcium and contractile force in stunned myocardium. Direct evidence for decreased myofilament Ca2+ responsiveness and altered diastolic function in intact ventricular muscle. Circ Res 1995; 76:1036–1048.
9. Gao WD, Liu Y, Mellgren R, et al. Intrinsic myofilament alterations underlying the decreased contractility of stunned myocardium. A consequence of Ca2+-dependent proteolysis? Circ Res 1996; 78:455–465.
10. Shen YT, Fallon JT, Iwase M, et al. Innate protection of baboon myocardium: effects of coronary artery occlusion and reperfusion. Am J Physiol 1996; 270:H1812–H1818.
11. Shen YT, Vatner SF. Differences in myocardial stunning following coronary artery occlusion in conscious dogs, pigs, and baboons. Am J Physiol 1996; 270: H1312–H1322.
12. Shen YT, Cervoni P, Claus T, et al. Differences in beta 3-adrenergic receptor cardiovascular regulation in conscious primates, rats and dogs. J Pharmacol Exp Ther 1996; 278:1435–1443.
13. Bellino FL, Wise PM. Nonhuman primate models of menopause workshop. Biol Reprod 2003; 68:10–18.
14. Smith AH, Wolfgang EA, Flynn DM, et al. Tachycardia-induced primate model of heart failure in cardiovascular drug discovery. J Pharmacol Toxicol Methods 2000; 43: 125–131.
15. Heyndrickx GR, Amano J, Patrick TA, et al. Effects of coronary artery reperfusion on regional myocardial blood flow and function in conscious baboons. Circulation 1985; 71:1029–1037.
16. Lavallee M, Vatner SF. Regional myocardial blood flow and necrosis in primates following coronary occlusion. Am J Physiol 1984; 246:H635–H639.
17. Qiu H, Tian B, Resuello RG, et al. Sex-specific regulation of gene expression in the aging monkey aorta. Physiol Genomics 2007; 29:169–180.
18. Sato N, Kiuchi K, Shen YT, et al. Adrenergic responsiveness is reduced, while baseline cardiac function is preserved in old adult conscious monkeys. Am J Physiol 1995; 269:H1664–H1671.
19. Shen YT, Vatner DE, Gagnon HE, et al. Species differences in regulation of alpha-adrenergic receptor function. Am J Physiol 1989; 257:R1110–R1116.
20. Takagi G, Asai K, Vatner SF, et al. Gender differences on the effects of aging on cardiac and peripheral adrenergic stimulation in old conscious monkeys. Am J Physiol Heart Circ Physiol 2003; 285:H527–H534.
21. Vatner SF. Effects of exercise and excitement on mesenteric and renal dynamics in conscious, unrestrained baboons. Am J Physiol 1978; 234:H210–H214.

22. Vatner SF, Franklin D, Higgins CB, et al. Coronary dynamics in unrestrained conscious baboons. Am J Physiol 1971; 221:1396–1401.
23. Vatner SF, Franklin D, Higgins CB, et al. Backpack telemetry. In: McCutcheon EP, ed. Chronically Implanted Cardiovascular Instrumentation. New York, NY: Academic Press, 1973.
24. Vatner SF, Patrick TA, Higgins CB, et al. Regional circulatory adjustments to eating and digestion in conscious unrestrained primates. J Appl Physiol 1974; 36:524–529.
25. Vatner SF, Patrick TA, Knight DR, et al. Effects of calcium channel blocker on responses of blood flow, function, arrhythmias, and extent of infarction following reperfusion in conscious baboons. Circ Res 1988; 62:105–115.
26. Zimpfer M, Vatner SF. Effects of acute increases in left ventricular preload on indices of myocardial function in conscious, unrestrained and intact, tranquilized baboons. J Clin Invest 1981; 67:430–438.
27. Van itters RL, Franklin DL. Telemetry of blood pressure in free-ranging animals via an intravascular gauge. J Appl Physiol 1966; 21:1633–1636.
28. Kudej RK, Vatner SF. Nitric oxide-dependent vasodilation maintains blood flow in true hibernating myocardium. J Mol Cell Cardiol 2003; 35:931–935.
29. Nishizawa T, Shen YT, Rossi F, et al. Altered autonomic control in conscious transgenic rabbits with overexpressed cardiac Gsalpha. Am J Physiol Heart Circ Physiol 2007; 292:H971–975.
30. Shen YT, Knight DR, Vatner SF, et al. Responses to coronary artery occlusion in conscious dogs with selective cardiac denervation. Am J Physiol 1988; 255:H525–533.
31. Shen YT, Vatner SF. Effects of a K+ATP channel opener, lemakalim, on systemic, coronary and regional vascular dynamics in conscious dogs: comparison with nifedipine, adenosine, nitroglycerin and acetylcholine. J Pharmacol Exp Ther 1993; 265: 1026–1037.
32. Shen YT, Vatner SF. Mechanism of impaired myocardial function during progressive coronary stenosis in conscious pigs. Hibernation versus stunning? Circ Res 1995; 76: 479–488.
33. Manders WT, Pagani M, Vatner SF. Depressed responsiveness to vasoconstrictor and dilator agents and baroreflex sensitivity in conscious, newborn lambs. Circulation 1979; 60:945–955.
34. Young MA, Knight DR, Vatner SF. Parasympathetic coronary vasoconstriction induced by nicotine in conscious calves. Circ Res 1988; 62:891–895.
35. Asai K, Kudej RK, Shen YT, et al. Peripheral vascular endothelial dysfunction and apoptosis in old monkeys. Arterioscler Thromb Vasc Biol 2000; 20:1493–1499.
36. Franklin DE, Watson NW, Pierson KE, et al. Technique for radio telemetry of blood-flow velocity from unrestrained animals. Am J Med Electron 1966; 5:24–28.
37. Vatner SF, Franklin D, Van Citters RL, et al. Effects of carotid sinus nerve stimulation on blood-flow distribution in conscious dogs at rest and during exercise. Circ Res 1970; 27:495–503.
38. Vatner SF, Higgins CB, Braunwald E. Effects of norepinephrine on coronary circulation and left ventricular dynamics in the conscious dog. Circ Res. 1974; 34:812–823.
39. Vatner SF, Higgins CB, Franklin D, et al. Effects of a digitalis glycoside on coronary and systemic dynamics in conscious dogs. Circ Res 1971; 28:470–479.
40. Vatner SF, McRitchie RJ. Interaction of the chemoreflex and the pulmonary inflation reflex in the regulation of coronary circulation in conscious dogs. Circ Res 1975; 37: 664–673.

41. Higgins CB, Vatner SF, Franklin D, et al. Effects of experimentally produced heart failure on the peripheral vascular response to severe exercise in conscious dogs. Circ Res 1972; 31:186–194.

42. Millard RW, Higgins CB, Franklin D, et al. Regulation of the renal circulation during severe exercise in normal dogs and dogs with experimental heart failure. Circ Res 1972; 31:881–888.

43. Vatner SF, Higgins CB, White S, et al. The peripheral vascular response to severe exercise in untethered dogs before and after complete heart block. J Clin Invest 1971; 50:1950–1960.

44. Buckberg GD, Luck JC, Payne DB, et al. Some sources of error in measuring regional blood flow with radioactive microspheres. J Appl Physiol 1971; 31:598–604.

45. Utley J, Carlson EL, Hoffman JI, et al. Total and regional myocardial blood flow measurements with 25 micron, 15 micron, 9 micron, and filtered 1–10 micron diameter microspheres and antipyrine in dogs and sheep. Circ Res 1974; 34:391–405.

46. Rudy LW Jr., Heymann MA, Edmunds LH Jr. Distribution of systemic blood flow during cardiopulmonary bypass. J Appl Physiol 1973; 34:194–200.

47. Rushmer RF, Franklin D, Ellis RM. Left ventricular dimensions recorded by sono-cardiometry. Circ Res 1956; 4:684–688.

48. Pagani M, Baig H, Sherman A, et al. Measurement of multiple simultaneous small dimensions and study of arterial pressure-dimension relations in conscious animals. Am J Physiol 1978; 235:H610–H617.

49. Patrick TA, Vatner SF, Kemper WS, et al. Telemetry of left ventricular diameter and pressure measurements from unrestrained animals. J Appl Physiol 1974; 37:276–281.

50. Heyndrickx GR, Millard RW, McRitchie RJ, et al. Regional myocardial functional and electrophysiological alterations after brief coronary artery occlusion in conscious dogs. J Clin Invest 1975; 56:978–985.

51. Hittinger L, Patrick T, Ihara T, et al. Exercise induces cardiac dysfunction in both moderate, compensated and severe hypertrophy. Circulation 1994; 89:2219–2231.

52. Theroux P, Ross J Jr., Franklin D, et al. Regional Myocardial function in the conscious dog during acute coronary occlusion and responses to morphine, propranolol, nitroglycerin, and lidocaine. Circulation 1976; 53:302–314.

53. Vatner SF. Correlation between acute reductions in myocardial blood flow and function in conscious dogs. Circ Res 1980; 47:201–207.

54. Vatner SF, Braunwald E. Effects of chronic heart failure on the inotropic response of the right ventricle of the conscious dog to a cardiac glycoside and to tachycardia. Circulation 1974; 50:728–734.

55. Vatner SF, Higgins CB, Franklin D, et al. Extent of carotid sinus regulation of the myocardial contractile state in conscious dogs. J Clin Invest 1972; 51:995–1008.

56. Prinzmetal M, Kennamer R, Merliss R, et al. Angina pectoris. I. A variant form of angina pectoris: preliminary report. Am J Med 1959; 27:375–388.

57. Hillis LD, Braunwald E. Coronary-artery spasm. N Engl J Med. 1978; 299:695–702.

58. Maseri A, L'Abbate A, Baroldi G, et al. Coronary vasospasm as a possible cause of myocardial infarction. A conclusion derived from the study of "preinfarction" angina. N Engl J Med 1978; 299:1271–1277.

59. Vatner SF, Pagani M, Manders WT. Alpha adrenergic constriction of coronary arteries in conscious dogs. Trans Assoc Am Physicians 1979; 92:229–238.

60. Vatner SF, Pagani M, Manders WT, et al. Alpha adrenergic vasoconstriction and nitroglycerin vasodilation of large coronary arteries in the conscious dog. J Clin Invest 1980; 65:5–14.
61. Van Citters RL, Franklin DL, Vatner SF, et al. Cerebral hemodynamics in the giraffe. Trans Assoc Am Physicians 1969; 82:293–304.
62. Baig H, Patrick TA, Vatner SF. Implantable pressure gauges for use in chronic animals. In: Fleming DG, Ko WH, Neuman MR, eds. Indwelling and Implantable Pressure Transducers. Cleveland, OH: CRC, 1977:35–43.
63. Franklin D, Vatner SF, Higgins CB, et al. Measurement and radiotelemetry of cardiovascular variables in conscious animals: techniques and applications. In: Harmison IT, ed. Research Animals in Medicine. Washington, DC: US Government Printing Office, 1973:1119–1133.
64. Vatner SF, Franklin D, Higgins CB, et al. Left ventricular response to severe exertion in untethered dogs. J Clin Invest 1972; 51:3052–3060.
65. Franklin D, Patrick TA, Kemper S, et al. A system for radiotelemetry of blood pressure, blood flow, and ventricular dimensions from animals: a summary report. Paper presented at: Proceedings of the International Telemetry Conference, 1971; Washington, DC.
66. Franklin D, Vatner SF, Van Citters RL. Studies on peripheral vascular dynamics using animals models. In: Animal Models for Biomedical Research. Vol. 4. Washington, DC: National Academy of Sciences, 1971:74–84.
67. Vatner SF, Patrick TA. Radio telemetry of blood flow and pressure measurements in untethered conscious animals. Bibl Cardiol 1974 34:1–11.
68. Asai K, Kudej RK, Takagi G, et al. Paradoxically enhanced endothelin-B receptor-mediated vasoconstriction in conscious old monkeys. Circulation 2001; 103: 2382–2386.
69. Reindardt V, Liss C, Stevens C. Restraint methods of laboratory non-human primates: a critical review. Animal Welfare 1995; 4:221–238.
70. Doebelin EO. Measurements Systems: Application and Design. 4th ed. New York, NY: McGraw-Hill, 1990.
71. Doebelin EO. System Dynamics: Modeling and Response. Columbus, OH: Merrill, 1972.
72. Harvey GF. ISA Transducer Compendium—Part 1. 2nd ed. New York, NY: Plenum, 1969.
73. Behzad R. Principles of Data Conversion System Design. Los Alamitos, CA: Wiley-IEEE Press, 1994.
74. Johns DA, Martin K. Analog Integrated Circuit Design. Mississauga, Canada: John Wiley & Sons Inc, 1997.
75. Jerri AJ. The Shannon sampling theorem—its various extensions and applications: a tutorial review. Proceedings of the IEEE. 1977; 65:1565–1596.
76. Ghaleh B, Shen YT, Vatner SF. Spatial heterogeneity of myocardial blood flow presages salvage versus necrosis with coronary artery reperfusion in conscious baboons. Circulation 1996; 94:2210–2215.
77. Shen YT, Yan L, Peppas A, et al. Activation of a cell survival program during post-ischemic heart failure in monkeys. Circulation. 2005; 111:1721.
78. Larosa G, Armstrong PW, Seeman P, et al. Beta adrenoceptor recovery after heart failure in the dog. Cardiovasc Res 1993; 27:489–493.

79. Moe GW, Stopps TP, Howard RJ, et al. Early recovery from heart failure: insights into the pathogenesis of experimental chronic pacing-induced heart failure. J Lab Clin Med 1988; 112:426–432.

80. Damiano RJ Jr., Tripp HF Jr., Asano T, et al. Left ventricular dysfunction and dilatation resulting from chronic supraventricular tachycardia. J Thorac Cardiovasc Surg 1987; 94:135–143.

81. McLaran CJ, Gersh BJ, Sugrue DD, et al. Tachycardia induced myocardial dysfunction. A reversible phenomenon? Br Heart J 1985; 53:323–327.

82. Packer DL, Bardy GH, Worley SJ, Smith MS, Cobb FR, Coleman RE, Gallagher JJ, German LD. Tachycardia-induced cardiomyopathy: a reversible form of left ventricular dysfunction. Am J Cardiol 1986; 57:563–570.

83. Shen YT, Lynch JJ, Shannon RP, et al. A novel heart failure model induced by sequential coronary artery occlusions and tachycardiac stress in awake pigs. Am J Physiol. 1999; 277(1 pt 2):H388–98.

84. Shen YT, Vatner SF, Morgans DJ, et al. Activating cardiac myosin, a novel inotropic mechanism to improve cardiac function in conscious dogs with congestive Heart Failure 2006; 114:II276 (1439).

6

Cardiovascular Toxicity of Antimicrobials

Daniel P. Healy

James L. Winkle College of Pharmacy, University of Cincinnati Health Science Center, Cincinnati, Ohio, U.S.A.

INTRODUCTION

Despite the rapid proliferation of novel anti-infective agents beginning in the 1960s and continuing through the 1980s, infectious diseases remain the third leading cause of death in the United States and the second leading cause of death worldwide (1). Community-acquired pneumonia alone affects approximately 4.5 million adults annually in the United States (2). Therefore, it is not surprising that antimicrobial agents continue to be among the most commonly prescribed drug classes. Fortunately, with the exception of life-threatening immediate hypersensitivity reactions, the toxicity profile of most antimicrobial compounds is relatively unremarkable. This may be attributed, at least in part, to the relatively short courses (e.g., ≤2 weeks) of antibiotics given for most common infections. Indeed, with longer courses of antibiotics required for infrequently encountered chronic infections or in critically ill patients, the risk of renal, hepatic, hematologic, and other types of serious toxicity significantly increases. Overall, the incidence of direct cardiovascular toxicity associated with antimicrobial therapy is very low. While certain antimicrobial compounds may possess direct cardiodepressant activity, generally this has only been demonstrated when using supraphysiologic concentrations in vitro or in anesthetized animals (3). Clinically, such cardiovascular toxicity associated with antimicrobial administration would not be expected to manifest unless one or more risk factors or conditions are present such as, but not limited to, diminished cardiac reserve (e.g., congestive heart failure, circulatory shock), the presence of cardiac arrhythmias, administration in an immunocompromised host, use of general anesthesia, presence of sepsis or septic shock, drug overdose, pharmacokinetic drug interactions resulting in elevated plasma levels of the antibiotic, and additive or synergistic pharmacodynamic effects when used in combination with other drugs possessing inherent depressant activity on the heart or vasculature (4–6). It is due to these many potential clinical factors that have not been thoroughly studied in the context of cardiovascular drug toxicity that warrants discussion of the mechanisms underlying the cardiotoxicity of antimicrobials.

This chapter will focus on clinically relevant cardiac toxicity secondary to QT-interval prolongation that has been described with macrolides/ketolides, fluoroquinolones, azole antifungals, and other agents. In addition, the chapter will attempt to briefly summarize a wealth of earlier information, much of which was published before 1980, that was detailed in the previous edition on the direct cardiovascular actions of aminoglycoside antibiotics (3). For an authoritative review of the influence of aminoglycosides on Ca^{2+} channel blockade in vascular smooth muscle and the myocardium, and their negative inotropic actions, the reader is referred to the third edition of this text (3). Since an exhaustive review of all related cardiovascular toxicity associated with miscellaneous or infrequently used antibiotics in clinical and veterinary medicine is beyond the scope of this chapter, the reader will be referred to authoritative reviews when pertinent.

TORSADES De POINTES AND QT-INTERVAL PROLONGATION

Torsades de pointes (TdP), often translated as a "twisting of the points," is a syndrome of polymorphic ventricular tachyarrhythmia characterized electrocardiographically by a gradual change in the amplitude and twisting of wide and variable QRS complexes around the isoelectric line (Fig. 1). While this syndrome often terminates spontaneously, it frequently recurs and can lead to syncope, ventricular fibrillation, and sudden death (5,6). Prolongation of the QT interval or heart rate-corrected QT interval (QTc) underlies most cases of TdP and can be due to congenital or acquired (e.g., drug therapy) causes. Inherited forms of long QT syndrome (LQTS) are due to various mutations in genes that control expression of sodium and potassium channels involved in cardiac

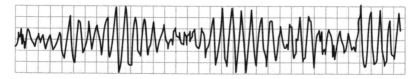

Figure 1 Characteristic electrocardiograph associated with the polymorphic ventricular tachyarrhythmia termed "torsades de pointes" (twisting of the points). This tracing depicts the characteristic changing amplitude and "twisting" of wide and variable QRS complexes around the isoelectric line.

repolarization (5). To date, seven genotypes have been identified, each with distinct symptoms, cardiac triggers, mortality risks, and treatment (7).

Most acquired causes of LQTS are related to drug therapy. Antimicrobial classes with a potential for causing LQTS, and therefore a higher theoretical risk of developing TdP, include the macrolides/ketolides, fluoroquinolones, azole antifungals, trimethoprim/sulfamethoxazole, and pentamidine. A comprehensive up-to-date registry of drugs, stratified by risk category based on a critical analysis of the published literature, is maintained by the Arizona Center for Education and Research on Therapeutics (ArizonaCERT) at http://www. QTdrugs.org (8). Table 1 lists the antimicrobials associated with some risk of causing TdP as currently assessed by ArizonaCERT.

Table 1 Risk Assessment of Antimicrobials Causing TdP

Level 1 risk: antimicrobials generally accepted to have a risk of causing TdP
- Macrolides: erythromycin, clarithromycin
- Fluoroquinolones: sparfloxacin, grepafloxacin—both removed from the U.S. market
- Pentamidine

Level 2 risk: antimicrobials with a possible risk of TdP based on availability of some reports showing an association with TdP and/or QT prolongation, but at this time lack substantial evidence for causing TdP.
- Fluoroquinolones: gatifloxacin, gemifloxacin, levofloxacin, moxifloxacin, ofloxacin
- Macrolides/azalides/ketolides: azithromycin, roxithromycin, telithromycin
- Azole antifungals: voriconazole
- Miscellaneous: amantadine, foscarnet

Level 3 risk: drugs to be avoided by patients with diagnosed or suspected congenital LQTS
- Fluoroquinolones: ciprofloxacin, gatifloxacin, gemifloxacin, levofloxacin, moxifloxacin, ofloxacin, sparfloxacin
- Macrolides/azalides/ketolides: erythromycin, clarithromycin, azithromycin, telithromycin
- Azole antifungals: fluconazole, itraconazole, ketoconazole, voriconazole
- Miscellaneous: amantadine, chloroquine, foscarnet, pentamidine, trimethoprim-sulfamethoxazole

Level 4 risk: drugs unlikely to cause TdP when used in recommended dosages and in patients without other risk factors[a]
- Fluoroquinolones: ciprofloxacin
- Azole antifungals: itraconazole, ketoconazole
- Miscellaneous: trimethoprim-sulfamethoxazole

---

[a]Risk factors such as concomitant QT-prolonging drugs, bradycardia, electrolyte disturbances, congenital long QT syndrome, concomitant drugs that inhibit metabolism. (Adapted from registry maintained by ArizonaCERT, http://www.QTdrugs.org; information as of 01 March 2006.) Accessed 20 June 2007.
Abbreviations: TdP, torsades de pointes; LQTS, long QT syndrome.
Source: From Ref. 8.

RISK FACTORS

Table 2 lists some of the identified risk factors associated with QT prolongation and TdP. Most cases of drug-induced TdP are associated with multiple clinical risk factors in susceptible individuals, suggesting that many drug-induced causes occur in those with inherited forms of LQTS (4,9). In addition, the concept of "reduced repolarization reserve" has been suggested to explain the variable risk associated with the development of TdP among susceptible individuals (5,9). In essence, the concept suggests that as multiple risk factors for TdP (Table 2) accumulate, the repolarization reserve becomes depleted, resulting in electrical instability within the ventricle.

Table 2 Risk Factors Associated with Drug-Induced QT Prolongation and Torsades de Pointes

Patient-related risk factors
- Congenital LQTS (QTc >500 milliseconds)
- Ion-channel polymorphisms
- Family history of sudden death
- Female gender
- Elderly
- Heart disease (congestive heart failure or hypertrophy, myocardial ischemia/infarction)
- Bradycardia
- Electrolyte imbalances especially hypokalemia, hypomagnesemia, hypocalcemia
- Recent conversion from atrial fibrillation, especially with a QT-prolonging drug
- Impaired drug metabolism and clearance without proper dosage reduction
- Endocrine disorders (e.g., hypothyroidism, diabetes mellitus)
- Cerebrovascular disease (e.g., stroke, subarachnoid hemorrhage)
- CNS infection or tumor
- Miscellaneous disorders (e.g., anorexia nervosa, "liquid protein" diets, hepatic failure, pheochromocytoma, hypothermia)

Drug-related risk factors
- QTc interval prolongation >60 milliseconds from pretreatment value
- Concomitant use of class I or III antiarrhythmics or other agents with intrinsic ability to prolong QT interval through blockade of potassium or other cardiac ion current channels
- High drug concentrations (e.g., determine by dose, dosing interval, route of administration, and rate of infusion relative to host's ability to metabolize/eliminate the drug)
- Potassium-wasting diuretics without adequate supplementation
- Pharmacokinetic drug interactions especially those involving CYP3A4 inhibitors (e.g., macrolides, azole antifungals) with agents known to prolong the QT interval
- Arsenic, organophosphates (insecticides, nerve gas) exposure

Abbreviation: CNS, central nervous system.
Source: Adapted from Refs. 5, 10–13.

In a study of 249 patients with TdP caused by noncardiac drugs, including 69 cases associated with antibiotic administration, the most commonly identified risk factor was female gender (71% overall, 65% for antibiotics) (10). Other risk factors were heart disease (53%), hypokalemia (31%), drug interactions with impairment of metabolism of a QT-prolonging drug or concomitant use of two or more QT-prolonging medications concomitantly (32%), presence of a LQTS before drug administration (16%) and excessive dose (9%). Importantly, all patients had at least one identifiable risk factor, and 71% had two or more risk factors (10). These results also support the reduced repolarization reserve concept (5,9).

It is important to note that the use of drugs known to prolong the QT interval is not generally associated with the development of TdP or other forms of ventricular arrhythmias unless high dosages, especially given by rapid intravenous injection, are used (11). Similarly, normal dosages given in the presence of a metabolic inhibitor can also result in excessive drug concentration in the plasma, which can also increase the risk for the development of arrhythmias (12).

ELECTROPHYSIOLOGIC MECHANISMS LEADING TO QT PROLONGATION (6,14–16)

Ventricular repolarization is a complex physiologic process governed by many membrane ion channels and transporters. The QRS complex of the surface electrocardiogram (ECG) represents the depolarization phase of the action potential, whereas the QT interval encompasses both the depolarization and repolarization phases. The lengthening of the QT interval, measured from the beginning of the QRS complex to the end of the T wave, represents the prolongation of the individual action potentials in certain cardiac myocytes. The action potential duration and thus the QT interval is controlled by a delicate balance of outward (primarily K+) and inward (primarily Ca++ and Na+) ion currents in the early, plateau, and late repolarization phases. These ion channels and transporters maintain normal electrical cardiac conduction.

The mechanism thought to be responsible for antibiotic and other drug-induced QT prolongation is the inhibition of the human ether-à-go-go-related gene (hERG), which encodes the rapid component of the delayed rectifier potassium (I_{Kr}) current (17–19). Blockade of the I_{Kr} current results in accumulation of potassium within the ventricular myocyte, which delays repolarization. Prolongation of the action potential may be followed by a second action potential termed an "early afterdepolarization," which may result in a premature ventricular complex (PVC). If this process becomes self-sustaining, it can form the triggering event for TdP. Certain cell types such as Purkinje fibers and mid-myocardial M cells appear likely to develop early afterdepolarizations, which can result in a myocardium that is susceptible to reentrant excitation and the development of TdP (5). It should be noted that while virtually all drugs known to cause QT prolongation and TdP are inhibitors of I_{kr}, many drugs that do not appear to cause TdP also block this potassium channel (17).

As previously mentioned, the inherited forms of LQTS are associated with mutations in one of at least seven genes known to modulate cardiac repolarization (5,7). Certain antibiotics and other drugs that block I_{kr} may, along with other risk factors (e.g., hypokalemia, structural heart defects, bradycardia), predispose a patient to the development of TdP. It is estimated that a significant number of individuals harbor a subclinical form of the congenital syndrome or carry subtle polymorphisms, which only becomes clinically apparent on exposure to I_{kr}-blocking drugs in the presence of other risk factors. The unmasking of the abnormal ion currents may result in a symptomatic ventricular arrhythmia such as TdP (13,20,21).

ASSESSMENT OF CARDIOTOXICITY

Since 1998, the single most common reason for a marketed pharmaceutical to be withdrawn or severely restricted has been prolongation of the QT interval associated with TdP (5). In addition to notable drugs such as terfenadine (Seldane), astemizole (Hismanal), cisapride (Propulsid) that were removed for this reason, this has also been the case with sparfloxacin and grepafloxacin, two fluoroquinolone antibiotics. As a result, most members of the fluoroquinolone class now carry precautions or warnings in their product information.

Given the previous discussion about the influence of the many risk factors associated with QT prolongation and the development of TdP, an attempt has been made to ensure a more standardized approach to the cardiotoxicity assessment of pharmaceuticals including antibiotics. The Safety and Efficacy Expert Working Groups of the International Conference on Harmonization (ICH) have developed final guidelines for the nonclinical and clinical evaluation of a pharmaceutical on QT/QTc prolongation (22,23). These guidelines have been recommended for adoption to the regulatory bodies of the European Union, Japan, and the United States. This guidance represents the U.S. Food and Drug Administration's (FDA) current thinking on the topic.

Since no single test exhibits adequate sensitivity and specificity for predicting the drug-induced QT-interval prolongation and proarrhythmic potential, it is recommended that preclinical testing include both in vitro and in vivo evaluation of four functional levels, including (*i*) ionic currents measured in isolated myocytes, tissues, cell lines, or expression systems; (*ii*) action potential parameters in isolated intact cardiac preparations; (*iii*) ECG parameters measured in conscious or anesthetized animals; and (*iv*) proarrhythmic effects in isolated cardiac preparations or animals (22). For further reading on the specifics of the nonclinical assays used to determine drug-related cardiac toxicity in this area, the reader is referred to excellent reviews by De Ponti et al. (12,24), Owens (11), and Fenichel et al. (25).

As previously discussed, the number of non-antiarrhythmic drugs removed from the market because of QT prolongation and the development of both nonfatal and fatal arrhythmias has heightened the sensitivity and need for rigorous premarketing assessment of cardiac safety. To that end, the development of clinical guidelines through the ICH E14 document now serves as a valuable resource to guide the drug development process to establish whether the drug has a threshold pharmacologic effect on cardiac repolarization, as determined by QT/QTc prolongation (23). In essence, the guidance strongly recommends a "thorough QT study" for any new agent under development. Typically, such a dedicated study for an antimicrobial is conducted as part of phase I investigation using healthy volunteers. The recommended studies are randomized, blinded, and controlled for all known sources of variation in QT/QTc measurement and employ a crossover design with an adequate washout between the investigational agent, placebo, and an active positive control (e.g., an agent known to cause QT/QTc prolongation). Various planned dosages given as single or multiple doses as well as supraphysiologic doses of the drug under investigation are studied. The pharmacokinetics of the drug and its metabolites, if any, will dictate the exact study design. The thorough QT evaluation study must be able to differentiate between a small mean change in QT/QTc from natural variability in placebo-treated patients. A negative study is one in which the largest mean difference between drug and placebo for the QT/QTc interval is approximately 5 milliseconds or less (23). Needless to say, a successful and thorough QT study requires careful planning, design, quality control, and execution. A good example of a newer agent following the established guidance for its effect on cardiac repolarization is the "thorough QT study" conducted by Barriere et al. on the new glycopeptide, telavancin (26). It is hoped that incorporation of this type of investigation early in the drug development process will minimize the number of new pharmaceuticals with a heightened potential for severe cardiotoxicity thereby preventing unexpected postmarketing occurrences of nonfatal and fatal arrhythmias leading to eventual withdrawal from the marketplace.

MACROLIDE AND RELATED ANTIBIOTICS

The macrolide antibiotics, in particular, erythromycin and clarithromycin, appear to be associated with the greatest risk of TdP as a result of QT prolongation. This is likely due to two reasons: their intrinsic concentration-dependent ability to block hERG K+ currents (27,28) and their ability to significantly inhibit the hepatic metabolism (especially CYP3A4) of other compounds, resulting in supratherapeutic levels and a greater torsadogenic potential (29). As previously mentioned, the registry maintained by ArizonaCERT (http://www.QTdrugs.org) lists drugs based on risk level (8). Erythromycin and clarithromycin are classified at the highest risk level since they are drugs generally accepted to carry a risk for causing TdP. Telithromycin, a chemically similar ketolide, and azithromycin, which is a chemically distinct azalide, are both listed as antimicrobials with a "possible risk of TdP"; however, both lack substantial evidence for causing TdP (8). Indeed, a retrospective evaluation of the U.S.

FDA's Adverse Event Reporting System (AERS) database revealed that of noncardiac drugs, macrolides accounted for the majority (77%) of reported cases of TdP (30). Although erythromycin and clarithromycin accounted for 53% and 36%, respectively, of all reports the rank order when corrected for the estimated number of outpatient prescriptions was clarithromycin > erythromycin > azithromycin (30).

An extensive study of the Tennessee Medicaid cohort involving 1,249,943 person-years of follow-up found the multivariate adjusted rate of sudden death from cardiac causes to be twice as high among patients who had received oral erythromycin as those who had not and five times higher in those who had received concurrent erythromycin and a CYP3A4 inhibitor than those who had not (31). In contrast, there was no increase in the risk of sudden death among those who had concurrently received oral amoxicillin and a CYP3A4 inhibitor. On the basis of these and other supporting in vitro, animal, and clinical data, the concurrent use of erythromycin and inhibitors of CYP3A4 should be avoided. This warning would also be prudent for clarithromycin since it is also a potent inhibitor of CYP3A4 metabolism and is associated with TdP (29,32). In general, concomitant administration of these two macrolides with other drugs that are metabolized by CYP3A4 and that can also cause QTc prolongation (e.g., astemizole, terfenadine, cisapride), increases the risk for a pharmacokinetic interaction resulting in TdP. All three of these agents are no longer marketed.

Macrolides have been shown to possess differential potency with respect to inhibition of I_{Kr} encoded by hERG. Volberg and colleagues (27) compared six macrolides on hERG currents expressed in HEK-293 cells and found the following concentrations resulting in 50% inhibition (IC_{50}): clarithromycin (32.9 μM), roxithromycin (36.5 μM), erythromycin (72.2 μM), josamycin (102.4 μM), erythromycylamine (273.9 μM), and oleandomycin (339.6 μM). In addition, desmethyl erythromycin, the primary metabolite of erythromycin, also inhibited hERG current with an IC_{50} of 147.1 μM. In a similar study by Stanat and colleagues (28), erythromycin and clarithromycin both inhibited hERG current in a concentration-dependent manner with IC_{50} values of 38.9 μM and 45.7 μM, respectively. Information presented to the FDA's Anti-infective Drug Products Advisory Committee Meeting on behalf of telithromycin, a ketolide, chemically related to macrolides, indicated an IC_{50} value of 42.5 μM, which is remarkably similar to both erythromycin and clarithromycin (33). Collectively, these results indicate that clinically achievable plasma concentrations of erythromycin (especially when given intravenously), clarithromcyin, and telithromycin can produce a significant level of hERG channel blockade. These data are also consistent with those obtained from animal models in which erythromycin and clarithromycin, but not azithromycin, demonstrated a torsadogenic potential and proarrhythmic profile (34,35).

The concentration dependency found in the in vitro experiments corresponds to the clinical reports of macrolide-associated TdP. The majority of cases implicating erythromycin involved the intravenous formulation given in relatively high dosages (e.g., 4 g/day) (36,37). These dosages given intravenously result in peak plasma concentrations approximately 5-fold to 30-fold higher than the typical 500-mg oral dose (38). The margin of safety between the typical unbound plasma concentrations relative to the hERG/I_{kr} IC_{50} values is only about 10-fold with the intravenous formulation of erythromycin (4 g/day), whereas this ratio is about 200-fold with typical oral dosing (39). The margin for clarithromycin was estimated to be about 30-fold, which is right on the line of demarcation between the majority of drugs associated with TdP and those that are not (39). The ratio of free plasma concentrations of telithromycin to IC_{50} values is about 50, suggesting a relatively large degree of safety in the absence of other risk factors for QT prolongation (33).

Most cases involving TdP associated with clarithromycin administration have occurred in patients concurrently receiving contraindicated drugs such as cisapride, terfenadine, astemizole and pimozide, highlighting the importance of a probable pharmacokinetic drug interaction leading to supratherapeutic levels and the development of TdP (11). In support of this hypothesis, a study conducted in healthy volunteers showed a mean increase of 6 milliseconds in QTc interval with both clarithromycin and cisapride when given alone and an increase of 25 milliseconds when administered concurrently (40). Similarly, ketoconazole (an azole antifungal) and telithromycin (chemically similar to clarithromycin) caused mean changes in the QTc interval of 6.4 and 3.3 milliseconds, respectively, when administered alone, and 10.5 milliseconds ($p = 0.004$) when given concomitantly (33). This change was associated with a 95% increase in the exposure level of telithromycin as measured by the area under the plasma concentration-time curve over the 24-hour dosing interval (AUC_{0-24}). Both ketoconazole and telithromycin are known to act as both substrates for and inhibitors of P450 metabolism.

In contrast to erythromycin, clarithromycin, and telithromycin, azithromycin, a chemically distinct azalide antibiotic, does not appear to significantly inhibit hERG K+ channels or CYP3A4 metabolism (29,30). The number of case reports associated with cardiac toxicity attributed to azithromycin are noteworthy for their infrequency and most are potentially explained by other known risk factors such as comorbid diseases (e.g., cardiac, renal, hepatic), electrolyte derangements (e.g., hypokalemia, hypomagnesemia) and/or the concomitant administration of agents known to prolong the QT interval (30). The most recent case reported in a patient developing TdP while receiving azithromycin is typical of the complexity in trying to establish causality (41). Despite the authors' claim of the absence of other known precipitating factors for QTc prolongation and development of TdP, the patient was a 55-year-old female with intermittent symptomatic bradycardia who developed sepsis and renal failure requiring dialysis prior to adding azithromycin. The patient also received moxifloxacin and ciprofloxacin within the same time frame prior to the development of QTc prolongation and TdP, which occurred on day 7 of azithromycin therapy. While azithromycin may indeed have contributed to the development of TdP, it is difficult to establish a true cause and effect relationship.

FLUOROQUINOLONES

Fluoroquinolone antimicrobials are arguably the most widely prescribed class of antibiotics on the planet. They were the most widely prescribed class of antibiotics in adults in the United States from 1995 to 2002, and their prescribing increased threefold during that period (42). While more than a dozen have been developed over the past two decades, only a few remain for widespread clinical use in the treatment of systemic infections: ciprofloxacin, levofloxacin, moxifloxacin, and gemifloxacin. Many have been voluntarily withdrawn or removed from the worldwide market because of various problems including hepatotoxicity (e.g., temafloxacin, trovafloxacin), glucose derangements (e.g., gatifloxacin), phototoxicity (e.g., fleroxacin, sparfloxacin) and cardiac (e.g., sparfloxacin, grepafloxacin).

Although grepafloxacin was contraindicated in patients with known QTc prolongation and in patients receiving other agents known to inhibit hERG, it was associated with seven cardiac-related fatalities, including three cases of TdP resulting in its voluntary removal from the market in 1999 (43). With the removal of sparfloxacin and grepafloxacin because of the relatively high incidence of both nonfatal and fatal arrhythmias secondary to QT prolongation, many now consider this to be a class effect (44–46). As a result of this historical perspective, all new fluoroquinolones under development must undergo extensive in vitro, animal, and clinical testing to determine their propensity for causing QT prolongation and affect on cardiac repolarization. Older agents such as norfoxacin, ciprofloxacin, ofloxacin, and levofloxacin (levo isomer of ofloxacin) have been used extensively for many years largely without significant problems. Despite the possibility of a "class effect," most authorities clearly agree that differences exist among agents with respect to potency of hERG K+ channel blockade and QT prolongation (6,11,18,19,37,43,46–51).

Bischoff and coworkers investigated the effect of four quinolones on hERG-mediated K+ currents using Chinese hamster ovary (CHO) cells by patch clamp technique (18). Their results showed that ciprofloxacin did not interact with hERG channels at any tested concentration (e.g., $IC_{50} > 100$ µg/ml), whereas grepafloxacin ($IC_{50} = 37.5$ µg/ml) and moxifloxacin ($IC_{50} = 41.2$ µg/ml) showed an equal potency in hERG K+ current inhibition, in comparison to sparfloxacin ($IC_{50} = 13.5$ µg/ml) that displayed the greatest potency of the four agents studied (18).

Anderson et al. (48) studied both the in vitro (I_{Kr} inhibition) and in vivo (e.g., QTc interval prolongation and occurrence of tachyarrhythmias) effects of four quinolones. Similar to the results of the study by Bischoff et al. (18), they also found sparfloxacin to be the most potent inhibitor of I_{Kr} with an IC_{50} value of 0.23 µM while moxifloxacin, gatifloxacin, and grepafloxacin had mean IC_{50}

values of 0.75, 26.5, and 27.2 µM, respectively. In addition, all agents increased the maximum QT interval from baseline (241 milliseconds) to a mean of 370 milliseconds, 270 milliseconds, 280 milliseconds, and 255 milliseconds, respectively, for sparfloxacin, moxifloxacin, grepafloxacin, and gatifloxacin (48). During an extended 60-minutes observation period, sparfloxacin induced ventricular tachycardia in three of six animals and TdP in one of six animals while none of the other agents caused arrhythmias. The investigators found a good correlation between I_{Kr} antagonism, QT/QTc prolongation, and the development of arrhythmias for sparfloxacin and moxifloxacin, but not for grepafloxacin and gatifloxacin (48).

Kang and coinvestigators conducted the most extensive comparison of quinolones on both hERG K+ and KvLQT1/mink K+ channels (19). The latter channel is responsible for the slow component of the delayed rectifier current (I_{Ks}) in the human heart. While none of the tested quinolones inhibited the KvLQT1/mink K+ channel, sparfloxacin once again was the most potent agent inhibiting hERG channel currents with an IC_{50} value of 18 µM, followed by grepafloxacin (50 µM), moxifloxacin (129 µM), gatifloxacin (130 µM), levofloxacin (915 µM), ciprofloxacin (966 µM), and ofloxacin (1420 µM). Since they found over a 100-fold difference between the most (sparfloxacin) and least (ofloxacin) potent fluoroquinolones, they argued against a class effect. When comparing maximum free plasma concentrations of each agent to their respective IC_{50} values, they found very low safety ratios for sparfloxacin, intermediate margins for grepafloxacin, moxifloxacin, and gatifloxacin and high, desirable ratios for the least potent inhibitors, levofloxacin and ofloxacin (19). They further suggested that the C_5 and C_8 positions are important with respect to structure-activity relationships for cardiotoxicity and potency against hERG and QTc prolongation since both sparfloxacin and grepafloxacin have C5 substituents whereas levofloxacin, ofloxacin, and ciprofloxacin do not. They also point out that the equipotency of gatifloxacin and moxifloxacin with respect to hERG inhibition may correspond to the OMe substitution at C_8 (19).

Consistent with the data from the studies evaluating the effect of quinolones on I_{Kr} inhibition, various quinolones have been evaluated for their effect on cardiac action potential duration. Patmore and colleagues (52) compared the effects of sparfloxacin, grepafloxacin, moxifloxacin, and ciprofloxacin on the action potential duration recorded from canine isolated cardiac Purkinje fibers. The rank order of potency was sparfloxacin > grepafloxacin = moxifloxacin > ciprofloxacin (52).

There have been a number of randomized clinical trials, mostly conducted in healthy volunteers, comparing various quinolones with respect to their effect on QT-interval prolongation (53–57). Several trials have demonstrated small, but statistically significant increases in the QTc interval, primarily when large doses were administered (53–55), but without the occurrence of arrhythmias. Tsikouris et al. (57) found that moxifloxacin administered at a standard 400-mg/day dose for seven days prolonged the QTc interval by 6 milliseconds from baseline, whereas standard doses of levofloxacin (500 mg) and ciprofloxacin (500 mg) over the same time period did not. Noel et al. (55) found a dose-response relationship with levofloxacin with QTc changes of statistical significance at the higher dose levels. The same investigative group also found that high doses of moxifloxacin (800 mg), levofloxacin (1000 mg), and ciprofloxacin (1500 mg) all resulted in small, but statistically significant increases in the QTc interval compared with placebo with moxifloxacin causing the greatest QTc prolongation (54).

Consistent with the above data, a retrospective database analysis found ciprofloxacin and levofloxacin to be associated with the least cardiac toxicity among the quinolones, 0.3 cases and 5.4 cases per 10 million prescriptions, respectively; whereas gatifloxacin was associated with 27 cases per 10 million prescriptions (58). While several case reports of levofloxacin-associated QTc prolongation and TdP have been published, most have occurred in patients possessing other risk factors (59–61). The few cases of ciprofloxacin associated with the development of an arrhythmia are noteworthy because for their infrequency over the 20 years the drug has been extensively prescribed globally (62–64). Collectively, the currently available data suggest that ciprofloxacin is the fluoroquinolone with the highest margin of cardiac safety followed by levofloxacin and moxifloxacin. Both moxifloxacin and gemifloxacin bear more specific warnings in their product information, which seems reasonable pending the availability of more extensive postmarketing surveillance data. The fluoroquinolones as a class appear to have a lower potential for QTc prolongation and arrhythmias as compared with the macrolides (e.g., erythromycin and clarithromycin); however, as with all antimicrobials, the degree of repolarization reserve in a given patient, based on host and drug risk factors, will determine the influence an agent like a fluoroquinolone will have on QTc prolongation (5,9,65).

IMIDAZOLE AND TRIAZOLE ANTIFUNGALS

Ketoconazole, fluconazole, itraconazole, voriconazole, and posaconazole are azole antifungals that are widely prescribed for numerous infections ranging in both type and severity from mild superficial dermatophytic infections to vaginal candidiasis to life-threatening systemic fungal infections. All but the very newest member (posaconazole) has been associated with QT-interval prolongation and the development of TdP. While limited data are published concerning their differential potencies of this class on hERG K+ channel inhibition, ketoconazole has been shown to block I_{Kr} with an IC_{50} value of 49 μM (66), which is remarkably similar to those reported for the torsadogenic macrolides, erythromycin (38.9 μM) and clarithromycin (45.7 μM) (28). Most of the published case reports involving azoles and the development of QT prolongation with TdP have involved apparent pharmacokinetic interactions involving CYP3A4 metabolic inhibition of agents no longer available because of cardiac toxicity such as astemizole, terfenadine, and cisapride (37). Thus, all of the currently available azole antifungals have the potential for causing QT prolongation and TdP from two mechanisms: their intrinsic ability to inhibit hERG K+ channels and their ability to significantly inhibit the hepatic metabolism of others via CYP3A4, −2C9, and −2C19 pathways. Clinical reports suggest a greater propensity for cardiac toxicity associated with ketoconazole and itraconazole administration than with fluconazole or voriconazole; however, few comparative data exist to support this contention. A recent report by Philips and coworkers (67) involved the development of voriconazole-associated TdP in two patients with leukemia. While these two patients had other risk factors present (e.g., anthracycline therapy, acute cardiomyopathy, electrolyte disturbances), the apparent precipitation of a ventricular arrhythmia by voriconazole underscores the need for close ECG monitoring in all patients with other risk factors for QTc prolongation when receiving an azole antifungal (67). Given the widespread use of these drugs and the continued development of new agents in the same chemical class, the scientific community looks forward to published post-marketing surveillance evaluations of existing azoles using the FDA's AERS database with particular attention to drug-drug interactions as well as results from "thorough QT studies" from azoles in early stages of drug development.

MISCELLANEOUS ANTIMICROBIALS

Pentamidine is an antiprotozoal agent commonly used to treat *Pneumocystis jiroveci* (formerly *P. carinii*) pneumonia in immunocompromised patients, especially those with the acquired immunodeficiency syndrome (AIDS). Case reports of pentamidine-associated QT prolongation and TdP have been reported for two decades (68); however, the exact mechanism(s) involved is unclear. It should be noted that pentamidine shares some chemical structure similarities with procainamide, an agent with noted proarrhythmic potential (4).

In stably transfected HEK-293 cells, pentamidine was found to be a relatively weak inhibitor of I_{Kr}/hERG current with an IC_{50} of 252 μM (69); however, investigators found a significant downregulation in the membrane expression of the hERG channel densities at clinically achievable concentrations, suggesting a slightly different mechanism for causing QT prolongation and cardiac arrhythmias (69). A separate investigation confirmed pentamidine being an ineffective blocker (e.g., $IC_{50} > 300$ μM) as well as its inability to induce any significant effect on QT-interval prolongation in the isolated perfused rabbit heart model even at concentrations up to 30 μM (70). However, in a prospective evaluation of patients with AIDS who were given pentamidine in the standard intravenous dose of 4 mg/kg/day infused over one hour found a mean ± S.D. increase in QTc of 120 ± 30 milliseconds in 5 of 14 evaluable patients of whom three developed TdP (71). This is noteworthy since exclusion criteria included many of the known patient risk factors for QTc prolongation. However, two of the three patients who developed TdP and 9 of the 14 total patients also received an azole antifungal, agents now known to prolong QTc. In addition, some azoles also inhibit CYP2C19, and pentamidine is a known substrate for that isoform. Therefore, the dozen or so cases of TdP involving pentamidine over the past 20 years suggest that any arrhythmogenic activity is either related to a decrease in membrane expression of hERG channels in patients receiving chronic administration of pentamidine, a pharmacokinetic drug interaction resulting in elevated pentamidine or azole concentrations, and/or other mechanisms unrelated to hERG blockade.

Traebert and colleagues studied the effects of several antimalarial compounds on hERG K+ currents in stably transfected human embryonic kidney (HEK) cells (72). As a class, these agents are remarkably potent with respect to hERG inhibition with IC_{50} values ranging from 0.04 µM for halofantrine to 2.5 µM and 2.6 µM, respectively, for chloroquine and mefloquine (72). On the basis of these IC_{50} values relative to typical free (unbound) plasma concentrations, the order of the safety margin was mefloquine > lumefantrine > chloroquine > halofantrine (72). This ranking parallels clinical trials in that both halofantrine and chloroquine have been associated with significant QT prolongation whereas mefloquine and lumefantrine have not (73).

Sulfonamides in general and trimethoprim-sulfamethoxazole (cotrimoxazole) specifically have been among the most widely prescribed drugs worldwide over the past four decades. In general, they are not thought to possess a toxicity profile affecting the cardiac conduction system. Indeed, the limited number of cases of cotrimoxazole-associated TdP would suggest nothing more than background noise and the lack of a real effect on cardiac repolarization (74,75). However, a recent landmark investigation found a small subset of patients among those who developed QT prolongation and drug-induced arrhythmias who harbored a single nucleotide polymorphism (SNP) in the MiRP1 gene that encodes a peptide subunit of the I_{Kr} channel (21). One such patient developed QT prolongation (>600 milliseconds) following administration of cotrimoxazole. When investigated in vitro, the sulfamethoxazole component in clinically achievable concentrations inhibited the expressed mutant I_{Kr} channels, but not the wild-type channels. Trimethoprim did not significantly block I_{Kr} in clinically relevant concentrations in either the wild-type or mutant channels suggesting that the sulfamethoxazole moiety was responsible for that patient's QT prolongation. Furthermore and in support of a unique patient population with increased susceptibility to drug-induced arrhythmias, the two case reports in which there was an absence of confounding risk factors demonstrated a recurrence of TdP following rechallenge with trimethoprim-sulfamethoxazole (74,75). Taken together, Sesti and coinvestigators estimated that these data suggest that a small percentage of the population (1–2%) may possess the SNP increasing their risk for drug-induced arrhythmias (21).

SUMMARY

Several classes of antimicrobials such as the macrolides, fluoroquinolones, azoles, and antimalarials as well as individual agents (e.g., pentamidine) are known to inhibit hERG/I_{Kr} and therefore have the potential to significantly prolong QTc interval and cause arrhythmias such as TdP. Overall however, the risk of such antimicrobial-induced cardiac arrhythmias is relatively uncommon and can be minimized by paying strict attention to host- and drug-related risk factors, which appear to be common in almost all clinical cases that have been reported (10–12). In addition, since most drugs that inhibit hERG and delay the action potential do so in a concentration-dependent manner, clinicians must recognize situations leading to supratherapeutic concentrations of these and other agents especially as a result of inhibition of hepatic metabolism, which is common to the macrolides and azoles. The heightened sensitivity of noncardiac drugs causing QTc prolongation and TdP along with preclinical and clinical regulatory guidance for new drug development and the requirement for post-marketing surveillance of higher-risk compounds will hopefully decrease the future probability of antimicrobial-induced cardiotoxicity. Patients with known LQTS, structural heart defects, electrolyte derangements, those receiving Class Ia or III antiarrhythmics, or receiving other drugs known to prolong the QTc interval independently are at the greatest risk for cardiac toxicity mediated by macrolide, fluoroquinolone, or azole antibiotics. The risk-benefit ratio of antibiotic selection should therefore be decided on an individualized basis with a prospective ECG monitoring plan in place to avert serious toxicity. Avoidance of these antimicrobials in high-risk situations, when feasible, is the safest recommendation. Finally, the rapidly growing knowledge base concerning the genetic predisposition and related polymorphisms associated with drug- and antibiotic-induced QTc prolongation may help to prospectively identify patients at risk for cardiac toxicity and enhanced monitoring.

REFERENCES

1. Fauci AS. Infectious diseases: considerations for the 21st century. Clin Infect Dis 2001; 32:675.
2. Niederman MS, McCombs JS, Unger AN, et al. The cost of treating community-acquired pneumonia. Clin Ther 1998; 20:820.
3. Kerzee JK, Ramos KS, Parker JL, et al. Cardiovascular toxicity of antibacterial antibiotics. In: Acosta D Jr., ed. Cardiovascular Toxicology. 3rd ed. New York, NY: Taylor & Francis, 2002: 187–221.
4. De Ponti F, Poluzzi E, Montanaro N. QT-interval prolongation by noncardiac drugs: lessons to be learned from recent experience. Eur J Clin Pharmacol 2000; 56:1.
5. Roden DM. Drug-induced prolongation of the QT interval. New Engl J Med 2004; 350:1013.
6. Owens RC Jr., Ambrose PG. Antimicrobial safety: focus on fluoroquinolones. Clin Infect Dis 2005; 41:S144.

7. Priori SG, Schwartz PJ, Napolitano C, et al. Risk stratification in the long-QT syndrome. New Engl J Med 2003; 348:1866.

8. Arizona Center for Education and Research on Therapeutics. Available at: http://www.torsades.org/medical-pros/drug-lists/list-01.cfm?sort=Generic_name. Accessed June 13, 2007; information as of 3/01/06.

9. Roden DM. Taking the "idio" out of "idiosyncratic": predicting torsades de pointes. Pacing Clin Electrophysiol 1998; 21:1029.

10. Zeltser D, Justo D, Halkin A, et al. Torsade de pointes due to noncardiac drugs. Most patients have easily identifiable risk factors. Medicine 2003; 82:282.

11. Owens RC Jr. QT prolongation with antimicrobial agents. Understanding the significance. Drugs 2004; 64:1091.

12. De Ponti F, Poluzzi E, Cavalli A, et al. Safety of non-antiarrhythmic drugs that prolong the QT interval or induce torsade de pointes. Drug Saf 2002; 25:263.

13. Viskin S. Long QT syndromes and torsade de pointes. Lancet 1999; 354:1625.

14. Morganroth J. Relations of QTc prolongation on the electrocardiogram to torsades de pointes: definitions and mechanisms. Am J Cardiol 1993; 72:10B.

15. Moss AJ. Measurement of the QT interval and the risk associated with QTc interval prolongation: a review. Am J Cardiol 1993; 72:23B.

16. Shryock JC, Song Y, Wu L, et al. A mechanistic approach to assess the proarrhythmic risk of QT-prolonging drugs in preclinical pharmacologic studies. J Electrocardiol 2004; 37(suppl.):34.

17. Sanguinetti MC, Jiang C, Curran ME, et al. A mechanistic link between an inherited and an acquired cardiac arrhythmia: HERG encodes the I_{kr} potassium channel. Cell 1995; 81:299.

18. Bischoff U, Schmidt C, Netzer R, et al. Effects of fluoroquinolones on HERG currents. Eur J Pharmacol 2000; 406:341.

19. Kang J, Wang L, Chen XL, et al. Interactions of a series of fluoroquinolone antibacterial drugs with the human cardiac K+ channel HERG. Mol Pharmacol 2001; 59:122.

20. Napolitano C, Schwartz PJ, Brown AM, et al. Evidence for a cardiac ion channel mutation underlying drug-induced QT prolongation and life-threatening arrhythmias. J Cardiovasc Electrophysiol 2000; 11:691.

21. Sesti F, Abbott GW, Wei J, et al. A common polymorphism associated with antibiotic-induced cardiac arrhythmia. Proc Natl Acad Sci U S A 2000; 97:10613.

22. International Conference on Harmonization. Guidance for Industry. S7B Nonclinical evaluation of the potential for delayed ventricular repolarization (QT interval prolongation) by human pharmaceuticals, U.S. Department of Health and Human Services, Food and Drug Administration, 2005. Available at: http://www.fda.ove/cer/gd/ns/ichqt.htm. Accessed July 18, 2007.

23. International Conference on Harmonization. Guidance for Industry. E14 Clinical evaluation of QT/QTc interval prolongation and proarrhythmic potential for non-antiarrhythmic drugs, U.S. Department of Health and Human Services, Food and Drug Administration, 2005. Available at: http://www.fda.ove/cer/gd/ns/ichqt.htm. Accessed July 18, 2007.

24. De Ponti F, Poluzzi E, Montanaro N. Organizing evidence on QT prolongation and occurrence of torsades de pointes with non-antiarrhythmic drugs: a call for consensus. Eur J Clin Pharmacol 2001; 57:185.

25. Fenichel RR, Malik M, Antzelevitch C, et al. Drug-induced torsades de pointes and implications for drug development. J Cardiovasc Electrophysiol 2004; 15:475.

26. Barriere S, Genter F, Spencer E, et al. Effects of a new antibacterial, telavancin, on cardiac repolarization (QTc interval duration) in healthy subjects. J Clin Pharmacol 2004; 44:689.
27. Volberg WA, Koci BJ, Su W, et al. Blockade of human cardiac potassium channel human ether-a-go-go-related gene (HERG) by macrolide antibiotics. J Pharmacol Exp Ther 2002; 302:320.
28. Stanat SJ, Carlton CG, Crumb WJ Jr., et al. Characterization of the inhibitory effects of erythromycin and clarithromycin on the HERG potassium channel. Mol Cell Biochem 2003; 254:1.
29. Dresser GK, Spence JD, Bailey DG. Pharmacokinetic-pharmacodynamic consequences and clinical relevance of cytochrome P450 3A4 inhibition. Clin Pharmacokinet 2000; 38:41.
30. Shaffer D, Singer S, Korvick J, et al. Concomitant risk factors in reports of torsades de pointes associated with macrolide use: review of the United States Food and Drug Administration adverse event reporting system. Clin Infect Dis 2002; 35:197.
31. Ray WA, Murray KT, Meredith S, et al. Oral erythromycin and the risk of sudden death from cardiac causes. New Engl J Med 2004; 351:1089.
32. Lee KL, Jim MH, Tang SC, et al. QT prolongation and torsades de pointes associated with clarithromycin. Am J Med 1998; 104:395.
33. Aventis Pharmaceuticals, Ketek (telithromycin) briefing document for the FDA Anti-Infective Drug Products Advisory Committee Meeting, 2001. Available at: http://www.fda.gov/ohrms/dockets/ac/01/briefing/3746b_01_aventis.pdf. Accessed July 18, 2007.
34. Milberg P, Eckardt L, Bruns HJ, et al. Divergent proarrhythmic potential of macrolide antibiotics despite similar QT prolongation: fast phase 3 repolarization prevents early afterdepolarizations and torsade de pointes. J Pharmacol Exp Ther 2002; 303:218.
35. Eckardt L, Breithardt G, Haverkamp W. Electrophysiologic characterization of the antipsychotic drug sertindole in a rabbit heart model of torsade de pointes: low torsadogenic potential despite QT-prolongation. J Pharmacol Exp Ther 2002; 300:64.
36. Tschida SJ, Guay DR, Straka RJ, et al. QTc-interval prolongation associated with slow intravenous erythromycin lactobionate infusions in critically ill patients: a prospective evaluation and review of the literature. Pharmacotherapy 1996; 16:663.
37. Owens RC Jr., Nolin TD. Antimicrobial-associated QT interval prolongation: points of interest. Clin Infect Dis 2006; 43:1603.
38. Sivapalasingam S, Steigbigel NH. Macrolides, clindamycin, and ketolides. In: Mandell GL, Bennett JE, Dolin R, eds. Mandell, Douglas and Bennett's Principles and Practice of Infectious Diseases, 6th ed. Philadelphia, PA: Elsevier, 2005: 396–417.
39. Redfern WS, Carlsson L, Davis AS, et al. Relationships between preclinical cardiac electrophysiology, clinical QT interval prolongation and torsade de pointes for a broad range of drugs: evidence for a provisional safety margin in drug development. Cardiovasc Res 2003; 58:32.
40. Van Haarst AD, van 't Klooster GA, van Gerven JM, et al. The influence of cisapride and clarithromycin on QT intervals in healthy volunteers. Clin Pharmacol Ther 1998; 64:542.
41. Kezerashvili A, et al. Azithromycin as a cause of QT-interval prolongation and torsade de pointes in the absence of other known precipitating factors. J Interventional Cardiol Electrophysiol 2007; 18:243.

42. Linder JA, Huang ES, Steinman MA, et al. Fluoroquinolone prescribing in the United States: 1995 to 2002. Am J Med 2005; 118:259.
43. Rubenstein E, Camm J. Cardiotoxicity of fluoroquinolones. J Antimicrob Chemother 2002; 49:593.
44. Iannini PB, Doddamani S, Byazrova E, et al. Risk of torsades de pointes with non-cardiac drugs. Prolongation of QT interval is probably a class effect of fluoroquinolones. BMJ 2001; 322:46.
45. Ball P. Quinolone-induced QT interval prolongation: a not-so-unexpected class effect. J Antimicrob Chemother 2000; 45:557.
46. Ball P, Mandell L, Niki Y, et al. Comparative tolerability of the newer fluoroquinolone antibacterials. Drug Saf 1999; 21:407.
47. Bertino JS Jr., Fish D. The safety profile of the fluoroquinolones. Clin Ther 2000; 22:798.
48. Anderson ME, Mazur A, Yang T, et al. Potassium current antagonist properties and proarrhythmic consequences of quinolone antibiotics. J Pharmacol Exp Ther 2001; 296:806.
49. Leone R, Venegoni M, Motola D, et al. Adverse drug reactions related to the use of fluoroquinolone antimicrobials: An analysis of spontaneous reports and fluoroquinolone consumption data from three Italian regions. Drug Saf 2003; 26:109.
50. Frothingham R. Ciprofloxacin associated with a much lower rate of torsades de pointes than levofloxacin, gatifloxacin, or moxifloxacin in the FDA spontaneous reporting database. In: Programs and Abstracts of the 45th Annual Interscience Conference on Antimicrobial Agents and Chemotherapy (Washington, DC). Am Soc Microbiol 2005; 392:L-589 (abstr).
51. Falagas ME, Rafailidis PI, Rosmarakis ES. Arrhythmias associated with fluoroquinolone therapy. Int J Antimicrob Agents 2007; 29:374.
52. Patmore L, Fraser S, Mair D, et al. Effects of sparfloxacin, grepafloxacin, moxifloxacin, and ciprofloxacin on cardiac action potential. Eur J Pharmacol 2000; 406:449.
53. Demolis J-L, Kubitza D, Tennezé L, et al. Effect of a single oral dose of moxifloxacin (400 mg and 800 mg) on ventricular repolarization in healthy subjects. Clin Pharmacol Ther 2000; 68:658.
54. Noel GJ, Natarajan J, Chien S, et al. Effects of three fluoroquinolones on QT interval in healthy adults after single doses. Clin Pharmacol Ther 2003; 73:292.
55. Noel GJ, Goodman DB, Chien S, et al. Measuring the effects of supratherapeutic doses of levofloxacin on healthy volunteers using four methods of QT correction and periodic and continuous ECG recordings. J Clin Pharmacol 2004; 44:464.
56. Makaryus AN, Byrns K, Makaryus MN, et al. Effect of ciprofloxacin and levofloxacin on the QT interval: is this a significant "clinical" event? South Med J 2006; 99:52.
57. Tsikouris JP, Peeters MJ, Cox CD, et al. Effects of three fluoroquinolones on QT analysis after standard treatment courses. Ann Noninvasive Electrocardiol 2006; 11:52.
58. Frothingham R. Rates of torsades de pointes associated with ciprofloxacin, ofloxacin, levofloxacin, gatifloxacin, and moxifloxacin. Pharmacother 2001; 21:1468.
59. Samaha FF. QTc interval prolongation and polymorphic ventricular tachycardia in association with levofloxacin. Am J Med 1999; 107:528.
60. Paltoo B, O'Donoghue S, Mousavi MS. Levofloxacin induced polymorphic ventricular tachycardia with normal QT interval. Pacing Clin Electrophysiol 2001; 21:895.
61. Gandhi PJ, Menezes PA, Vu HT, et al. Fluconazole- and levofloxacin-induced torsades de pointes in an intensive care unit patient. Am J Health Syst Pharm 2003; 60:2479.

62. Daya SK, Gowda RM, Khan IA. Ciprofloxacin- and hypocalcemia-induced torsade de pointes triggered by hemodialysis. Am J Ther 2004; 11:77.
63. Prabhakar M, Krahn AD. Ciprofloxacin-induced acquired long QT syndrome. Heart Rhythm 2004; 1:624.
64. Singh H, Kishore K, Gupta MS, et al. Ciprofloxacin-induced QTc prolongation. J Assoc Physicians India 2002; 50:430.
65. Amankwa K, Krishnan SC, Tisdale JE. Torsades de pointes associated with fluoroquinolones: importance of concomitant risk factors. Clin Pharmacol Ther 2004; 75:242.
66. Dumaine R, Roy M-L, Brown AM. Blockade of HERG and Kv1.5 by ketoconazole. J Pharmacol Exp Ther 1998; 286:727.
67. Philips JA, Marty FM, Stone RM, et al. Torsades de pointes associated with voriconazole use. Transpl Infect Dis 2007; 9:33.
68. Wharton JM, Demopulos PA, Goldschlager N. Torsade de pointes during administration of pentamidine isethionate. Am J Med 1987; 83:571.
69. Cordes JS, Sun Z, Lloyd DB, et al. Pentamidine reduces hERG expression to prolong the QT interval. Br J Pharmacol 2005; 145:15.
70. Katchman AN, Koerner J, Tosaka T, et al. Comparative evaluation of HERG currents and QT intervals following challenge with suspected torsadogenic and non-torsadogenic drugs. J Pharmacol Exp Ther 2006; 316:1098.
71. Eisenhauer MD, Eliasson AH, Taylor AJ, et al. Incidence of cardiac arrhythmias during intravenous pentamidine therapy in HIV-infected patients. Chest 1994; 105:389.
72. Traebert M, Dumotier B, Meister L, et al. Inhibition of hERG K+ currents by antimalarial drugs in stably transfected HEK293 cells. Eur J Pharmacol 2004; 484:41.
73. Touze JE, Heno P, Fourcade L, et al. The effects of antimalarial drugs on ventricular repolarization. Am J Trop Med Hyg 2002; 67:54,.
74. Weiner I, Rubin DA, Martinez E, et al. QT prolongation and paroxysmal ventricular tachycardia occurring during fever after trimethoprim-sulfamethoxazole administration. Mt Sinai J Med 1981; 48:53.
75. Lopez JA, et al. QT prolongation and torsade de pointes after administration of trimethoprim-sulfamethoxazole. Am J Cardiol 1987; 59:376.

7

Cardiotoxicity of Anthracyclines and Other Antineoplastic Agents

Jane Pruemer

University of Cincinnati College of Pharmacy, Cincinnati, Ohio, U.S.A.

INTRODUCTION

The treatment of malignant disease with antineoplastic agents has become more widespread with the availability of additional active drugs and treatment regimens. Adjuvant treatment programs attempting to eradicate microscopic disease are now commonplace for breast, colorectal, lung, osteosarcoma, and testicular tumors, and investigational in a number of other solid tumors. Neoadjuvant chemotherapy regimens preceding definitive local treatment are now used in the therapy of locally advanced breast cancer, osteosarcomas, head and neck tumors, and, in some cases, non–small cell lung cancer. Patients with advanced testicular tumors, small cell lung cancer, lymphomas, myeloma, and leukemias can experience prolonged survival and, in some cases, are cured with chemotherapy as the primary treatment. Many patients with metastatic and/or advanced disease will receive successful palliative treatment with antineoplastics. The gains of these treatment programs are not without risks of complications because of the toxic nature of the agents used. Late abnormalities of left ventricular performance have been reported in survivors of childhood cancers (1–6). Late cardiotoxicity has been observed in bone marrow transplant patients who received anthracyclines (7). Cardiac failure and dysrhythmias have occurred from 6 to 19 years after anthracycline therapy in some patients (8). Table 1 provides an overview of the cardiotoxicity of various antineoplastic agents.

Table 1 Cardiotoxicity of Antineoplastic Agents

Antitumor class/ drug	Toxicity	Comment
Antitumor antibiotics		
Anthracyclines		Mechanism: oxidative damage via lipid peroxidation; increased risk of cardiotoxicity with cumulative dosing >400 mg/m^2; dexrazoxane or liposomal formulation can reduce toxicity
Daunorubicin	Cardiomyopathy	
Doxorubicin	Myopericarditis	
Epirubicin	SVT	
Idarubicin	Ventricular ectopy	
Anthraquinones	CHF	Increased risk with cumulative dose >160 mg/m^2
Mitoxantrone	Arrhythmias	
Bleomycin	Pericarditis; myocardial ischemia/infarction	
Mitomycin	CHF	Increased risk with cumulative dose >30 mg/m^2
Topoisomerase inhibitors		
Etoposide	Vasospasm Myocardial ischemia/ infarction	Case reports only
Alkylating agents		
Cyclophosphamide	Heart block Tachyarrhythmias CHF Hemorrhagic myopericarditis	Mechanism: endothelial capillary damage; observed at doses >120–170 mg/kg; cardiac failure usually resolves over 3–4 wk and is treated with supportive care
Ifosfamide	Atrial ectopy Bradycardia CHF	Observed at doses >6.25–10 g/m^2
Cisplatin	Arrhythmias Heart block CHF Myocardial ischemia/ infarction	Mechanism may be related to drug-induced electrolyte abnormalities; von Willebrand's factor concentration can predict arterial occlusive events; vast majority of cardiac toxicity is seen in combination with chemotherapy
Busulfan	Endocardial fibrosis	Single autopsy finding
Microtubule-targeting drugs		
Vinca alkaloids	Myocardial ischemia/ infarction	Mechanism: vasoconstriction

Table 1 Cardiotoxicity of Antineoplastic Agents (*Continued*)

Antitumor class/ drug	Toxicity	Comment
Taxanes	Bradycardia/AV block Atrial and ventricular arrhythmias CHF Myocardial ischemia	Typically reversible; may potentiate anthracycline toxicity
Antimetobolites		
Fluorouracil	Cardiac failure Atrial or ventricular ectopy Myocardial ischemia/ infarction	Likely mechanism is coronary vasospasm; ischemic events more common when used in combination with cisplatin; β-blocker, calcium channel blocker, or nitrates may decrease risk
Capecitabine	Same as above	Not as well studied as infusional fluorouracil
Methotrexate	Arrhythmias Myocardial ischemia/ infarction	Case reports only
Fludarabine	Hypotension Angina	
Cytarabine	Angina Pericarditis with effusion	Corticosteroids seem to be beneficial for pericarditis
Biologic response modifiers		
Interferons	Atrial and ventricular arrhythmias AV block CHF Myocardial ischemia/ infarction	Toxicity is usually indirect and a result of altered cellular physiology; toxicity is typically reversible
Interleukin-2	CHF Arrhythmias Myocardial ischemia/ infarction	Toxicity related to capillary leak syndrome; decreased vascular resistance may not return for up to 6 days after discontinuation; treatment is supportive
Differentiation agents		
All-transretinoic acid	Myocardial ischemia/ infarction Pericardial effusion	Retinoic acid syndrome occurs in 10–15% of patients and may respond to corticosteroids
Arsenic trioxide	Prolonged QT torsades de pointes	Treatment is magnesium and potassium; these patients may also develop retinoic acid syndrome and are treated as above
Antibodies		
Trastuzumab	Cardiomyopathy Cardiac failure	Increased incidence when combined with chemotherapy, especially anthracyclines; toxicity is not dose related

(*Continued*)

Table 1 Cardiotoxicity of Antineoplastic Agents (*Continued*)

Antitumor class/ drug	Toxicity	Comment
Rituximab Bevacizumab	Arrhythmias Myocardial infarction, CVA	Few reported infusion-related deaths secondary to cardiogenic shock; risk factors: age >65 yr, prior myocardial infarction, CVA
Hormones Diethylstilbestrol	Vasospasm	Seen at doses ≥5 mg/day

Abbreviations: SVT, superficial venous thrombosis; CHF, congestive heart failure; AV, atrioventricular; CVA, cerebrovascular accident. *Source*: From Ref. 228.

The incidence and severity of cardiotoxicity of antineoplastic agents is dependent on several factors: (*i*) the type of drug, (*ii*) dose, (*iii*) schedule, (*iv*) age of patient, (*v*) presence of coexisting cardiac disease, and (*vi*) previous mediastinal irradiation. Patients who have been recognized to be at an increased risk of developing doxorubicin cardiotoxicity include the elderly, those with prior cardiac disease, children, and those who have had previous mediastinal irradiation (9–12).

This chapter is a review of the cardiotoxic effects of the commonly used anthracyclines, a discussion of possible mechanisms of action and prevention, as well as additional discussion of other antineoplastics with cardiotoxic effects.

ANTHRACYCLINES

Doxorubicin and Daunorubicin

The anthracyclines doxorubicin and daunorubicin are among the most widely used antineoplastics, with established response rates in leukemias as well as in a variety of solid tumors (13,14). Doxorubicin is active against lymphomas, gastric cancer, small cell lung cancer, sarcomas, and breast cancer. Daunorubicin has a more limited spectrum of activity, primarily being used in acute leukemias. Unfortunately, these agents have the most well-recognized cardiotoxic profile of cancer treatments.

Three distinct types of anthracycline-induced cardiotoxicity have been described. First, acute or subacute injury can occur immediately after treatment. This rare form of cardiotoxicity may cause transient arrhythmias (15,16), a pericarditis-myocarditis syndrome, or acute failure of the left ventricle (17). Second, anthracyclines can induce chronic cardiotoxicity that results in cardiomyopathy. This is a more common form of damage and is clinically the most important (18–20). Finally, late-onset ventricular dysfunction (10,21,22) and arrhythmias (4,23,24) that manifest years to decades after anthracycline treatment has been completed are increasingly recognized.

Electrocardiographic (EKG) changes noted in association with the administration of the anthracyclines include ST-T wave changes, sinus tachycardia, ventricular and atrial ectopy, atrial tachyarrhythmia, and low-voltage QRS complex (18,25,26). The most common EKG finding noted in studies using continuous EKG recording devices is ventricular ectopy (16,27). In general, EKG changes are reversible and of little clinical consequence; however, cardiac arrest, presumably due to a dysrhythmia, has been reported (28).

The more serious toxicity of the anthracyclines and their dose-limiting effect is a dose-dependent cardiomyopathy. The overall incidence of cardiomyopathy has ranged from 0.4% to 10%, with an associated mortality rate of 28% to 61% (9,25,29,30). On the basis of a number of studies, the onset of symptoms of congestive heart failure (CHF) following the last dose of anthracycline ranged from 2 days to 10.3 years (4,9,31). One study (25) reported a shorter median time (25 days) to CHF in fatal cases than in nonfatal cases (56 days). However, more recent data suggest that the incidence of cardiomyopathy may be higher and may occur even years after treatment and at a much lower cumulative dose (11,32). Part of this increase may be explained by increased awareness of cardiotoxicity with improved screening as well as better long-term survival, especially in the pediatric population. The definition of cardiotoxicity has expanded beyond the clinical events of cardiac failure and now includes predefined laboratory values, such as left ventricular ejection fraction (LVEF) based on radionuclide ventriculography or two-dimensional echocardiography, even when patients are asymptomomatic.

As opposed to the adult population in whom the majority of clinical cardiotoxicity events appear to develop within the first year of treatment, childhood cancer survivors who have received anthracycline-based chemotherapy remain at risk for developing cardiomyopathy even years later (10). In their analysis of 201 long-term survivors of pediatric malignancies, abnormal cardiac systolic function (defined by echocardiography) was detected in almost 25% of the patients 4 to 20 years after completion of the anthracycline treatment. The frequency of subclinical cardiotoxicity in published data varies from 0% to 57%, while the rate of clinical cardiac failure is 0% to 16% (1,2). Other than cumulative anthracycline dose and mediastinal irradiation, which are recognized risks in adults, age at diagnosis and female gender have also been shown to be independent risk factors for the development of cardiomyopathy in the pediatric population (33).

Risk factors for the development of anthracycline cardiomyopathy have been identified. For both doxorubicin and daunorubicin, a dose-response relationship exists between the total dose of anthracycline and the development of CHF. Initial studies reporting doxorubicin cardiotoxicity identified a dose of 600 mg/m^2 as the cardiotoxic threshold above which CHF was more likely to occur (34,35). In large retrospective reviews of over 4000 patients, Von Hoff and colleagues identified an increasing probability of developing CHF as the dose of the anthracycline was increased. The cumulative probability of developing CHF

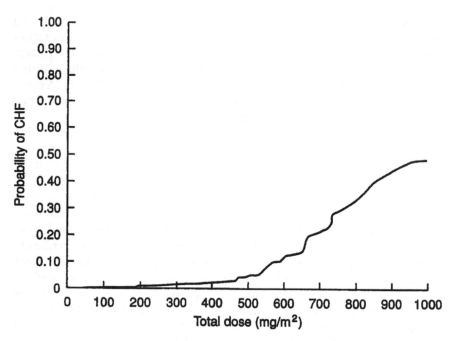

Figure 1 Cumulative probability of developing doxorubicin-induced CHF versus total cumulative dose of doxorubicin in 3941 patients receiving doxorubicin. *Abbreviation*: CHF, congestive heart failure. *Source*: From Ref. 9.

with doxorubicin was 3% at 400 mg/m^2 and 7% at 550 mg/m^2. The greatest increase in the slope of the curve was noted at the 550-mg/m^2 total dose level (9) (Fig. 1). The majority of patients developed cardiomyopathy within the first year of completion of treatment and had a mortality rate of greater than 40%. For daunorubicin, the incidence of CHF at 600 mg/m^2 was 1.5%, with an increase to 12% at a total dose of 1000 mg/m^2 (18). More recently, a study of escalating doses of doxorubicin in patients with advanced breast cancer noted significant decreases in left ventricular function by radionuclide multigated blood pool scans (MUGA) at a mean dose of 459 mg/m^2 (SD + 165 mg/m^2) (36). These data continue to support an approximate dose of 550 mg/m^2 as a threshold for increased risk for the development of cardiotoxicity, as identified by Von Hoff and colleagues.

The Early Breast Cancer Trialists' Collaborative Group conducted a meta-analysis of 40 randomized studies comparing surgery alone versus surgery plus adjuvant radiotherapy in women with breast cancer (12). They found the majority of non–breast cancer-related deaths were due to cardiovascular mortality secondary to the effects of irradiation in the heart and the great vessels. This occurred with old treatment techniques. In contrast, the Danish Breast

Cancer Cooperative Group used modern techniques that minimized the degree of radiation exposure to the heart (37).

The schedule of doxorubicin administration has been shown to influence the incidence of both drug-induced noncardiac as well as cardiotoxicity. Multiple studies have shown that weekly administration or prolonged infusions of doxorubicin decrease the incidence of drug-induced cardiomyopathy without sacrificing efficacy (38–42). Other risk factors frequently associated with the development of anthracycline-induced CHF include advanced age of the patient (9,43), preexisting cardiac disease (25,35), prior mediastinal radiation (25,35,44), and concomitant administration of other cytotoxic agents (25,26,45–48). Prospective evaluation of cardiac function during treatment with anthracyclines has become standard practice. Noninvasive methods in use include serial EKGs for change in QRS voltage (49), rest and exercise radionuclide angiography for measurement of LVEF (50–52), exercise and Doppler echocardiographic analysis of left ventricular function (53–55), and QRS-Korotkoff interval (56).

The gold standard for measurement of cardiac damage due to anthracyclines is endomyocardial biopsy with the designated pathologic changes, rated 1 to 3, correlating with the degree of toxicity. A pathologic score of zero denotes no changes; 1 denotes early myofibrillar dropout and/or swelling of the sarcoplasmic reticulum; 2 reveals progressive myofibrillar dropout with cytoplasmic vacuolization, or both; and 3 reveals diffuse myocyte damage with marked cellular changes in mitochondria, nuclei, and sarcoplasmic reticulum and cell necrosis (57). Despite some evidence of lack of correlation between cardiac biopsy scores and radionuclide measurement of LVEF, of the noninvasive methods radionuclide angiography appears to be the most practical and reliable method of serial assessment of cardiac function (58,59). Recommendations for discontinuation of anthracycline therapy include ejection fractions (EFs) less than 45% at rest, failure to increase the EF with exercise, or greater than 10% decrease from a normal pretreatment level (52,60,61).

The actual mechanism of anthracycline cardiotoxicity remains elusive. No single theory adequately explains or integrates our current understanding of the clinical, biochemical, and molecular effects of these agents on cardiac structure and function. Similarly, the cytotoxicity of the anthracyclines has undergone extensive scrutiny over the years. A variety of biochemical effects are known, including inhibition of nucleic acid metabolism as a result of intercalation with DNA, chelation of transition metal ions, participation in oxidation-reduction reactions, and binding to cell membranes (62–64). Unfortunately, the precise mechanism of the cytotoxic action of anthracyclines has yet to be defined. There is emerging evidence, however, that the cytotoxic/antitumor effect may be related to the activation of topoisomerase II-mediated DNA cleavage rather than the DNA intercalation itself (65). The ultrastructural changes seen with anthracycline therapy are well documented and reproducible in a variety of laboratory animals as well as in humans (66–69). As mentioned earlier, these changes reveal several cellular abnormalities linking myofibrillar loss and cytoplasmic vacuolization due to swelling of the sarcotubular system, structural abnormalities in the mitochondria with deposits of electron-dense bodies, and increased numbers of lysosomes (17,70).

Multiple researchers have attempted to explain the ultrastructural changes seen in myocardial cells after treatment with anthracyclines in terms of a unifying theory of action. There are several leading hypotheses of anthracycline cardiotoxicity. These include (*i*) free radical formation with subsequent membrane damage and interference with energy metabolism; (*ii*) interference with calcium metabolism; (*iii*) the effect of histamine and other catecholamines; and (*iv*) toxicity due to a cardiotoxic metabolite.

Free radical formation by doxorubicin and the resulting cardiac DNA and membrane damage have been extensively studied and considered critical in the evolution of anthracycline-induced cardiotoxicity (67,71,72). The quinone-containing anthracyclines (doxorubicin, daunorubicin, epirubicin) were first noted to produce free radicals in the mid-1970s. Under aerobic conditions such as those in the myocardium, the quinone can be reduced to a free radical (semiquinone) by several electron-donating enzyme systems, such as NADPH and cytochrome P450 reductase and NADH dehydrogenase. The semiquinone free radicals subsequently react with molecular oxygen to form superoxide, hydrogen peroxide, and hydroxyl radicals and, in turn, result in lipid peroxidation of cell membranes with continued generation of additional free radicals. Interaction with and damage to the cell membrane then influences cell permeability and function. The generation of these free radicals with accumulation of lipid peroxides is well documented (67,73). In addition, it is clear that free radical formation occurs at a variety of sites including the cytosol, mitochondria, and sarcoplasmic reticulum and possibly explains the ultrastructural lesions commonly seen (74). Free radicals also impair sequestration of calcium by the sarcoplasmic reticulum and ultimately may result in decreased calcium stores, resulting in impaired contractility and relaxation of cardiac muscle (75,76). Increased calcium influx and myocardial calcium content have also been described in treatment with doxorubicin (70,77). Free radicals may also be generated by nonenzymatic reactions of iron with doxorubicin with similar consequences. Although little free iron is present within the myocardium, there is evidence that doxorubicin can abstract iron from ferritin (78). Interference with calcium metabolism may be a direct result of effects on cellular membranes rather than on the inciting event in anthracycline-induced cardiotoxicity. Early on, it was thought that increased levels of intracellular calcium were responsible for mitochondria dysfunction, with resultant depletion of high-energy phosphate stores and contractile dysfunction. The electron-dense bodies seen in mitochondria were found to contain calcium (79). Accumulation of calcium was well documented in vivo in mitochondria in a variety of organs in the rabbit treated with chronic administration of doxorubicin (70,80). Recent data, however, point more toward an initial deficiency of intracellular calcium and its resultant effects on calcium flux and muscle contraction (81). Studies with combinations of calcium channel–blocking drugs thought to prevent calcium accumulation with anthracycline treatment have provided conflicting data regarding their influence on cardiotoxic effects (82–84).

Another theory of anthracycline cardiotoxicity revolves around the involvement of histamine and other vasoactive substances as causative agents. Support for this theory comes from experiments examining histopathologic lesions produced in rabbits after histamine infusions, which were found to be similar to doxorubicin-induced lesions (85). These same authors were able to show that histamine release was stimulated in vitro by doxorubicin. Additional studies by others have supported these findings as well as documented prevention of histamine release with the use of inhibitors such as theophylline and disodium cromoglycate and with the free radical scavenger *N*-acetylcysteine (NAC), which was also found to inhibit the release of histamine (86). Klugman and colleagues also noted the absence of typical histopathologic cardiac lesions in the animals treated with the inhibitors.

The possibility of a metabolite of doxorubicin as the offending cardiotoxic agent has also been previously suggested (87–89). Olson and colleagues compared the in vitro cardiotoxic effects of doxorubicin and doxorubicinol, the carbon-13 alcohol metabolite of doxorubicin. In their study, doxorubicinol was found to be a more potent inhibitor of contractile function, of membrane-associated ion pumps, and greatly decreased calcium loading within the sarcoplasmic reticulum vesicles. In addition, the authors noted intracardiac conversion of doxorubicin to doxorubicinol, further supporting previous evidence of accumulation in cardiac tissue in a time-dependent fashion (87,90). Of interest, these authors found that doxorubicin maintained greater cytotoxicity in three pancreatic adenocarcinoma cell lines over the metabolite, suggesting separation of cytotoxic and cardiotoxic effects.

Cardioprotectants

Perhaps one of the more enlightening aspects providing some insight into mechanisms of cardiotoxicity has been the various agents tested to prevent cardiotoxicity. These agents include coenzyme Q (CoQ 10) (91), NAC (92), prenylamine (93), and the bispiperazinedione ICRF-187 (94), which is now known as dexrazoxane and is Food and Drug Administration (FDA) approved for the prevention of anthracylcine-induced cardiotoxicity. Inhibition of CoQ 10, a mitochondrial enzyme involved in oxidative phosphorylation, results in cardiac lesions in the rat similar to those seen with doxorubicin cardiotoxicity (95). Investigators described the prevention of experimental cardiotoxicity by doxorubicin with the addition of CoQ 10 (ubiquinone) in the isolated rabbit heart model (96). These same investigators administered ubiquinone to rabbits and were able to demonstrate prevention of doxorubicin cardiotoxicity in vivo (97). More recently, CoQ 10 has been studied for its therapeutic effect in dilated cardiomyopathy, with evidence of efficacy (98). Prenylamine is a calcium channel–blocking agent that has undergone investigation in Argentina. After obtaining laboratory evidence of cardioprotection in animals, investigators proceeded with a small randomized trial in patients (93,99). Cardiotoxicity as evidenced by congestive cardiomyopathy and supraventricular dysrhythmia was seen in the untreated patients. There were no cardiac events in the group treated with prenylamine. As mentioned earlier, other studies have not revealed a benefit with the use of other calcium channel blockers.

NAC is a sulfhydryl compound shown, in mice, to confer cardiac protection from doxorubicin treatment theoretically through increased sulfhydryl content in the heart (92). However, when a randomized trial with the oral form was conducted in cancer patients, treatment with NAC did not confer significant cardioprotection (100). Of all these agents, only dexrazoxane has been studied in a randomized, prospective fashion and has shown consistent evidence of modulating cardiotoxicity due to anthracyclines (94).

Dexrazoxane (Zinecard™)

Dexrazoxane, previously known as ICRF-187, is an iron-chelating agent whose chelating properties were first noted during phase I testing of the compound as an antineoplastic agent (101). It is a bisdioxopiperazine compound that hydrolyzes to an open ring form, which in turn chelates intracellular iron generated by doxorubicin, thereby inhibiting the subsequent production of free radicals responsible for the cardiac damage. Anthracycline cardiotoxicity is thought to be prevented by the binding of dexrazoxane to ferrous ions at intracellular sites that would normally complex with doxorubicin. It is the iron-doxorubicin complex that is thought to be responsible for the generation of free radicals, with the subsequent cascade of events leading to cardiac damage (67,102).

Dexrazoxane was studied extensively in women with advanced breast cancer receiving doxorubicin as well as epirubicin therapy (94,103,104). Dexrazoxane has a significant cardioprotectant effect, as measured by non-invasive testing and clinical CHF when given with doxorubicin, but has been implicated in causing a lower response rate than doxorubicin alone (104). For this reason, many clinicians are reluctant to use this agent in patients who are responding to anthracycline therapy. The FDA has approved the agent for use in women with metastatic breast cancer who have previously received a total of 300 mg/m^2 of doxorubicin and who are continuing to respond to therapy. It is not approved for use in the adjuvant treatment of breast cancer. Dexrazoxane has also been studied in the prevention of cardiotoxicity associated with epirubicin (105). In summary, there are several theories of the mechanism of anthracycline cardiotoxicity without an all-encompassing theory to explain the myriad properties and effects of this class of antineoplastic agent. Further investigation and elucidation are required and are ongoing. Dexrazoxane continues to show promise as a clinically useful agent in the prevention of doxorubicin cardiotoxicity.

Liposomal Doxorubicin, Pegylated Liposomal Doxorubicin, and Liposomal Daunorubicin

The rationale of encapsulating doxorubicin within liposomes is to allow the sequestration of the drug from organs, such as the heart and gastrointestinal tract, which have tight capillary junctions, while enhancing delivery of the cytotoxic agent to tumor sites lined by compromised vasculature. Liposomal production of doxorubicin results in a prolongation of the plasma half-life and alteration in its tissue distribution. Doxorubicin has been administered to patients in a liposome-encapsulated form with a suggestion of less cardiotoxicity, as determined by radionuclide EF and, in a few patients, Billingham score on endomyocardial biopsy (106,107). Liposomal doxorubicin has been studied extensively in the treatment of acquired immunodeficiency syndrome (AIDS)-associated Kaposi's sarcoma (108,109), as well as in the treatment of refractory ovarian cancer.

One form of liposomal doxorubicin was found to produce a significantly reduced cardiotoxicity rate (defined both clinically and on radionuclide veno-cardiography scan) at 6% compared with 21% for doxorubicin, while maintaining comparable tumor response (110). Another study of this compound compared with doxorubicin as single agent in 244 women with metastatic breast cancer resulted in cardiotoxicity in 2% of those in the liposomal doxorubicin arm versus 8% in the doxorubicin arm (111). In a phase III trial of 509 women with metastatic breast cancer, pegylated liposomal doxorubicin resulted in 11% cardiac events versus 40% for conventional doxorubicin at a cumulative dose of greater than 500 to 550 mg/m^2 (112). Liposomal daunorubicin is approved for the treatment of human immunodeficiency virus (HIV)-associated Kaposi's sarcoma with similar potential for cardiac effects.

Anthracycline Analogs

Over 1000 anthracycline derivatives have been synthesized with the hope of retaining therapeutic efficacy with less toxicity of both myelosuppression and cardiotoxicity (113). Studies of correlations between structure and activity demonstrate that changes at the 4 position of the amino sugar moiety affect toxicity and indicate that cardiotoxicity can be separated from therapeutic effect (114). Only compounds with cytotoxicity that preclinically is at least equal to doxorubicin are then tested further to ascertain their toxicity profile. Determining whether these analogs are beneficial and less toxic than doxorubicin continues to be an active area of investigation. The following briefly reviews the cardiotoxicity seen with several of the compounds in clinical use or undergoing clinical evaluation (Fig. 2).

Esorubicin (Deoxydoxorubicin)

Esorubicin is an anthracycline analog synthesized by the removal of the hydroxyl group from the 4 carbon of the sugar moiety of the parent compound

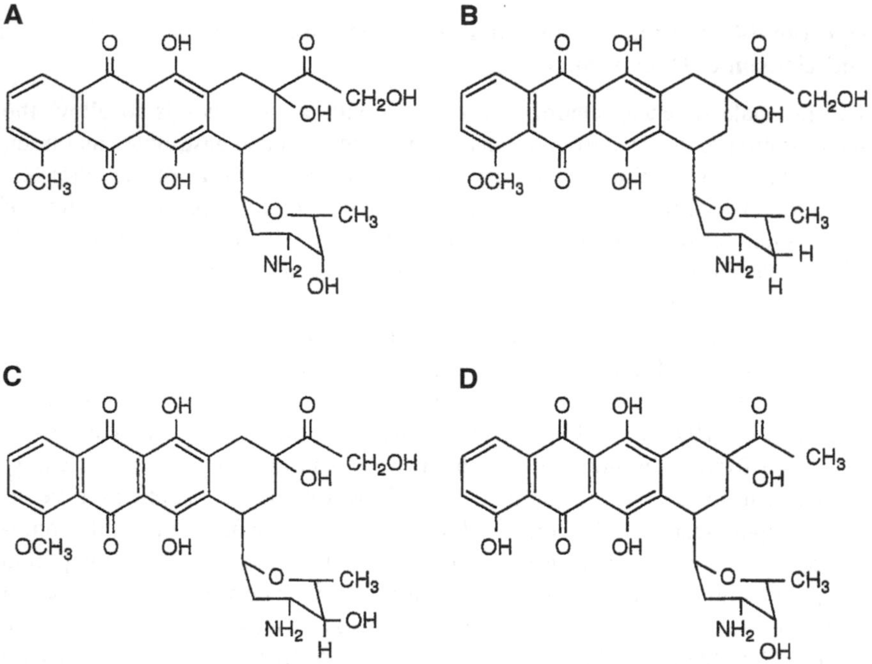

A

B

C

D

Figure 2 Anthracyclines. (**A**) Doxorubicin. (**B**) Epirubicin. (**C**) Esorubicin. (**D**) Idarubicin.

doxorubicin. Recent follow-up of 136 patients treated with esorubicin on one of two Cancer and Leukemia Group B (CALGB) phase II protocols has been reported (115). Serial MUGA scans were obtained in 36 of 44 patients who received more than four cycles of therapy. Decreases in LVEF of more than 5% were noted at doses of 240 mg/m^2 and of more than 10% at doses of 480 mg/m^2. Overall, cardiotoxicity was observed in 11 patients (8%) without previous anthracycline or history of cardiovascular disease. The cardiotoxicity described included overt CHF asymptomatic decreases in LVEF, sinus tachycardia, and one myocardial infarction.

Epirubicin

Epirubicin is a stereoisomer of doxorubicin with a different configuration of the hydroxyl group in the 4 position of the sugar moiety. It was introduced into clinical practice in the 1980s. Cardiotoxicity similar in scope to that reported for doxorubicin has been reported with epirubicin. In two studies of patients with advanced breast cancer without prior treatment with an anthracycline, CHF was reported in four patients who received cumulative doses of epirubicin greater that 1000 mg/m^2 (116) and in one patient who received a total dose of 797 mg/m^2 (117).

There have been several studies reported that have included endomyocardial biopsies as part of the evaluation documenting cardiotoxicity due to epirubicin (118–120). In all these studies, the type and severity of histologic abnormalities were similar to those seen with doxorubicin and correlated with increasing doses of epirubicin. Dardir and colleagues noted a statistically significant correlation ($p = 0.0006$) between the total dose of epirubicin and pathologic changes quantified by the use of the Billingham scale (100). In one study, doses smaller than 500 mg/m^2 were not associated with cardiotoxicity. However, at doses of 500 to 1000 mg/m^2, 2% of the patients developed CHF, with an increase to 35% of the patients developing CHF at cumulative doses greater than 1000 mg/m^2 (101). A similar degree of clinical cardiotoxicity was reported at cumulative doses of 900 to 1000 mg/m^2 (121). Nair and colleagues evaluated the efficacy and toxicity of epirubicin and doxorubicin in 211 patients with non-Hodgkin's lymphoma. In their study, the maximum dose of epirubicin was 480 mg/m^2 (75 mg/m^2 per dose) and that of doxorubicin was 300 mg/m^2 (50 mg/m^2 per dose). The MUGA scan indicated a similar reduction in the global EF, peak ejection, and peak flow rates in the two arms. Thus, epirubicin was found to have the same cardiotoxicity at the subclinical level as doxorubicin (122). This was supported by a retrospective analysis of epirubicin cardiotoxicity in 469 patients with metastatic breast cancer (123). This analysis confirmed a significantly increasing risk of CHF in patients who receive cumulative doses greater than 950 mg/m^2 of epirubicin.

In a study comparing FAC (fluorouracil, doxorubicin, cyclophosphamide) with FEC (fluorouracil, epirubicin, cyclphosphamide) in women with advanced breast cancer, the Italian Multicentre Breast Study Group found the mean reduction in LVEF was 6.6% in the epirubicin arm compared with 17.6% in the doxorubicin arm (124).

Idarubicin (4-Demethoxydaunorubicin)

Idarubicin differs from the parent compound doxorubicin in substitution of the C-4 methoxyl group with a hydrogen atom. During phase I testing with the agents, the significant cardiotoxicity described was limited to patients who had received previous treatment with anthracyclines. Therefore, postulating a direct cause and effect was not possible (125–127). The cardiotoxicity described ranged from asymptomatic EKG changes to overt CHF requiring therapy and discontinuation of the idarubicin. In phase II studies, decreases in LVEF without clinical signs of cardiac failure were seen infrequently and were limited to patients who had received prior anthracyclines (128–132). In these studies, cumulative doses of 800 mg/m^2 orally and 169 mg/m^2 intravenously were tolerated without signs of clinical CHF. Anderlini and colleagues performed a retrospective review of idarubicin cardiotoxicity in patients with acute myeloid leukemia or myelodysplasia. They analyzed a group of 127 patients who received idarubicin-based induction and postremission or salvage therapy and who achieved a complete remission. They determined that the probability of idarubicin-related cardiomyopathy was 5% at a cumulative idarubicin dose of 150 to 290 mg/m^2 and that cardiomyopathy was uncommon with cumulative doses greater than this (133).

Mitoxantrone (Novantrone^{TM})

Mitoxantrone, a substituted anthraquinone, was developed in an attempt to achieve similar antitumor activity to the anthracyclines but with less toxicity. Despite modifications, mitoxantrone has been reported to have cardiac effects, although on a lesser scale than the anthracyclines. Described cardiotoxicity includes decreases in LVEF and CHF (134). Dysrhythmias have been noted infrequently (135). In a large series including a randomized study comparing cyclophosphamide, doxorubicin, and 5-fluorouracil (5-FU) with cyclophosphamide, mitoxantrone, and 5-FU in patients with metastatic breast cancer, the incidence of CHF was less than 2% (125,136,137). The majority of patients experiencing CHF have received more than 120 mg/m^2 of mitoxantrone, but similar toxicity has been reported at lower doses in patients both with and without prior exposure to an anthracycline (126,138,139). Treatment of CHF related to mitoxantrone therapy usually responds to management with digoxin, diuretics, and discontinuation of mitoxantrone, with the possibility of eventual return to a baseline cardiac status (129). A small number of endomyocardial biopsies have been carried out and revealed changes consistent with anthracycline-induced cardiomyopathy (140,141).

Predisposing factors to mitoxantrone cardiotoxicity include prior anthracycline therapy, mediastinal irradiation, and prior cardiovascular disease; prior anthracycline therapy is the most important factor (142). In patients previously treated with anthracyclines, the incidence of CHF is negligible up to doses of 100 mg/m^2. In patients without previous treatment with anthracyclines, doses up to 160 mg/m^2 appear to be tolerated without significant cardiotoxicity (143). Careful monitoring of cardiac EF at cumulative doses greater than 100 mg/m^2 is recommended, especially in those at risk for development of cardiotoxicity. Toxicology studies performed in beagle dogs did not reveal clinical manifestations of CHF or EKG changes (144). Abnormalities on endomyocardial biopsies in dogs were limited to dilatation of the sarcoplasmic reticulum (145). In one study, mitoxantrone was shown to be an antioxidant inhibiting both basal and drug-induced peroxidation of lipids (146). It follows that as lipid peroxidation is important in the development of cardiotoxicity of anthracyclines and anthracycline-like drugs, mitoxantrone theoretically has the potential for causing less cardiotoxicity. To date, this has also been shown to be the case clinically.

OTHER ANTITUMOR AGENTS

Arsenic Trioxide

Currently approved for the treatment of acute promyelocytic leukemia, arsenic trioxide is an agent that induces differentiation. Patients treated in clinical trials with arsenic trioxide have been reported to develop prolongation of the QT interval as well as torsades de points (147–150). Arsenic-induced arrhthymias may best be managed with the use of parenteral potassium and magnesium, maintaining high normal levels. Patients receiving this agent should be closely monitored with serial EKGs and serum electrolytes.

Cyclophosphamide

Severe hemorrhagic cardiac necrosis has been reported in the transplant setting at doses of 120 to 240 mg/kg given over one to four days (151–153). The presenting symptoms are tachycardia and refractory CHF. EKG changes reveal sinus tachycardia, low-voltage QRS complex, ST segment elevation, and non-specific ST–T wave changes. Left ventricular systolic function, as assessed by echocardiographic fractional shortening, has been shown to be significantly decreased from baseline in patients with and without clinical symptoms of heart failure (154). Significant increases in lactate dehydrogenase (LDH) and creatine phosphokinase (CPK) suggesting myocardial damage are seen in approximately one-half of the patients. Symptoms of cardiac necrosis may not become evident until two weeks after dosing, but are rapidly fatal when present (155). Pathologic findings at autopsy include dilated heart, patchy transmural hemorrhages, focal areas of fibrinous pericarditis, and myocardial necrosis, and interstitial lesions consisting of hemorrhage, edema, and fibrin deposition (141,142). There are emerging data that the intracellular thiol glutathione may play a role in the protection against cardiac injury caused by cyclophosphamide (156).

There is some evidence that cyclophosphamide in combination with other agents, particularly bischloroethylnitrosourea (BCNU), 6-thioguanine, cytosine arabinoside (Ara-C), and total body irradiation, may be more cardiotoxic than cyclophosphamide alone (157). In one study, 4 of 15 patients died of acute myopericarditis after using the combination of BCNU, cyclophosphamide, 6-thioguanine, and Ara-C (138). Another study reported a 9% incidence of fatal cardiomyopathy and/or pericarditis with this same combination or high-dose cyclophosphamide and total body irradiation (158). An additional 22% of patients experienced nonfatal CHF. The majority of patients in each of these studies had received prior anthracyclines, possibly compounding their risk of developing cardiotoxicity from these regimens. A more recent study has evaluated the cardiotoxicity of cyclophosphamide in a twice-daily higher dose compared with a lower daily-dose schedule (159). LVEFs did not change significantly in either group; however, four of the five patients who developed clinical cardiotoxicity (four pericarditis and one CHF) were in the higher-dose group. The conclusion of the authors was that the twice-daily dosing schedule, although not completely without cardiotoxicity, resulted in less ventricular dysfunction. As more experience is gained in bone marrow transplantation, it will be important to identify regimens and dosing schedules that allow for efficacy without excessive toxicity.

Cisplatin

Cisplatin, a bifunctional alkylating agent with a broad spectrum of activity, is associated with rare reports of cardiotoxicity. Cisplatin-induced bradycardia (160) and paroxysmal supraventricular tachycardia have also been reported (161,162). Ischemic vascular events with myocardial infarctions in young patients with and without mediastinal radiation who were treated with cisplatin-based combination chemotherapy are among the most serious toxicities reported with the agent (163,164). Coronary artery spasm was documented in one patient at cardiac catheterization in the absence of atherosclerotic disease. Two cases of severe coronary artery atherosclerosis and one case of fibrous intimal proliferation in young males with testicular cancer after cisplatin-based chemotherapy have been documented (165,166). None of the patients were considered to have had significant risk factors for coronary artery disease; only one patient had received thoracic irradiation.

5-Fluorouracil

The reported incidence of cardiac side effects with 5-FU, a widely used antimetabolite, is low at approximately 1.6% (167). However, with high-dose continuous infusion 5-FU, the incidence has been reported to be as high as 7.6% (168). Angina with ischemic EKG changes is the most frequent cardiotoxicity noted (169). The first reports of chest pain associated with ischemic EKG changes in patients receiving 5-FU occurred in 1975. All three patients failed to have subsequent evidence of a myocardial infarction; EKG abnormalities resolved with discontinuation of the drug (170). Ischemic EKG changes, left ventricular dysfunction, and hypotension with dyspnea associated with infusions of 5-FU alone and in combination with cisplatin have been reported previously (171,172). Severe but reversible heart failure with global hypokinesis and cardiogenic shock has been reported in association with continuous infusions of 5-FU (173–175). Extensive cardiac evaluations have been performed in a small number of these patients without documentation of significant coronary artery disease or clear evidence of vasospasm (155–157,176,177). The episodes of severe heart failure and cardiogenic shock resolved with aggressive support following discontinuation of the 5-FU infusion in most reported cases. Conflicting evidence exists regarding the efficacy of nitrates and/or calcium channel–blocking agents in preventing anginal episodes, which suggests that mechanisms other than coronary vasospasm may be involved in the cardiac effects of 5-FU (178–180). Myocardial infarctions have been reported in a small number of patients as well as deaths in patients refractory to supportive therapy (157–159,167). The mechanism by which 5-FU causes cardiotoxicity is unknown. Possible etiologies include vasospasm, a direct cardiotoxic effect either from 5-FU or one of its metabolites, or some other metabolic derangement, leading to either an increase in metabolic demands or a decrease in the available energy to meet those demands. Comparisons have been made to the "stunned myocardium," a syndrome of reversible postischemic ventricular dysfunction (181). Few animal data exist to support any particular theory at the present time. There is laboratory evidence of persistent radioactivity in the myocardium of mice injected with 14C-labeled 5-FU 96 hours after injection, suggesting delayed metabolism in the heart (182). In addition, both the pharmacokinetics and the toxicity profiles of oral, bolus intravenous, and prolonged intravenous administration of 5-FU are known to differ. Lower but sustained plasma levels and less myelosuppression and greater mucositis are noted with the prolonged infusion (183). These differences may ultimately provide insight into the mechanism of 5-FU cardiotoxicity.

Today, 5-FU is often combined with leucovorin (folinic acid) in an effort to improve its antitumor effect. Grandi and colleagues have reported a non-invasive evaluation of the cardiotoxicity of this combination in patients with colorectal cancer. They evaluated blood pressure, EKG, and two-dimensional and digitized M-mode echocardiograms before and after several doses and cycles of the combination. They concluded that 5-FU and low-dose folinic acid treatment induced a decrease of left ventricular systolic function and an impairment of diastolic function, which developed without symptoms and were transient and reversible (184).

Cytosine Arabinoside

Cytarabine, a nucleoside analog effective in treating acute leukemia, rarely causes cardiotoxicity. There are, however, case reports of a cardiac dysrhythmia (185) and acute pericarditis (186) encountered during high-dose therapy. At the time of the pericarditis, the patient was in complete clinical remission from acute lymphocytic leukemia. Pericardial fluid analysis was negative for tumor or an infectious agent. No evidence of myocardial damage either clinically or by laboratory studies was noted during the episode of pericarditis.

Imatinib (Gleevec™)

Imatinib mesylate is a small molecule inhibitor of the fusion protein Bcr-Abl, the causal agent in chronic myelogenous leukemia. Severe CHF and left ventricular dysfunction have been reported in patients taking imatinib. In an international randomized phase III study in over 1000 patients with newly diagnosed chronic myelogenous leukemia in chronic phase, cardiotoxicity was observed in 0.7% of patients taking imatinib (187). Patients with increased age, cardiac disease, or risk factors for cardiac failure should be monitored carefully while receiving imatinib. Ten patients have been reported who developed severe CHF while on imatinib (188). Transmission electron micrographs showed mitochondrial abnormalities and accumulation of membrane whorls in both vacuoles and the endoplasmic reticulum.

Taxanes: Paclitaxel (Taxol™) and Docetaxel (Taxotere™)

As single agents, paclitaxel and docetaxel have negligible cardiotoxicity when compared with the anthracyclines. Paclitaxel, a taxane derived from the Pacific yew tree, has become a major agent in the treatment of breast cancer, ovarian cancer, and non–small cell lung cancer. In the early clinical development of paclitaxel, the drug was recognized to have a unique toxicity profile. In addition to the more routine side effects observed with antineoplastic agents (bone marrow suppression, alopecia, etc.), hypersensitivity reactions were observed. Patients were also found to develop cardiac arrhythmia, particularly bradycardia, and episodes of sudden cardiac death were reported (189–192).

In a retrospective review of gynecologic cancer patients treated with paclitaxel, with or without a platinum agent, Markman and colleagues found 15 patients had major cardiac risk factors before therapy. These risk factors included preexisting CHF, severe coronary artery disease, angina, and patients who were being treated for rhythm disturbances with agents such as β-blockers. There was no deterioration in cardiac function observed in these patients subsequent to paclitaxel therapy (193). It is now recognized that much of the initial concern for the cardiac effects of paclitaxel were related to severe hypersensitivity reactions and that with appropriate premedication patients are unlikely to experience these dysrhythmias. Early phase II studies confirmed that a combination of paclitaxel and anthracyclines resulted in an unacceptably high incidence of CHF in greater than 20% of patients. In the doxorubicin plus paclitaxel trials of Gianni et al. (194) and Gehl et al. (195), an alarming incidence of cardiac dysfunction and clinical CHF (about 20%) was observed. However, in the randomized phase II trial of Sledge et al. (196), there was no increased incidence of cardiotoxicity in the group of patients receiving doxorubicin plus paclitaxel compared with the group receiving doxorubicin alone. It should be noted that the combination of doxorubicin plus paclitaxel used by Sledge et al. (196) differed from that used by both Gianni et al. (194) and Gehl et al. (195) with regard to dose, duration of administration, interval between administration of doxorubicin and paclitaxel, and dose of doxorubicin. Subsequently, Gianni et al. (197) studied the pharmacokinetic interference between paclitaxel and doxorubicin, which results in nonlinear doxorubicin plasma disposition and increased concentrations of doxorubicin and its metabolite doxorubicinol. Therefore, it is believed that the exposure of the patients to higher concentrations of doxorubicin could be responsible for the increased cardiotoxicity when given with paclitaxel. There was an increase in total doxorubicin plasma exposure by 30% when the paclitaxel infusion immediately followed doxorubicin, compared with a delay of 24 hours between the two infusions. Similarly, doxorubicin clearance is also reduced by one-third when the paclitaxel infusion precedes doxorubicin.

Trastuzumab (Herceptin™)

Trastuzumab is a recombinant, humanized monoclonal antibody against human epidermal growth factor recept-2 (HER-2) protein. HER-2 protein is overexpressed in about one-third of breast cancers (198). The pivotal trial showed that trastuzumab combined with chemotherapy for patients with HER-2–positive metastatic breast cancer resulted in a significant increase in response rate but an unexpected disproportionate percentage of patients (27%) developed cardiotoxicity. There were 16% who had New York Heart Association (NYHA) class III or class IV heart failure compared with 3% in the single-agent anthracycline arm (199). Cardiotoxicity also occurred in 13% of the trastuzumab plus paclitaxel arm compared with only 1% in the paclitaxel alone arm. An additional retrospective review of seven phase I and phase II trials using trastuzumab confirmed the additive cardiotoxicity with anthracyclines (200). Trastuzumab, as a single agent, is associated with a cardiotoxicity rate of 3% to 7% and does not appear to be dependent on either cumulative dose or treatment duration.

The pathogenesis of trastuzumab cardiotoxicity has been proposed to include immune-mediated toxicity, drug-drug interaction, and direct toxicity. It is postulated that the mechanism for recovery of cardiac damage induced by anthracyclines may be impaired by trastuzumab.

Amsacrine

This drug is an acridine orange derivative with documented activity in acute leukemia and lymphoma. Reported cardiotoxicity with this agent has included dysrhythmias (201–203), ventricular dysfunction (204), and acute myocardial necrosis (205), although the last effect occurred after administration of multiple drugs and in the setting of progressive disease. Significant QT prolongation may be the initial effect resulting in increased vulnerability to ventricular dysrhythmias, as noted by some authors (206,207). The presence of hypokalemia may compound the risk of developing a dysrhythmia (160,183,208). One study of heavily pretreated patients concluded that an anthracycline dose greater than 400 mg/m^2 and administration of more than 200 mg/m^2 of amsacrine (AMSA) over 48 hours were related to an increased risk of cardiac effects associated with the AMSA therapy (164). Four of the six patients who developed clinical CHF in that study were in this high-risk group. To date, a cumulative dose effect and its relationship to cardiotoxicity have not been demonstrated for this agent (167).

Studies in rabbits at high doses and in dogs using toxic doses of high, lethal, and supralethal doses of AMSA revealed marked effects of atrioventricular and intraventricular conduction systems (209). First- and second-degree atrioventricular block, prolongation of QRS and QT intervals, ventricular premature contractions, atrial flutter, and ventricular tachycardia were among the noted effects.

BIOLOGICS

Interferon

The incidence of cardiovascular toxicity associated with interferon therapy has been in the range of 5% to 12% (210). Increasing dose, increasing age, and a prior history of cardiovascular disease appear to be risk factors for the development of cardiotoxicity with the interferons (211). The most frequently reported cardiotoxicities are primarily hypotension and tachycardia and may be related to the febrile reaction commonly seen rather than a direct cardiotoxic effect (212). Nonfatal dysrhythmias, predominantly supraventricular tachyarrhythmias, have been described in patients receiving interferon therapy (209). Early clinical trials in France were temporarily halted because of four deaths from myocardial infarctions in patients treated with interferon (210). Myocardial infarctions in patients with and without prior cardiac histories have been reported previously (205,215–217). Infrequent reports of CHF with short-term and prolonged administration of interferons have been described by Cooper et al. (218), Lindpainter et al. (205), Brown et al. (219), and Deyton et al. (220). The report of three patients with Kaposi's sarcoma and HIV-positive status suggests a possible synergism between interferon and the HIV virus. Postmortem findings in one case revealed four-chamber enlargement without evidence of coronary artery disease, fibrosis, or amyloid or inflammatory infiltrates, suggesting a drug-related etiology of the cardiomyopathy (221). Although the reports of cardiovascular toxicities with interferon treatment overall are infrequent, older patients and those with a history of previous cardiac events may be at increased risk for the development of cardiotoxicity from interferons.

Interleukin-2/Lymphokine-Activated Killer Cells

Significant cardiotoxicity with interleukin-2 (IL-2) alone and in combination with (LAK) cells has been documented by all centers involved in these investigations. The incidence of hypotension requiring pharmacologic support with vasopressors was 65% in 317 patients treated at the National Cancer Institute (NCI) (222). Dysrhythmias, primarily supraventricular tachyarrhythmias, occurred in 9.7% of cases. Angina or ischemic changes were noted in 2.6% of patients and myocardial infarction in 1.5%.

Hemodynamic changes seen in patients receiving IL-2/LAK therapy consisted of a decrease in mean arterial pressure and systemic vascular resistance with an increase in heart rate and cardiac index (215,223). Cardiac dysfunction with significantly decreased stroke index and left ventricular stroke work associated with a reduction in LVEF was also noted in the NCI study. Complete heart block has been documented in one patient (224). Severe myocarditis with lymphocytic and eosinophilic infiltrates with areas of myocardial necrosis on autopsy has been documented in one patient on high-dose IL-2 therapy (225). The hemodynamic changes seen are consistent with those seen in early septic shock (226). The etiology of the hypotension is thought to be due to an increase in vascular permeability (capillary leak phenomenon), leading to both a decrease in intravascular volume and a reduction in systemic vascular resistance (218,227). The actual mechanism by which this high-output/low-resistance state occurs is currently unknown. Leading possibilities include a direct effect of IL-2 or an indirect effect mediated by another cytokine or substance released by IL-2. Investigational studies with IL-2 in various schedules and doses are ongoing.

SUMMARY

Cardiotoxicity, primarily due to treatment with anthracyclines, continues to provide a fertile area of research for scientists and physicians. Further research is required to unravel the precise mechanism of anthracycline cardiotoxicity. The search for a less cardiotoxic but equivalent cytotoxic anthracycline analog continues to be an active focus of preclinical and clinical research. With the increasing use of antineoplastics in the treatment of malignant disease, there has been increased recognition of varied cardiac effects with multiple agents. Undoubtedly, this body of knowledge will continue to grow and result in additional research questions over the coming years.

REFERENCES

1. Kremer L, van Dalen E, Offringa M, et al. Frequency and risk factors of anthracycline-induced clinical heart failure in children: a systematic review. Ann Oncol 2002; 13:503–512.
2. Kremer L, van der Pal H, Offringa M, et al. Frequency and risk factors of subclinical cardiotoxicity after anthracycline therapy in children: a systematic review. Ann Oncol 2002; 13:819–829.
3. Hancock SL, Donaldson SS, Hoppe RT. Cardiac disease following treatment of Hodgkin's disease in children and adolescents. J Clin Oncol 1993; 11:1208–1215.
4. Lipshultz SE, Colan SD, Gelber RD, et al. Late cardiac effects of doxorubicin therapy for acute lymphoblastic leukemia in childhood. N Engl J Med 1991; 324: 808–815.
5. Sorensen K, Levitt G, Bull C, et al. Anthracycline dose in childhood acute lymphoblastic leukemia: issues of early survival versus late cardiotoxicity. J Clin Oncol 1997; 15:61–68.

6. Nysom K, Holm K, Lipsitz SR, et al. Relationship between cumulative anthracy-cline dose and late cardiotoxicity in childhood acute lymphoblastic leukemia. J Clin Oncol 1998; 16:545–550.

7. Lele SS, Durrant STS, Atherton JJ, et al. Demonstration of late cardiotoxicity following bone marrow transplantation by assessment of exercise diastolic filling characteristics. Bone Marrow Transplant 1996; 17:1113–1118.

8. Steinherz LJ, Steinherz PG, Tan C. Cardiac failure and dysrhythmias 6–19 years after anthracycline therapy: a series of 15 patients. Med Pediatr Oncol 1995; 24:352–361.

9. Von Hoff DD, Laylard MW, Basa P, et al. Risk factors for doxorubicin-induced congestive heart failure. Ann Intern Med 1979; 91:710–717.

10. Steinherz LJ, Steinherz PG, Tan CT, et al. Cardiac toxicity 4 to 20 years after completing anthracycline therapy. J Am Med Assoc 1991; 266:1672–1677.

11. Hequet O, Le QH, Moullet I, et al. Subclinical late cardiomyopathy after doxor-ubicin therapy for lymphoma in adults. J Clin Oncol 2004; 22:1864–1871.

12. Early Breast Cancer Trialists' Collaboratovie Group. Favourable and unfavourable effect on long-term survival of radiotherapy for early breast cancer: an overview of the randomized trials. Lancet 2000; 355:1757–1770.

13. Blum RH, Carter SK. Adriamycin: a new anticancer drug with significant clinical activity. Ann Intern Med 1974; 80:249–259.

14. Young RC, Ozols RF, Myers CE. The anthracycline antineoplastic drugs. N Engl J Med 1981; 205:139–153.

15. Lenaz L, Page JA. Cardiotoxicity of adriamycin and related anthracyclines. Cancer Treat Rev 1976; 3:111–120.

16. Steinberg JS, Cohen AJ, Wasserman AG, et al. Acute arrhythmogenicity of dox-orubicin administration. Cancer 1987; 60:1213–1218.

17. Ferrans VJ. Overview of cardiac pathology in relation to anthracycline cardiotox-icity. Cancer Treat Rep 1978; 62:955–961.

18. Von Hoff DD, Rozenoweig M, Layard M, et al. Daunomycin-induced cardiotoxicity in children and adults. A review of 110 cases. Am J Med 1977; 62:200–208.

19. Bristow MR, Billingham ME, Mason JW, et al. Clinical spectrum of anthracycline antibiotic cardiotoxicity. Cancer Treat Rep 1978; 62:873–879.

20. Freidman MA, Bozdech MJ, Billingham ME, et al. Doxorubicin cardiotoxicity. Serial endomyocardial biopsies and systolic time intervals. J Am Med Assoc 1978; 240:1603–1606.

21. Haq MM, Legha SS, Choksi J, et al. Doxorubicin-induced congestive heart failure in adults. Cancer 1985; 56:1361–1365.

22. Schwartz RG, McKenzie WB, Alexander J, et al. Congestive heart failure and left ventricular dysfunction complicating doxorubicin therapy. Seven-year experience using serial radionuclide angiocardiography. Am J Med 1987; 82:1109–1118.

23. Yeung ST, Yoong C, Spink J, et al. Functional myocardial impairment in children treated with anthracyclines for cancer. Lancet 1991; 337:816–818.

24. Larsen RL, Jakacki RI, Vetter VL, et al. Electrocardiographic changes and arrhythmias after cancer therapy in children and young adults. Am J Cardiol 1992; 70:73–77.

25. Minow RA, Benjamin RS, Gottleib JA. Adriamycin (NSC-123127) cardiomyop-athy—an overview with determination of risk factors. Cancer Chemother Rep 1975; 6:195–201.

26. Praga C, Beretta G, Vigo PL, et al. Adriamycin cardiotoxicity: a survey of 1273 patients. Cancer Treat Rep 1979; 63:827–834.
27. Freiss GG, Boyd JF, Geer MR, et al. Effects of first-dose doxorubicin on cardiac rhythm as evaluated by continuous 24-hour monitoring. Cancer 1985; 56:2762–2764.
28. Wortman JE, Lucas JS. Schuster E, et al. Sudden death during doxorubicin administration. Cancer 1979; 44:1588–1591.
29. Halazun JF, Wagner HR, Gaeta JF, et al. Daunorubicin cardiac toxicity in children with acute lymphocytic leukemia. Cancer 1974; 33:545–554.
30. LaFrak EA, Pitha J, Rosenheim S, et al. Adriamycin (NSC 123127) cardiomyopathy. Cancer Chemother Rep 1975; 6:203–208.
31. Freter CE, Lee TC, Billingham ME, et al. Doxorubicin cardiac toxicity manifesting seven years after treatment. Am J Med 1986; 80:483–485.
32. Swain S, Whaley F, Ewer M. Congestive heart failure in patients treated with doxorubicin: a retrospective analysis of three trials. Cancer 2003; 97:2869–2879.
33. Lipschultz SE, Lipsitz SR, Mone SM, et al. Female sex and higher drug dose as risk factors for late cardiotoxic effects of doxorubicin therapy for childhood cancer. N Engl J Med 1995; 332:1738–1743.
34. Bonadonna G, Beretta B, Tancini G, et al. Adriamycin (NSC-123127) studies at the Instituto Nazionale Tumori, Milan. Cancer Chemother Rep 1975; 6:231–245.
35. Cortes EP, Lutman G, Wanka J, et al. Adriamycin (NSC-123127) cardiotoxicity: a clinicopathologic correlation. Cancer Chemother Rep 1975; 6:215–225.
36. Jones RB, Holland JF, Bhardwaj S, et al. A phase I–II study of intensive-dose adriamycin for advanced breast cancer. J Clin Oncol 1987; 5:172–177.
37. Overgaard M, Jensen MB, Overgaard J, et al. Postoperative radiotherapy in high-risk postmenopausal breast-cancer patients given adjuvant tamoxifen: Danish Breast Cancer Cooperative Group DBCG 82C randomized trial. Lancet 1999; 353: 1641–1648.
38. Weiss AJ, Metter GE, Fletcher WS, et al. Studies on adriamycin using a weekly regimen demonstrating its clinical effectiveness and lack of cardiac toxicity. Cancer Chemother Rep 1976; 60:813–822.
39. Chelbowski R, Pugh R, Paroly W, et al. Adriamycin on a weekly schedule: clinically effective with low incidence of cardiotoxicity. Clin Res 1979; 27:53A.
40. Legha SS, Benjamin RS, Mackay B, et al. Reduction of doxorubicin cardiotoxicity by prolonged continuous intravenous infusion. Ann Intern Med 1982; 96:133–139.
41. Lum BL, Svee JM, Torti FM. Doxorubicin: alteration of dose scheduling as a means of reducing cardiotoxicity. Drug Intell Clin Pharm 1985; 19:259–264.
42. Gundersen S, Kvinnsland S, Klepp O, et al. Weekly adriamycin versus VAC in advanced breast cancer. A randomized trial. Eur J Cancer Clin Oncol 1986; 22:1431–1434.
43. Bristow MR, Mason JW, Billingham ME, et al. Doxorubicin cardiomyopathy: evaluation by phonocardiography, endomyocardial biopsy, and cardiac catheterization. Ann Intern Med 1978; 88:168–175.
44. Merril J, Greco FA, Zimbler H, et al. Adriamycin and radiation: synergistic cardiotoxicity. Ann Intern Med 1975; 82:122–123.
45. Kushner JP, Hansen WL, Hammar SP. Cardiomyopathy after widely separated courses of adriamycin exacerbated by actinomycin-D and mithramycin. Cancer 1975; 36:1577–1584.

46. Smith PJ, Ekert H, Waters KD, et al. High incidence of cardiomyopathy in children treated with adriamycin and DTIC in combination chemotherapy. Cancer Treat Rep 1977; 61:1736–1738.
47. Buzdar AV, Legha SS, Tashima CK, et al. Adriamycin and mitomycin-C: possible synergistic cardiotoxicity. Cancer Treat Rep 1978; 62:1005–1008.
48. Watts RG. Severe and fatal anthracycline cardiotoxicity at cumulative doses below 400 mg/m 2: evidence for enhanced toxicity with multiagent chemotherapy. Am J Hematol 1991; 36:217–218.
49. Minow RA, Benjamin RS, Leo ET, et al. Adriamycin cardiomyopathy—risk factors. Cancer 1977; 39:1397–1402.
50. Singer JW, Narahara KA, Ritchie JL, et al. Time and dose-dependent changes in ejection fraction determined by radionuclide angiography after anthracycline therapy. Cancer Treat Rep 1978; 62:945.
51. Alexander J, Dainiak N, Berger HJ, et al. Serial assessment of doxorubicin cardiotoxicity with quantitative radionuclide angiocardiography. N Engl J Med 1979; 300:278–283.
52. Palmeri ST, Bonow RO, Myers CE, et al. Prospective evaluation of doxorubicin cardiotoxicity by rest and exercise radionuclide angiography. Am J Cardiol 1986; 58:607–613.
53. Bloom KR, Bini RM, Williams CM, et al. Echocardiography in adriamycin cardiotoxicity. Cancer 1978; 41:1265–1269.
54. Marchandise B, Schroeder E, Boslv A, et al. Early detection of doxorubicin cardiotoxicity: interest of Doppler echocardiographic analysis of the left ventricular filling dynamics. Am Heart J 1989; 118:92–98.
55. Weesner KM, Bledsoe M, Chauvenet A, et al. Exercise echocardiography in the detection of anthracycline cardiotoxicity. Cancer 1991; 68:435–438.
56. Greco FA. Subclinical adriamycin cardiotoxicity: detection by timing the arterial sounds. Cancer Treat Rep 1978; 62:901–905.
57. Billingham ME, Bristow MR, Glatstein E, et al. Adriamycin cardiotoxicity: endomyocardial biopsy evidence of enhancement by irradiation. Am J Surg Pathol 1977; 1:17–23.
58. Marshall RC, Berger HJ, Reduto LA, et al. Variability in sequential measures of left ventricular performance assessed with radionuclide angiocardiography. Am J Cardiol 1978; 41:531–536.
59. Ewer MS, Ali MK, Mackay B, et al. A comparison of cardiac biopsy grades and ejection fraction estimations in patients receiving adriamycin. J Clin Oncol 1984; 2:112–117.
60. Piver MS, Marchetti DL, Parthasarathy KL, et al. Doxorubicin hydrochloride (adriamycin) cardiotoxicity evaluated by sequential radionuclide angiocardiography. Cancer 1985; 56:76–80.
61. Steinberg JS, Wasserman AG. Radionuclide ventriculography for evaluation and prevention of doxorubicin cardiotoxicity. Clin Ther 1985; 7:660–667.
62. Pigram WJ, Fuller W, Amilton LDH. Stereochemistry of intercalation: interaction of daunomycin with DNA. Nature 1972; 253:17–19.
63. Murphree SA, Cunningham LS, Hwang KM, et al. Effects of adriamycin on surface properties of sarcoma 180 ascites cells. Biochem Pharmacol 1976; 25:1227–1231.
64. Sinha BK. Binding specificity of chemically and enzymatically activated anthracycline anticancer agents to nucleic acids. Chem Biol Interact 1980; 30:67–77.

65. Tewey KM, Chen GI, Nelson EM, et al. Intercalative antitumor drugs interfere with the breakage-reunion of mammalian DNA topoisomerase II. J Biol Chem 1984; 259:9182–9187.

66. Janke RA. An anthracycline antibiotic-induced cardiomyopathy in rabbits. Lab Invest 1974; 30:292–303.

67. Meyers CE, McGuire WP, Liss RH, et al. Adriamycin: the role of lipid peroxidation in cardiac toxicity and tumor response. Science 1977; 197:165–167.

68. Billingham ME. Some recent advances in cardiac pathology. Hum Pathol 1979; 10:367–386.

69. Singal PK, Segstro RJ, Singh RP, et al. Changes in lysosomal morphology and enzyme activities during the development of adriamycin-induced cardiomyopathy. Can J Cardiol 1985; 1:139–147.

70. Olson HM, Young DM, Prieur DJ, et al. Electrolyte and morphologic alterations of myocardium in adriamycin-treated rabbits. Am J Pathol 1974; 77:439–454.

71. Doroshow JH. Effect of anthracycline antibiotics on oxygen radical formation in rat heart. Cancer Res 1983; 43:460–472.

72. Rajagopalan S, Politi PM, Sinha BK, et al. Adriamycin-induced free radical formation in the perfused rat heart: implications for cardiotoxicity. Cancer Res 1988; 48: 4766–4769.

73. Singal PK, Pierce GN. Adriamycin stimulates low-affinity Ca 2+ binding and lipid peroxidation but depresses myocardial function. Am J Physiol 1986; 250:H419–H425.

74. Doroshow JH. Role of reactive oxygen production in doxorubicin cardiac toxicity. In: Hacker MP, Lazo JS, Tritton TR, eds. Organ Directed Toxicities of Anticancer Drugs. The Hague, the Netherlands: Martinus Nijhoff, 1988:31–40.

75. Abramson JJ, Salama G. Sulfhydryl oxidation and calcium release from sarcoplasmic reticulum. Mol Cell Biochem 1988; 82:81–84.

76. Olson RD, Mushlin PS. Doxorubicin cardiotoxicity: analysis of prevailing hypotheses. FASEB J 1990; 4:3076–3086.

77. Azuma J, Sperelakis N, Hasegawa H, et al. Adriamycin cardiotoxicity: possible pathogenic mechanisms. J Mol Cell Cardiol 1981; 13:381–397.

78. Zweier JL, Gianni L, Muindi J, et al. Differences in O2 reduction by the iron complexes of adriamycin and daunomycin: the importance of side chain hydroxyl group. Biochim Biophys Acta 1986; 884:326–336.

79. Singal PK, Forbes MS, Sperelakis N. Occurrence of intramitochondrial Ca 2+ granules in a hypertrophied heart exposed to adriamycin. Can J Physiol Pharmacol 1983; 62:1239–1244.

80. Revis N, Marusic N. Effects of doxorubicin and its aglycone metabolite on calcium sequestration by rabbit heart, liver, and kidney mitochondria. Life Sci 1979; 25: 1055–1064.

81. Jensen RA. Doxorubicin cardiotoxicity: contractile changes after long term treatment in the rat. J Pharmacol Exp Ther 235: 1986; 197–203.

82. Suzuki T, Kanda H, Kawai Y, et al. Cardiotoxicity of anthracycline antineoplastic drugs—clinicopathological and experimental studies. Jpn Circ J 1979; 43:1000–1008.

83. Rabkin SW. Interaction of external calcium concentrations and verapamil on the effects of doxorubicin (adriamycin) in the isolated heart preparation. J Cardiovasc Pharmacol 1983; 5:848–855.

84. Maisch B, Gregor O, Zuess M, et al. Acute effect of calcium channel blocks on adriamycin exposed adult cardiocytes. Basic Res Cardiol 1985; 80:626–635.

85. Bristow MR, Kantrowitz NE, Harrison WD, et al. Mediation of subacute anthracycline cardiotoxicity in rabbits by cardiac histamine release. J Cardiovasc Pharmacol 1983; 5:913.

86. Klugman FB, Decorti G, Candussio L, et al. Inhibitors of adriamycin-induced histamine release *in vitro* limit adriamycin cardiotoxicity *in vivo*. Br J Cancer 1986; 54:743–748.

87. Del Tacca M, Danesi R, Ducci M, et al. Might adriamycinol contribute to adriamycin-induced cardiotoxicity? Pharmacol Res Commun 1985; 17:1073–1084.

88. Boucek RJ, Olson RD, Brenner DE, et al. The major metabolite of doxorubicin is a potent inhibitor of membrane-associated ion pumps: a correlative study of cardiac musclewith isolated membrane fractions. J Biol Chem 1987; 262:15851–15856.

89. Olson RD, Mushlin PS, Brenner DE, et al. Doxorubicin cardiotoxicity may be due to its metabolite, doxorubicinol. Proc Natl Acad Sci U S A 1988; 85:3585–3589.

90. Peters JH, Gordon GR, Kashiwase D, et al. Tissue distribution of doxorubicin and doxorubicinol in rats receiving multiple doses of doxorubicin. Cancer Chemother Pharmacol 1981; 7:65–70.

91. Cortes EP. Adriamycin cardiotoxicity: early detection by systolic time interval and possible prevention by coenzyme Q10. Cancer Treat Rep 1978; 62:887.

92. Doroshow JH, Locker GY, Ifrim I, et al. Prevention of doxorubicin cardiotoxicity in the mouse by N-acetylcysteine. J Clin Invest 1981; 68:1053–1064.

93. Milei J, Marantz A, Ale J, et al. Prevention of adriamycin-induced cardiotoxicity by prenylamine: a pilot double blind study. Cancer Drug Deliv 1987; 4:129–136.

94. Speyer JL, Green MD, Jacquotte AZ, et al. ICRF-187 permits longer treatment with doxorubicin in women with breast cancer. J Clin Oncol 1992; 10:117–127.

95. Combs AB, Kishi T, Poter TH, et al. Models for clinical disease. I. Biochemical cardiotoxicity of coenzyme Q 10 inhibitor in rats. Res Commun Chem Pathol Pharmacol 1976; 13:333–339.

96. Bertazzoli C, Sala L, Tosano MG. Antagonistic action of ubiquinone on experimental cardiotoxicity of adriamycin in isolated rabbit heart. Int Res Commun Sys Med Sci 1975; 3:367.

97. Bertazzoli C, Sala L, Socia E, et al. Experimental adriamycin cardiotoxicity prevented by ubiquinone *in vivo*. Int Res Commun Sys Med Sci 1975; 3:468.

98. Langsjoen PH, Langsjoen PH, Folkers K. A six-year clinical study of therapy of cardiomyopathy with coenzyme Q 10. Int J Tissue React 1990; 12:169–171.

99. Milei J, Vazquez A, Boveris A, et al. The role of prenylamine in the prevention of adriamycin-induced cardiotoxicity. A review of experimental and clinical findings. J Int Med Res 1988; 16:19–30.

100. Myers CE, Bonow R, Palmeri S, et al. A randomized controlled trial assessing the prevention of doxorubicin cardiomyopathy by N-acetylcysteine. Semin Oncol 1983; 10(suppl 1):53–55.

101. Von Hoff DD, Howser D, Lewis B, et al. Phase I study of ICRF-187 using a daily for 3 days schedule. Cancer Treat Rep 1981; 65:249–252.

102. Hasinoff BB. The interaction of the cardioprotective agent ICRF-187 ((+)-1,2-bis (3,5-dioxopiperazinyl-1-yl)propane): its hydrolysis product (ICRf-198); and other chelating agents with the Fe(III) and Cu(II) complexes of adriamycin. Agents Actions 1990; 29:374–381.

103. Venturini M, Michelotti A, Del Mastro L, et al. Multicenter randomized controlled clinical trial to evaluate cardioprotection of dexrazoxane versus no cardioprotection

in women receiving epirubicin chemotherapy for advanced breast cancer. J Clin Oncol 1996; 14:3112–3120.

104. Swain SM, Whaley FS, Gerber MC, et al. Cardioprotection with dexrazoxane for doxorubicin-containing therapy in advanced breast cancer. J Clin Oncol 1997; 15:1318–1332.

105. Lopez M, Vici P, Di Lauro L, et al. Randomized prospective clinical trial of high-dose epirubicin and dexrazoxane in patients with advanced breast cancer and soft tissue sarcomas. J Clin Oncol 1998; 16:86–92.

106. Balazsovits JA, Mayer LD, Bally MG, et al. Analysis of the effect of liposome encapsulation on the vesicant properties, acute and cardiac toxicities, and antitumor efficacy of doxorubicin. Cancer Chemother Pharmacol 1989; 23:81–86.

107. Treat J, Greenspan A, Forst D, et al. Anti-tumor activity of liposome-encapsulated doxorubicin in advanced breast cancer: Phase II study. J Natl Cancer Inst 1990; 82:1706–1710.

108. Wagner D, Kern WV, Kern P, et al. Liposomal doxorubicin in AIDS-related Kaposi's sarcoma: long-term experience. Clin Invest 1994; 72:417–423.

109. Harrison M, Tomlinson D, Stewart S, et al. Liposomal-entrapped doxorubicin: an active agent in AIDS-related Kaposi's sarcoma. J Clin Oncol 1995; 13:914–920.

110. Batist G, Ramakrishnan G, Rao C, et al. Reduced cardiotoxicity and preserved antitumour efficacy of liposome-encapsulated doxorubicin and cyclophosphamide compared with conventional doxorubicin and cyclophosphamide in a randomized, multicenter trial of metastatic breast cancer. J Clin Oncol 2001; 19:1444–1454.

111. Harris L, Batist G, Belt R, et al. Liposome-encapsulated doxorubicin compared with conventional doxorubicin in a randomized multicenter trial as first-line therapy of metastatic breast carcinoma. Cancer 2002; 94:25–36.

112. O'Brien M, Wigler N, Inbar N, et al. Reduced cardiotoxicity and comparable efficacy in a phase III trial of pegylated liposomal doxorubicin HCl (CAELYX/ Doxil) versus conventional doxorubicin for first-line treatment of metastatic breast cancer. Ann Oncol 2004; 15:440–449.

113. Weiss RB, Sarosy B, Clagett-Carr K, et al. Anthracycline analogs: the past, present, and future. Cancer Chemother Pharmacol 1986; 18:185–197.

114. Casazza AM. Experimental evaluation of anthracycline analogs. Cancer Treat Rep 1979; 63:835–844.

115. Ringenberg QS, Propert KJ, Muss HB, et al. Clinical cardiotoxicity of esorubicin (4-deoxydoxorubicin, DxDx): prospective studies with serial gated heart scans and reports of selected cases. Invest New Drugs 1990; 8:221–226.

116. Jain KK, Casper ES, Geller NL, et al. A prospective randomized comparison of epirubicin and doxorubicin in patients with advanced breast cancer. J Clin Oncol 1985; 3:818–826.

117. Havsteen H, Brynjolf I, Svahn T, et al. Prospective evaluation of chronic cardiotoxicity due to high-dose epirubicin of combination chemotherapy with cyclophosphamide, methotrexate, and 5-fluorouracil. Cancer Chemother Pharmacol 1989; 23:101–104.

118. Dardir MD, Ferrans VJ, Mikhael YS, et al. Cardiac morphologic and functional changes induced by epirubicin chemotherapy. J Clin Oncol 1989; 7:947–958.

119. Macchiarini P, Danesi R, Mariotti R, et al. Phase II study of high-dose epirubicin in untreated patients with small-cell lung cancer. Am J Clin Oncol 1990; 13:302–307.

120. Nielsen D, Jensen NB, Dombernowsky O, et al. Epirubicin cardiotoxicity: a study of 135 patients with advanced breast cancer. J Clin Oncol 1990; 8:1806–1810.

121. Jensen B, Skovsgaard T, Nielsen S, et al. Functional monitoring of anthracycline cardiotoxicity. A prospective, blinded, long-term observational study of outcome in 120 patients. Ann Oncol 2002; 13:699–707.

122. Nair R, Ramakrishnan G, Nair NN, et al. A randomized comparison of the efficacy and toxicity of epirubicin and doxorubicin in the treatment of patients with non-Hodgkin's lymphoma. Cancer 1998; 82:2282–2288.

123. Ryberg M, Nielsen D, Skovsgaard T, et al. Epirubicin cardiotoxicity: an analysis of 469 patients with metastatic breast cancer. J Clin Oncol 1998; 16:3502–3508.

124. Italian Multicentre Breast Study with Epirubicin. Phase III randomoized study of fluorouracil, epirubicin, and cyclophosphamide *v* fluorouracil, doxorubicin, and cyclophosphamide in advanced breast cancer: an Italian multicentre trial. J Clin Oncol 1998; 6:976–982.

125. Berman E, Wittes RE, Leyland-Jones B, et al. Phase I and clinical pharmacology studies of intravenous and oral administration of 4-demethoxydaunorubicin in patients with advanced cancer. Cancer Res 1983; 43:6096–6101.

126. Daghestani AN, Arlin ZA, Leyland-Jones B, et al. Phase I and II clinical and pharmacological study of 4-demethoxydaunorubicin (idarubicin) in adult patients withacute leukemia. Cancer Res 1985; 45:1408–1412.

127. Tan CTC, Hancock C, Steinherz P, et al. Phase I clinical pharmacological study of 4-demethoxydaunorubicin (idarubicin) in children with advanced cancer. Cancer Res 1987; 47:2990–2995.

128. Kris MG, Gralla RJ, Kelsen DP, et al. Phase II trial of oral 4-demethoxydaunorubicin in patients with non-small cell lung cancer. Am J Clin Oncol 1985; 8:377–379.

129. Martoni A, Pacciarini MA, Pannuti F. Activity of 4-demthoxydaunorubicin by the oral route in advanced breast cancer. Eur J Cancer Clin Oncol 1985; 21:803–806.

130. Chisesi T, Capnist G, De Dominicis E, et al. A phase II study of idarubicin (4-demethoxydaunorubicin) in advanced myeloma. Eur J Cancer Clin Oncol 1988; 24:681–684.

131. Gillies H, Lian R, Rogers H, et al. Phase II trial of idarubicin in patients with advanced lymphoma. Cancer Chemother Pharmacol 1988; 21:261–264.

132. Villani F, Galimberti M, Comazzi R, et al. Evaluation of cardiac toxicity of idarubicin (4-demethoxydaunorubicin). Eur J Cancer Clin Oncol 1989; 25:13–18.

133. Anderlini P, Benjamin RS, Wong FC, et al. Idarubicin cardiotoxicity: a retrospective study in acute myeloid leukemia and myelodysplasia. J Clin Oncol 1995; 13:2827–2834.

134. Shenkenberg TD, Von Hoff DD. Mitoxantrone: a new anticancer drug with significant clinical activity. Ann Intern Med 1986; 105:67–81.

135. Gams RA, Wesler MJ. Mitoxantrone cardiotoxicity: results from Southeastern Cancer Study Group. Cancer Treat Symp 1984; 3:31–33.

136. Clark GM, Tokaz KL, Von Hoff DD, et al. Cardiotoxicity in patients treated with mitoxantrone on Southwest Oncology Group phase II protocols. Cancer Treat Symp 1984; 3:25–30.

137. Bennett JM, Muss HD, Doroshow JH, et al. A randomized multicenter trial comparing mitoxantrone, cyclophosphamide, and fluorouracil in the therapy of metastatic breastcarcinoma. J Clin Oncol 1988; 6:1611–1620.

138. Coleman RE, Maisey MN, Khight RK, et al. Mitoxantrone in advanced breast cancer—a phase II study with special attention to cardiotoxicity. Eur J Cancer Clin Oncol 1982; 20:771–776.
139. Schell FC, Yap HY, Blumenschein G, et al. Potential cardiotoxicity with mitoxantrone. Cancer Treat Rep 1982; 66:1641–1643.
140. Aapro MS, Alberts DS, Woolfenden JM, et al. Prospective study of left ventricular function using radionuclide scans in patients receiving mitoxantrone. Invest New Drugs 1983; 1:341–347.
141. Unverferth DV, Bashore TM, Magrien RD, et al. Histologic and function characteristics of human heart after mitoxantrone therapy. Cancer Treat Symp 1984;3:47–53.
142. Crossley RJ. Clinical safety and tolerance of mitoxantrone. Semin Oncol 1984; 11(suppl 1):54–58.
143. Posner LE, Dukart G, Goldberg J, et al. Mitoxantrone: an overview of safety and toxicity. Invest New Drugs 1985; 3:123–132.
144. Henderson BM, Dougherty WJ, James VC, et al. Safety assessment of a new anticancer compound, mitoxantrone, in beagle dogs: comparison with doxorubicin. I. Clinical observations. Cancer Treat Rep 1982; 66:1139–1143.
145. Sparano BM, Gordon G, Hall C, et al. Safety assessment of a new anticancer compound, mitoxantrone, in beagle dogs: comparison with doxorubicin. II. Histologic and ultrastructural pathology. Cancer Treat Rep 1982; 66:1145–1158.
146. Kharasch ED, Novak RF. Inhibition of adriamycin-stimulated microsomal lipid peroxidation by mitoxantrone and ametantrone, two new anthracenedione antineoplastic agents. Biochem Biophys Res Commun 1982; 108:1346–1352.
147. Unnikrishnan D, Dutcher J, Varshneya N, et al. Torsades de pointes in 3 patients with leukemia treated with arsenic trioxide. Blood 2001; 97:1514–1516.
148. Barbey J, Pezzullo J, Soignet S. Effect of arsenic trioxide on QT interval in patients with advanced malignancies. J Clin Oncol 2003; 21:3609–3615.
149. Ohnishi K, Yoshida H, Shigeno K, et al. Prolognation of the QT interval and ventricular tachycardia in patients treated with arsenic trioxide for acute promyelocytic leukemia. Ann Intern Med 2000; 133:881–885.
150. Soignet S, Frankel S, Douer D, et al. United States multicenter study of arsenic trioxide in relapsed acute promyelocytic leukemia. J Clin Oncol 2001; 19:3852–3860.
151. O'Connell TX, Berenbaum MC. Cardiac and pulmonary effects of high doses of cyclophosphamide and isophosphamide. Cancer Res 1974; 34:1586–1591.
152. Applebaum FR, Strauchen JA, Graw BR Jr., et al. Acute lethal carditis caused by high dose combination chemotherapy. Lancet 1976; 1:58–62.
153. Goldberg MA, Antin JH, Guinan EC, et al. Cyclophosphamide cardiotoxicity: an analysis of dosing as a risk factor. Blood 1986; 68:1114–1118.
154. Gottdiener JS, Applebaum FR, Ferrans VJ, et al. Cardiotoxicity associated with high-dose cyclophosphamide therapy. Arch Intern Med 1981; 141:758–763.
155. Slavin RE, Millan JC, Mullins CM. Pathology of high dose intermittent cyclophosphamide therapy. Hum Pathol 1975; 6:693–709.
156. Friedman HS, Colvin OM, Aisaka K, et al. Glutathione protects cardiac and skeletal muscle from cyclophosphamide-induced toxicity. Cancer Res 1990; 50:2455–2462.
157. Trigg ME, Finlay JL, Bozdech M, et al. Fatal cardiac toxicity in bone marrow transplant patients receiving cytosine arabinoside, cyclophosphamide, and total body irradiation. Cancer 1987; 59:38–42.

158. Cazin B, Gorin NC, Laporte JP, et al. Cardiac complications after bone marrow transplantation. Cancer 1986; 57:2061–2069.
159. Braverman AC, Antin JH, Plappert MT, et al. Cyclophosphamide cardiotoxicity in bone marrow transplantation: a prospective evaluation of new dosing regimens. J Clin Oncol 1991; 9:1215–1223.
160. Schlaeffer F, Tovi F, Leiberman A. Cisplatin-induced bradycardia. Drug Intell Clin Pharm 1983; 17:899–901.
161. Hashimi LA, Khalyl MF, Salem PA. Supraventricular tachycardia: a probable complication of platinum treatment. Oncology 1984; 41:174–175.
162. Fassio T, Canobbio L, Gasparini G, et al. Paroxysmal supraventricular tachycardia during treatment with cisplatin and etoposide combination. Oncology 1986; 43:219–220.
163. Doll DC, List AF, Greco FA, et al. Acute vascular ischemic events after cisplatin-based combination chemotherapy for germ-cell tumors of the testis. Ann Intern Med 1986; 105:48–51.
164. Talcott JA, Herman TS. Acute ischemic vascular events and cisplatin. Ann Intern Med 1987; 107:121–122.
165. Edwards BS, Lane M, Smith FE. Long-term treatment with cis-dichloro-diamineplatinum(II)-vinblastine-bleomycin: possible association with severe coronary artery disease. Cancer Treat Rep 1979; 63:551–552.
166. Bodensteiner DC. Fatal coronary artery fibrosis after treatment with bleomycin, vincristine, and cisplatinum. South Med J 1981; 74:898–899.
167. La Bianca R, Berretta G, Clerici M, et al. Cardiac toxicity of 5-fluorouracil: a study of 1083 patients. Tumori 1982; 68:505–510.
168. de Forni M, Malet-Martino MC, Jaillais P, et al. Cardiotoxicity of high-dose continuous infusion fluorouracil: a prospective clinical study. J Clin Oncol 1992; 10:1795–1801.
169. Freeman NJ, Costanza ME. 5-Fluorouracil-associated cardiotoxicity. Cancer 1988; 61:36–45.
170. Dent RG, McCall I. 5-Fluorouracil and angina. Lancet 1975; 1:347–348.
171. Jakubowski AA, Kemeny N. Hypotension as a manifestation of cardiotoxicity in three patients receiving cisplatin and 5-fluorouracil. Cancer 1988; 62:266–269.
172. Rezkalla S, Kloner RA, Enslev J, et al. Continuous ambulatory ECG monitoring during fluorouracil therapy: a prospective study. J Clin Oncol 1989; 7:509–514.
173. Chaudary S, Song SYT, Jaski BE. Profound yet reversible heart failure secondary to 5-fluorouracil. Am J Med 1988; 85:454–456.
174. McKendall GR, Shurman A, Anamur M, et al. Toxic cardiogenic shock associated with infusion of 5-fluorouracil. Am Heart J 1988; 118:184–186.
175. Martin M, Diaz-Rubio E, Furio V, et al. Lethal cardiac toxicity after cisplatin and 5-fluoruracil chemotherapy. Am J Clin Oncol 1989; 12:229–234.
176. Collins C, Weiden PL. Cardiotoxicity of 5-fluorouracil. Cancer Treat Rep 1987; 71:733–736.
177. Ensley JF, Patel B, Kloner R, et al. The clinical syndrome of 5-fluorouracil cardiotoxicity. Invest New Drugs 1989; 7:101–109.
178. Kleiman NS, Lehane DE, Geyer CE, et al. Prinzmetal's angina during 5-fluorouracil chemotherapy. Am J Med 1987; 82:566–568.
179. Patel B, Kloner RA, Ensley J, et al. 5-Fluorouracil cardiotoxicity: left ventricular dysfunction and effect of coronary vasodilators. Am J Med Sci 1987; 294:238–243.

180. Oleksowicz L, Bruckner HW. Prophylaxis of 5-fluorouracil induces coronary vasospasm with calcium channel blockers. Am J Med 1988; 85:750–751.
181. Braunwal E, Kloner RA. The stunned myocardium: prolonged postischemic ventricular dysfunction. Circulation 1982; 66:1146–1149.
182. Liss RH, Chadwick M. Correlation of 5-fluorouracil (NSC-19893) distribution in rodents with toxicity and chemotherapy in man. Cancer Chemother Rep 1974; 58:777–786.
183. Fraile RJ, Baker LH, Buroker TR, et al. Pharmacokinetics of 5-fluorouracil administered orally, by rapid intravenous and by slow infusion. Cancer Res 1980; 20:2223–2228.
184. Grandi AM, Pinotti G, Morandi E, et al. Noninvasive evaluation of cardiotoxicity of 5-fluorouracil and low doses of folinic acid: a one-year follow-up study. Ann Oncol 1997; 8:705–708.
185. Willemze R, Zwaan FE, Colpin G, et al. High dose cytosine arabinoside in the management of refractory acute leukemia. Scand J Haematol 1982; 29:141–146.
186. Vaickus L, Letendre L. Pericarditis induced by high-dose cytarabine therapy. Arch Intern Med 1984; 144:1868–1869.
187. Drucker B, Guilhot F, O'Brien SG, et al. Five-year follow-up of patients receiving imatinib for chronic myeloid leukemia. N Eng J Med 2006; 355:2408–2417.
188. Kerkela R, Grazette L, Yacobi R, et al. Cardiotoxicity of the cancer therapeutic agent imatinib mesylate. Nat Med 2006; 12:908–916.
189. Kris MG, O'Connell JP, Gralla RJ, et al. Phase I trial of Taxol given as a 3-hour infusion every 21 days. Cancer Treat Rep 1986; 70:605–607.
190. Rowinsky EK, McGuire WP, Guarnieri T, et al. Cardiac disturbances during the administration of Taxol. J Clin Oncol 1991; 9:1704–1712.
191. Rowinsky EK, Donehower RC. Paclitaxel (Taxol). N Engl J Med 1995; 332: 1004–1014.
192. Shek TW, Luk ISC, Ma L, et al. Paclitaxel-induced cardiotoxicity: an ultrastructural study. Arch Pathol Lab Med 1996; 120:89–91.
193. Markman M, Kennedy A, Webster K, et al. Paclitaxel administration to gynecologic cancer patients with major risk factors. J Clin Oncol 1998; 16:3483–3485.
194. Gianni L, Munzone E, Capri G, et al. Paclitaxel by 3-hour infusion in combination with bolus doxorubicin in women with untreated metastatic breast cancer: high antitumor efficacy and cardiac effects in a dose-finding and sequence-finding study. J Clin Oncol 1995; 13:2688–2699.
195. Gehl J, Boesgaard M, Paaske T, et al. Combined doxorubicin and paclitaxel in advanced breast cancer: effective and cardiotoxic. Ann Oncol 1996; 7:687–693.
196. Sledge GW, Neuberg D, Ingle J, et al. Phase II trial of doxorubicin vs. paclitaxel vs. doxorubicin + paclitaxel as first-line therapy for metastatic breast cancer: an intergroup trial. Proc Am Soc Clin Oncol 1997; 16:1a.
197. Gianni L, Vigano L, Locatelli A, et al. Human pharmacokinetic characterization and in vitro study of the interaction between doxorubicin and paclitaxel in patients with breast cancer. J Clin Oncol 1997; 15:1906–1915.
198. Slamon D, Clark G, Wong S, et al. Human breast cancer: Correlation of relapse and survival with amplification of the HER-2/neu oncogene. Science 1987; 235: 177–182.

199. Slamon D, Leyland-Jones B, Shak S, et al. Use of chemotherapy plus a monoclonal antibody against HER2 for metastatic breast cancer that overexpresses HER2. N Engl J Med 2001; 344:783–792.
200. Seidman A, Hudis C, Pierri MK, et al. Cardiac dysfunction in the trastuzumab clinical trials experience. J Clin Oncol 2002; 20:1215–1221.
201. Von Hoff DD, Elson D, Polk G, et al. Acute ventricular fibrillation and death during infusion of 4(9-acridinylamino)methanesulfon-m-anisidide (AMSA). Cancer Treat Rep 1980; 64:356–358.
202. McLaughlin P, Salvador PG, Cabanillas F, et al. Ventricular fibrillation following AMSA. Cancer 1983; 52:557–558.
203. Dhaliwal HS, Shannon MS, Barnett MJ, et al. Treatment of acute leukemia with m-AMSA in combination with cytosine arabinoside. Cancer Chemother Pharmacol 1986; 18:59–62.
204. Steinherz LJ, Steinherz PG, Mangiacasale D, et al. Cardiac abnormalities after AMSA administration. Cancer Treat Rep 1982; 66:483–488.
205. Lindpainter K, Lindpainter LS, Wentworth M, et al. Acute myocardial necrosis during administration of amsacrine. Cancer 1986; 57:1284–1286.
206. Weiss RB, Moquin D, Adams JD, et al. Electrocardiogram abnormalities after AMSA administration. Cancer Chemother Pharmacol 1983; 10:133–134.
207. Shinar E, Hasin Y. Acute electrocardiographic changes induced by amsacrine. Cancer Treat Rep 1984; 68:1169–1172.
208. Weiss RB, Grillo-Lopez AJ, Marsoni S, et al. Amsacrine-associated cardiotoxicity: an analysis of 82 cases. J Clin Oncol 1986; 4:918–928.
209. D'Alessandro N, Gebbia N, Crescimanno M, et al. Effects of amsacrine (m-AMSA), a new aminoacridine antitumor drug, on the rabbit heart. Cancer Treat Rep 1983; 67:467–474.
210. Kirkwood JM, Ernstoff MS. Interferons in the treatment of human cancer. J Clin Oncol 1984; 2:336–352.
211. Quesada JR, Talpaz M, Rios A, et al. Clinical toxicity of interferons in cancer patients: a review. J Clin Oncol 1986; 4:234–243.
212. Martino S, Ratanatharathorn V, Karanes C, et al. Reversible arrhythmias observed in patients treated with recombinant alpha 2 interferon. J Cancer Res Clin Oncol 1987; 113:376–378.
213. Dickson D. Death halts interferon trials in France. Science 1982; 218:772.
214. Sarna G, Figlin R, Callaghan M. Alpha (human leukocyte)-interferon as treatment for non-small cell carcinoma of the lung: a phase II trial. J Biol Response Mod 1983; 2:343–347.
215. Foon KA, Shervwin SA, Abrams PG, et al. Treatment of advanced non-Hodgkin's lymphoma with recombinant leukocyted interferon in human malignancy. N Engl J Med 1984; 311:1148–1152.
216. Grunberg SM, Kempf RA, Itri LM, et al. Phase II study of recombinant alpha interferon in the treatment of advanced non-small cell lung carcinoma. Cancer Treat Rep 1985; 70:1031–1032.
217. Cooper MR, Fefer A, Thompson J, et al. Alpha 2 interferon/melphalan/prednisone in previously untreated patients with multiple myeloma: a phase I–II trial. Cancer Treat Rep 1986; 70:473–476.
218. Brown TD, Koeller J, Beougher K, et al. A phase I clinical trial of recombinant DNA gamma interferon. J Clin Oncol 1987; 5:790–798.

219. Deyton LR, Walker RE, Kovacs JA, et al. Reversible cardiac dysfunction associated with interferon alpha therapy in AIDS patients with Kaposi's sarcoma. N Engl J Med 1989; 321:1246–1249.
220. Cohen MC, Huberman MS, Nesto RW. Recombinant alpha 2 interferon-related cardiomyopathy. Am J Med 1988; 85:549–551.
221. Lee RE, Lotze MT, Skibber JM, et al. Cardiorespiratory effects of immunotherapy with interleukin-2. J Clin Oncol 1989; 7:7–20.
222. Gaynor ER, Vitek L, Sticklin L, et al. The hemodynamic effects of treatment with interleukin-2 and lymphokine-activated killer cells. Ann Intern Med 1988; 109:953–958.
223. Vaitkus PT, Grossman D, Fox KR, et al. Complete heart block due to interleukin-2 therapy. Am Heart J 1990; 119:978–980.
224. Samlowski WE, Ward JH, Craven CM, et al. Severe myocarditis following high-dose interleukin-2 administration. Arch Pathol Lab Med 1989; 113:838–841.
225. Ognibene FP, Rosenberg SA, Lotze M, et al. Interleukin-2 administration causes reversible hemodynamic changes and left ventricular dysfunction similar to those seen in septic shock. Chest 1988; 94:750–754.
226. Nora R, Abrams JS, Tait NS, et al. Myocardial toxic effects during recombinant interleukin-2 therapy. J Natl Cancer Inst 1989; 81:59–63.
227. Floyd JD, Nguyn DT, Lobins RL, et al. Cardiotoxicity of cancer therapy. J Clin Oncol 2005; 23:7685–7696.
228. Spiegel RJ. The alpha interferons: clinical overview. Semin Oncol 1987; 14:1–12.

8

Pathogenesis of Catecholamine-Induced Cardiomyopathy

Naranjan S. Dhalla, Melissa R. Dent, and Amarjit S. Arneja

Institute of Cardiovascular Sciences, St. Boniface General Hospital Research Centre, and Departments of Physiology and Internal Medicine, Faculty of Medicine, University of Manitoba, Winnipeg, Canada

INTRODUCTION

Activation of the sympathetic nervous system (SNS) in response to stress releases catecholamines from the sympathetic nerve endings and adrenal medulla. Catecholamines, such as epinephrine, norepinephrine, and dopamine, are the major components that are released endogenously because of stressful stimuli, whereas isoproterenol is a synthetic catecholamine that simulates the actions of SNS activation on the heart. The adrenergic receptors in the heart that are stimulated by catecholamines are the α-adrenoceptors and β-adrenoceptors (β_1 and β_2); however, the β_2-adrenoceptors are found chiefly in extracardiac sites, such as arterioles, where they cause dilation. On the other hand, the α-adrenoceptors present in the vascular smooth muscle are mainly concerned with the maintenance of blood vessel tone. SNS activation results in increased cardiac contraction, increased heart rate, increased systolic blood pressure, and decreased diastolic pressure. Catecholamines at low concentration are beneficial in regulating heart function by exerting a positive inotropic action on the myocardium (1), whereas high concentrations of catecholamines or chronic exposure to catecholamines over a prolonged period produce deleterious effects on the cardiovascular system.

It has been known for many years that epinephrine, norepinephrine, and isoproterenol cause cardiac hypertrophy and/or myocardial lesions (2–5). The lesions caused by epinephrine, norepinephrine, and isoproterenol were qualitatively similar, but the lesions that were seen after isoproterenol treatment were more severe than those produced by epinephrine or norepinephrine (6,7). In fact, isoproterenol was found to be 29 to 72 times more potent in producing myocardial lesions of equal severity than epinephrine or norepinephrine. Large doses of exogenously administered norepinephrine in humans and animals were observed to produce myocardial lesions that include focal necrosis and degeneration as well as mononuclear leukocytic infiltration (8). Typical pathological findings of catecholamine-induced myocardial damage are hypertrophy and contraction band necrosis of myofibers accompanied by a moderate inflammatory reaction; fibrous replacement of the myocardium can sometimes occur (9). These myocardial lesions and damage are considered to represent "catecholamine-induced myocardial cell damage," "catecholamine-induced myocarditis," or "myocardial infarction (MI)" and are now designated as "catecholamine-induced cardiomyopathy." The activation of SNS has been observed in patients suffering from acute MI as well as during percutaneous transluminal coronary angioplasty; the levels of catecholamines were found to correlate with the degree of injury. Catecholamine-induced cardiomyopathy is also associated with several pathological conditions such as pheochromocytoma (4,10–12), subarachnoid hemorrhage, and various other intracranial lesions (13–16) as well as following electrical stimulation of the stellate ganglion (17,18) or hypothalamus (19) in experimental animals showing high levels of plasma catecholamines. These studies not only demonstrate that catecholamines are capable of producing myocardial necrosis but also suggest that myocardial cell damage seen in patients may be the result of high levels of circulating catecholamines for a prolonged period. It should be pointed out that reversible catecholamine-induced cardiomyopathy has also been reported (20–24).

Catecholamines are known to produce a wide variety of direct and indirect pharmacological actions on cardiovascular hemodynamics and metabolism. As a consequence of these complex effects, it has been difficult to determine whether catecholamines exert a direct toxic influence on the myocardium or whether myocardial cell damage is in some way secondary to other actions of catecholamines (5,25–30). Up until now, several mechanisms such as cardiovascular hemodynamic and metabolic changes, alterations in the sarcolemmal (SL) permeability, formation of oxidation products of catecholamines, and accumulation of catecholamine metabolites during the monoamine oxidase (MAO) reaction are thought to be involved in the pathogenesis on catecholamine-induced cardiomyopathy (31–43). Although there is no clear-cut implication of any one of these mechanisms, an attempt has been made in this review to formulate a unifying concept regarding the pathophysiology and clinical significance of catecholamine-induced cardiomyopathy.

CARDIOTOXICITY OF CATECHOLAMINES

Epinephrine-Induced Cardiomyopathy

The main effects of epinephrine are increased cardiac output, heart rate, and limb blood flow as well as decreased systolic and disastolic blood pressure (1). Repetitive infusions of high doses of epinephrine induce cardiomyopathy with progressive hemodynamic deterioration, left ventricular (LV) dilation and hypertrophy, depressed systolic function, and different stages of neurohormonal compensation (44). In 1905, it was first reported that epinephrine caused cardiac lesions (2); the epinephrine-induced lesions were visible to the naked eye and occurred in about 60% of the animals, whereas microscopic examination revealed further lesions in a still larger percentage. It has been reported that an injection of sparteine sulfate or caffeine sodium benzoate followed by epinephrine provided an easy and certain method of producing myocardial lesions (45–48), whereas sparteine sulfate alone did not produce myocardial lesions (49). Not only relatively high dose levels of epinephrine but also a continuous infusion of epinephrine for 120 to 289 hours, at a rate considered to be well below the maximum physiological rate of secretion by the adrenal gland, could cause small endocardial lesions in the left ventricle (50). Epinephrine-induced cardiomyopathy has also been shown to be associated with fibrosis as well as reduction in left atrial and LV responses to isoproterenol; however, responses to Ca^{2+} were normal or enhanced but the densities of both α- and β-adrenoceptors were reduced.

Norepinephrine-Induced Cardiomyopathy

Infusion of norepinephrine was found to result in increased heart rate, reduced limb blood flow, and increased systolic and diastolic blood pressures; the reasons for the difference in effects between norepinephrine and epinephrine is the fact that norepinephrine, unlike epinephrine, stimulates both the myocardial β-adrenergic receptors and vascular α-adrenergic receptors (1). Early studies have shown that norepinephrine caused focal myocarditis in association with subendocardial and subepicardial hemorrhages (51,52). In a quantitative study on the pathological effects of norepinephrine, it was observed that dosages that are considered physiological and indeed harmless when administered for short periods of time may become lethal after prolonged infusion (53). Thus, the duration of infusion appears to be an important factor in determining whether a particular dose of norepinephrine is likely to produce myocardial lesions. In addition to myocardial cell damage, norepinephrine was also demonstrated to produce derangements of metabolic processes in the heart such as fatty degeneration (54). In subsequent studies (55,56), remarkable similarities were found in cardiac triglyceride (TG) content and serum enzyme levels after large doses of epinephrine and norepinephrine as well as following MI produced by coronary artery occlusion. From these studies it seems reasonable to suggest that cardiac injury due to catecholamines may be due to coronary constriction leading to ischemic damage. It has also been shown that high doses of norepinephrine increase matrix metalloproteinase (MMP)-9 activity and cause extracellular matrix disruption, LV dilation, and cardiac dysfunction (57). Oxidative stress is also likely to contribute to the development of norepinephrine-induced cardiomyopathy; this view is supported by the observation that allopurinol reduced the myocyte damage due to norepinephrine, as a consequence of scavenging the free radicals and preservation of the adenine nucleotide pool (58). Although cardiac denervation has been shown to protect myocytes against ischemia reperfusion injury due to a decrease in norepinephrine content, such a protection by cardiac denervation was considered not to be associated with a decrease in norepinephrine-derived free radicals (59). Thus, mechanisms other than formation of oxyradicals due to the availability of norepinephrine may be important for inducing cardiotoxicity.

Isoproterenol-Induced Cardiomyopathy

Administration of isoproterenol depletes the energy reserve of cardiac muscle cells and causes complex biochemical and structural changes that eventually lead to cell damage and necrosis (60). Isoproterenol can also cause severe oxidative stress in the myocardium, resulting in infarct-like necrosis of the heart myocardium (43). In fact, it was discovered that relatively low and nonlethal doses of isoproterenol can cause severe myocardial necrosis (5,61). Although the LD_{50} of isoproterenol in rats was reported to be 680 mg/kg, doses as low as 0.02 mg/kg were observed to produce microscopic focal necrotic lesions. The severity of myocardial damage was closely related to the dosage of isoproterenol used and varied from focal lesions affecting single cells to massive infarcts involving large portions of the myocardium. Isoproterenol-induced myocardial lesions were generally found to be localized in the apex as well as in the LV subendocardium, and were observed less frequently in the papillary muscle and the right ventricle. Isoproterenol was also found to produce apical lesions and disseminated focal necrosis (62); however, these lesions were frequently fatal and the median lethal dosage was much lower. Isoproterenol has been observed to produce a number of biochemical or electrophysiological alterations, which precede the histopathological changes in the heart. It is believed that isoproterenol-induced myocardial necrosis is related to altered myocardial energy generation, which may be related to Ca^{2+}-overload.

   Ca^{2+}-influx after isoproterenol in rats shows two phases: a rapid process occurring immediately, followed by a delayed slower influx of Ca^{2+}. The initial phase is associated with histopathological alterations of the myocardium (mitochondrial swelling and Z-disk thickening due to hypercontraction). Thus, the initial phase is thought to be the key event during isoproterenol-induced myocardial necrosis (63). Another study suggests that there are three stages of isoproterenol-induced cardiotoxicity: preinfarction, which occurs before

12 hours; infarction, which occurs from 12 to 24 hours; and postinfarction, which occurs after 24 hours following isoproterenol admistration (64). 17-β-estradiol inhibited the stimulatory action of isoproterenol on Ca^{2+}-influx via the L-type Ca^{2+} channel in the ventricular myocytes. This inhibition may lead to reductions in the heart rate and contraction, therefore reducing oxygen consumption and producing cardioprotection (65). Estrogen also inhibited the augmented cyclic adenosine monophosphate (cAMP) production on isoproterenol administration (66). When Ca^{2+}-influx was inhibited, there was only a reduction in isoproterenol-myocardial necrosis, suggesting factors other than Ca^{2+} may be involved. Isoproterenol can also increase the levels of serum and myocardial lipids, leading to coronary heart disease (67) and stimulate lipid peroxidation, leading to irreversible damage to the myocardial membrane (67). Specifically, damage to the myocardium could be due to the induction of free radical–mediated lipid peroxidation. Recently, some studies have shown that certain treatments may improve the negative effects of isoproterenol. For example, pretreating isoproterenol cardiotoxic hearts with naringin, a predominant flavanone found in grapefruit, significantly decreased the levels of thiobarbituric acid–reactive substances and cardiac tissue lipid peroxides in plasma and heart, in addition to increased activities of superoxide dismutase (SOD), catalase, reduced glutathione (GSH), GSH-dependent enzymes glutathione peroxidase (GPx) and glutathione-S-transferase (GST) in the heart (43). Isoproterenol also decreased the levels of antioxidants, vitamin C and vitamin E; however, pretreatment with naringin increased the antioxidant levels (43).

In one study, isoproterenol was observed to induce GSH oxidation and conjugation, but this effect decreased at subphysiological Ca^{2+} concentrations. Simultaneous incubation with copper increased isoproterenol oxidation and GSH oxidation but decreased GSH conjugation (68). Vitamin C (69,70) has shown protection from myocardial lipid peroxidation, and likewise, vitamin E pretreatment protected the myocardium against isoproterenol-induced injury (71). In another study, S-allylcysteine lowered the lipid peroxidation end products and increased the levels of SOD, catalase, GSH, GPx, GST, and ascorbic acid (67). Also, mangiferin, a pharmacologically active phytochemical, has demonstrated hypolipidemic activity in isoproterenol-induced rats (67). Isoproterenol was shown to result in diffuse areas of fibrosis; however, when treated with phenytoin, the fibrosis was less severe (72). Some studies have shown a marked increase in cholesterol, free fatty acids, and TGs in both serum and heart in isoproterenol-induced cardiomyopathy; aspirin showed a marked reversal of these metabolic changes induced by isoproterenol (73). Isoproterenol can also produce an accumulation of neutral fat droplets in the sarcoplasm; γ-hydroxybutyrate either abolished or reduced the accumulation of fat and completely prevented myofiber death (74). In isoproterenol-treated rats, there was a decrease in diagnostic marker enzymes of MI, which are creatine kinase, lactate dehydrogenase (LDH), aspartate transaminase, alanine transaminase; this change may be due to membrane leakage caused by isoproterenol-induced damage to the SL membrane.

Oral S-allycysteine administration restored these activities in isoproterenol-treated rats (60). From these studies, it appears that the isoproterenol-induced cardiomyopathy may be due to oxidative stress and free radical damage, myocardial hypoperfusion, glycogen depletion, electrolyte imbalance, and lipid accumulation.

CHARACTERISTICS OF CATECHOLAMINE-INDUCED CARDIOMYOPATHY

Several early events such as ultrastructural, histological, biochemical, electrolyte, and membrane changes occur less than 48 hours after the injection of catecholamines for the production of myocardial necrosis. These alterations during the development of catecholamine-induced cardiomyopathy are described below.

Ultrastructural Changes

Table 1 shows the time –course of ultrastructural changes following iso-proterenol injections in rats reported previously (15,75–79). It has been observed that there is no correlation between mitochondrial damage and disruption of myofilaments seen 10 minutes after the isoproterenol injection, normal appearing mitochondria being found among fragmented filaments and swollen mitochondria with ruptured cristae and electron-dense deposits among apparently undamaged sarcomeres (76–80). Within 30 to 60 minutes, there also occurs a

Table 1 Ultrastructural Changes During the Development of Catecholamine-Induced Cardiomyopathy

Time after isoproterenol injection	Findings
A. Within 4–6 min	Disorientation of myofilament, irregular sarcomere length, occasional regions of contracture, rupture of myofilaments, and slight dilatation of sarcoplasmic reticulum.
B. Within 10 min	Swelling of mitochondria, occasional occurrence of electron-dense bodies, and disorganization as well as fragmentation of myofibrils.
C. Within 30–60 min	Electron-dense granular deposits in mitochondria, numerous lipid droplets, margination of nuclear chromatin, disappearance of glycogen granules, and swelling as well as disruption of transverse and longitudinal tubles.
D. Within 1–24 hr	Interstitial and intercellular edema, extensive inflammation, herniation of cellular discs, and extensive vacuolization.

spectrum of damage to the contractile filaments, ranging from irregular bands of greater or less than normal density in sarcomeres of irregular length to fusion of sarcomeres into confluent masses and granular disintegration of the myofilaments (75–78). The effects of norepinephrine, epinephrine, and isoproterenol are qualitatively identical at the cellular level (78–83), with the exception that glycogen depletion (78,81) and fat deposition (83) were much more extensive with epinephrine than with isoproterenol or norepinephrine. From the foregoing discussion it appears that alterations of the contractile filaments begin with irregularities in length and misalignment of the sarcomeres, which are usually associated with an increased thickness and density of the Z-band. Contracture ensues, with the Z-bands becoming indistinct, actin and myosin filaments can no longer be distinguished. Granular disintegration of the sarcomeres follows with the appearance of large empty spaces within the muscle cells, and this fragmentation likely contributes to swelling of the cell. The tubular elements and mitochondria commence swelling soon after catecholamine injection, and the mitochondrial matrix is subsequently decreased in electron density. However, it is pointed out that swelling of the transverse tubules and sarcoplasmic reticulum (SR) is not as consistent a finding as the mitochondrial swelling and may not be evident with certain fixatives. Rupture of the cristae and deposition of electron-dense material in mitochondria represent the final stage in the disruption of these organelles. Accumulation of lipid droplets and disappearance of glycogen granules is not usually evident until these other changes have occurred to some degree and are probably due to the well-known metabolic effects of catecholamines. Herniation of intercalated discs and vacuolization are probably secondary to the swelling and disruption of subcellular organelles and the disintegration of myofilaments.

Histological Changes

Histological changes in catecholamine-induced cardiomyopathy are generally characterized by degeneration and necrosis of myocardial fiber, accumulation of inflammatory cells such as leukocytes, interstitial edema, lipid droplet (fat deposition), and endocardial hemorrhage. Table 2 shows the time course of histological changes following isoproterenol injection (5,30,31,62,78, 80,82,84,85). Interstitial edema is usually associated with subendocardial and subepicardial hemorrhages following administration of catecholamines and is characteristically present in damaged areas of the myocardium even after 72 hours (5,62,78,80,84). Interstitial edema and inflammation are much more prominent following epinephrine or norepinephrine injections even though isoproterenol is more potent in producing cellular damage (78). Accordingly, it has been suggested that edema and inflammation result from mechanisms different from those causing necrotic tissue damage during the development of catecholamine-induced cardiomyopathy. Histochemical alterations subsequent to administration of lesion producing doses of catecholamines have also been

Table 2 Histological Changes During the Development of Catecholamine-Induced Cardiomyopathy

Time after isoproterenol injection	Findings
A. Within 10 min	Darkly stained contraction bands in thin sections from Araldite-embedded ventricule pieces.
B. Within 2–6 hr[a]	Focal myocardial degeneration including loss of striations with sarcoplasmic smudging, lipid accumulation, margination of nuclear chromatin and increased cytoplasmic eosinophilia, capillary dilatation, interstitial edema, subendocardial and subepicardial hemorrhage, opacity and fuchsinorrhagia of the muscle fiber, myocytolysis, vacuolization, and aggregation of lymphomononuclear cells.
C. Within 12–24 hr	Fibers with highly eosinophilic cytoplasm (mottled appearance); fibers show swelling, fragmentation and hyalinization; fibers are hemogenous, strongly eosinophilic, peroxidase acid-Schiff (PAS)-positive, stain pink or deep red with Cason's trichrome, and exhibit fat deposition (lipid droplet).

[a]Changes similar to these have also been reported within 4 to 5 hours after norepinephrine injection.

reported in detail (78,79,81,83). A marked loss of glycogen is seen within 30 minutes, and is most marked following epinephrine administration. Accumulation of peroxidase acid-Schiff (PAS)-positive material is seen at one hour and in an increasing number of fibers over the next 24 hours. This is associated with loss of normal striations and appearance of clear vacuoles. A metachromatic substance is usually observed in areas of interstitial edema and inflammation.

All three catecholamines have been shown to produce biphasic changes in the activities of different oxidative enzymes (Table 3). There is a rapid increase in the activities of enzymes; this is evident within five minutes in various individual fibers, followed by a gradual decline in the activities during 6 to 12 hours. Certain areas of the myocardium having markedly diminished oxidative enzyme activities are interspersed with fibers of normal activities. Decline in oxidative enzyme activities of certain fibers progresses until frank necrosis is evident and there is complete loss of the activities. In each case the degree of change of the enzyme activities is proportional to the normal level of activity of the enzyme involved. Cytochrome oxidase activity is unchanged until evidence of early necrosis is seen after 6 to 12 hours, at which time the activity of this enzyme decreases as well. An increased number of lipid droplets are observed at 30 minutes. Fatty change is more evident in the endocardial region than elsewhere and has been reported by Ferrans et al. (78) to be least apparent with epinephrine; this is in direct contradiction of the findings of Lehr et al. (83). The

Table 3 Biochemical Changes During the Development of Catecholamine-Induced Cardiomyopathy

A.	Cardiac oxidative enzymes	Biphasic (↑↓) changes in succinic dehydrogenase, NAD diaphorase, lactic dehydrogenase, isocitric dehydrogenase, malic dehydrogenase, β-hydroxybutyric dehydrogenase, α-glycerophosphate dehydrogenase, glutamic dehydrogenase, and ethanol dehydrogenase
B.	Blood (serum) contents	Glucose ↑, TG ↑, nonesterified fatty acid ↑, cholesterol ~, total protein ↓, aldosterone ↑, glucocorticoid ↓, total steroid ↓, GOT/AST ↑, GPT ↑, LDH ↑, CPK ↑
C.	Myocardial contents	Glycogen ↓ then ↑, lactate ↓, nonesterified fatty acid ↓, TG ↑, free fatty acids ~ (LV, epi), phospholipids ~ (LV, epi), TG uptake↑, TG synthesis from acetate or palmitate ~, hexosamine ↑ (iso), mucopolysaccharide ↑ (iso), GOT activity ↓ (iso), LDH activity ↓ (iso), ratio of H to M isozyme ↓

Abbreviations: ↑, increase; ~, no change; ↓, decrease; iso, by isoproterenol; epi, by epinephrine; TG, triglyceride; GOT, glutamate-oxalacetate transferase; AST, aspartate amino transferase; GPT, glutamate-pyruvate transferase; LDH, lactate dehydrogenase; CPK, creatine phosphokinase.

reason for this discrepancy is not clear; however, fibers, which contain large lipiddroplets, show decreased activities of the oxidative enzymes, including cytochrome oxidase. Furthermore, all three catecholamines cause a slight increase in the staining of cytoplasm for lysosomal esterase activity (83). It has been reported that ATPase and acid phosphatase were also increased in norepinephrine-induced cardiomyopathy (85).

Biochemical Changes

Following catecholamine administration, the coronary blood flow, myocardial oxygen uptake, and cardiac respiratory quotient were increased (86). Table 3 shows some biochemical changes in catecholamine-induced cardiomyopathy (35,86–95). Glycogen content of the heart decreased rapidly after an injection of isoproterenol and then rose above control level during subsequent five hours (90). Serum glutamate-oxaloacetate transaminase (GOT), aspartate aminotransferase (AST), glutamate-pyruvate transaminase (GPT), LDH, and creatine phosphokinase (CPK) were all greatly elevated during the acute phase of necrotization following catecholamine administration (86,88,89,91). Cardiac AST and GOT activities decreased in a time- and dose-dependent manner following isoproterenol injection (94). Such a decrease in the enzyme activities correlated well with the occurrence and severity of macroscopic lesions. Total cardiac LDH activity fell as well following isoproterenol injection (95); this depression of activity was of long duration, lasting several days and appeared to be due to a decrease in the ratio of its H:M isoenzymes. These findings are consistent with the loss of enzymes from the heart as reflected by an increase in plasma concentrations of transaminases and LDH. There was no significant increase in the contents of free fatty acids or phospholipids in the left ventricle, while there was a significant increase in the TG content of every layer of the LV wall, following epinephrine infusion; the greatest increase in TG content occurred in the endocardium (33). Furthermore, increased TG uptake and unchanged TG synthesis from acetate or palmitate are consistent with the appearance of numerous lipid droplets reported in histological and ultrastructural studies (92). The myocardial content of hexosamines became greatly elevated within 24 hours after an injection of isoproterenol, and this increase in mucopolysaccharide could not be attributed to fibroblasts or other infiltrating cells (93).

It was reported that a single, large subcutaneous dose of epinephrine, norepinephrine, or isoproterenol produced uncoupling of oxidative phosphorylation in rat heart mitochondria (42); however, these catecholamines did not affect normal rat heart mitochondria under in vitro conditions. A reduced respiratory control index (RCI) of heart mitochondria 24 hours after isoproterenol injection has also been reported (96,97). The results of several studies on cardiac adenine nucleotides following isoproterenol injection in rats are somewhat contradictory. A decrease in the levels of all adenine nucleotides has been reported (98) but no change in the relative amount of ATP, ADP, and AMP was evident. On the other hand, a decrease in ATP and creatine phosphate (CrP) levels and a decrease in both ATP/ADP and ATP/AMP ratios without any significant difference in the levels of ADP, AMP, glycogen, lactate, pyruvate, lactate/pyruvate ratio, TG, cholesterol, or phospholipids have been reported (99). Studies of this sort are difficult to evaluate; firstly because the results are expressed in terms of gram wet heart weight, which increases because of a large increase in extracellular fluid volume, following catecholamine administration (99,100) and secondly because the scattered portions of the myocardium undergoing necrotic change are "diluted" within a very large mass of cardiac tissue that has been affected only slightly or not at all. When both ATP and CrP stores of the myocardium were decreased on injecting catecholamines, it was evident that the high-energy phosphate stores in the heart were depressed (101,102); a large increase in the orthophosphate content of the myocardium was also observed. These results suggest lowering of the energy state of myocardium because of high doses of catecholamines, and these changes appear to be at least partly due to an impairment in the process of energy production. On the other hand, relatively little information regarding changes in the process of energy use during catecholamine-induced myocardial cell damage is available in the literature. In this regard, it has been found that myosin extracted from rat hearts following isoproterenol injections contained a large component consisting of a stable aggregated form of myosin (103,104), whereas only the monomeric form of myosin was extracted from control animals. The first phase of aggregation involved a low polymer, probably a dimer, and the aggregated form of myosin did not possess any ATPase activity; there was no evidence of proteolytic damage to the myosin. It has been reported that injection of a "lesion-producing" dose of isoproterenol caused an elevation of cardiac myofibrillar ATPase activity and decreased high-energy phosphate stores (105). However, studies in our laboratory (106) did not reveal any change in myofibrillar Ca^{2+}-stimulated ATPase, while the basal ATPase activity was depressed. Thus, it appears that further investigations are needed for making a meaningful conclusion regarding changes in the process of energy use in hearts of animals treated with toxic doses of catecholamines. Isoproterenol-induced cardiac dysfunction is associated with elevated endothelin-1 and altered cardiomyocyte response to endothelin-1 (107). Administration of isoproterenol also upregulates inducible nitric oxide synthase expression and increases nitric oxide production in the heart leading to enhanced formation of reactive nitrogen species or peroxynitrite (108).

Electrolyte Changes

Tissue Cation Contents

Table 4 shows electrolyte changes in catecholamine-induced cardiomyopathy (82,83,101,102,109,110). The sodium content of the myocardium did not change until about 24 hours, at which time it was increased; this may be a reflection of an increased interstitial fluid volume (82,83,109,110). On the other hand, alterations of myocardial potassium content are less certain. Although a transient loss of myocardial potassium has been frequently reported (100,111–113), this is a short-term phenomenon not lasting more than one to five minutes and may be a result of the increased frequency of contraction (114). In this regard, it has been

Table 4 Electrolyte Changes During the Development of Catecholamine-Induced Cardiomyopathy

Time after injection	Electrolyte changes
A. Changes in tissue cation content	
3–24 hr	Mg^{2+} ↓, phosphate ↓,
6 hr	Ca^{2+} ↑, Ca^{2+} uptake ↑ (iso) (6- to 7-fold),
24 hr	Na^+ ~ or ↑
B. Serum levels of electrolytes	
3 hr	Mg^{2+} ↑ (iso), Na^+ ↓ (iso), Ca^{2+} ↓ (iso)
7 hr	Mg^{2+} to control K^+ ↑, Na^+ ↓, Ca^{2+} ↓
24 hr	All of electrolytes became normal with the exception of Ca^{2+}

Abbreviations: ↑, increase; ~, no change; ↓, decrease; iso, by isoproterenol.

reported that norepinephrine caused a dose-dependent uptake of potassium (115). In studies concerned with the cardiotoxicity of epinephrine, both an increase (83) and a decrease (33) in the potassium content of the myocardium have been reported. A decrease of myocardial potassium content following isoproterenol injection has also been reported (96). As mentioned previously, myocardial cation content determinations are complicated by both the increase of interstitial fluid volume, which accompanies necrosis, and by the admixture of necrotic and normal fibers, which characterizes "multifocal disseminated" necrosis.

Serum Levels of Electrolytes

By 24 hours all serum electrolyte levels returned to normal with the exception of calcium, which remained slightly low. It has been reported that, after an initial period of uptake of potassium and phosphate, loss of these ions was evident (86). Thus, serum electrolyte measurements appear to confirm the loss of magnesium and phosphate from the heart and the uptake of calcium as early, important events in the etiology of catecholamine-induced necrosis. Since both net increases and decreases of myocardial and serum potassium have been found at different times, it is possible that potassium may be taken up by more or less undamaged myocardial cells while it is being released from fibers undergoing necrotic changes.

Membrane Changes

By virtue of their ability to regulate Ca^{2+} movements in the myocardial cell, different membrane systems such as SL, SR, and mitochondria are considered to determine the status of heart function in health and disease (116–119). Accordingly, alterations in SR, mitochondrial, and SL membranes were observed in myocardium from animals treated with high doses of catecholamines (120,121). To investigate the role of these membrane changes in the development of contractile dysfunction and myocardial cell damage due to catecholamines, rats were injected intraperitoneally with high doses of isoproterenol (40 mg/kg) and the hearts were removed at 3, 9, and 24 hours post injection (106,122–128). The cardiac hypertrophy as measured by the heart or body weight ratio and depression in contractile function were seen at 9 and 24 hours, whereas varying degrees of myocardial cell damage occurred within 3 to 24 hours of isoproterenol injection (Table 5). Alterations in heart membranes were evident from the fact that phospholipid contents in SL and mitochondria were increased at 3 and 9 hours, whereas the SR phospholipid contents increased at 3, 9, and 24 hours after injecting isoproterenol. It was interesting to observe that phospholipid N-methylation, which has been shown to medulate the Ca^{2+}-transport activities (123), exhibited an increase at 3 hours and a decrease at 24 hours in both SL and SR, while no changes were observed in mitochondria (Table 5). These studies (106,122–124) suggest that changes in heart

Table 5 Cardiac Contractile Function, Structure, and Membrane Phospholipid Changes at Different Times of Injecting High Doses of Isoproterenol (40 mg/kg, i.p.) in Rats

	Time after isoproterenol injection		
	3 hr	9 hr	24 hr
Heart/body weight ratio	no change	increase	increase
Contractile force development	no change	decrease	decrease
Myocardial cell damage	slight	moderate	severe
Sarcolemmal phospholipid contents	increase	increase	no change
Sarcoplasmic reticular phospholipid contents	increase	increase	increase
Mitochondrial phospholipid contents	increase	increase	no change
Sarcolemmal phospholipid methylation	increase	no change	decrease
Sarcoplasmic reticular phospholipid methylation	increase	no change	decrease
Mitochondrial phospholipid methylation	no change	no change	no change

Source: From Refs. 106,122,123,124.

membranes during the development of catecholamine-induced cardiomyopathy are of crucial importance in determining the functional and structural status of the myocardium.

An analysis of results described in various investigations (106, 125–127) revealed that the activity of the SL Ca^{2+}-pump (ATP-dependent Ca^{2+}-uptake and Ca^{2+}-stimulated ATPase), which is concerned with the removal of Ca^{2+} from the cytoplasm, was increased at 3 hours and decreased at 24 hours following isoproterenol injection (Table 6). On the other hand, Na^+-dependent

Table 6 Sarcolemmal Changes in Myocardium at Different Times of Injecting High Doses of Isoproterenol (40 mg/kg, i.p.) in Rats

	Time after isoproterenol injection		
	3 hr	9 hr	24 hr
ATP-dependent Ca^{2+} uptake	increase	no change	decrease
Ca^{2+}-stimulated ATPase	increase	no change	decrease
Na^+-dependent Ca^{2+} uptake	decrease	decrease	decrease
Na^+-induced Ca^{2+} release	no change	no change	no change
ATP-independent Ca^{2+} binding	no change	increase	increase
Sialic acid content	no change	increase	increase
Nitrendipine binding	no change	no change	no change
Na^+/K^+ ATPase	no change	no change	no change
Ca^{2+}/Mg^{2+} ecto-ATPase	no change	no change	no change

Source: From Refs. 106,125–127.

Ca^{2+}-uptake, unlike the Na^+-induced Ca^{2+}-release, was decreased at 3, 9, and 24 hours of isoproterenol administration. The SL ATP-independent Ca^{2+}-binding, which is considered to reflect the status of superficial stores of Ca^{2+} at the cell membrane, and SL sialic acid residues, which bind Ca^{2+}, were increased at 9 and 24 hours (Table 6). These SL alterations were not associated with any changes in the nitrendipine binding (an index of Ca^{2+}-channels), Na^+-K^+ ATPase (an index of Na^+-pump), and Ca^{2+}/Mg^{2+} ecto-ATPase (an index of Ca^{2+}-gating mechanism). An early increase in SL Ca^{2+}-pump may help the cell to remove Ca^{2+}, whereas depressed Na^+-Ca^{2+} exchange can be seen to contribute toward the occurrence of intracellular Ca^{2+}-overload. Likewise, an increase in the entry of Ca^{2+} from the elevated SL superficial Ca^{2+} stores as well as depressed SL Ca^{2+}-pump may contribute toward the occurrence of intracellular Ca^{2+}-overload at late stage catecholamine-induced cardiomyopathy.

It is now well known that relaxation of the cardiac muscle is mainly determined by the activity of Ca^{2+}-pump located in the SR, whereas the interaction of Ca^{2+} with myofibrils determines the ability of myocardium to contract. On the other hand, mitochondria, which are primarily concerned with the production of ATP, are also known to accumulate Ca^{2+} to lower the intracellular concentration of Ca^{2+} under pathological conditions. Data from different studies (106,122,124) as summarized in Table 7 indicate biphasic changes in the sarcoplasmic reticular Ca^{2+}-pump (ATP-dependent Ca^{2+}-uptake and Ca^{2+}-stimulated ATPase) activities during the development of catecholamine-induced cardiomyopathy. Mitochondrial Ca^{2+}-uptake, unlike mitochondrial ATPase activity, was increased at 9 and 24 hours of isoproterenol injection. Although no change in myofibrillar Ca^{2+}-stimulated ATPase activity was apparent, the myofibrillar Mg^{2+} ATPase activity was depressed at 9 and 24 hours of isoproterenol injection (Table 7). Time-dependent changes in the adrenergic receptor mechanisms

Table 7 Subcellular Alterations in Myocardium at Different Times of Injecting High Doses of Isoproterenol (40 mg/kg; i.p.) in Rats

	Time after isoproterenol injection		
	3 hr	9 hr	24 hr
Sarcoplasmic reticular Ca^{2+} uptake	increase	no change	decrease
Sarcoplasmic reticular Ca^{2+}-stimulated ATPase	increase	no change	decrease
Mitochondrial Ca^{2+} uptake	no change	increase	increase
Mitochondrial ATPase	no change	no change	no change
Myofibrillar Ca^{2+}-stimulated ATPase	no change	no change	no change
Myofibrillar Mg^{2+} ATPase	no change	decrease	decrease

Source: From Refs. 106,122,124.

Table 8 Changes in Adrenergic Receptor Mechanisms in Myocardium at Different Times of Injecting High Doses of Isoproterenol (40 mg/kg; i.p.) in Rats

	Time after isoproterenol injection		
	3 hr	9 hr	24 hr
β-adrenergic receptors	no change	decrease	no change
α-adrenergic receptors	no change	no change	decrease
Adenylyl cyclase activity	no change	no change	no change
Epinephrine-stimulated adenylyl cyclase	decrease	decrease	no change
Gpp(NH)p-stimulated adenylyl cyclase	decrease	decrease	decrease
NaF-stimulated adenylyl cyclase	decrease	decrease	decrease

Source: From Refs. 128.

(128), which are also concerned with the regulation of Ca^{2+} movements in myocardium, were also seen during the development of catecholamine-induced cardiomyopathy (Table 8). In particular, the number of γ-adrenergic receptors was decreased at 9 hours, whereas the number of α-adrenergic receptors decreased at 24 hours of isoproterenol injection. In another study it was found that norepinephrine increased myocardial β_1-adrenoceptor density at one and four hours post norepinephrine treatment (129); in contrast, chronic administration of norepinephrine for eight weeks has been shown to reduce β_1-adrenoceptor density (130,131). The basal adenylyl cyclase activities were not changed, whereas stimulation of adenylyl cyclase by epinephrine was depressed at three and nine hours. Activation of adenylyl cyclase by a non-hydrolyzable analog of guanine nucleotide (Gpp(NH)p) and NaF was decreased at 3, 9, and 24 hours of isoproterenol injection (Table 8). Chronic infusion of isoproterenol has also been associated with an increase in cardiac β-adrenergic receptor kinase content (132). Recently in another study, early changes in intracellular Ca^{2+}-overload were observed to occur two minutes following isoproterenol injection. During the preinfarction period (before 12 hours) there was a significant increase in Ca^{2+} levels in cardiac mitochondrial and microsomal fractions. Enhanced mitochondrial Ca^{2+}-uptake, decreased ryanodine binding and Na^+/Ca^{2+} exchanger activity, as well as activation of PMCA and SERCA have also been reported. These changes lead to failed compensation and failed recuperation of Ca^{2+} dynamics during the first six hours post isoproterenol treatment (64). Accordingly, it is suggested that subcellular mechanisms concerned with the regulation of Ca^{2+} movements are altered in catecholamine-induced cardiomyopathy.

In summary, it appears that some of the changes in heart membranes are adaptive in nature, whereas others contribute toward the pathogenesis of myocardial cell damage and contractile dysfunction. The early increase in

SL and SR Ca^{2+}-pump mechanisms as well as late changes in mitochondrial Ca^{2+}-uptake seems to help the myocardial cell in lowering the intracellular concentration of Ca^{2+}. On the other hand, the early depression in SL Na^{+}-Ca^{2+} exchange and late decrease in SL and SR Ca^{2+}-pump may lead to the development of intracellular Ca^{2+}-overload. This change may result in the redistribution and activation of lysosomal enzymes (133) and other mechanisms for the disruption of the myocardial cell due to high levels of circulating catecholamines. It should be mentioned that genes such as UCP2 and FHL1 have been identified to play a role in the development of cardiomyopathy induced by β-adrenergic signaling (134). Increased protein amounts of the tumor suppressor PTEN in response to isoproterenol stimulation may negatively regulate PI3 kinase activity (135). PI3 kinase γ was found to be critical for inducing myocardial hypertrophy, interstitial fibrosis, and cardiac dysfunction in response to β-adrenergic stimulation (136). P110g -/- mice, which are deficient for the catalytic subunit for pI3 kinase γ, have shown resistance to the effects of isoproterenol on cardiac structure and function; however, these animals did not show any change in the induction of hypertrophy markers in response to isoproterenol (136).

Coronary Spasm and Catecholamines

Under a wide variety of stressful conditions, where circulating levels of catecholamines are markedly elevated, the occurrence of coronary spasm and arrhythmia has been well recognized (137). In fact, coronary spasm is considered to result in arrhythmia, myocardial ischemia, and myocardial cell damage because of catecholamines. To understand the mechanisms of coronary spasm, changes in coronary resistance were monitored upon infusion of norepinephrine in the isolated perfused rat heart preparations (138). A biphasic change in coronary resistance was evident; however, when norepinephrine infusion was carried out in the presence of a β-adrenergic blocking agent, propranolol, only a marked increase in coronary resistance (coronary spasm) was evident. This coronary spasm was dependent on the extracellular concentration of Ca^{2+} and was prevented by α-adrenergic blocking agents as well as Ca^{2+} antagonists (138). On the other hand, indomethacin and acetylsalicylic acid, which interfere with prostaglandin metabolism, did not modify the norepinephrine-induced coronary spasm (138). In another set of experiments, intravenous injection of epinephrine in rats was observed to elicit varying degrees of arrhythmias, depending on the time and dose of the hormone (139,140). Pretreatment of animals with vitamin E, reducing agent (cysteine), or oxygen-free radical scavenger (SOD) was found to markedly reduce the incidence of arrhythmia due to epinephrine. These results indicate the importance of free radicals in the generation of cardiotoxic effects of high concentrations of catecholamines.

MECHANISMS OF CATECHOLAMINE-INDUCED CARDIOMYOPATHY

Although excessive amounts of circulating catecholamines are known to induce cardiomyopathy, the mechanisms are not clearly understood. Various theories have been proposed to suggest the cause and mechanisms for the development of catecholamine-induced cardiomyopathy. The major hypotheses include: (*i*) a relative cardiac hypoxemia due to increased cardiac work and myocardial oxygen demands, aggravated by hypotension in the case of isoproterenol (30,62); (*ii*) coronary arterial vasoconstriction (spasm) causing endocardial ischemia (27,28); (*iii*) inadequate perfusion of the endocardium due to impaired venous drainage of the heart (141); (*iv*) hypoxia due to direct oxygen-wasting effects of catecholamines or their oxidation products (41); (*v*) interference with mitochondrial oxidative phosphorylation by free fatty acids (142,143); (*vi*) occurrence of intracellular Ca^{2+}-overload due to massive calcium influx (102); (*vii*) formation of adrenochromes and other oxidation products including oxyradicals (124,138,140); (*viii*) potassium depletion (144) and altered permeability of the myocardial cell membrane through elevation of plasma nonesterified–free fatty acids (145); and, (*ix*) depletion of intracellular magnesium required for many ATP-dependent enzymatic processes (109,146).

This section is devoted to discussion of different mechanisms, which have been suggested to explain the cardiotoxic effects of catecholamines.

Relative Hypoxia and Hemodynamic Changes

Figure 1 shows the concept of relative cardiac hypoxemia and hemodynamic changes, which have been shown to occur as a consequence of an injection of isoproterenol. It was found that both high and low doses of isoproterenol increased heart rate similarly, but the cardiac lesion–producing doses of isoproterenol resulted in a fall in blood pressure. It was suggested that the fall in aortic blood pressure was of such a degree that a reduced coronary flow could be inferred. It was further postulated that the necrotic lesions are the ischemic infarcts due to a decreased coronary flow during a time when both amplitude and frequency of cardiac contractions are increased. Thus, the greater damage to myocardium by isoproterenol as compared with epinephrine or norepinephrine was attributed to the dramatic hypotension. Various factors, such as previous myocardial damage, previous isoproterenol injections, or activation of metabolic processes were considered to provide cardiac muscle cells with an adaptation to withstand the increased oxygen demand and relative hypoxia produced by isoproterenol (147). On the other hand, it was found that dl-ephedrine and d-amphetamine produced lesions in less than 50% of animals, although these agents increase blood pressure, while ephedrine and amphetamine have a positive inotropic effect (34). Accordingly, it was suggested that drugs with both positive inotropic and chronotropic actions might not produce cardiac lesions. In fact, methoxamine, which has no positive inotropic effect, was found to produce

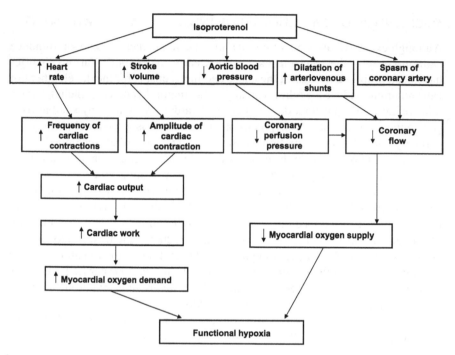

Figure 1 Myocardial functional hypoxia due to isoproterenol.

cardiac lesions. In another study (35), the hemodynamic effects of "pharmacologic" and lesion-producing doses of sympathomimetics were compared. It was found that lesion-producing doses of isoproterenol decreased aortic flow and heart rate as compared with pharmacological doses, but these were still above the control values. Stroke work was greater with lesion-producing doses as compared with pharmacological doses, but the mean aortic pressure, which determines the coronary perfusion pressure, was not reduced by the lesion-producing doses of isoproterenol. Thus, there is evidence of impaired function of the myocardium, but the hemodynamic change does not appear adequate to produce insufficient myocardial perfusion. As a result of these findings, it was suggested that the effects of isoproterenol were due to some direct action on the myocardial cell and not solely due to the hemodynamic effects. Furthermore, the coronary flow could not have been greatly reduced by isoproterenol because the blood pressure remained above that in shock and the cardiac output was increased (31), and thus it was concluded that hypotension is nonessential for the production of cardiac necrosis by isoproterenol. This view was supported by the finding that verapamil was effective in protecting the heart from isoproterenol-induced necrosis even though blood pressure fell almost twice as much when verapamil was administered together with isoproterenol as it did following administration of isoproterenol alone (148).

Coronary Spasms and Hemodynamic Effects

Another hypothesis closely related to that of coronary insufficiency of hemo-dynamic origin is that of a relative ischemia resulting from coronary vascular changes. It was found that isoproterenol changed the distribution of uniform coronary flow in the endomyocardium (27). These results suggest that dilatation of arteriovenous shunts might be responsible for the endocardial ischemia because coronary flow is usually increased with isoproterenol. On the other hand, a marked occlusion of coronary vessels was observed in 69% of animals at 30 minutes and 33% of animals at 60 minutes, but almost no occlusion was seen at 24 hours following isoproterenol injection (149). It was thought that these results occurred due to spasm of the coronary vessels. Changes in peripheral resistance due to catecholamines were also important because it was possible to reproduce essentially similar pathological changes by surgical occlusion of the efferent vessels (141). On this basis it was suggested that impairment of venous drainage via venospasm largely accounts for the adverse effects of catecholamines.

Blood flow to the LV subendocardial muscle has been suggested to be compromised during systole and to occur mainly during diastole because intramyocardial compressive force is greatest in this region (150,151). Further-more, it has been shown (152) that when aortic diastolic pressure was lowered or diastole shortened (by pacing) and myocardial oxygen demands simultaneously raised, myocardial performance was found to be impaired. Scintillation counting of the distribution of ^{141}Ce-, ^{85}Sr-, or ^{46}Sc-labeled microspheres was used to determine the coronary flow distribution during isoproterenol infusion (153). When isoproterenol was infused at a rate, which failed to maintain the increase in contractile force, it was found that subendocardial flow fell by 35%, while subepicardial flow increased by 19%. Thus, although spasm of coronary arteries and/or veins may well occur, it is possible that increased cardiac activity, reduced aortic pressure, and greatly decreased diastole could also be responsible for an under perfusion of the endocardium.

A serious challenge to the concept of impaired ventricular perfusion as the primary cause of necrosis was presented by employing the ^{85}Kr clearance method to study perfusion of the ventricle during epinephrine infusion (33). Evidence of myocardial necrosis was obtained 75 minutes after the start of epinephrine infusion, but ^{85}Kr clearance studies showed no difference in the rate of clearance from inner, middle, and outer layers of the left ventricle in either the control or epinephrine-treated hearts. Thus, there was no evidence for ischemia of subendocardial tissue as a causal factor in the epinephrine-induced necrosis. On the other hand, a decreased passage of the trace substance horseradish per-oxidase from the capillaries to the myocardial interstitium was observed in a study in which isoproterenol was infused at a low concentration (25). Thus, this controversy still remained to be resolved. The hypothesis that the vascular factors are the primary cause of necrotic lesions was also tested using the turtle heart as a unique model in which perfusion of the endocardium is not vascular (32). In the turtle heart, the internal spongy musculature is supplied by diffusion from the ventricular lumen via intertrabecular spaces, while the outer compact layer is supplied by the coronary artery branching off the aorta. Isoproterenol injections were found to produce necrotic lesions in the spongy layer of the turtle heart, which does not support the concept that isoproterenol-induced cardiac necrosis is due to a vascular mechanism.

Metabolic Effects

Figure 2 shows the concept involving metabolic and hemodynamic changes in the development of catecholamine-induced cardiomyopathy. It was pointed out that the catecholamine-induced myocardial necrosis must be considered to be of a mixed pathogenesis involving both direct metabolic actions in the cardiac muscle as well as factors secondary to vascular and hemodynamic effects (154). Cardiac lesions due to epinephrine and isoproterenol are of a mixed type in which both hypoxia secondary to vascular and hemodynamic effects as well as direct metabolic effects in the heart muscle have a role in their development. It is not, then, unreasonable to regard vascular and hemodynamic effects as complicating factors, which greatly aggravate some more direct toxic influence of catecholamines on myocardial cells. Accordingly, it can be readily understood

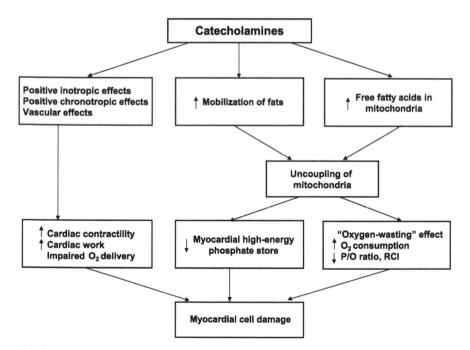

Figure 2 Cardiac and lipid mobilization in catecholamine-induced cardiomyopathy.

how a reduction in the extent and severity of catecholamine-induced lesions is brought about by interventions, which specifically block the peripheral vascular change, prevent the positive inotropic and chronotropic effects of these drugs on the heart, or improve the delivery of oxygen to the myocardium.

Many years ago Raab (41) attributed the cardiotoxic actions of catecholamines to their oxygen-wasting effect. According to him: "The most conspicuous reaction of myocardial metabolism to the administration of adrenaline is an intense enhancement of local oxygen consumption which, in certain dosages, by far exceeds the demand of simultaneously increased myocardial muscular work, and which is only partially compensated by a simultaneous increase of coronary blood flow. In this respect adrenaline is able, so to speak, to mimic the anoxiating effects of coronary insufficiency in the absence of any real coronary anomaly. It should be emphasized, however, that the tissue anoxia resulting from the administration of adrenaline is probably not caused by adrenaline itself but by an oxidation product of adrenaline (Bruno Kisch's omega), which acts as an oxidation catalyst even in very high dilutions." It was found that identical electrocardiographic changes occurred during cardiac sympathetic nerve stimulation, electrically induced muscular exercise, or intravenous injection of norepinephrine or epinephrine, when coronary artery dilatability is impaired and during exogenous anoxia or partial occlusion of the coronary arteries (155). This was taken as evidence that the increased O_2 consumption caused by catecholamines produced a relative hypoxia if coronary flow could not be sufficiently increased.

A crucial point in the concept of oxygen wasting concerns the origin of the increased O_2 consumption with catecholamines—whether it is due to a decreased efficiency of oxygen use or an increased oxygen demand. It was found that the oxygen consumption of resting papillary muscle was not increased by catecholamines even in concentrations 10 times higher than those effective in stimulating O_2 consumption of contracting papillary muscles (156). This study concluded that the increased O_2 consumption of the intact heart following administration of epinephrine or norepinephrine is secondary to the increased contractility. On the other hand, it was reported that low dose norepinephrine exerted a maximal inotropic effect with little or no increase of O_2 consumption, while larger doses had no further inotropic effect but did increase O_2 consumption, indicating that it is excessive catecholamine concentrations which cause oxygen wasting (157).

It was observed that the increase of O_2 consumption of the potassium-arrested heart caused by catecholamines was 5% to 20% of that found in the beating heart (158); this study concluded that most, but not all, of the increased O_2 consumption was secondary to hemodynamic alterations and increased cardiac work. In a similar comparison of the effects of epinephrine on O_2 consumption in beating and arrested hearts, it was found that about one-third of the increment in O_2 consumption in beating hearts was accounted for by a metabolic effect dissociable from the increased work (159). Furthermore, it was reported that this effect could be blocked by dichloroisoproterenol but not by phentol-amine (160). From these studies it is evident that catecholamines can cause an increase in O_2 consumption that is not related to increased cardiac work or activity and the concept of decreased efficiency or oxygen wasting is therefore justified. It has been suggested that this oxygen-wasting effect was actually due to an oxidation product of epinephrine (41), and one such oxidation product, adrenochrome, was shown to uncouple mitochondria (161). The uncoupling of mitochondria by adrenochrome was antagonized by GSH in high concentration, probably due to a direct reduction of adrenochrome, since the characteristic red color of adrenochrome was lost when GSH was added in the presence or absence of mitochondria, whereas oxidized GSH did not affect this uncoupling by adrenochrome.

It was found the P:O ratio of heart mitochondria by norepinephrine, epi-nephrine, or isoproterenol was significantly low (42). RCI and QO_2 were similar to control, but unfortunately the control RCI values in these experiments were very low. A good relationship between elevation of myocardial catecholamine content and depression of P:O ratio in mitochondria was observed. Whereas propranolol pretreatment enhanced the increase in myocardial catecholamines and caused a more marked depression of mitochondrial P:O ratios, dibenzyline and reserpine inhibited both the increase in catecholamine contents and the decrease in the mitochondrial P:O ratio. Since catecholamines under in vitro conditions did not affect the P:O ratio of mitochondria at a concentration of 1 mM, it was concluded that this was not a direct action of the catecholamines on the mitochondria, but instead adrenochrome or one of its metabolites might be responsible for the observed effect (42). In one experiment studying the oxida-tive phosphorylation of heart mitochondria from isoproterenol-treated rats revealed that the RCI was reduced without affecting the P:O ratio (96). It is not possible to draw any definite conclusions from these studies with respect to the effects of catecholamines on mitochondrial respiration, although uncoupling of oxidative phosphorylation is certainly indicated and would explain both the oxygen-wasting effect and the depletion of myocardial high-energy phosphate stores caused by large doses of catecholamines.

Having found that heart mitochondria from catecholamine-treated rats were uncoupled, the level of free fatty acids in the mitochondria was determined because free fatty acids are known to uncouple mitochondria (42). No difference in mitochondrial-free fatty acid content or composition was found, and it was concluded that the observed uncoupling might not be due to the accumulation of fatty acids. Furthermore, ephedrine, which produced no significant changes in plasma nonesterified–free fatty acids, was observed to cause cardiac lesions (145). Nevertheless, it was found that inhibition of lipolysis by nicotinic acid, β-pyridyl carbonyl, or high plasma glucose concentrations during infusion of isoproterenol could substantially reduce the increase in myocardial oxygen consumption. This may be possibly due to the prevention of the uncoupling action of high intracellular concentrations of free fatty acid in the heart, following catecholamine administration (142). A casual relationship between the increase in plasma-free fatty acids following norepinephrine administration and the occurrence of cardiac lesions has also been postulated (143). The evidence fails to implicate elevated levels of free fatty acids as primary agents in mitochondrial uncoupling following administration of catecholamines. But it was suggested that metabolism of free fatty acids in some way aggravate the cardiotoxic effects of catecholamines (142) as well as the correlation of severity of lesions with the amount of body fat (162).

Electrolytes Shifts and Intercellular Ca^{2+}-Overload

Figure 3 shows the concept of electrolyte shifts in the genesis of catecholamine-induced cardiomyopathy. In view of the close relationship between electrolyte shifts and the occurrence of necrotic lesions, it has been suggested that changes in myocardial electrolyte contents initiated by altered cationic transfer ability of myocardial cells at the plasma membrane and subcellular membrane sites by catecholamines contribute to irreversible failure of cell function (109). Critical in the pathogenesis of irreversible damage was the loss of cellular Mg^{2+} (146). In

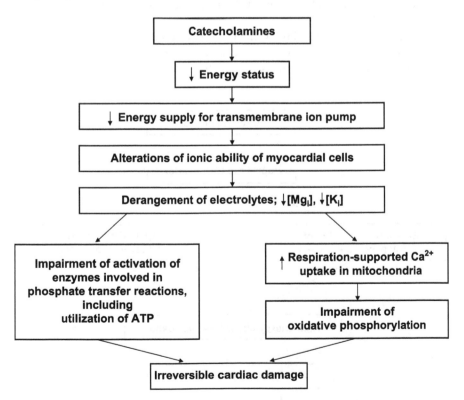

Figure 3   Energy status and electrolyte shifts in catecholamine-induced cardiomyopathy.

this regard, it was pointed out that Mg^{2+} is an important activator cation participating in the function of many enzymes involved in phosphate transfer reactions, including use of ATP. Unfortunately, this mechanism cannot be considered adequate to explain the reduction of high-energy phosphate content in the myocardium (102), since interference with energy use would have the opposite effect. On the other hand, Mg^{2+} is reported to cause a decrease in the respiration-supported uptake of Ca^{2+} by isolated heart mitochondria (163) and could thus be important in regulating the mitochondrial function in terms of oxidative phosphorylation. It has been similarly argued that it is the derangement of myocardial electrolyte balance, specifically the loss of K^+ and Mg^{2+} ions from the myocardium, which is the central mechanism in a variety of cardiomyopathies (144). But this derangement of electrolyte balance was considered to be secondary to an inadequate supply of energy for transmembrane cation pumps required for the maintenance of electrolyte equilibrium, which occurs with oxygen deficiency or impaired energy production. It has also been suggested that electrolyte shifts are an important component in the development of irreversible damage produced by both direct and indirect pathogenic mechanisms, and that myocardial resistance is related to the ability of the heart to maintain a normal electrolyte balance in the face of potentially cardiotoxic episodes (154).

Figure 4 shows the involvement of intracellular Ca^{2+}-overload in the pathogenesis of catecholamine-induced cardiomyopathy. It was observed that the isoproterenol-induced necrosis and decline in high-energy phosphates were

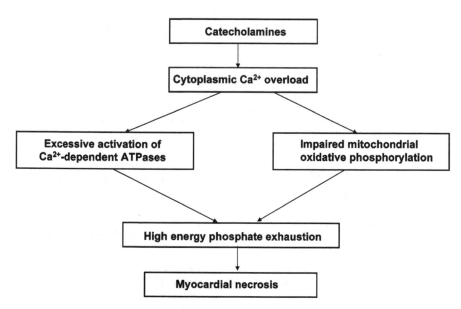

Figure 4 Intracellular Ca^{2+}-overload in catecholamine-induced cardiomyopathy.

associated with a six- to sevenfold increase in the rate of radioactive Ca^{2+}-uptake and a doubling of net myocardial Ca^{2+} content (102). This finding suggested that isoproterenol causes a greatly increased influx of Ca^{2+}, which overloads the cardiomyocytes. It was postulated that the intracellular Ca^{2+}-overload initiates a depression in high-energy phosphate stores by excessive activation of Ca^{2+}-dependent ATPases and impairing mitochondrial oxidative phosphorylation. When high-energy phosphate exhaustion reaches a critical level, fiber necrosis results. This hypothesis attempts to explain why the myocardium is sensitized to isoproterenol-induced necrosis by factors, such as 9-α-fluorocortisol acetate, dihydrotachysterol, NaH_2PO_4, high extracellular Ca^{2+}, or increased blood pH, which favors intracellular Ca^{2+}-overload. Consistent with this hypothesis, K^+ and Mg^{2+} salts, low extracellular Ca^{2+}, thyrocalcitonin, low blood pH, or specific blockers of transmembrane Ca^{2+} fluxes protect the heart against isoproterenol, presumably by preventing the occurence of intracellular Ca^{2+}-overload. In support of the central role for Ca^{2+}-overload in the pathogenesis of catecholamine-induced necrosis is the observation that spontaneous necrotization of cardiac tissue in myopathic hamsters, which exhibit high levels of circulating catecholamines, is prevented by treatment with a Ca^{2+}-channel blocker, verapamil (164,165). It was also shown that propranolol could completely block the increase of Ca^{2+} content of the myocardium but would only reduce the incidence of lesions rather than preventing them. Also, necrosis of skeletal muscle fibers can be induced through mechanical injury of the cell membrane, permitting increased amount of Ca^{2+}-influx, which can be prevented by elimination of Ca^{2+} from the Ringer solution or by an outward electric current, which blocks Ca^{2+}-influx (166). Unfortunately, there is no direct evidence that it is in fact Ca^{2+}, which produces the decline of high-energy phosphate in the hearts of animals given isoproterenol, and a causal relationship has not yet been established. Furthermore, it has been found that myocardial Ca^{2+} content increased on increasing the dose of isoproterenol in the range from 0.1 to 10 μg/kg, but it did not increase further with higher dose levels required to produce myocardial lesions (167). It has also been shown that increased cystolic Ca^{2+} in the myocytes may be due to leakage from the SR through dysfunctional ryanodine receptors (168). Thus, it was suggested that the inotropic response to catecholamines is related to Ca^{2+} entry but that the necrosis may be due to some other factor, possibly the intracellular metabolism of Ca^{2+}. Nonetheless, the dramatic modification of necrosis by factors influencing transmembrane Ca^{2+} fluxes clearly suggests the involvement of Ca^{2+} at some level in the etiology of necrosis caused by catecholamines (167).

Figure 5 shows the concept involving MAO and other oxidation processes in the development of catecholamine-induced cardiomyopathy. On the basis of coincidence of localization of isoproterenol-induced myocardial lesions and the highest myocardial MAO activity, it has been suggested that the accumulation of products metabolically formed during deamination of catecholamines may be the cause of necrosis in the heart (169). It is further pointed out that the lower

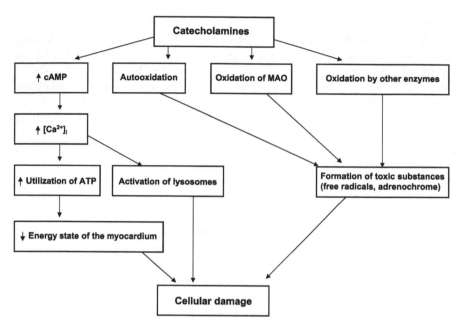

Figure 5 Increase cyclic AMP and oxidation of catecholamines in catecholamine-induced cardiomyopathy. *Abbreviation*: MAO, monoamine oxidase.

sensitivity to isoproterenol may be due to the lesser MAO activity in the hearts of young rats in comparison with the older rats. These observations as well as the protective effect of monoamine oxidase inhibitors (MAOI) do not appear to be consistent with the hypothesis of intracellular Ca^{2+}-overload. Likewise, no specific explanation has been offered for the changes in contractile proteins, which are seen to occur in catecholamine-induced necrotic lesions except for the suggestion that a direct interaction of catecholamine or some metabolite with the heavy meromyosin region of the myosin molecule is involved (104). It is possible that MAOI may reduce the oxidation of catecholamines and thus decrease the formation of toxic substance such as free radicals and adrenochrome and subsequent myocardial necrosis. It may very well be that lysosomes (133) are activated because of intracellular Ca^{2+}-overload, and this may produce cellular damage due to catecholamines. Furthermore, catecholamines are known to markedly increase the concentration of cAMP in the heart, and it is likely that this agent in high concentrations may represent an important factor for causing catecholamine-induced myocardial necrosis in association with changes due to the oxidation products of catecholamines (Fig. 5).

In summary, the majority of the factors found to influence the severity of catecholamine-induced lesions can be understood in terms of their effects on hemodynamic factors, delivery of oxygen to the myocardium, electrolyte balance, metabolism of calcium, and mobilization of lipids. It would thus appear

Table 9 Possible Mechanisms for Cardiotoxic Effects of High Levels of Circulating Catecholamines

1. Functional hypoxia	a.	Increased cardiac work
	b.	Excessive demand for O_2
2. Coronary insufficiency	a.	Coronary spasm
	b.	Hemodynamic effects
3. Increased membrane permeability	a.	Electrolyte shift
	b.	Loss of intracellular contents
4. Decreased levels of high energy phosphate stores	a.	Excessive hydrolysis of ATP
	b.	Uncoupling of mitochondrial oxidative phosphorylation
5. Alterations in lipid metabolism	a.	Increased lipolysis
	b.	Increased accumulation of fatty acids
6. Intracellular Ca^{2+} overload	a.	Excessive Ca^{2+} entry and intracellular release
	b.	Depressed Ca^{2+} efflux and intracellular uptake
7. Oxidative stress	a.	Formation of free radicals
	b.	Formation of adrenochrome

that hemodynamic and coronary vascular factors contribute significantly to the severity of myocardial damage following catecholamine administration, but that some primary pathogenic mechanism acting directly on the myocardial cell is probably involved as well. Furthermore, it is clear that the exhaustion of high-energy phosphate store and disruption of electrolyte balance are crucial events in the etiology of irreversible cell damage. Although mobilization of lipids and the occurrence of intracellular Ca^{2+}-overload may be involved, the nature of the direct pathogenic influence following injection of catecholamines is yet unknown. Some of the possible mechanisms, which have been proposed to explain the cardiotoxic effects of catecholamines, are given in Table 9.

Adrenochrome and Related Oxidation Products

Catecholamines can easily undergo oxidation with production of unstable catecholamine o-quinones that in turn give rise to the respective adrenochromes and subsequent production of oxygen-free radicals like superoxide radicals. These superoxide radicals can then be reduced by SOD to hydrogen peroxide (129). Auto-oxidation products of catecholamines, such as adrenochrome, acting in conjuction with catecholamines, are critical factors in inducing cardiomyopathy and in initiating myocardial necrosis. This effect may be mediated through generation of free radical and their interaction with the sulfhydryl groups. In addition to the spontaneous oxidation of epinephrine to adrenochrome by an autocatalytic process (170), adrenochrome is enzymatically formed in mammalian tissues. These enzymes include tyrosinases (171–176) and polyphenol oxidases from various sources (176–180), particularly in guinea pig and rat muscles (180). Other enzyme systems shown to actively convert epinephrine to adrenochrome are xanthine oxidase (181), leukocyte myeloperoxidase (182,183), heart muscle cytochrome C oxidase (184–186), cyanide insensitive system present in the heart and skeletal muscle (187), cytochrome-indophenol oxidase system present in all tissues (187,188), and an unidentified enzyme in the cat salivary gland (189). The oxidation of epinephrine has also been reported to be catalyzed by cytochrome C and methamyoglobin (190), which stabilizes the formation of adrenochrome in the presence of bicarbonate buffer regardless of the oxidizing system used (191), and has been reported to occur in blood (192,193). Much of the work in the literature dealing with the physiological and pharmacological effects of the oxidation products of epinephrine was carried out before the structure of adrenochrome was known, and has been discussed in a review article on this subject (194). Furthermore, in view of the inherent instability of adrenochrome in solution, one can not be certain whether the specific effects or the absence of certain effects can truly be considered as an accurate assessment of the adrenochrome activity. Nevertheless, it is worth reviewing the broad spectrum of physiological activities, which have been attributed to adrenochrome or at least to some closely related products of adrenochrome.

Table 10 shows the effects of adrenochrome, adrenoxyl, and oxidized epinephrine. Oxidized epinephrine solutions have been found to inhibit cardiac

Table 10 Effects of Adrenochrome, Adrenoxyl, and Oxidized Epinephrine

A. Adrenochrome	blood pressure $\downarrow$, vasoconstriction, powerful hemostatic agents, capillary permeability $\downarrow$, blood sugar $\downarrow$ (anti-insulinase), O_2 consumption $\downarrow$ (?), oxygen uptake $\sim$ or $\downarrow$, lactic acid production $\downarrow$, uncoupling of mitochondria oxidation phosphorylation, P/O ratio $\downarrow$, pyruvate oxidation $>$ succinate oxidation
B. Adrenoxyl	mitochondrial K^+ $\downarrow$, ATPase activity $\downarrow$, alteration of P/O ratio
Adrenochrome (Inhibition) glucose (Stimulation)	phosphorylation, glycolysis, hexokinase, phosphofrucktokinase glycogen synthesis, hexose monophosphate shunt
Adrenochrome + Adrenoxyl (Inhibition)	myosin ATPase activity
Adrenochrome + oxidized epinephrine (Inhibition)	monoamine oxidase, the enzyme alkaline phosphatase
Adrenochrome + Adrenoxyl	antimitotic activity $\downarrow$, coenzyme A $\downarrow$, antihistaminic effect $\downarrow$, mitochondrial material $\uparrow$

inotropism and chronotropism (172,173,177,195–197) and to increase rather than decrease the tone of rabbit intestinal strips (198). Adrenochrome has been reported to increase blood pressure (199,200), to be effective as a vasoconstrictor (201), to be a powerful hemostatic agent, and to diminish the capillary permeability (202,203). Adrenochrome has frequently been reported to reduce blood sugar levels and potentiate the effects of insulin and has been described as an anti-insulinase (194,204), although this claim has been disputed (205). Administration of adrenochrome either by injection or by feeding has been reported to increase oxygen consumption in humans and guinea pigs (206,207) as well as tissue oxygen consumption in vitro (208,209). On the other hand, some investigators have observed that adrenochrome may stimulate, inhibit, or have no effect on tissue oxygen consumption, depending on the metabolic substrate used (210) or the adrenochrome concentration (211). Reports are also available to show that adrenochrome did not affect the oxygen uptake in rat muscle (212) but inhibited oxygen uptake and lactic acid production in dog heart slices (213). Adrenochrome has been observed to uncouple mitochondrial oxidative phosphorylation and depress P:O ratios (161,214,215). It has been suggested that adrenochrome may act as a hydrogen carrier between substrate and molecular oxygen with the formation of water and regeneration of adrenochrome after each cycle (214).

Adrenochrome was reported to be much more effective in inhibiting pyruvate oxidation than succinate oxidation (215). Adrenoxyl, a closely related epinephrine oxidation product, has been found to lower mitochondrial potassium content, decrease mitochondrial ATPase activity, and alter mitochondrial P:O ratio (216). Adrenochrome also inhibited hexokinase and phosphofructokinase, thus inhibiting glucose phosphorylation and glycolysis, while stimulating glycogen synthesis (187,217–220) and the hexose monophosphate shunt (221,222). Adrenochrome and adrenoxyl have both been found to be inhibitors of myosin ATPase activity in the heart and smooth muscle (223–226). Adrenochrome and oxidized epinephrine solutions were also observed to inhibit MAO in a variety of tissues (227–229) and alkaline phosphatase activity (230). It was thought that inhibition of different enzymes is due at least partly to the reversible oxidation of sulfhydryl groups in the enzymes (225,227). Other effects attributed to adrenochrome and adrenoxyl include antimitotic activity (231), reduction of coenzyme A levels in the heart, kidneys, and brain (232), antihistaminic properties (194), and an increase in mitochondrial material of cultured cells (233). Thus, it is evident that adrenochrome is a highly reactive molecule chemically and it not only is capable of oxidizing protein sulfhydryl groups but is also a dynamic catalyst for the deamination of a variety of amines and amino acids (234–238). Furthermore, it functions as an oxidative hydrogen carrier acting on either metabolic substrates (214) or $NADP^+$ (222) and thus altering or disrupting essential metabolic pathways. The metabolism of adrenochrome and related epinephrine oxidation products has been studied in rabbits, cats, and dogs (239–241). Adrenochrome injected into rabbits rapidly disappeared from the blood, transformed to adrenolutin in the liver, and then removed from the system via the kidney (239). Most of the adrenochrome was excreted in the urine as adrenolutin (both free and conjugated), or in the form of a fluorescent brown pigment, while a small amount was excreted unchanged. In cats and dogs, approximately 70% was excreted in the form of a variety of adrenochrome reduction products and other indoles (240). An unstable yellow pigment has been observed in the urine of rats after the injection of ^{14}C-labeled adrenochrome (242).

In view of the foregoing discussion, it can be appreciated that there is evidence both for the presence of and the formation of adrenochrome in mammalian tissues. Furthermore, adrenochrome has been shown to be capable of producing a wide variety of metabolic changes by interfering with numerous enzyme systems. Thus, adrenochrome and/or other catecholamine oxidation products may be regarded as possible candidates that are involved in toxic manifestation occurring in conjunction with catecholamine excess or altered catecholamine metabolism. The injection of catecholamines into animals can be conceived to result in the formation of oxidation products such as adrenochrome in the circulating blood as well as in the myocardial cell. The accumulation of these oxidation products in myocardium could then directly or indirectly, acting by themselves or in conjunction with other effects of catecholamines, initiate processes leading to myocardial necrosis. Accordingly, experiments were undertaken to understand the problem of whether or not catecholamines, their oxidation products, or metabolites are indeed capable of a direct toxic influence on the heart (243). When the isolated rat hearts were perfused with high concentrations of isoproterenol for one hour, no depression in contractile activity or myocardial cell damage was evident (243). These observations were confirmed by other investigators (244). On the other hand, perfusion of the isolated hearts with oxidized isoproterenol produced dramatic cardiac contractile, morphological, and subcellular alterations (243,245). Toxic effects of isoproterenol on cultured cardiac muscle cells were also shown to be due to its oxidation (246). In fact, the contractile dysfunction and myocardial cell damage in the isolated perfused rat hearts due to adrenochrome were observed to depend on its concentration as well as time of perfusion (247). Various pharmacological agents and cations, which prevent the occurrence of intracellular Ca^{2+}-overload, were observed to reduce the cardiac contractile failure and cell damage due to adrenochrome (248,249). Adrenochrome was suggested to affect Ca^{2+} movements in the myocardial cell because of its action on the SL, sarcoplasmic reticular, and mitochondrial membranes (250–253). In fact, adrenochrome was found to accumulate in the myocardium and localize at different subcellular organelles (253,254). Adrenochrome was also shown to be a potent coronary artery constrictor in the isolated rat heart preparations (255). Although administration of adrenochrome to rats was found to induce arrhythmia, myocardial cell damage, and heart dysfunction under in vivo conditions (256–258), oxidation products other than adrenochrome are also involved in the genesis of catecholamine-induced cardiotoxicity (259).

A number of mechanisms have been suggested to explain the pathogenesis of myocardial injury caused by catecholamine exposure. One possibility is that catecholamine cardiotoxicity is induced by free radicals derived from catecholamine autooxidation (260). Since the oxidation of catecholamines results in the formation of aminochromes (such as adrenochrome) and free radicals, it is possible that adrenochrome in addition to free radicals may also be involved in the development of catecholamine-induced cardiotoxicity. It is pointed out that the GSH/GSSG ratio, which is a good estimation of redox state and oxidative stress in the cell, was decreased within 1 hour to 30 days following norepinephrine administration. GSH was eventually depleted, which may be due to conjugation with o-quinone and/or oxidation to GSSG. There was also increase in GPx activity four hours after norepinephrine administration, which may contribute to GSH consumption and GSSG formation due to its action on hydrogen peroxide. The activities of both SOD and GSH reductase were increased eight hours after norepinephrine treatment. This delay in the increase of antioxidant activity may explain the accumulation of superoxide-free radical and GSSG after four hours. Since malondialdehyde was increased in norepinephrine-treated rats despite the increased antioxidant activity, it is evident that reactive oxygen species were not sufficiently neutralized (129). We have also found that rats treated with high dose isoproterenol resulted in increased malondialdehyde content as well as increased formation of conjugated dienes and low GSH redox ratio (261). Not only depressed cardiac SL ATP-dependent Ca^{2+}-uptake, Ca^{2+}-stimulated ATPase activity, and Na^+-dependent Ca^{2+} accumulation were observed in iso-proterenol-treated hearts, but such changes were also seen in rat hearts perfused with adrenochrome. All of the catecholamine-induced changes were attenuated with vitamin E treatment. Furthermore, incubation of SL membrane with different concentrations of adrenochrome decreased the ATP-dependent and Na^+-dependent Ca^{2+}-uptake activities. These findings support the occurrence of oxidative stress, which may depress the SL Ca^{2+} transport and result in the development of Ca^{2+}-overload and heart dysfunction in catecholamine-induced cardiomyopathy (261). Vitamin E was also found to prevent the isoproterenol-induced arrhythmia, lipid peroxidation, myocardial cell damage, and loss of high-energy phosphates, whereas vitamin E deficiency was shown to increase the sensitivity of animals to the cardiotoxic actions of isoproterenol (140,262,263). Freedman et al. (264) reported a correlation between myocardial susceptibility to oxidative stress due to isoprenaline-induced injury and magnesium-deficient as well as vitamin E-deficient diets. Isoproterenol-induced cardiomyopathy in rats fed vitamin E or zinc showed reduced levels of lipid peroxidation (262,263). Treatment with vitamin E, selenium, and zinc rendered protection against lesions produced in stressed pigs with high blood levels of catecholamines (265). Other antioxidants such as ascorbic acid and sodium bisulfate have also been shown to prevent the cytotoxic effects of isoproterenol in cultured rat myocardial cells (266–268). Ferulic acid, a natural antioxidant, in combination with ascorbic acid synergistically improves the mitochondrial dysfunction during isoproterenol-induced cardiotoxicity (269). Exercise training, which is considered to increase the antioxidant reserve, was reported to decrease the myocardial cell damage due to catecholamines (270,271). Probucol, a clinically used cholesterol-lowering drug with antioxidant properties, inhibited oxidative stress, enhanced endogenous antioxidant reserve (GPx), and increased ATP content (272). The mechanism by which the activation of SNS may induce oxidative stress appears to be the auto-oxidation of catecholamines; this oxidation results in the formation of cyclized o-quinones, two protons and two electrons, whereas o-semiquinones, when oxidized, result in the formation of superoxide radicals. This may start a chain reaction of hydroxide radical generation, lipid peroxidation, and protein oxidation (273). It is therefore likely that antioxidant therapy may prove highly beneficial in preventing the cardiovascular problems where the circulating levels of catecholamines are elevated markedly. In this regard, it should be pointed out that oxygen-free radials have been shown to exert cardiotoxic effects such as myocardial cell damage, contractile failure, subcellular alterations, and intracellular Ca^{2+}-overload (274–282). Thus, it appears that the generation of oxyradicals, in addition to the formation of aminochromes, may play an important role in the pathogenesis of cardiotoxicity under conditions associated with high levels of circulating catecholamines. A scheme indicating the involvement of both free radicals and adrenochrome in the development of catecholamine-induced arrhythmias, coronary spasm, contractile failure, and myocardial cell damage is depicted in Figure 6.

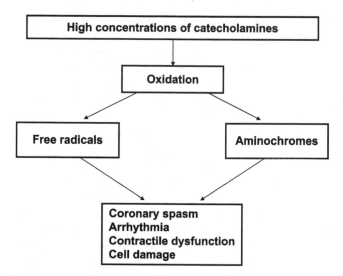

Figure 6 Schematic representation of the mechanism for the genesis of cardiotoxic effects of high concentrations of catecholamines.

MODIFICATION OF CATECHOLAMINE-INDUCED CARDIOMYOPATHY

Pharmacological Interventions

Monoamine Oxidase Inhibitors

Table 11 shows the effects of different types of drugs, including MAOIs, on catecholamine-induced cardiomyopathy. MAOI of the hydrazine type has been found to decrease the incidence and severity of myocardial lesions following catecholamine administration (90,96,162,283–286) and to antagonize increases in myocardial water, sodium, and chloride as well as loss of potassium (96). The hydrazine type inhibitors investigated include isocarboxazide, iproniazide, pivaloylbanzhydrazine, and phenylzine. On the other hand, the nonhydrazine type MAOI such as tranylcypromine, pargyline, and RO5-7071 have been reported by some workers to be ineffective (90,285,286), although a reduction of the severity of isoproterenol-induced lesions with pargyline and another nonhydrazine MAOI identified as E-250 has been reported (287). It was also found that hydrazine-type inhibition is longlasting, whereas tranylcypromine is a competitive blocker, with an intensive but transient effect and thus the inhibition produced by the nonhydrazine-type drugs may be of insufficient duration to afford protection (169).

β-Adrenergic Blocking Agents

The β-receptor blocking compounds (Table 11), propranolol, pronethalol, and dichloroisoproterenol, were found to reduce the incidence and severity of myocardial lesions induced by isoproterenol (109,110,162,167,288). While some studies (95) have reported that pronethalol was ineffective, others (94) have reported that pronethalol afforded some protection against the loss of myocardial AST activity caused by epinephrine, norepinephrine, and high doses of isoproterenol but potentiated the loss of AST activity with moderate lesion-producing doses of isoproterenol. Propranolol has also been found to ameliorate or completely prevent electrolyte shifts (increased myocardial Ca^{2+}) associated with the isoproterenol-induced necrosis (110,167), thus producing an apparent dichotomy between the occurrence of lesions and electrolyte shifts, since less severe myocardial lesions were still seen. In one study propanolol only partially prevented the cardiotoxic effects of epinephrine (289). In view of the proportion of the ventricle not undergoing necrotic damage in these experiments, it is difficult to know whether the alterations of electrolytes are truly and completely prevented. It has been reported that propranolol reduced the amount by which myocardial ATP declined following the isoproterenol-induced damage (290). Propranolol appears to have a more selective action on endocardial versus midmyocardial or epicardiac changes in metabolism due to catecholamines (291). One can thus conclude that the β-adrenergic blocking agents are capable of modifying certain cardiotoxic effects of catecholamines.

Table 11 The Effects of Some Pharmacological Agents in Catecholamine-Induced
Cardiomyopathy

	Drugs	Effects
A. Monoamine oxidase inhibitors		
a. hydrazine type	isocarboxazide	decrease
	iproniazide	decrease
	pivaloylbanzhydrazine	decrease
	phenylzine	decrease
b. nonhydrazine type	tranilcypromine	no change
	pargyline	no change
	R05-707	no change or decrease (iso)
	E-250	decrease
B. β-adrenergic blocking agents	popranolol	decrease (iso)
	pronethalol	decrease or no change (iso, epi, nor)
	dicloroisoproterenol	decrease (iso)
C. α-adrenergic blocking agents	azapetine	decrease (phe, epi, nor) no change (iso)
	phentolamine	decrease (phe, epi, nor) no change (iso)
	diberanamine	decrease (phe, epi, nor) no change (iso)
	dihydroergocryptin	decrease (phe, epi, nor) no change (iso)
	phenoxybenzamine	decrease (phe, epi, nor) no change (iso)
	tolazoline	decrease (phe, epi, nor) no change (iso)
D. Postganglionic blockers	guanethidine	no change (iso)
	isocaramidine	no change (iso)
	reserpine	no change (iso)
	pyrogallol	no change (iso)
	serotonin + nialimide	decrease
E. Calcium channel blocker	verapamil	decrease (iso)
	D600	decrease (iso)
	phenylamine	decrease (iso)
	vascoril	decrease (iso)
	diltiazem	decrease (iso)
	clentiazem	decrease (epi)
F. Angiotensin converting enzyme inhibitor	captopril	decrease
G. Antiarrhythmic drug	propafenone	decrease (epi)

Abbreviations: decrease, decrease in the severity of myocardial lesion; no change, no change
of the severity of myocardial lesion; iso, isoproterenol; epi, epinephrine; nor, norepinephrine; phe,
phenylephrine.

α-Adrenergic Blocking Agents

The α-adrenergic blocking compounds (Table 11), such as azapetine, phentolamine, dibenamine, dihydroergocryptin, phenoxybenzamine, and tolazoline were ineffective against isoproterenol (90,95,288,292,293) but reduced somewhat the incidence and severity of lesions caused by α-receptor agonists, such as phenylephrine (109,293), epinephrine (95,109,293,294), and norepinephrine (95,293). The α-blockers also ameliorated the loss of myocardial AST and LDH activities as well as the shift of electrolytes caused by epinephrine and norepinephrine (83,95,295). These agents were usually more effective against epinephrine lesions when used in combination with a β-blocker (83,109,289,293).

Postganglionic Blockers and Others

The postganglionic blocker (Table 11), guanethidine, has been reported to be ineffective (90,292) or to increase the severity (287) of necrosis caused by isoproterenol. Isocaramidine has also been found to have no effect on the isoproterenol-induced necrosis (90). Reserpine, which is known to decrease catecholamine stores, has been reported to be without effect (90,286) or to increase the severity (169,287) of isoproterenol-induced lesions. Pyrogallol, a catechol-O-methyl transferase inhibitor, increased the severity of lesions (169). Serotonin and nialimide administered together reduced the severity and incidence of myocardial lesions (296). Other drugs that were found to influence the production of lesions by isoproterenol are the vasodilators such as sodium nitrite, aminophylline, dipyridamole, and hexobenzine and the psychosedative drugs such as chlorpromazine, chlordiazepoxide, meprobamate, amitriptyline, and creatinol-O-phosphate, as well as antioxidants such as zinc (90,297,298). In this regard, it is worth mentioning that most of these drugs are not specific with respect to their site of action, and conclusions drawn from such studies should be interpreted with some caution. Inhibition of lipolysis by nicotinic acid or β-pyridyl carbonyl decreased the amount by which isoproterenol infusion increased the myocardial oxygen consumption (142). Chronic administration of nicotine in high doses tended to increase the severity and incidence of lesions produced by isoproterenol (299).

Calcium Channel Blockers

The calcium channel blockers (Table 11), verapamil, D-600, phenylamine, and vascoril reduced the severity of lesions and prevented the decrease in high-energy phosphate stores and accumulation of Ca^{2+} by the myocardium caused by isoproterenol injections (101,102,300). Another Ca^{2+} antagonist, diltiazem, also prevented the isoproterenol-induced changes in myocardial high-energy phosphate stores in rats and afforded significant protection of LV function following norepinephrine administration (301,302). Furthermore, it has been reported that clentiazem prevented epinephrine-myocardial lesions in addition to reducing the mortality (303).

Angiotensin Converting Enzyme Inhibitors and Angiotensin Type 1 Receptor Blockers

It has been reported that trandolapril, an angiotensin converting enzyme (ACE) inhibitor, prevented both cardiac hypertrophy and increased the angiotensin II content by isoproterenol (304). It has also been reported that captopril, another ACE inhibitor (Table 11), attenuated cardiomyopathy associated with phenochromocytoma (305,306). Captopril decreased blood pressure and heart rate without changing the ventricular weight:body weight ratio or collagen accumulation. In other studies, ramipril also had no influence on the collagen accumulation in isoproterenol-induced cardiac fibrosis (307). However, when spironolactone-200, a mineralcorticoid receptor antagonist, was given, it prevented cardiac remodeling and fibrosis but did not reduce the blood pressure and heart rate. This study suggests that neither blood pressure elevation nor tachycardia cause hypertrophy or fibrosis in the isoproterenol-induced cardiac hypertrophy model (308). AT_1 receptor blockers such as losartan and candesartan have also been studied. Losartan has shown to reduce fibrosis and candesartan has shown to accelerate Ca^{2+}- uptake but prevent protein kinase A phosphorylation of ryanodine receptor therefore making the SR less susceptible to oxidative stress–induced Ca^{2+} leak (309).

Hormonal, Electrolyte, and Metabolic Interventions

Table 12 shows the effects of hormonal, electrolyte, and metabolic interventions on catecholamine-induced cardiomyopathy. The mineralocorticoids, such as deoxy-corticosterone and 9-α-fluorocortisol, increased the severity of myocardial lesions (102,162,283,310,311), the level of Ca^{2+} accumulation (101,102), and the depletion of high-energy phosphate stores (85) caused by isoproterenol. Administration of KCl, $MgCl_2$, or NH_4Cl reduced the severity of lesions (84,102,146) and protected against the electrolyte shifts and reduction of high-energy phosphate store (92,102,146). On the other hand, when plasma Mg^{2+}, K^+, and H^+ concentrations were low, the isoproterenol-induced lesions were potentiated (312). Administration of K^+-Mg^{2+} aspartate together with isoproterenol has also been found to prevent or reduce the changes in myofibrillar ATPase activity, Ca^{2+} accumulation by mitochondria and microsomes, and high-energy phosphates stores (105), in addition to decreasing the severity of ultrastructural damage in the myocardium (313). Calciferol and another antirachitic agent, dihydrotachysterol, increased the severity of necrotic lesions, as did Na_2HPO_4 (101,102,162). The increased severity of the lesions was associated with a further increase in Ca^{2+}-uptake and a greater fall of high-energy phosphate stores in the heart. Likewise, thyrocalcitonin as well as reduction of plasma

Table 12   Effects of Some Hormonal, Electrolytes, and Metabolic Interventions in Catecholamine-Induced Cardiomyopathy

	Effects
A. Steroids	
deoxycorticosterone	increase
9-α-fluorocortisol	increase
estrone	increase
testosterone	increase
estrogen	no change
progesterone	no change
glucocorticoids	no change
cortisone	no change
B. Thyroid hormones	
thyroxine, hyperthyroidism	increase
thyroidectomy, thiouracil, propylthiouracil	decrease
anthracitic agents	increase
(dihydrotachysterol, calfenil)	
thyrocalcitonin	decrease
C. Electrolytes	
low serum Ca^{2+} concentration	decrease
$NaHPO_4$	increase
high sodium, low potassium diets	increase
low sodium, high potassium diets	decrease
administration of KCl, $MgCl_2$, NH_4Cl	decrease
low plasma Mg^{2+}, K^+, H^+ concentrations	increase
administration of K^+ + Mg^{2+}-aspartate	decrease
D. Others	
glucose, lactate, pyruvate	no change
sex, breed	no change
increased body weight, excess body fat	increase
starvation, restricted food intake	decrease
previous myocardial damage	decrease
previous isoproterenol injection	decrease
coronary arteriosclerosis	decrease
cardiac hypertrophy, simultaneous hypoxia	increase
higher ambient temperature	increase
high altitude acclimation, hyperbaric oxygen	decrease
isolation stress, cold exposure	increase

Abbreviations: increase, increased the severity of myocardial lesion; decrease, decreased the severity of myocardial lesion; no change, no change in the severity of myocardial lesion.

calcium with EDTA decreased the extent of both lesions and electrolyte shifts (102).

     The severity of myocardial damage due to catecholamines was increased with increased body weight and excess body fat (162,283,314,315). The severity of lesions did increase with age, but this was probably an indirect effect as a consequence of an increase in body weight with age (316). It has also been reported that the pattern of catecholamine-induced cardiomyopathy may not be uniform but instead may depend strictly on the stage of cardiac growth (6). Previous myocardial damage markedly reduced the severity of lesions produced by high doses of isoproterenol (317–319); this protective effect disappeared with time and did not result from necrosis of the extracardiac tissue. A higher ambient temperature also potentiated the necrotic effect of isoproterenol, possibly due to the increased workload on the heart during thermoregulatory vasodilation (320) as well as changes in the Ca^{2+} transport mechanisms (120). Isolation stress or cold exposure both increased the severity of isoproterenol-induced lesion and electrolyte shifts (162,283,314,321,322), although this may be an indirect result of increased mineralocorticoid production, which occurs under these conditions (321–323).

It appears that factors that increase the workload on the heart also increase the metabolic rate, interfere with oxygen supply to myocardial cells, favor the electrolyte change or the mobilization of lipids, and aggravate the necrotic influence of catecholamines. On the other hand, factors that block the stimulatory effects of catecholamines, thereby reducing cardiac work, or otherwise reduce myocardial metabolic rate, aid in the supply of oxygen to the myocardium, limit the mobilization of lipids, or counteract the ionic shifts to reduce the severity of necrotic changes. In particular, the interventions, which promote the occurrence of intracellular Ca^{2+}-overload, have been shown to aggravate, and those, which reduce the intracellular Ca^{2+}-overload, have been reported to prevent the catecholamine-induced cardiotoxicity. Although the protective effect of MAOI compounds is still enigmatic, it is clear from the above discussion that an imbalance between oxygen availability and work, the metabolism of lipids and the alteration of electrolyte balance are all crucial factors contributing to the etiology of catecholamine lesions.

SUMMARY AND CONCLUSIONS

It is well known that massive amounts of catecholamines are released from the sympathetic nerve endings and adrenal medulla under stressful situations. Initially, these hormones produce beneficial effects on the cardiovascular system to meet the energy demands of various organs in the body, and their actions on the heart are primarily mediated through the stimulation of β-adrenergic receptors, G protein, adenylate cyclase, and cAMP system in the myocardium. However, prolonged exposure of the heart to high levels of catecholamines results in coronary spasm, arrhythmias, contractile dysfunction, cell damage, and myocardial necrosis. Different pharmacological, hormonal, and metabolic interventions, which are known to reduce the occurrence of intracellular Ca^{2+}-overload, have been shown to prevent the cardiotoxic actions of catecholamines. Several mechanisms such as relative hypoxia, hemodynamic alterations, coronary insufficiency, changes in lipid mobilization and energy metabolism, electrolyte imbalance, and membrane alterations have been suggested to explain the cardiotoxic effects of high concentrations of catecholamines. Recent studies have shown that oxidation of catecholamines results in the formation of highly toxic substances such as aminochromes (e.g., adrenochrome) and free radicals and these then, by the virtue of their actions on different types of heart membranes, cause intracellular Ca^{2+}-overload and myocardial cell damage. Hemodynamic and metabolic actions of catecholamines may aggravate toxic effects of the oxidation products of catecholamines. Thus, it appears that antioxidant therapy in combination with some Ca^{2+} antagonist and/or metabolic intervention may be most effective in preventing the catecholamine-induced cardiomyopathy.

ACKNOWLEDGMENTS

The work reported in this article was supported by a grant from the Heart and Stroke Foundation of Manitoba. Melissa R. Dent is a predoctoral fellow with the Heart and Stroke Foundation of Canada.

REFERENCES

1. Opie LH. The Heart: Physiology, from Cell to Circulation. 3rd ed. Philadephia, PA: Lippincott-Raven, 1998.
2. Ziegler K. Uber die Wirkung intravenoser Adrenalin injection auf das Gefasssystem und ihre Beziehungen zur Arterisclerose. Beitr Z Path Anat uz allg Path 1905; 38:229–254.
3. Pearce RM. Experimental myocarditis: A study of the histological changes following intravenous injections of adrenaline. J Exp Med 1906; 8:400–409.
4. Szakacs JE, Cannon A. l-norepinephrine myocarditis. Am J Clin Path 1958; 30:425–430.
5. Rona G, Chappel CI, Balazs T, et al. An infarct-like myocardial lesion and other toxic manifestations produced by isoproterenol in the rat. Arch Path 1959; 67: 443–455.
6. Ostadal B, Pelouch V, Ostadalova I, et al. Structural and biochemical remodeling in catecholamine-induced cardiomyopathy: comparative and ontogenetic aspects. Mol Cell Biochem 1995; 147:83–88.
7. Ostadal B, Muller E. Histochemical studies on the experimental heart infarction in the rat. Naunyn-Schmiedebergs Arch Pharmok u exp Path 1966; 254:439–447.
8. Sato Y, Tanaka M, Nishikawa T. Reversible catecholamine-induced cardiomyopathy by subcutaneous injections of epinephrine solution in an anesthetized patient. Anesthesiology 2000; 92:615–619.
9. Brilakis ES, Young WF, Wilson JW, et al. Reversible catecholamine-induced cardiomyopathy in a heart transplant candidate without persistent or paroxysmal hypertension. J Heart Lung Transpl 1999; 4:376–380.
10. Kline IK. Myocardial alterations associated with pheochromocytoma. Am J Path 1961; 38:539–551.

11. Szakacs JE, Dimmette RM, Cowart EC Jr. Pathologic implication of the catecholamines, epinephrine and norepinephrine. US Armed Forces Med J 1959; 10:908–925.
12. van Vliet PD, Burchell HB, Titus JL. Focal myocarditis associated with pheochromocytoma. New Eng J Med 1966; 274:1102–1108.
13. Connor RCR. Focal myocytolysis and fuchsinophilic degeneration of the myocardium of patients dying with various brain lesions. Ann N Y Acad Sci 1969; 156:261–270.
14. Greenhoot JH, Reichenbach DD. Cardiac injury and subarachnoid hemorrhage. A clinical, pathological and physiological correlation. J Neurosurg 1969; 30:521–526.
15. Reichenbach DD, Benditt EP. Catecholamines and cardiomyopathy: The pathogenesis and potential importance of myofibrillar degeneration. Human Path 1970; 1:125–150.
16. Smith RP, Tomlinson BE. Subendocardial hemorrhages associated with intra cranial lesions. J Path Bact 1954; 68:327–334.
17. Kaye MP, McDonald RH, Randall WC. Systolic hypertension and subendocardial hemorrhages produced by electrical stimulation of the stellate ganglion. Circ Res 1961; 9:1164–1170.
18. Klouda MA, Brynjolfson G. Cardiotoxic effects of electrical stimulation of the stellate ganglia. Ann N Y Acad Sci 1969; 156:271–279.
19. Melville KI, Garvey HL, Sluster HE, et al. Central nervous system stimulation cardiac ischemic change in monkeys. Ann N Y Acad Sci 1969; 156:241–260.
20. Wood R, Commerford PJ, Rose AG, et al. Reversible catecholamine-induced cardiomyopathy. Am Heart J 1991; 121:610–613.
21. Hicks RJ, Wood B, Kalff V, et al. Normalization of left ventricular ejection fraction following resection of pheochromocytoma in a patient with dilated cardiomyopathy. Clin Nucl Med 1991; 16:413–416.
22. Hamada N, Akamatsu A, Joh T. A case of phlochromocytoma complicated acute renal failure and cardiomyopathy. Jpn Circ J 1993; 57:84–90.
23. Elian D, Harpaz D, Sucher E, et al. Reversible catecholamine-induced cardiomyopathy presenting as acute pulmonary edema in a patient with pheochromocytoma. Cardiology 1993; 83:118–120.
24. Powers FM, Pifarre R, Thomas JX Jr. Ventricular dysfunction in norepinephrine-induced cardiomyopathy. Circ Shock 1994; 43:122–129.
25. Boutet M, Huttner I, Rona G. Aspect microcirculatoire des lesions myocardiques provoquees par l'infusion de catecholamines, Etude ultra structural a l'aide de traceurs de diffusion, I. Isoproterenol. Pathologie-Biologie 1973; 21:811–825.
26. Boutet M, Huttner I, Rona G. Aspect microcirculatoire des lesions myocardiques provoquees par l'infusion de catecholamines. Etude ultra structural a l'aide traceurs de diffusion. II. Norepinephrine. Pathologie-Biologie 1974; 22:377–387.
27. Handforth CP. Isoproterenol-induced myocardial infarction in animals. Arch Path 1962; 73:161–165.
28. Handforth CP. Myocardial infarction and necrotizing arteritis in hamsters produced by isoproterenol (Isuprel). Med Serv J Can 1962; 18:506–512.
29. Rona G, Boutet M, Hutter I, et al. Pathogenesis of isoproterenol induced myocardial alterations: Functional and morphological correlates. In: Dhalla NS, ed. Recent Advances in Studies on Cardiac Structure and Metabolism. Baltimore: University Park Press, 1973:507–525.

30. Rona G, Kahn DS, Chappel CI. Studies on infarct-like myocardial necrosis produced by isoproterenol: A review. Rev Can Biol 1963; 22:241–255.

31. Maruffo CA. Fine structural study of myocardial changes induced by isoproterenol in Rhesus monkeys (Macaca mulatta). Am J Path 1967; 50:27–37.

32. Ostadal B, Rychterova V, Poupa O. Isoproterenol-induced acute experimental cardiac necrosis in the turtle. Am Heart J 1968; 76:645–649.

33. Regan TJ, Markov A, Kahn MI, et al. Myocardial ion and lipid exchanges during ischemia and catecholamine induced necrosis: Relation to regional blood flow. In: Bajusz E, Rona G, eds. Recent Advances in Studies in Cardiac Structure and Metabolism. Baltimore: University Park Press, 1972:656–664.

34. Rosenblum I, Wohl A, Stein AA. Studies in cardiac necrosis I. Production of cardiac lesions with sympathomimetic amines. Toxicol Appl Pharmacol 1965; 7:1–8.

35. Rosenblum I, Wohl A, Stein AA. Studies in cardiac necrosis. II. Cardiovascular effects of sympathomimetic amines producing cardiac lesions. Toxicol Appl Pharmacol 1965; 7:9–17.

36. Bhagat B, Sullivan JM, Fisher VW, et al. cAMP activity and isoproterenol-induced myocardial injury in rats. In: Kobayashi T, Ito Y, Rona G, eds. Recent Advances in Studies on Cardiac Structure and Metabolism. Baltimore: University Park Press, 1978:465–470.

37. Todd GL, Baroldi G, Pieper GM, et al. Experimental catecholamine-induced myocardial necrosis. I. Morphology, quantification and regional distribution of acute contraction band lesions. J Mol Cell Cardiol 1985; 17:317–338.

38. Todd GL, Baroldi G, Pieper GM, et al. Experimental catecholamine-induced myocardial necrosis. II. Temperal development of isoproterenol-induced contraction band lesions correlated with ECG, hemodynamic and biochemical changes. J Mol Cell Cardiol 1985; 17:647–656.

39. Boutet M, Huttner I, Rona G. Permeability alterations of sarcolemmal membrane in catecholamine-induced cardiac muscle cell injury. Lab Invest 1976; 34:482–488.

40. Todd GL, Cullan GE, Cullan GM. Isoproterenol-induced myocardial necrosis and membrane permeability alterations in the isolated perfused rabbit heart. Exp Mol Pathol 1980; 33:43–54.

41. Raab W. Pathogenic significance of adrenalin and related substances in heart muscle. Exp Med Surg 1943; 1:188–225.

42. Sobel B, Jequier E, Sjoerdsma A, et al. Effect of catecholamines and adrenergic blocking agents on oxidative phosphorylation in rat heart mitochondria. Circ Res 1966; 19:1050–1061.

43. Rajadurai M, Stanely Mainzen Prince P. Preventive effect of naringin on lipid peroxides and antioxidants in isoproterenol-induced cardiotoxicity in Wistar rats: biochemical and histopathological evidences. Toxicology 2006; 228:259–268.

44. Muders F, Friedrich E, Luchner A, et al. Hemodynamic changes and neurohormonal regulation during development of congestive heart failure in a model of epinephrine-induced cardiomyopathy in conscious rabbits. J Card Fail 1999; 5:109–116.

45. Fleisher MS, Loeb L. Experimental myocarditis. Arch Int Med 1909; 3:78–91.

46. Fleisher MS, Loeb L. The later stages of experimental myocarditis. J Am Med Assoc 1909; 53:1561–1571.

47. Fleisher MS, Loeb L. Uber experimentelle myocarditis. Central bl f allg Path u path Anat 1909; 20:104–106.

48. Fleisher MS, Loeb L. Further investigations in experimental myocarditis. Arch Int Med 1910; 6:427–438.
49. Christian HA, Smith RM, Walker IC. Experimental cardiorenal disease. Arch Int Med 1911; 8:468–551.
50. Samson PC. Tissue changes following continuous intravenous injection of epinephrine hydrochloride into dogs. Arch Path 1932; 13:745–755.
51. Hackel DB, Catchpole BN. Pathologic and electrocardiographic effects of hemorrhagic shock in dogs treated with l-norepinephrine. Lab Invest 1958; 7:358–368.
52. Vishnevskaya OP. Reflex mechanisms in the pathogenesis of adrenaline myocarditis. Bull Exp Biol Med 1956; 41:27–31.
53. Szakacs JE, Mehlman B. Pathologic change induced by l-norepinephrine. Quantitative aspects. Am J Cardiol 1960; 5:619–627.
54. Maling HM, Highman B. Exaggerated ventricular arrhythmia and myocardial fatty changes after large doses of norepinephrine and epinephrine in unanaesthetized dogs. Am J Physiol 1958; 194:590–596.
55. Highman B, Maling HM, Thompson EC. Serum transaminase and alkaline phosphates levels after large doses of norepinephrine and epinephrine in dogs. Am J Physiol 1959; 196:436–440.
56. Maling HM, Highman B, Thompson EC. Some similar effects after large doses of catecholamine and myocardial infarction in dogs. Am J Cardiol 1960; 5:628–633.
57. Chiu YT, Cheng CC, Lin NN, et al. High-dose norepinephrine induces disruption of myocardial extracellular matrix and left ventricular dilatation and dysfunction in a novel feline model. J Chin Med Assoc 2006; 69:343–350.
58. Jiang JP, Chen V, Downing SE. Modulation of catecholamine cardiomyopathy by allopurinol. Am Heart J 1991; 122:115–121.
59. Nonomura M, Nozawa T, Matsuki A, et al. Ischemia-induced norepinephrine release, but not norepinephrine-derived free radicals, contributes to myocardial ischemia-reperfusion injury. Circ J 2005; 69:590–595.
60. Padmanabhan M, Stanely Mainzen Prince P. Preventive effect of S-allylcysteine on lipid peroxides and antioxidants in normal and isoproterenol-induced cardiotoxicity in rats: a histopathological study. Toxicology 2006; 224:128–137.
61. Chappel CI, Rona G, Balazs T, et al. Severe myocardial necrosis produced by isoproterenol in the rat. Arch Int Pharmacodyn 1959; 122:123–128.
62. Rona G, Zsoter T, Chappel C, et al. Myocardial lesions, circulatory and electro cardiographic changes produced by isoproterenol in the dog. Rev Can Biol 1959; 18:83–94.
63. Mohan P, Bloom S. Lipolysis is an important determinant of isoproterenol-induced myocardial necrosis. Cardiovasc Pathol 1999; 8:255–261.
64. Diaz-Munoz M, Alvarez-Perez MA, Yanez L, et al. Correlation between oxidative stress and alteration of intracellular calcium handling in isoproterenol-induced myocardial infarction. Mol Cell Biochem 2006; 289:125–136.
65. Meyer R, Linz KW, Surges R, et al. Rapid modulation of L-type calcium current by acutely applied oestrogens in isolated cardiac myocytes from human, guinea pig and rat. Exp Physiol 1998; 83:305–321.
66. Li HY, Bian JS, Kwan YW, et al. Enhanced responses to 17β-estradiol in rat hearts treated with isoproterenol: involvement of cyclic AMP-dependent pathway. J Pharmacol Exp Ther 2000; 293:592–598.

67. Nair PS, Devi CS. Efficacy of mangiferin on serum and heart tissue lipids in rats subjected to isoproterenol induced cardiotoxicity. Toxicology 2006; 228:135–139.

68. Remiao F, Carmo H, Carvalho F, et al. Copper enhances isoproterenol toxicity in isolated rat cardiomyocytes: effects on oxidative stress. Cardiovasc Toxicol 2001; 1:195–204.

69. Higuchi Y. Changes of lipid peroxides and alpha-tocopherol in rats with experimentally induced myocardial necrosis. Acta Med Okayama 1982; 36:113–124.

70. Namikawa K, Okazaki Y, Nishida S, et al. Studies on early stage changes of peroxide lipid in isoproterenol-induced myocardial injury. Yakugaku Zasshi 1992; 112:557–562.

71. Singal PK, Dhillon KS, Beamish RE, et al. Protective effects of zinc against catecholamine-induced myocardial changes. Electrocardiographic and ultrastructural studies. Lab Invest 1981; 44:426–433.

72. Besbasi FS, Hamlin RL. Influence of phenytoin on isoproterenol-induced myocardial fibrosis in rats. Am J Vet Res 1990; 51:36–39.

73. Manjula TS, Geetha A, Ramesh TG, et al. Reversal of changes of myocardial lipids by chronic administration of aspirin in isoproterenol-induced myocardial damage in rats. Indian J Physiol Pharmacol 1992; 36:47–50.

74. Kolin A, Brezina A, Mamelak M, et al. Cardioprotective action of sodium gamma-hydroxybutyrate against isoproterenol induced myocardial damage. Int J Exp Pathol 1993; 74:275–281.

75. Bloom S, Cancilla PA. Myoctyolysis and mitochondrial calcification in rat myocardium after low doses of isoproterenol. Am J Path 1969; 54:373–391.

76. Csapa Z, Dusek J, Rona G. Early alterations of cardiac muscle cells in isoproterenol induced necrosis. Arch Path 1972; 93:356–365.

77. Kutsuna F. Electron microscopic studies on isoproterenol-induced myocardial lesions in rats. Jap Heart J 1972; 13:168–175.

78. Ferrans VJ, Hibbs RG, Walsh JJ, et al. Histochemical and electron mircorsopic studies on the cardiac necrosis produced by sympathomimetic agents. Ann N Y Acad Sci 1969; 156:309–332.

79. Ferrans VJ, Hibbs RG, Black WC, et al. Isoproterenol-induced myocardial necrosis. A histochemical and electron microscopic study. Am Heart J 1964; 68:71–90.

80. Ferrans VJ, Hibbs RG, Cipriano PR, et al. Histochemical and electron microscopic studies of norepinephrine-induced myocardial necrosis in rats. In: Bajusz E, Rona G, eds. Recent Advances in Studies on Cardiac Structure and Metabolism. Baltimore: University Park Press, 1972:495–525.

81. Ferrans VJ, Hibbs RG, Weiley HS, et al. A histochemical and electron microscopic study of epinephrine-induced myocardial necrosis. J Mol Cell Cardiol 1970; 1:11–22.

82. Lehr D. Healing of myocardial necrosis caused by sympathomimetic amines. In: Bajusz E, Rona G, eds. Recent Advance in Studies on Cardiac Structure and Metabolism. Baltimore: University Park Press, 1972:526–550.

83. Lehr D, Krukowski M, Chau R. Acute myocardial injury produced by sympathomimetic animes. Israel J Med Sci 1969; 5:519–524.

84. Schenk EA, Moss AJ. Cardiovascular effects of sustained norepinephrine infusions. II. Morphology. Circ Res 1966; 18:605–615.

85. Khullar M, Datta BN, Wahi PL, et al. Catecholamine-induced experimental cardiomyopathy- a histopathological, histochemial and ultrastructural study. Indian Heart J 1989; 41:307–313.

86. Regan TJ, Moschos CB, Lehan PH, et al. Lipid and carbohydrate metabolism of myocardium during the biphasic inotropic response to epinephrine. Circ Res 1966; 19:307–316.

87. Wexler BC, Judd JT, Kittinger GW. Myocardial necrosis induced by isoproterenol in rats: Changes in serum protein, lipoprotein, lipids and glucose during active necrosis and repair in arteriosclerotic and nonarteriosclerotic animals. Angiology 1968; 19:665–682.

88. Wexler BC, Judd JT, Lutmer RF, et al. Pathophysiologic change in arteriosclerotic and nonarteriosclerotic rats following isoproterenol-induced myocardial infarction. In: Bajusz E, Rona G, eds. Recent Advances in Studies on Cardiac Structure and Metabolism. Baltimore: University Park Press, 1972:463–472.

89. Wexler BC, Kittinger GW. Myocardial necrosis in rats: Serum enzymes, adrenal steroid and histopathological alterations. Circ Res 1963; 13:159–171.

90. Zbinden G, Moe RA. Pharmacological studies on heart muscle lesions induced by isoproterenol. Ann N Y Acad Sci 1969; 156:294–308.

91. Wexler BC. Serum creatine phosphokinase activity following isoproterenol-induced myocardial infarction in male and female rats with and without arteriosclerosis. Am Heart J 1970; 79:69–79.

92. Regan TJ, Passannante AJ, Oldewurtel HA, et al. Metabolism of ^{14}C labeled triglycerides by the myocardium during injury induced by norepinephrine. Circulation 1968; 38(suppl 6):162 (abstr).

93. Judd JT, Wexler BC. Myocardial connective tissue metabolism in response to injury: Histological and chemical studies of nucopolysaccharids and collagen in rat hearts after isoproterenol-induced infarction. Circ Res 1969; 25:201–214.

94. Wenzel DG, Chau RYP. Dose-time effect of isoproterenol on aspartate aminotransferase and necrosis of the rat heart. Toxicol Appl Pharmacol 1966; 8:460–463.

95. Wenzel DG, Lyon JP. Sympathomimetic amines and heart lactic dehydrogenasee isoenzymes. Toxicol Appl Pharmacol 1967; 11:215–228.

96. Stanton HC, Schwartz A. Effects of hydrazine monoamine oxidase inhibitor (phenelzine) on isoproterenol-induced myocardiopathies in the rat. J Pharmacol Exp Ther 1967; 157:649–658.

97. Vorbeck ML, Malewski EF, Erhart LS. Membrane phospholipid metabolism in the isoproterenol-induced cardiomyopathy of the rat. In: Fleckenstein A, Rona G, eds. Recent Advances in Studies on Cardiac Structure and Metabolism. Baltimore: University Park Press, 1975:175–181.

98. Hattori E, Yatsaki K, Miyozaki T, et al. Adenine nucleotides of myocardium from rats treated with isoproterenol and/or Mg- or K-deficiency. Jpn Heart J 1969; 10:218–224.

99. Kako K. Biochemical changes in the rat myocardium induced by isoproterenol. Can J Physiol Pharmacol 1965; 43:541–549.

100. Robertson WVB, Peyser P. Changes in water and electrolytes of cardiac muscle following epinephrine. Am J Physiol 1951; 166:277–283.

101. Fleckenstein A. Specific inhibitors and promoters of calcium action in the excitation-contraction coupling of heart muscle and their role in the prevention or production of myocardial lesions. In: Harris P, Opie LH, eds. Calcium and the Heart. London and New York: Academic Press, 1971:135–188.

102. Fleckenstein A, Janke J, Doering HJ. Myocardial fiber necrosis due to intracellular Ca-overload. A new principle in cardiac pathophysiology. In: Dhalla NS, ed. Recent

Advances in Studies on Cardiac Structure and Metabolism. Baltimore: University Park Press, 1974:563–580.

103. Pelouch V, Deyl Z, Poupa O. Experimental cardiac necrosis in terms of myosin aggregation. Physiol Bohemoslov 1968; 17:480–488.

104. Pelouch V, Deyl Z, and Poupa O. Myosin aggregation in cardaic necrosis induced by isoproterenol in rats. Physiol Bohemoslov 1970; 19:9–13.

105. Fedelesova M, Ziegelhoffer A, Luknarova O, et al. Prevention by K^+, Mg^{++}-aspartate of isoproterenol-induced metabolic changes in myocardium. In: Fleckenstein A, Rona G, eds. Recent Advances in Studies on Cardiac Structure and Metabolism. Baltimore: University Park Press, 1975:59–73.

106. Dhalla NS, Dzurba A, Pierce GN, et al. Membrane changes in myocardium during catecholamine-induced pathological hypertrophy. In: Alpert NR, ed. Perspectives in Cardiovascular Research. New York, NY: Raven Press, 1983:527–534.

107. Suzuki M, Ohte N, Wang ZM, et al. Altered inotropic response of endothelin-1 in cardiomyocytes from rats with isoproterenol-induced cardiomyopathy. Cardiovasc Res 1998; 39:589–599.

108. Hu, A., Jiao, X., Gao, E., et al. 2006. Chronic beta-adrenergic receptor stimulation induces cardiac apoptosis and aggravates myocardial ischemia/reperfusion injury by provoking inducible nitric-oxide synthase-mediated nitrative stress. J Pharmacol Exp Ther 318: 469–75.

109. Lehr D. Tissue electrolyte alteration in disseminated myocardial necrosis. Ann N Y Acad Sci 1969; 156:344–378.

110. Lehr D, Krukowski M, Colon R. Correlation of myocardial and renal necrosis with tissue electrolyte changes. J Am Med Assoc 1966; 197:105–112.

111. Melville KI, Korol B. Cardiac drug responses and potassium shifts. Studies on the interrelated effects of drugs on coronary flow, heart action and cardiac potassium movement. Am J Cardiol 1958; 2:81–94.

112. Melville KI, Korol B. Cardiac drug responses and potassium shifts. Studies on the interrelated effect of drugs on coronary flow, heart action and cardiac potassium movement. Am J Cardiol 1958; 2:189–199.

113. Nasmyth PA. The effect of corticosteroids on the isolated mammalian heart and its response to adrenaline. J Physiol 1957; 139:323–136.

114. Langer GA. Ion fluxes in cardiac excitation and contraction and their relation to myocardial contractility. Physiol Rev 1968; 48:708–757.

115. Daggett WM, Mansfield PB, Sarnoff SJ. Myocardial K^+ changes resulting from inotropic agents. Fed Proc 1964; 23:357.

116. Dhalla NS, Ziegelhoffer A, Harrow JAC. Regulation role of membrane systems in heart function. Can J Physiol Pharmacol 1977; 55:1211–1234.

117. Dhalla NS, Das PK, Sharma GP. Subcellular basis of cardiac contractile failure. J Mol Cell Cardiol 1978; 10:363–385.

118. Dhalla NS, Pierce GN, Panagia V, et al. Calcium movements in relation to heart function. Basic Res Cardiol 1982; 77:117–139.

119. Dhalla NS, Dixon IMC, Beamish RE. Biochemical basis of heart function and contractile failure. J Appl Cardiol 1991; 6:7–30.

120. Varley KG, Dhalla NS. Excitation-contraction coupling in heart. XII. Subcellular calcium transport in isoproterenol-induced myocardial necrosis. Exptl Mol Pathol 1973; 19:94–105.

121. Fedelesova M, Dzurba A, Ziegelhoffer A. Effect of isoproterenol on the activity of Na^+-K^+ adenosine triphosphatase from dog heart. Biochem Pharmacol 1974; 23:2887–2893.

122. Panagia V, Pierce GN, Dhalla KS, et al. Adaptive changes in subcellular calcium transport during catecholamine-induced cardiomyopathy. J Mol Cell Cardiol 1985; 17:411–420.

123. Okumura K, Panagia V, Beamish RE, Biphasic changes in the sarcolemmal phopshatidylethanolamine N-methylation in catecholamine-induced cardiomyopathy. J Mol Cell Cardiol 1987; 19:357–366.

124. Dhalla NS, Ganguly PK, Panagia V, et al. Catecholamine-induced cardiomyopathy: Alterations in Ca^{2+} transport systems. In: Kawai C, Abelman WH, eds. Pathogenesis of Myocarditis and Cardiomyopathy. Tokyo: University of Tokyo Press, 1987:135–147.

125. Makino N, Dhruvarajan R, Elimban V, et al. Alterations of sarcolemmal Na^+-Ca^{2+} exchange in catecholamine-induced cardiomyopathy. Can J Cardiol 1985; 1:225–232.

126. Makino N, Jasmin G, Beamish RE, et al. Sarcolemmal Na^+-Ca^{2+} exchange during the development of genetically determined cardiomyopathy. Biochem Biophys Res Commun 1985; 133:491–497.

127. Panagia V, Elimban V, Heyliger CE, et al. Sarcolemmal alterations during catecholamine induced cardiomyopathy. In: Beamish RE, Panagia V, Dhalla NS, eds. Pathogenesis of Stress-induced Heart Disease. Boston: Martinus Nijhoff, 1985: 121–131.

128. Corder DW, Heyliger CE, Beamish RE, et al. Defect in the adrenergic receptor-adenylate cyclase system during development of catecholamine-induced cardiomyopathy. Am Heart J 1984; 107:537–542.

129. Neri M, Cerretani D, Fiaschi A, et al. Correlation between cardiac oxidative stress and myocardial pathology due to acute and chronic norepinephrine administration in rats. J Cell Mol Med 2007; 11:156–170.

130. Vatner DE, Vatner SF, Nejima J, et al. Chronic norepinephrine elicits desensitization by uncoupling the beta-receptor. J Clin Invest 1989; 84:1741–1748.

131. Dong E, Yatani A, Mohan A, et al. Myocardial beta-adrenoceptor down-regulation by norepinephrine is linked to reduced norepinephrine uptake activity. Eur J Pharmacol 1999; 384:17–24.

132. Iaccarino G, Tomhave ED, Lefkowitz RJ, et al. Reciprocal in vivo regulation of myocardial G protein-coupled receptor kinase expression by beta-adrenergic receptor stimulation and blockade. Circulation 1998; 98:1783–1789.

133. Roman S, Kutryk MJB, Beamish RE, et al. Lysosomal changes during the development of catecholamine-induced cardiomyopathy. In: Beamish RE, Panagia V, Dhalla NS, eds. Pathogenesis of Stress-induced Heart Disease. Boston: Martinus Nijhoff, 1985:270–280.

134. Vatner SF, Millard RW, Patrick TA, et al. Effects of isoproterenol on regional myocardial function, electrogram, and blood flow in conscious dogs with myocardial ischemia. J Clin Invest 1976; 57:1261–1271.

135. Crackower MA, Oudit GY, Kozieradzki I, et al. Regulation of myocardial contractility and cell size by distinct PI3K-PTEN signaling pathways. Cell 2002; 110:737–749.

136. Oudit GY, Crackower MA, Eriksson U, et al. Phosphoinositide 3-kinase gamma deficient mice are protected from isoproterenol-induced heart failure. Circulation 2003; 108:2147–2152.
137. Selye H. The Pluicausal Cardiopathies. Springfield, IL: Charles C Thomas, 1961.
138. Beamish RE, Dhalla NS. Involvement of catecholamines in coronary spasm under stressful conditions. In: Beamish RE, Singal PK, Dhalla NS, eds. Stress and Heart Disease. Boston: Martinus Nijhoff, 1985:129–141.
139. Lown B. Clinical management of ventricular arrhythmias. Hospital Practice 1982; 17:73–86.
140. Singal PK, Kapur N, Beamish RE, et al. Antioxidant protection against epinephrine-induced arrhythmias. In: Beamish RE, Singal PK, Dhalla NS, eds. Stress and Heart Disease. Boston: Martinus Nijhoff, 1985.
141. Jasmin G. Morphologic effects of vasoactive drugs. Can J Physiol Pharamcol 1966; 44:367–372.
142. Mjos DD. Effect of inhibition of lipolysis on myocardial oxygen consumption in the presence of isoproterenol. J Clin Invest 1971; 50:1869–1873.
143. Hoak JC, Warner ED, Connor WE. New concept of levarterenol-induced acute myocardial ischemic injury. Arch Pathol 1969; 87:332–338.
144. Raab W. Myocardial electrolyte derangement: Crucial feature of plusicausal, so-called coronary, heart disease. Ann N Y Acad Sci 1969; 147:627–686.
145. Rosenblum I, Wohl A, Stein A. Studies in cardiac necrosis. III. Metabolic efects of sympathomimetic amines producing cardiac lesions. Toxicol Appl Pharamcol 1965; 7:344–351.
146. Lehr D, Chau R, Kaplan J. Prevention of experimental myocardial necrosis by electrolyte solutions. In: Bajusz B, Rona G, eds. Recent Advances in Studies on Cardiac Structure and Metabolism. Baltimore: University Park Press, 1972:684–698.
147. Rona G, Dusek J. Studies on the mechanism of increased myocardial resistance. In: Bajusz B, Rona G, eds. Recent Advances in Studies on Cardiac Structure and Metabolism. Baltimore: University Park Press, 1972:422–429.
148. Strubelt O, Siegers CP. Role of cardiovacular and ionic changes in pathogenesis and prevention of isoprenaline-induced cardiac necrosis. Pathophysiology and morphology of myocardial cell alteration. In: Fleckenstein A, Rona, G, eds. Recent Advances in Studies on Cardiac Structure and Metabolism. Baltimore: University Park Press, 1975:135–142.
149. Ostadal B, Poupa O. Occlusion of coronary vessels after administration of iso-prenoline, adrenalin and noradrenalin. Physiol Bohemoslov 1967; 16:116–119.
150. Brandi G, McGregor M. Intramural pressure in the left ventricle of the dog. Cardiovasc Res 1969; 3:472–475.
151. Cutarelli R, Levy MN. Intraventricular pressure and the distribution of coronary blood flow. Circ Res 1963; 12:322–327.
152. Buckberg GD, Fixler DE, Archie JP, et al. Experimental subendocardial ischemia in dogs with normal coronary arteries. Circ Res 1972; 30:67–81.
153. Buckberg GD, Ross G. Effects of isoprenaline on coronary blood flow: Its distribution and myocardial performance. Cardiovasc Res 1973; 7:429–437.
154. Bajusz E. The terminal electrolyte-shift mechanism in heart necrosis: Its significance in the pathogenesis and prevention of necrotizing cardiomyopathies. In: Bajusz E, ed. Electrolytes and Cardiovascular Diseases. Basel, Switzerland: S. Karger, 1975.

155. Raab W, van Lith P, Lepeschkin E, et al. Catecholamine-induced myocardial hypoxia in the presence of impaired coronary dilatability independent of external cardiac work. Am J Cardiol 1962; 9:455–470.

156. Lee KS, Yu DH. Effects of epinephrine on metabolism and contraction of cat papillary muscle. Am J Physiol 1964; 206:525–530.

157. Wesifeldt ML, Gilmore JP. Apparent dissociation of the inotropic and O_2 consumption effects of norepinephrine. Fed Proc 1964; 23:357 (abstr).

158. Klocke FJ, Kaiser GA, Ross J Jr., et al. Mechanism of increase of myocardial oxygen uptake produced by catecholamines. Am J Physiol 1965; 209:913–918.

159. Challoner DR, Steinberg D. Metabolic effect of epinephrine on the QO_2 of the arrested isolated perfused rat heart. Nature 1965; 205:602–603.

160. Hauge A, Oye I. The action of adrenaline in cardiac muscle. II. Effect on oxygen consumption in the asystolic perfused rat heart. Acta Physiol Scand 1966; 68:295–303.

161. Park JH, Meriwether BP, Park CR, et al. Gluthathione and ethylenediamine-tetraacetate antagonism of uncoupling of oxidative phosphorylation. Biochim Biophys Acta 1956; 22:403–404.

162. Kahn DS, Rona G, Chappel CI. Isoproterenol-induced cardiac necrosis. Ann N Y Acad Sci 1969; 156:285–293.

163. Sordahl LA, Sliver BB. Pathological accumulation of calcium by mitochondria: Modulation by magnesium. In: Fleckenstein A, Rona G, eds. Recent Advances in Studies on Cardiac Structure and Metabolism. Baltimore: University Park Press, 1975:85–93.

164. Lossnitzer K, Janke J, Hein B, et al. Disturbed myocardial calcium metabolism: A possible pathogenetic factor in the hereditary cardiomyopathy of the Syrian hamster. In: Fleckenstein A, Rona G, eds. Recent Advances in Studies on Cardiac Structure and Metabolism. Baltimore: University Park Press, 1975:207–217.

165. Jasmin G, Bajusz E. Prevention of myocardial degeneration in hamsters with hereditory cardiomyopathy. In: Fleckenstein A, Rona G, eds. Recent Advances in Studies on Cardiac Structure and Metabolism. Baltimore: University Park Press, 1975:219–229.

166. Fleckenstein A, Janke J, Doering HJ, et al. Key role of Ca in the production of noncoronarogenic myocardial necroses. In: Recent Advances in Studies on Cardiac Structure and Metabolism. Baltimore: University Park Press, 1975:21–32.

167. Bloom S, Davis D. Isoproterenol myocytolysis and myocardial calcium. In: Dhalla NS, ed. Recent Advances in Studies on Cardiac Structure and Metabolism. Baltimore: University Park Press, 1974:581–590.

168. Ellison G, Torella D, Karakikes I, et al. Acute beta-adrenergic overload produces myocyte damage through calcium leakage from the ryanodine receptor 2(RyR2) but spares cardiac stem cells. J Bio Chem 2007; 282:11397–11407.

169. Muller E. Histochemical studies on the experimental heart infarction in the rat. Naunyn-Schmiedebergs Arch Pharmok u exp Path 1966; 254:439–447.

170. Kisch B. Die autokatalyse der adrenalinoxydation. Biochem Z 1930; 220:84–91.

171. Okagawa M, Ichitsubo H. Oxidation and reduction of adrenaline in the body. Proc Jap Pharmacol Soc 1935; 9:155.

172. Heirman P. L'adrenoxine, adrenaline oxydee inhibitrice. Compt Rend Soc Biol 1937; 126:1264–1266.

173. Heirman P. Action de la tyrosinase sur l'oxidation et les effets cardiaques de l'adrenaline et de la tyramine. Compt Rend Soc Biol 1937; 124:1250–1251.

174. Hogeboom GH, Adams MH. Mammalian tyrosinase and dopa oxidase. J Biol Chem 1942; 145:272–279.
175. Mason HS. The chemistry of melanin. II. The oxidation of dihydroxyphenylalanine by mammalian dopa oxidase. J Biol Chem 1947; 168:433–438.
176. von Euler US. Noradrenaline - Chemistry, Physiology, Pharmacology and Clincial Aspects. Springfield, IL: Charles C. Thomas, 1956.
177. Heirman P. Modifications of the cardiac action of adrenaline in the course of its oxidation by phenolases. Arch Intern Physiol 1938; 46:404–415.
178. Blaschko H, Schlossman H. The inactivation of adrenaline by phenolases. J Physiol 1940; 98:130–140.
179. Derouaux G. The in vitro oxidation of adrenaline and other diphenol amines by phenol oxidase. Arch Intern Pharmacodyn Therap 1943; 69:205–234.
180. Wajzer J. Oxydation de l'adrenaline. Bull Soc Chim Biol 1946; 28:341–345.
181. Valerno DM, McCormack JJ. Xanthine oxidase-mediated oxidation of epinephrine. Biochem Pharmacol 1971; 20:47–55.
182. Vercauteren R. Sur la cytochimie des granulocytes eosinophiles. Bull Soc Chim Biol 1951; 33:522–525.
183. Odajima T. Myeloperoxidase of the leukocyte of normal blood. II. Oxidation-reduction reaction mechanism of the myeloperoxidase. Biochim Biophys Acta 1971; 235:52–60.
184. Philpot FJ. Inhibition of adrenaline oxidation by local anaesthetics. J Physiol 1940; 97:301–307.
185. Slater EC. The measurement of the cytochrome oxidase activity of enzyme preparations. Biochem J 1949; 44:305–318.
186. Iisalo E, Rekkarinen A. Enzyme action on adrenaline and noradrenaline. Studies on heart muscle in vitro. Acta Pharmacol Toxicol 1958; 15:157–174.
187. Green DE, Richter D. Adrenaline and adrenochrome. Biochem J 1937; 31:596–616.
188. Bacq ZM. Metabolism of adrenaline. Pharmacol Rev 1949; 1:1–26.
189. Axelrod J. Enzymic oxidation of epinephrine to adrenochrome by the salivary gland. Biochim Biophys Acta 1964; 85:247–254.
190. Falk JE. The formation of hydrogen carriers by haemitin-catalyzed peroxidations. Biochem J 1949; 44:369–373.
191. Chaix P, Pallaget C. Comparative characteristics of the oxidation of adrenaline and noradrenaline. Congr Intern Biochim, Resumes Communs 1952; 2nd Congr, Paris 54 (Chem Abstracts 1954; 48:12851).
192. Chikano M, Kominami M. Uber die spaltung des adreanlins im serum Biochem Z 1929; 205:176–179.
193. Hoffer A. Adrenochrome and adrenolutin and their relationship to mental disease. In: Garattini S, Ghetti V, eds. Psychotropic Drugs. Amsterdam: Elsevier, 1957: 10–25.
194. Osmond H, Hoffer A. Schizophrenia: A new approach continued. J Mental Sci 1959; 105:653–673.
195. Schweitzer A. Comparative investigations of the action of p-benzo-quinone and omega on the function of the frog heart. Arch Ges Physiol 1931; 228:568–585.
196. Sanders E. The inhibiting effect of oxidized adrenalin. Arch Exptl Path Pharmakol 1939; 193:572–575.

197. Webb WR, Dodds RP, Unal MO, et al. Suspended animation of the heart with metabolic inhibitors. Effect of magnesium sulfate or fluoride and adrenochrome in rats. Ann Surg 1966; 164:343–350.
198. Yen T. The reversal of the effect of adrenaline upon the rabbit intestine and the toad limb vessels. Tohoku J Exptl Med 1930; 14:415–465.
199. Raab W, Lepeschkin E. Pressor and cardiac effects of adrenochrome (omega) in the atropinized cat. Exptl Med Surg 1950; 8:319–329.
200. Titaev AA. Relation of some metabolites to the sympathetic nervous system in newborn animals. Chem Abstracts 1964; 60:8438.
201. Green S, Mazur A, Shorr E. Mechanism of catalytic oxidation of adrenalin by ferritin. J Biol Chem 1956; 220:237–255.
202. Parrot JL. Decrease of capillary permeability under the influence of adrenochrome. Compt Rend Soc Biol 1949; 143:819–822 (Chem Abstracts 1950; 44:5008).
203. Lecomte J, Fischer P. The effect of trihydroxy-1-methylindole on bleeding time and capillary permeability. Arch Int Pharmacodyn Therap 1951; 87:225–231.
204. Marquordt P. The pharmacology and chemistry of the adrenochromes. Z Ges Exptl Med 1944; 114:112–126 (Chem Abstracts 1950; 44:2657).
205. Snyder FH, Leva E, Oberst, FW. An evaluation of adrenochrome and iodoadrenochrome based on blood-sugar levels in rabbits. J Am Pharm Assoc 1947; 36:253–255.
206. Kaulla KNV. Uber die beeinflussung des O_2- Verbrauches durch adrenochrom beim meerschweinchen. Biochem Z 1949; 319:453–456.
207. Parrot JL, Cara M. Action of adrenochrome on oxygen consumption of man and guinea pig. Compt Rend Soc Biol 1951; 145:1829–2862 (Chem Abstracts 1952; 46:10415).
208. Kisch B. Katalytische wirkungen oxydierten adrenalins. Klin Wochshr 1930; 9:1062–1064.
209. Gaisinska MY Utevskii AM. Effect of catecholamines on oxidative processes under normal conditions and in experimental hypertension. Ukr Biokhim Zh 1962; 34:237–242 (Chem Abstracts 1962; 57:3986).
210. Radsma W, Golterman HL. Influence of adrenaline and adrenochrome on oxygen consumption of liver homogenates. Biochim Biophys Acta 1954; 113:80–86.
211. Kisch B, Leibowitz J. Die beeinflussung der gewebsatmung der omega und durch chinon. Biochem Z 1930; 220:97–116.
212. Issekutz B Jr., Lichtneckert I, Hetenyi G Jr., et al. Metabolic effects of noradrenaline and adrenochrome. Arch Int Pharmacodyn Therap 1950; 84:376–384.
213. Itasaka K. Tissue respiration and substrate utilization of heart muscle slices. Fukuoka Igaku Zasshi 1958; 49:3347–3367 (Chem Abstracts 1959; 53:7436).
214. Wieland O, Suyter M. Der stoffwechselwirkung des adrenochroms. Klin Wochschr 1956; 34:647–648.
215. Krall AR, Siegel GJ, Goznaski DM, et al. Adrenochrome inhibition of oxidative phosphorylation by rat brain mitochondria. Biochem Pharmacol 1964; 12:1519–1525.
216. Sudovtsov VE. Effect of adrenoxyl on the oxidative phosphorylation and potassium and sodium permeability of mitochondria. In: Severin Bioklium SE, ed. MitokhondriMoscow: Funkts, Sist Kletochnykh Organell, Mater, Simp, 1969:83–88. (Chem Abstracts 1971; 74:2436).
217. Wajzer J. 1946 Effect pasteur du muscle de grenouille et adrenochrome. Bull Soc Chim Biol 28:345–349.

218. Wajzer J. Synthese dur glycogene en presence d'adrenochrome. Bull Soc Chim Biol 1947; 29:237–239.
219. Meyerhof O, Randall LO. Inhibitory effects of adrenochrome on cell metabolism. Arch Biochem 1948; 17:171–182.
220. Walaas E Walaas O Jervell K. Action of adrenochrome on glucose phosphorylation in the rat diaphragm. Congr Intern Biochim, Resumes Communs, 1952; 2nd Congr, Paris 67 (Chem Abstracts 1955; 49:5632).
221. Pastan I, Herring B, Johnson P, et al Mechanisms by which adrenaline stimulates glucose oxidation in the thyroid. J Biol Chem 1962; 237:287–290.
222. Dumont JE, Hupka S. Action of neuromimetic amines on the metabolism of thyroid incubated in vitro. Compt Rend Soc Biol 1962; 156:1942–1946 (Chem Abstracts 1963; 59:5434).
223. Dickens F, Glock GE. Mechanism of oxidative inhibition of myosin. Biochim Biophys Acta 1951; 7:578–584.
224. Inchiosa MA. Jr, Van Demark NL. Influence of oxidation products of adrenaline on adenosinetriphosphatase activity of a uterine muscle preparation. Proc Soc Exptl Biol Med 1958; 97:595–597.
225. Denisov VM. Effect of the oxidation products of catecholamines on the ATPase activity of myosin. Ukr Biokhim Zh 1964; 36:711–717 (Chem Abstracts 1965; 62:2930).
226. Denisov VM, Rukavishnikova SM. Influence of adrenoxyl on the activity of heart adrenosine-triphosphatase and phosphorylase. Ukr Biokhim Zh 1968; 40:384–387 (Chem Abstracts 69:105000).
227. Friedenwald JS, Heniz, H. Inactivation of amine oxidase by enzymatic oxidative products of catechol and adrenaline. J Biol Chem 1942; 146:411–419.
228. Usdin E, Usdin VR. Effects of psychotropic compounds on enzyme systems. II. In vitro inhibition of monoamine oxidase (MAO). Proc Soc Exptl Biol Med 1961; 108:461–463.
229. Petryanik VD. Effect of adrenochrome and vikasol on monoamine oxidase of some rabbit organs. Ukr Biokhim Zh 1971; 43:225–228 (Chem Abstracts 1971; 75:47117).
230. Anderson AB. Inhibition of alkaline phosphatase by adrenaline and related dihydroxyphenols and quinones. Biochim Biophys Acta 1961; 54:110–114.
231. Heacock RA. The chemistry of adrenochrome and related compounds. Chem Rev 1959; 59:181–237.
232. Shebeko GS. Effect of adrenaline and adrenoxyl on the level of coenzyme A in some organs of albino rats. Ukr Biokhim Zh 1970; 42:596–599 (Chem Abstracts 1971; 74:72333).
233. Frederick J. Cytologic studies on the normal mitochondria and those submitted to experimental procedures in living cells cultured in vitro. Arch Biol 1958; 69:167–349.
234. Blix G. Adrenaline as an oxidation catalyzer. Oxidative deamination of amino acids by some means of adrenaline or some simple hydroxygenzenes. Skand Arch Physiol 1929; 56:131–172.
235. Kisch B, Leibowitz J. Die omegakatalyze der oxidativen glykokollspaltung. Biochem Z 1930; 220:370–377.
236. Kisch B. Die omegakatalyze der oxidativen glykokollspaltung. Neue untersuchungen. Biochem Z 1931; 236:380–386.

237. Kisch B. O-Chinone als fermentmodell. II. Mitteilung: Versuche mit verschiedened substraten. Biochem Z 1932; 244:440–450.

238. Aberhalden E, Baertich E. Deamination of glycine by "omega" (adrenaline oxidation product). Fermentforschung 1937; 15:342–347 (Chem Abstracts 1938; 32:3431).

239. Fischer P, Landtsheer L. The metabolism of adrenochrome and trihydrox-ymethylindole in the rabbit. Experientia 1950; 6:305–306.

240. Fischer P, Lecomte J. Metabolisme de l'adrenochrome, de ses produits de reuction et du trihydroxy-N-methylindol chez le lapin, le chat et le chien. Bull Soc Chim Biol 1951; 33:569–600.

241. Noval JJ, Sohler A, Stackhouse SP, et al. Metabolism of adrenochrome in experimental animals. Biochem Pharmacol 1962; 11:467–473.

242. Schayer RW, Smiley RL. The metabolism of epinephrine containing isotropic carbon. III. J Biol Chem 1953; 202:425–430.

243. Yates JC, Dhalla NS. Induction of necrosis and failure in the isolated perfused rat heart with oxidized isoproterenol. J Mol Cell Cardiol 1975; 7:807–816.

244. Steen EM, Noronha-Dutra AA, Woolf N. The response of isolated rat heart cells to cardiotoxic concentrations of isoprenaline. J Pathol 1982; 137:167–176.

245. Dhalla NS, Yates JC, Lee SL, et al. Functional and subcellular changes in the isolated rat heart perfused with oxidized isoproterenol. J Mol Cell Cardiol 1978; 10:31–41.

246. Severin S, Sartore S, Schiaffino S. Direct toxic effects of isoproterenol on cultured muscle cells. Experientia 1977; 33:1489–1490.

247. Yates JC, Beamish RE, Dhalla NS. Ventricular dysfunction and necrosis produced by adrenochrome metabolite of epinephrine: Relation to pathogensis of catecholamine cardiomyopathy. Am Heart J 1981; 102:210–221.

248. Yates JC, Taam GML, Singal PK, et al. Protection against adrenochrome-induced myocardial damage by various pharmacological interventions. Br J Exp Pathol 1980; 61:242–255.

249. Yates JC, Taam GML, Singal PK, et al. Modification of adrenochrome-induced cardiac contractile failure and cell damage by changes in cation concentrations. Lab Invest 1980; 43:316–326.

250. Takeo S, Fliegel L, Beamish RE, et al. Effects of adrenochrome on rat heart sarcolemmal ATPase activities. Biochem Pharmacol 1980; 29:559–564.

251. Takeo S, Taam GML, Beamish RE, et al. Effects of adrenochrome on calcium accumulating and adenosine triphosphate activities of the rat heart microsomes. J Pharmacol Exp Therap 1980; 214:688–693.

252. Takeo S, Taam GML, Beamish RE, et al. Effect of adrenochrome on calcium accumulation by heart mitochondria. Biochem Pharmacol 1981; 30:157–163.

253. Taam GML, Takeo S, Ziegelhoffer A, et al. Effect of adrenochrome on adenine nucleotides and mitochondrial oxidative phosphorylation in rat heart. Can J Cardiol 1986; 2:88–93.

254. Fliegel L, Takeo S, Beamish RE, et al. Adrenochrome uptake and subcellular distribution in the isolated perfused rat heart. Can J Cardiol 1985; 1:122–127.

255. Karmazyn M, Beamish RE, Fliegel L, et al. Adrenochrome-induced coronary artery constriction in the rat heart. J Pharmacol Exp Ther 1981; 219:225–230.

256. Singal PK, Dhillon KS, Beamish RE, et al. Myocardial cell damage and cardiovascular changes due to I.V. infusion of adrenochrome in rats. Br J Exp Pathol 1982; 63:167–176.

257. Beamish RE, Dhillon KS, Singal PK, et al. Protective effect of sulfinpyrazone against catecholamine metabolite adrenochrome-induced arrhythmias. Am Heart J 1981; 102:149–152.

258. Beamish RE, Singal PK, Dhillon KS, et al. Effects of sulfinpyrazone on adrenochrome-induced changes in the rat heart. In: Hirsch J, Steele PP, Verrier RL, eds. Effects of Platelet-active Drugs on the Cardiovascular System. Denver: University of Colorado Press, 1981:131–146.

259. Singal PK, Yates JC, Beamish RE, et al. Influence of reducing agents on adrenochrome-induced changes in the heart. Arch Pathol Lab Med 1981; 105:664–669.

260. Piper RD, Li FY, Myers ML, et al. Effects of isoproterenol on myocardial structure and function in septic rats. J Appl Physiol 1999; 86:993–1001.

261. Tappia PS, Hata T, Hozaima L, et al. Role of oxidative stress in catecholamine-induced changes in cardiac sarcolemmal Ca^{2+} transport. Arch Biochem Biophys 2001; 387:85–92.

262. Singal PK, Kapur N, Dhillon KS, et al. Role of free radicals in catecholamine-induced cardiomyopathy. Can J Physiol Pharmacol 1982; 60:1390–1397.

263. Singal PK, Beamish RE, Dhalla NS. Potential oxidative pathways of catecholamines in the formation of lipid peroxides and genesis of heart disease. In: Spitzer JJ, ed. Myocardial Injury. Plenum Publishing Corporation, 1983:391–401.

264. Freedman AM, Cassidy MM, Weglicki WB. Captopril protects against myocardial injury induced by magnesium deficiency. Hypertension 1991; 18:142–147.

265. Haggendal J, Jonsson L, Johansson G, et al. Catecholamine-induced free radicals in myocardial cell necrosis on experimental stress in pigs. Acta Physiol Scand 1987; 131:447–452.

266. Ramos K, Acosta D. Prevention by l(-)ascorbic acid of isoproterenol induced cardiotoxicity in primary culture of rat myocytes. Toxicology 1983; 26:81–90.

267. Ramos K, Combs AB, Acosta D. Cytotoxicity of isoproterenol to cultured heart cells: Effects of antioxidants on modifying membrane damage. Toxicol Appl Pharmacol 1983; 70:317–323.

268. Acosta D, Combs AB, Ramos K. Attenuation by antioxidants of Na^+/K^+ ATPase inhibition by toxic concentrations of isoproterenol in cultured rat myocardial cells. J Mol Cell Cardiol 1984; 16:281–284.

269. Yogeeta SK, Raghavedran HRB, Gnanapragasam A, et al. Ferulic acid with ascorbic acid synergistically extenuates the mitochondrial dysfunction during beta-adrenergic catecholamine induced cardiotoxicity in rats. Chemico-Biol Inter 2006; 163:160–169.

270. Rupp H, Bukhari AR., Jacob R. Modulation of catecholamine synthesizing and degrading enzymes by swimming and emotional excitation in the rat. In: Jacob R, ed. Cardiac Adaptation to Hemodynamic Overload, Training and Stress. Darmstardt: Dr. D. Steinkopff Verlag, 1983:267–273.

271. Mitova M, Bednarik B, Cerny E, et al. Influence of physical exertion on early isoproterenol-induced heart injury. Basic Res Cardiol 1983; 78:131–139.

272. El-Demerdash E, Awad AS, Taha RM, et al. Probucol attenuates oxidative stress and energy decline in isoproterenol-induced heart failure in rat. Pharmocol Res 2005; 51:311–318.

273. Dhalla NS, Temsah RM, Netticadan T. Role of oxidative stress in cardiovascular diseases. J Hypertens 2000; 18:655–673.

274. Burton KP, McCord JM, Ghai G. Myocardial alterations due to free radical generation. Am J Physiol 1984; 246:H1776–H1783.

275. Blaustein AS, Schine L, Brooks WW, et al. Influence of exogenously generated oxidant species on myocardial function. Am J Physiol 1986; 250:H595–H599.

276. Gupta M, Singal PK. Time course of structure, function and metabolic changes due to an exogenous source of oxygen metabolites in rat heart. Can J Physiol Pharmacol 1989; 67:1549–1559.

277. Kaneko M, Beamish RE, Dhalla NS. Depression of heart sarcolemmal Ca^{2+}-pump activity by oxygen free radicals. Am J Physiol 1989; 256:H368–H374.

278. Rowe GT, Manson NH, Caplan M, et al. Hydrogen peroxide and hydroxyl radical mediation of activated leukocyte depression of cardiac sarcoplasmic reticulum: Participation of cyclooxygenase pathway. Circ Res 1983; 53:584–591.

279. Hata T, Kaneko M, Beamish RE, et al. Influence of oxygen free radicals on heart sarcolemmal Na^+-Ca^{2+}exchange. Coronary Artery Dis 1991; 2:397–407.

280. Kaneko M, Hayashi H, Kobayashi A, et al. Stunned myocardium and oxygen free radicals - sarcolemmal membrane damage due to oxygen free radicals. Jap Circ J 1991; 55:885–892.

281. Matsubara T, Dhalla NS. Effect of oxygen free radicals on cardiac contractile activity and sarcolemmal Na^+-Ca^{2+}exchange. J Cardiovasc Pharmacol Therapeut 1996; 1:211–218.

282. Matsubara T, Dhalla NS. Relationship between mechanical dysfunction and depression of sarcolemmal Ca^{2+}-pump activity in hearts perfused with oxygen free radicals. Mol Cell Biochem 1996; 160/161:179–185.

283. Rona G, Chappel CI, Kahn DS. The significance of factors modifying the development of isoproterenol-induced myocardial necrosis. Am Heart J 1963; 66: 389–395.

284. Zbinden G. Inhibition of experimental myocardial necrosis by the monoamine oxidase inhibitor isocarboxazid (Marplan). Am Heart J 1960; 60:450–453.

285. Zbinden G. Effects of anoxia and amine oxidase inhibitors on myocardial necrosis induced by isoproterenol. Fed Proc 1961; 20:128.

286. Zbinden G, Bagdon RE. Isoproterenol-induced heart necrosis, an experimental model for the study of angina pectoris and myocardial infarct. Rev Can Biol 1963; 22:257–263.

287. Leszkovsky GP, Gal G. Observations on isoprenaline-induced myocadial necroses. J Pharm Pharmacol 1967; 19:226–230.

288. Dorigotti L, Gaetani M, Glasser AH, et al. Competitive antagonism of isoproterenol-induced cardiac necrosis by ß-adrenerecptor blocking agents. J Pharm Pharmacol 1969; 21:188–191.

289. Blaiklock RG, Hirsh EM, Dapson S., et al. Epinephrine induced myocardial necrosis: effects of aminophylline and adrenergic blockade. Res Commun Chem Pathol Pharmacol 1981; 34:179–192.

290. Kako K. The effect of beta-adrenerigc blocking agent on biochemical changes in isoproterenol-induced myocardial necrosis. Can J Physiol Pharamcol 1966; 44: 678–682.

291. Pieper GM, Clayton FC, Todd GL, et al. Temporal changes in endocardial energy metabolism following propranolol and the metabolic basis for protection against isoprenaline cardiotoxicity. Cardiovasc Res 1979; 13:207–214.

292. Mehes G, Rajkovits K, Papp G. Effect of various types of sympatholytics on iso-proterenol-induced myocardial lesions. Acta Physiol Acad Sci Hung 1966; 29:75–85.

293. Mehes G, Papp G, Rajkovits K. Effect of adrenergic- and ß-receptor blocking drugs on the myocardial lesions induced by sympathomimetic amines. Acta Physiol Acad Sci Hung 1967; 32:175–184.

294. Waters LL, de Suto-Nagy GI. Lesions of the coronary arteries and great vessels of the dog following injection of adrenaline. Their prevention by Dibenamine. Science 1950; 111:634–635.

295. Wenzel DG, Chau RY. Effect of adrenergic blocking agents on reduction of myocardial aspartate-amino transferase activity by sympathomimetics. Toxic Appl Pharmacol 1966; 9:514–520.

296. Bajusz E, Jasmin G. Protective action of serotonin against certain chemically and surgically induced cardiac necroses. Rev Canad Biol 1962; 21:51–62.

297. Okumura K, Ogawa K, Satake T. Pretreatment with chlorpromazine prevents phospholipid degradation and creatine kinase depletion in isoproterenol-induced myocardial damage in rats. J Cardiovasc Pharmacol 1983; 5:983–988.

298. Godfraind T, Strubois X. The prevention by creatinol O-phosphate of myocardial lesions evoked by isoprenaline. Arch Int Pharmacodyn Therap 1979; 237:288–297.

299. Wenzel, D.G., Stark, L.G. 1966. Effect of nicotine on cardiac necrosis induced by isoproterenol. Am Heart J 71: 368–370.

300. Sigel H, Janke J, Fleckenstein A. Restriction of isoproterenol-induced myocardial Ca uptake and necrotization by a new Ca-antagonistic compound (ethyl-4(3,4,5-trimethoxycinnamoyl) piperazinyl acetate (Vascoril). In: Fleckenstein A, Rona G, eds. Recent Advances in Studies on Cardiac Structure and Metabolism. Baltimore: University Park Press, 1975:121–126.

301. Jolly SR, Reeves WC, Mozingo S, et al. Effect of diltiazem on norepinephrine-induced acute left ventricular dysfunction. Int J Cardiol 1992; 36:31–40.

302. Takeo S, Takenaka F. Effects of diltiazem on high-energy phosphate content reduced by isoproterenol in rat myocardium. Arch Int Pharmacodyn Therap 1977; 228:205–212.

303. Deisher TA, Narita H, Zera P, et al. Protective effect of clentiazem against epinephrine-induced cardiac injury in rats. J Pharmacol Exp Ther 1993; 266:262–269.

304. Nagano M, Higaki J, Nakamura F, et al. Role of cardiac angiotensin II in iso-proterenol-induced left ventricular hypertrophy. Hypertension 1992; 19:708–771.

305. Hu ZW, Billingham M, Tuck M, et al. Captopril improves hypertension and car-diomyopathy in rats with pheochromocytoma. Hypertension 1990; 15:210–215.

306. Salathe M, Weiss P, Ritz R. Rapid reversal of heart failure in a patient with phaeochromocytoma and catecholamine-induced cardiomyopathy who was treated with captopril. Br Heart J 1992; 68:527–528.

307. Grimm D, Elsner D, Schunkert H, et al. Development of heart failure following iso-proterenol administration in the rat: role of the renin-angiotensin system. Cardiovasc Res 1998; 37:91–100.

308. Gallego M, Espina L, Vegas L, et al. Spironolactone and captopril attenuates isoproterenol-induced cardiac remodelling in rats. Pharmacol Res 2001; 44:311–315.

309. Tokuhisa T, Yano M, Obayashi M, et al. AT$_1$ receptor antagonist ryanodine receptor function rendering isoproterenol-induced failing heart less susceptible to Ca^{2+} leak induced by oxidative stress. Circ J 2006; 70:777–786.

310. Chappel CI, Rona G, Balazs T, et al. Comparison of cardiotoxic actions of certain sympathomimetic amines. Can J Biochem Physiol 1959; 37:35–42.

311. Rona G, Chappel CI, Gaudry R. Effect of dietary sodium and potassium content on myocardial necrosis elicited by isoproterenol. Lab Invest 1961; 10:892–897.

312. Janke J, Fleckenstein A, Hein B, et al. Prevention of myocardial Ca overload and necrotization by Mg and K salts or acidosis. In: Fleckenstein A, Rona G, eds. Recent Advances in Studies on Cardiac Structure and Metabolism. Baltimore: University Park Press, 1975:33–42.

313. Slezak J, Tribulova N. Morphological changes after combined administration of isoproterenol and K^+-Mg^{2+}-Aspartate as a Physiological Ca^{2+} antagonist. In: Fleckenstein A, Rona G, eds. Recent Advances in Studies on Cardiac Structure and Metabolism. Baltimore: University Park Press, 1975:75–84.

314. Balazs T. Cardiotoxicity of isoproterenol in experimental animals. Influence of stress, obesity, and repeated dosing. In: Bajusz B, Rona G, eds. Recent Advances in Studies on Cardiac Structure and Metabolism. Baltimore: University Park Press, 1972:770–778.

315. Balazs T, Sahasrabudhe MR, Grice HC. The influence of excess body fat on cardiotoxicity of isoproterenol rats. Tox Appl Pharamcol 1962; 4:613–620.

316. Rona G, Chappel CI, Balazs T, et al. The effect of breed, age and sex on myocardial necrosis produced by isoproterenol in the rat. J Gerontol 1959; 14:169–173.

317. Dusek J, Rona G, Kahn DS. Myocardial resistance. A study of its development against toxic doses of isoproterenol. Arch Pathol 1970; 89:79–83.

318. Dusek J, Rona G, Kahn DS. Myocardial resistance to isoprenaline in rats: Variatons with time. J Pathol 1971; 105:279–282.

319. Selye H, Veilleux R, Grasso S. Protection by coronary ligation against isoproterenol-induced myocardial necrosis. Proc Soc Exp Biol Med 1960; 104:343–345.

320. Faltova E, Poupa P. Temperature and experimental acute cardiac necrosis. Can J Physiol Pharmacol 1969; 47:295–299.

321. Balazs T, Murphy JG, Grice HC. The influence of environmental changes on the cardiotoxicity of isoprenaline in rats. J Pharm Pharmacol 1962; 14:750–755.

322. Raab W, Bajusz E, Kimura H, et al. Isolation, stress, myocardial electrolytes and epinephrine cardiotoxicity in rats. Proc Soc Exp Biol Med 1968; 127:142–147.

323. Hatch AM, Wiberg GS, Zawidzka Z, et al. Isolation syndrome in the rat. Toxicol Appl Pharmacol 1965; 7:737–745.

9

Adverse Cardiovascular Effects of Centrally Acting Psychiatric Medications

William F. Pettit

Department of Behavioral Medicine and Psychiatry; West Virginia Initiative for Innate Health and Robert C. Byrd Health Sciences Center, West Virginia University School of Medicine, Morgantown, West Virginia, U.S.A.

Donald Mishra and Mitchell S. Finkel[a]

Departments of Medicine; Behavioral Medicine and Psychiatry; Physiology and Pharmacology; Robert C. Byrd Health Sciences Center, West Virginia University School of Medicine, Morgantown, West Virginia and Louis A. Johnson VA Medical Center, Clarksburg, West Virginia, U.S.A.

INTRODUCTION

There has been a proliferation of new medications in every field of medicine over the past half-century. This has been particularly true in the area of psychopharmacology. Entirely new classes of psychotropic medications have been developed, resulting in improved efficacy and safety. Increased efficacy has led to widespread use of these medications to the benefit of literally millions of patients.

Fortunately, most psychotropic medications have minimal or no cardiotoxicity in healthy subjects at therapeutic blood levels. However, the patients for whom these medications are prescribed are not "healthy subjects" and often suffer from comorbid conditions. In addition, psychiatric patients are at

---

[a] Dr Mitchell S. Finkel is also associated with the Department of Physiology and Pharmacology, Robert C. Byrd Health Sciences Center of West Virginia University, Morgantown, West Virginia, U.S.A.

considerably higher risk for intentional and unintentional overdose. Thus, there are a number of factors that can lead to serious and potentially fatal adverse effects with these medications.

This chapter is designed to serve as a teaching text to introduce the unfamiliar reader to the subjects of cardiovascular toxicity and psychopharmacology. It is also written to serve as a reference text for the more experienced expert interested in cardiovascular toxicology. A dual approach is used to achieve these two objectives. A series of clinical vignettes are provided to expose the reader to the terms and concepts of cardiovascular and psychopharmacology. Tables summarizing the adverse cardiovascular effects of psychiatric medications are provided to serve as a rapid reference. The text, itself, is written in sections that can be read separately and in any order.

ANTIPSYCHOTICS

In 1952, chlorpromazine (Thorazine®) was introduced into psychiatric practice after clinical reports demonstrated the drug's favorable side-effect profile and its efficacy in treating acute psychosis. At the time of this writing, there are 20 antipsychotic drugs available for prescription in the United States. Fourteen of these, often referred to as typical antipsychotic agents, are thought to work primarily by blocking the dopamine (DA) receptor, D 2. The other seven atypical antipsychotic agents are thought to have their therapeutic effects primarily mediated via regulation of both D 2 and 5 hydroxytryptamine (5 HT_2; serotonin) antagonism.

Tables 1A and 1B include a representative sample of six typical, or first-generation antipsychotics. Tables 2A and 2B show the seven presently available atypical antipsychotic medications, including the six second-generation antipsychotics and the third-generation "dopamine system stabilizer," aripiprazole (Abilify).

Clinical Vignette

A 46-year-old obese woman with a history of schizophrenia was admitted to the hospital for overt psychosis. She had no history of heart disease and her only medical problem was hypertension. She regularly took risperidone 2 mg/day for her schizophrenia and hydrochlorothiazide (a diuretic) 12.5 mg/day for her hypertension. After admission, the patient was started on 4 mg of risperidone/day. On the second night after admission, she became agitated. At that time, she was tachycardic with a pulse of 126. Haloperidol 5 mg IV was administered. After 30 minutes, the patient was still agitated and tachycardic. Another 5 mg of IV haloperidol was given. An hour later, the patient was calm, but remained tachycardic with a pulse of 115. An echocardiogram (ECG) was done that showed sinus tachycardia with a QTc of 510 milliseconds. No such conduction delay was seen on an ECG done one month before. The patient was placed on telemetry and antipsychotics were discontinued. Labs, including electrolytes

(*text continues on page 272*)

Table 1A Antipsychotic Drugs

Typical first generation	Chemical classification	Approx. dosage equiv. (mg)	FDA approved	AzCERT class[a]	Major metabolism site(s) (4)	Enzyme(s) inhibited (4)	Enzyme(s) induced (4)
Pimozide (Orap®)	Diphenylbutyl-piperidine	1.5	Tics from Tourette's disorder not responsive to Haldol[b]	1	**3A4**[e], 1A2	2D6 3A4[f] 1A2	None known
Fluphenazine (Prolixin®)	Phenothiazine Piperazine cpd.	1.6	Acute and chronic psychoses[c] Acute mania or mixed episodes in bipolar disorder Prophylaxis of bipolar disorder	Not listed	**2D6**[e], 1A2	**2D6**[f], 1A2	None known
Haloperidol (Haldol®)	Butyrophenone	2	Tics associated with Tourette's Acute and chronic psychoses[c] Acute mania or mixed episodes in bipolar disorder Prophylaxis of bipolar disorder	1	**2D6**[e], **3A4**[e] 1A2	**2D6**[e]	None known
Mesoridazine (Serentil®)	Phenothiazine Piperidine cpd.	50	Refractory schizophrenia	1	2D6, 1A2	?	?
Thioridazine (Mellaril®)	Phenothiazine cpd.	100	Refractory schizophrenia	1	**2D6**[e], 1A2 2C19, FMO$_3$	**2D6**[f]	?3A4

(Continued)

Table 1A Antipsychotic Drugs (*Continued*)

Typical first generation	Chemical classification	Approx. dosage equiv. (mg)	FDA approved	AzCERT class[a]	Major metabolism site(s) (4)	Enzyme(s) inhibited (4)	Enzyme(s) induced (4)
Chlorpromazine (Thorazine®)	Phenothiazine aliphatic cpd.	100	Tics associated with Tourette's Acute and chronic psychoses[c] Acute mania or mixed episodes in bipolar disorder Prophylaxis of bipolar disorder Others[d]	1	**2D6**[e], 1A2, 3A4, UGT1A4, UGT1A3	**2D6**[f]	None known

[a]The Arizona Centers for Education and Research on Therapeutics, also known as Arizona CERT or AzCERT, maintains a list and classification of drugs that prolong the QT interval and/or induce torsades de pointes (see Ref. 1).

[b]Pimozide is also approved for refractory delusional parasitosis and severe tics.

[c]Schizophrenia, manic phase of bipolar disorder, delusional disorder, schizoaffective disorder.

[d]Chlorpromazine has many approved indications including nausea/vomiting, intractable hiccups, acute intermittent porphyria and as an adjunct in treatment of tetanus.

[e]Bold type indicates major pathway.

[f]Bold type indicates potent inhibition.

Note: Metabolism data presented relate to parent drug and metabolites combined. BOLD type indicates major metabolic pathway.

Abbreviations: FMO₃, flavin monooxygenase; UGT, uridine 5′-diphosphate glucuronosyltransferase.

Sources: Adapted from Refs. 3, 4, and 5.

Table 1B Antipsychotic Drugs

Typical or first-generation antipsychotics Generic name (trade name)	Important for therapeutic 5HT₂A/D2	Pharmacological effects of antipsychotics on neurotransmitters/receptors that have direct and indirect cardiovascular effects					Frequency percentage of adverse cardiovascular reaction to antipsychotics at therapeutic doses				
		H1 blockade Hypotension weight gain	M1 blockade Sinus tachycardia QRS changes	α₁ blockade Postural hypotension reflex tachycardia	5HT₂ blockade Hypotension	Summary Hypotensive effect	AzCERT class[a] degree of risk of TdP	Orthostatic hypotension	Tachycardia	ECG abnormalities	QTc prolongations >450 ms
Pimozide (Orap®)	5.2	+	+	+++	+++	+	1	>2	>2	>2[d]	>2[d]
Fluphenazine (Prolixin®)	24	+++	+	+++	++++	++	1	>2	>10	>2	<2[c]
Haloperidol (Haldol®)	9	+	+	+++	+++	+	1	>2	<2	<2	>2[c,e]
Mesoridazine (Serentil®)	1.26	++++	+++	++++	++++	++	1	>30	>10	>10[c]	>10[c]
Thioridazine (Mellaril®)	17.8	+++	++++	++++	++++	+++	1	>30	>10	>30[c]	>10[c]
Chlorpromazine (Thorazine®)	0.07	+++	+++	++++	++++	++ oral ++– IM	1	>30[b]	>10	>30[c]	>2[b]

Note: The ratio of K_i values between various neurotransmitters/receptors determines the pharmacological profile for any one drug key: K_i(M) 1000–10,000 = +; 100–1000 = ++; 10–100 = +++; 1–10 = ++++.

[a] The Arizona Centers for Education and Research on Therapeutics, also known as Arizona CERT or AzCERT, maintains a list and classification of drugs that prolong the QT interval and/or induce torsades de pointes (see Ref. 1).

[b] More frequent with rapid dose increase.

[c] Higher doses pose greater risk.

[d] Pimozide above 20 mg poses greater risk.

[e] >35m IV over ≤ 6 hr shown to have considerable propensity to QTc prolongation and TdP.

Sources: Adapted from Refs. 3, 4, and 5.

Table 2A Antipsychotic Drugs

A typical second-generation	Chemical classification[a]	Approx. dosage equiv. (mg)	FDA approved	AzCERT class[a]	Major metabolism site(s) (2)	Enzyme(s) inhibited (2)	Enzyme(s) induced (2)
Clozapine (Clozaril®)	Dibenzodiazapine	75	Treatment–resistant schizophrenia; Patients with schizophrenia or schizoaffective disorder who are judged to be at chronic risk for suicide	2	1A2, 3A4, 2D6, 2C19, UGT 1A3	2D6[e]	None known
Olanzapine (Zyprexa®)	Thienobenzodiazepine	1.7	Schizophrenia; Acute manic or mixed episodes of bipolar disorder[b]; Maintainance monotherapy in bipolar patients or combination therapy (with lithium or depakote); Acute agitation associated with schizophrenia and acute mania	Not listed	1A2, 2D6, UGT 1A4, Other ? UGTS,? FMO_3	None known	None known
Quetiapine (Seroquel®)	Dibenzothiazepine	67	Schizophrenia; Acute manic episodes of bipolar disorder[b]; Either as monotherapy or as adjunct therapy to lithium or divalproex; Monotherapy of bipolar depression	2	3A4, sulfation	None known	None known
Risperidone (Risperdal®)	Benzisoxazole	0.5	Schizophrenia; Acute mania or mixed episodes of bipolar disorder[b]	2	2D6, 3A4	2D6[d]	None

Ziprasidone (Geodon®)	Benzisothia-zolpiprazyiny-lindolone derivative	13	Schizophrenia Acute manic and mixed episodes of bipolar disorder[b] IM preparation: Acute agitation in schizophrenic patients	2	Aldehyde-oxidase 3A4, IA2	None known	None known
Paliperidone (Invega®)		1	Schizophrenia	Not listed		None known	None known
Aripiprazole (Abilify®)	Quinolinone derivative	2.5	Schizophrenia Acute manic and mixed episodes of bipolar disorder[b] IM preparation: Acute agitation in schizophrenic patients	Not listed	2D6, 3A4	None	None known

[a]The Arizona Centers for Education and Research on Therapeutics, also known as Arizona CERT or AzCERT, maintains a list and classification of drugs that prolong the QT interval and/or induce torsades de pointes (see Ref. 1).

[b]Schizophrenia, manic phase of bipolar disorder, delusional disorder, schizo affective disorder.

[c]Marked (bold type).

[d]Moderate.

[e]Mild.

Note: Metabolism data presented relate to parent drug and metabolites combined. Bold type indicates major metabolic pathway.

Abbreviations: DSS, dopamine system stabilizer; FMO(3), flavin monoxygenase; UGT, uridine 5′-diphosphate glucuronosyltransferase.

Sources: Adapted from Refs. 3, 4, and 5.

Table 2B Antipsychotics

| A typical or second-generation antipsychotics | | Pharmacological effects of antipsychotics on neurotransmitters/receptors which have direct and indirect cardiovascular effects | | | | | | Frequency percentage of adverse cardiovascular reaction to antipsychotics at therapeutic doses | | | | |
| | | H1 blockade | M1 blockade | α_1 blockade | $5HT_2$ blockade | Summary | AzCERT class[a] | | | | |
Generic name (trade name)	$5HT_{2A}$/D2 ratio	Hypotension Weight gain	Sinus tachycardia QRS changes	Postural Hypotension Reflex tachycardia	Hypotension	Hypotensive effect	Degree of risk of TdP	Orthostatic hypotension	Tachycardia	ECG abnormalities	QTc prolongations >450
Clozapine (Clozaril®)	0.01	++++	+++	+++	++++	+++	2	>10[b]	>10[b]	>30[d]	<2[e]
Olanzapine (Zyprexa®)	0.36	++++	++++	+++	++++	++	Not listed	>2	>2[f]	<2	<2
Quetiapine (Seroquel®)	1.84	+++	+	++++	+++	+++	2	>10	>10	<2	<2
Risperidone (Risperdal®)	0.05	+++	+−	++++	+++	+++	2	>10[b]	>10	<2	<2
Ziprasidone (Geodon®)	1	+++	−	+++	+++++	+	2	>2	>2	>30[d]	<2[d]

| Paliperidone (Invega®) Third-generation DDS | Not available | Not Available | Not available | Not available | Not available | Not listed | >2 | >10 | >2 | <2 |
| Aripiprazole (Abilify®) | 1 | ++ | − | ++++ | ++++ | 0/+ | Not listed | >2 | <2 | <2 |

[a] The Arizona Centers for Education and Research on Therapeutics, also known as Arizona CERT or AzCERT, maintains a list and classification of drugs that prolong the QT interval and/or induce torsades de pointes (see Ref. 1).

[b] May be higher at the start of therapy or with rapid dose increase.

[c] More frequent with rapid dose increase.

[d] Higher doses pose greater risk.

[e] Pimozide above 20 mg poses greater risk.

[f] Bradycardia frequent with IM olanzapine; often accompanied by hypotension.

Note: $5HT_{2}A/D2$ ratio indicates relative preference for D2 vs. $5HT_{2}A$ receptors.

Abbreviation: DDS, dopamine system stabilizer.

Sources: Adapted from Refs. 3, 4, and 5.

with magnesium, were within normal limits. During the next half-hour, the patient developed "torsades de pointes" (TdP) (French expression that literally translates to "twisting of the points"; irregular, wide complex tachycardia that appears to rotate around its axis). The rhythm deteriorated rapidly to ventricular fibrillation. Despite exhaustive resuscitation measures, the patient expired.

Discussion

Unexplained deaths have been reported with antipsychotic use since the early 1960s. Syncope and sudden death occur more frequently in people with schizophrenia (6). It has become generally accepted that antipsychotics can sometimes be a primary causal factor. In other cases, they are at least a contributing factor for sudden cardiac death. This became even more recognized when the U.S. Food and Drug Administration (FDA) application for sertindole (an atypical antipsychotic agent) was declined. Sertindole had been linked to multiple cases of sudden death, syncope, and QT prolongation (7). Sertindole was initially approved in the United Kingdom, but in 2000 was voluntarily suspended from use because of continued links to sudden cardiac death. Subsequent evaluation of the literature during the FDA's assessment of ziprasidone's (Geodon®) application (which was approved) led to restrictions in use and warnings for thioridazine (Mellaril®), mesoridazine (Serentil®), pimozide (Orap®), and droperidol (Inapsine®). All of these medications were found to produce significant lengthening of the QT interval on the ECG and have documented reports of sudden cardiac death and TdP arrythymia even at therapeutic doses.

QTc Prolongation and TdP

Antipsychotics may cause or contribute to sudden death by several potential mechanisms. Particular interest has centered on TdP, a polymorphic ventricular arrhythmia that can progress to ventricular fibrillation and sudden death. The corrected QT (QTc) interval is a heart rate–corrected value that represents the time between the onset of electrical depolarization of the ventricles and the end of repolarization. Prolongation of the QTc interval has become accepted as the surrogate marker for the potential of a drug to cause TdP. In individual patients, an absolute QTc interval of more than 500 milliseconds or an increase of 60 milliseconds from baseline is regarded as indicating an increased risk of TdP. Even so, it has been shown that TdP can occur with lower QTc values or changes.

The Arizona Centers for Education and Research on Therapeutics, also known as Arizona CERT, or AzCERT, maintains a list of drugs that prolong the QT interval and/or induce TdP. It utilizes information from the medical literature, the FDA approved drug labeling and reports submitted to the FDA's adverse events reporting system database. The list of drugs is divided into groups 1 to 4. Drugs in group 1 are generally accepted as having a risk of causing TdP. Group 2 drugs have been associated with the occurrence of TdP, but no substantial evidence to suggest a causal relationship. Group 3 drugs generally do not cause TdP unless coupled with preexisting risk factors. Group 4 drugs have been weakly associated with TdP but at normal levels carry very low risk for inducing the condition (www.torsades.org).

Antipsychotic Agents and Sudden Cardiac Death

All antipsychotic agents have the potential to produce QT interval prolongation on the ECG in a dose-dependent manner to varying degrees. Blockade of the human cardiac potassium (K^+) channel encoded by the human ether-a-go-go-related gene (hERG) has been shown to be a common factor in these and other classes of drugs that cause QT prolongation. As a result, hERG channel inhibition is now commonly used in drug development and assessment to predict the capacity of a drug to prolong the QT interval.

The relationship between K^+ channel inhibition and sudden cardiac death is modulated by a number of factors. These include effects on other ion channels, receptors, plasma protein binding, metabolic interactions, ion disturbances, and genetic changes in cardiac repolarization characteristics (8). Other arrhythmogenic disorders such as myocardial ischemia, diabetes, or adrenergic factors further obfuscate the relationship between the hERG channel, the risk of TdP, and sudden death. Clinical QT prolongation with typical antipsychotics is observed in approximately 10% of users. TdP or surrogates are reported with a frequency of about 1 in 10,000 users (0.01%). TdP is usually spontaneously self-terminating. The death rate is one-tenth of patients with TdP (0.00001 of all patients taking the drug).

There are indications in the general population that simple QTc prolongation in the absence of cardiac risk factors is not indicative of an increased risk of sudden death (9). In their 2004 review article Montanez et al. (9) viewed seven prospective cohort studies including over 36,000 individuals. Among these individuals, there were 2677 (8.7%) with a prolonged QTc interval, defined as 440 milliseconds or greater. They found no consistent evidence for increased risk for overall mortality, cardiovascular-related mortality, or sudden death, except perhaps for patients with prior cardiovascular disease.

Ion Channels and Cardiac Action Potential

The human ventricular action potential consists of five sequential phases (10–12). They are as follows:

Phase 0: The upstroke of the action potential is primarily a consequence of a rapid transient influx of Na^+ [sodium current (I_{Na})] through Na^+ channels.

Phase 1: The termination of the upstroke of the action potential and early afterdepolarization (EAD) phase result from the inactivation of the

Na^+ channels and the transient efflux of K^+ [transient outward K^+ current (I_{TO})] through K^+ channels.

Phase 2: The plateau of the action potential is a reflection of the balance between the influx of Ca^{2+} [calcium current (I_{Ca})] through L-type Ca^{2+} channels and outward repolarizing K^+ currents.

Phase 3: The sustained downward stroke of the action potential and the late repolarization phase result from the efflux of K^+ [rapidly activating delayed rectifier K^+ current (I_{Kr}) and slow activating delayed rectifier K^+ current (I_{Kr})] though delayed rectifier K^+ channels.

Phase 4: The resting potential is maintained by the inward rectifier K^+ current (I_{K1}).

Ion Channel Basis of QT Interval Prolongation

The prolongation of the QT interval in the ECG is caused by the prolongation of the action potential of the ventricular myocytes, brought about by a reduction of outward currents and/or enhancement of inward currents during phases 2 or 3 of the action potential. A reduction in the net outward current and/or increase in inward current can potentially facilitate the development of EADs (10,12,13). They occur preferentially in mid-myocardium and Purkinje cells. EADs are depolarizations occurring during phases 2 and 3 before repolarization is complete. Prolongation of the action potential allows reactivation of slow inward Na^+ and Ca^{2+} currents by reactivation of the L-type Ca^{2+} current and/or activation of the sodium-calcium exchange current. EADs may give rise to one or more premature action potentials. These interrupt early phase 3 repolarization and possibly result in multifocal ventricular extrasystoles and TdP.

In the inherited form of the long QT syndrome, prolongation of the cardiac repolarization phase has been shown to result from both K^+ and Na^+ channel defects. K^+ channel genes known to be involved include KVLQT1-I_{Ks}, hERG-I_{Kr} and KCNE1 and KCNE2 (minK)-I_{Ks} (encoding an auxiliary K^+ channel subunit). The Na^+ channel gene shown to affect the QT interval is SCN5A gene encoding 1Na. Drugs may prolong the QT interval by exerting effects on any of these known channels. However, the best studied of these is the hERG-I_{Kr} channel. Virtually all drugs known to cause TdP, including atypical and typical antipsychotics, block the rapidly activating component of this delayed rectifier K^+ current (8,10,12).

Repolarization Reserve

Roden have presented the concept of "repolarization reserve." This term refers to the normal function of the delayed rectifier currents I_{Ks} and I_{Kr} to contribute to a stable repolarization and a large repolarization reserve (14).

Multiple factors can reduce the repolarization reserve, thus increasing the risk for QT prolongation, TdP and sudden death. Factors that can contribute to a reduction in replorarization reserve include the following:

1. Congenital factors
    i. congenital polymorphism of ion channel regulation
    ii. congenital prolonged QT syndrome
    iii. congenital slow metabolizer status affecting primary route of metabolism of drugs that block the delayed rectifier currents [e.g., CYP450 2D6(pm) poor metabolizer]
    iv. female gender
2. Metabolic factors
    i. hypokalemia (a common contributing factor in case reports of TdP and sudden death)
    ii. hypomagnesmia
    iii. hypocalcemia
3. Drugs that have a high affinity for hERG receptor at therapeutic doses. Primary examples are the typical antipsychotics pimozide, droperidol, haloperidol, mesoridazine, chlorpromazine, thioridazine and the opiate agonist, methadone (AzCERT class 1).
4. Drugs that at therapeutic doses have a moderate affinity for hERG receptor that
    i. are taken in overdose;
    ii. are given in large doses intravenously (e.g., IV Haldol);
    iii. are given in combination with one or more other drugs which have affinity for the hERG receptor (pharmacodynamic effect) (e.g., anti-arrhythmic drugs classes 1a and 3, fluroquinolone antibiotics, macrolide antibiotics, imidazoline antifungals, and tricyclic and heterocyclic antidepressants (see www.torsades.org for updated classification of all medications implicated in QT prolongation and TdP); and
    iv. are given in combination with a medication that inhibits its metabolism, thus iatrogenetically creating "overdose" blood levels (i.e., pharmacokinetic effect).
5. Preexisting cardiac disease
    i. history of myocardial infarction (MI)
    ii. cardiac ischemia
    iii. congestive heart failure
    iv. valvulopathy
    v. cardiomyopathy
    vi. acquired prolonged QT interval (for women, >470 milliseconds; for men, >450 milliseconds) (15)
    vii. recent conversion from atrial fibrillation

    viii. digitalis therapy
      ix. diuretic therapy (even in the presence of normal plasma electrolytes)
       x. bradycardia

6. Miscellaneous contributing factors

       i. ↑ age (pharmodynamic and pharmacokinetic changes with advanced age)
      ii. heightened emotional state (increased adrenergic tone)
    iii. physical restraint
    iv. obesity (BMI > 27)
     v. depleted nutritional status
    vi. liver disease
   vii. renal disease
  viii. diabetes mellitus

Risk Factors for TdP

In a recent review article, Justo et al. (16) investigated the case reports of 70 patients with TdP induced with psychotropic drugs. On the basis of earlier reviews (14), these case reports were analyzed for the presence of six recognized risk factors for TdP prior to the initiation of the psychotropic drug. The identified risk factors that can lessen the repolarization reserve are female gender (70%), hypokalemia (14.2%), high dose of the offending drug (27.1%), concomitant use of a QT interval–prolonging agent (30.8%), advanced heart disease (34.2%), and a history of long QT syndrome (LQTS) (18.5%).

Of the associated psychotropic drugs, haloperidol and thioridazine were responsible for most of the cases, accounting for 37.1% and 30%, respectively. The remaining 23 (32.8%) miscellaneous cases included chlorpromazine (4), imipramine (3), amitriptyline (2), clomipramine (2), and maprotiline (2). One each took desipramine, doxepin, droperidol, fluoxetine, ketanserin, pimozide, promethazine, protriptyline, risperidone or trazodone.

Antipsychotic Dose–Related QTc Prolongation

QTc prolongation with antipsychotic drugs as with other drugs is dose related (17–21). Warner et al. showed that the QTc prolongation was significantly more likely to occur in patients receiving doses of antipsychotics above 2000 mg chlorpromazine equivalent per day. Reilly et al. (22) assessed the ECGs from 495 psychiatric patients to determine predictors of QTc lengthening (defined from a healthy group control as greater than 465 milliseconds). Antipsychotic dosage was defined as a standard 0 to 1000-mg chlorpromazine equivalent per day, high (1001–2000 mg chlorpromazine equivalent per day) and very high (>2000 mg chlorpromazine equivalent per day). From a logistic regression analysis, antipsychotic dosage emerged as a robust predictor of QTc lengthening [adjusted odds ratio (OR) for high dosage 5.3: 95% confidence interval (CI) 1.2–294.4: $p = 0.03$, adjusted OR for very high dosage 8.2: 95% CI 1.5–43.6; $p = 0.01$].

Antipsychotics and hERG Channel Inhibition (Experimental Animal Studies)

The effects of antipsychotics on K^+ channels have been explored by different patch clamp studies. Kongsamut et al. (23) compared hERG channel affinities for a series of antipsychotic drugs. Dose-response relationships generated from this protocol yielded IC_{50} values (IC_{50} = concentration that produces 50% inhibition of hERG) as follows: sertindole 2.7 nmol/L; pimozide 18 nmol/L; risperidone 167 nmol/L; ziprasidone 169 nmol/L; thioridazine 191 nmol/L; quetiapine 5765 nmol/L, and olanzapine 6013 nmol/L.

Two major comparative electrophysiological studies of antipsychotics have been published: one study by Adamantidis et al. (24) on Purkinje fibres and another by Drici et al. (25) on isolated feline heart. The data reported by Adamantidis et al. show a concentration-dependent increase of APD (action potential duration) induced by droperidol. For haloperidol and risperidone, the APD increased rapidly for concentrations >0.1 μmol/L. The effect on the APD was less marked for clozapine. In another report, Gluais et al. (26) investigated the effect of risperidone on potentials recorded on Purkinje fibres and ventricular myocardium and K^+ currents recorded from atrial and ventricular rabbit isolated myocytes. The results showed that risperidone (0.1–0.3 μmol/L) exerted potent lengthening effects on the APD in both tissues, with high potency in the Purkinje fibers, and caused the development of EADs at a low stimulation rate. The study by Drici et al. (25) investigated the potency of five antipsychotics (the atypicals risperidone and olanzapine and clozapine and sertindole (which did not receive FDA approval in the United States) and the typical antipsychotic haloperidol) in lengthening the QT interval of the perfused isolated heart. The hearts were infused with increasing concentrations of drug (0.1–20 mmol/L) for 40-minute intervals at each concentration. Data indicated that all tested drugs prolonged the QT interval in a concentration-dependent manner.

Human Clinical Studies

Many studies have compared the QTc interval in patients treated with antipsychotics with control patients. These studies show a lengthening of QTc interval with most antipsychotic drugs (22,27,28). Kitayama H et al. (27) demonstrated that long term treatment with antipsychotic drugs in conventional doses prolonged QTc dispersion but did not increase ventricular tachyarrythmias in patients with schizophrenia in the absence of cardiac disease. As in other studies, the antipsychotic drugs caused QTc lengthening in a dose-related manner. The effects are substantially more pronounced for thioridazine or droperidol than for other antipsychotics that have been shown to confer an increased risk of drug-induced arrhythmia. Cardiovascular mortality has been studied from data collected in a large North American study of nearly 100,000 outpatients with schizophrenia who were treated with antipsychotics (7). QTc data were corrected using the Fredericia's formula (QT/RR 1/3). The mean increases in QTc were 1.1% for olanzapine (Zyprexa®), 3% for risperidone (Risperdal®), 4.8%

for quetiapine (Seroquel®), 7.3% for haloperidol (Haldol®), 15.4% for ziprasidone (Geodon) and 29.6% for thioridazine (Mellaril) (7).

In conclusion, it has become apparent that the variability and susceptibility to drug induced long QT syndrome among patients is multifactorial. These factors include environmental, genetic, and disease determinants that affect the plasma concentration of a drug and the pharmacological effects on the hERG K^+ channel.

Antipsychotic Effects on Neurotransmitter Receptors

Tables 2A and 2B show the effects of antipsychotics on neurotransmitter receptors known to have direct and indirect cardiac effects.

Cardiac Effects of Typical Antipsychotics

The six conventional antipsychotic medications are a representative sample of the "typical" or "first-generation" antipsychotic medications available in the United States. Pimozide, fluphenazine, haloperidol, mesoridazine, thioridazine and chlorpromazine have all been associated with QTc prolongation, TdP and sudden death (29–42). These medications have less orthostatic hypotension when compared with the less potent typical antipsychotics mesoridazine, thioridazine, and chlorpromazine, which have a greater than 30% incidence of orthostatic hypotension. This effect is likely related to their more potent actions on H_1, α_1, and $5HT_2$ blockade when compared with the more potent (from an antipsychotic standpoint) neuroleptics. Mesoridazine, thioridazine, and chlorpromazine also have an increased incidence of tachycardia, which is related to their significant increase in M1 blockade when compared with pimozide, fluphenazine, and haloperidol. It is noted that fluphenazine does have a greater incidence of tachycardia (>10%), than pimozide and haloperidol. From the neurotransmitters, it appears that this is related to a greater effect at H1 blockade and $5HT_2A$ blockade, leading to a reflex tachycardia. The incidence of ECG abnormalities and QTc prolongation is low for pimozide at low doses. Many of the instances of fatal sudden death and TdP that have been reported with pimozide are related primarily to doses above 20 mg/day or have involved a pharmacokinetic interaction that has resulted in a blood level equivalent to or greater than a daily 20-mg dose.

Cardiac Effects Atypical Antipsychotics

The neurotransmitter receptor effects of the second-generation antipsychotics and the third-generation "dopamine system stabilizer" (aripiprazole) contribute to hypotension. The incidence of orthostatic hypotension is greatest with clozapine, quetiapine, and risperidone when compared with that of olanzapine, ziprasidone, and aripiprazole. It has been noted with clozapine and risperidone that the incidence of hypotension is higher at the start of therapy or with rapid dose increase. It is important to note that the hypotensive effect of these medications can be life-threatening in the presence of the frail elderly. This is particularly true when they are on other medications that lower blood pressure, particularly via α_1 blockade (e.g., Prazosin). These patients would be most susceptible to the α_1 blockade of quetiapine and risperidone.

Comparison of Atypical and Typical Antipsychotics

In their 2005 article, Liperoti et al. compared the cardiac related risk of hospitalization for ventricular arrhythmias or cardiac arrest, between the patients on conventional or typical antipsychotics and those with atypical antipsychotics. This involved a case-controlled study of residents of nursing homes in six U.S. states, who were hospitalized for ventricular arrhythmias or cardiac arrest between July 1998 and December 30, 1999. The sample consisted of 650 cases and 2962 controls. The use of conventional antipsychotics was associated with a nearly twofold increase in the risk of hospitalization for ventricular arrhythmias or cardiac arrests (OR 1.86; 95% CI, 1.27 to 2.74). There was no increased risk associated with the use of atypical antipsychotics (OR 0.87; 95% CI, 0.58 to 2.32). The risk of hospitalization for ventricular arrhythmias or cardiac arrests was highest among conventional users with cardiac disease (OR 3.27; 95% CI, 1.95 to 5.47) (43).

Adverse Metabolic Effects of Antipsychotics

There has been a growing concern about the metabolic effects of antipsychotic medications, especially with certain second-generation antipsychotics. Newcomer et al. (44) reviewed the current evidence that the treatment with antipsychotic medications may be associated with increased risk for weight gain, insulin resistance, hypoglycemia, dyslipidemia, and type 2 diabetes mellitus (44). Many of these items are risk factors for cardiovascular disease. This serves as an indirect causal pathway in which antipsychotics, mainly atypicals, can lead to coronary artery disease and sudden cardiac death.

Newcomer et al. conducted a meta-analytic review indicating that clozapine was consistently associated with an increased risk for diabetes compared with conventional antipsychotics (OR 1.37; 95% CI, 1.25–1.52) versus no antipsychotics (OR 7.44; 95% CI 1.59–34.75) (45). Olanzapine was also associated with increased risk for diabetes compared with conventional antipsychotics (OR 1.26; 95% CI, 1.10–1.46) versus no antipsychotics (OR 2.31, 95% CI, 0.98–5.46). Neither risperidone nor quetiapine compared to either conventional antipsychotic or no antipsychotics were associated with an increased diabetic risk. Newcomer et al. also compared the effects of conventional and atypical antipsychotics on glucose regulation in chronically treated nondiabetic patients with schizophrenia and untreated healthy control subjects. The patients in the control groups were carefully matched for adiposity and age. According to a modified oral glucose-tolerance test, patients receiving olanzapine ($N = 12$) and clozapine ($N = 9$) had significantly higher fasting and postprandial plasma glucose values compared with patients receiving conventional antipsychotics ($N = 17$) and untreated healthy control subjects ($N = 31$) $p < 0.01$ for all comparisons). The risperidone group had higher postprandial glucose levels compared with control subjects ($p < 0.01$), but not in comparison with the conventional antipsychotic group. Patients on olanzapine had higher calculated insulin resistance compared with those who received conventional antipsychotic agents ($p < 0.05$). Those who received risperidone, or typical antipsychotics did not differ from control subjects.

The use of some atypical antipsychotics (e.g., olanzapine, clozapine) is associated with an increased risk for weight gain and disordered glucose and lipid metabolism (46). Weight gain is not an absolute prerequisite for the development of insulin resistance, impaired glucose tolerance, dyslipidemia, or type 2 diabetes mellitus. These adverse metabolic effects on coronary artery risk factors may be causally related to the increased rates of cardiovascular morbidity and mortality seen in schizophrenia patients.

Clozapine: Myocarditis/Cardiomyopathy/Sudden Death

Clozapine is the only antipsychotic with established efficacy in patients with vigorously defined refractory schizophrenia and has shown significant reduction of suicidality in patients with schizophrenia.

Recently attention has focused on the association of myocarditis and cardiomyopathy with Clozapine. In some cases young people with no prior cardiac history have died (47,48).

Two hundred thirty-one cases of myocarditis or cardomyopathy have been reported with Clozapine; all other antipsychotics have totaled just 89 such reports. The onset of Clozapine associated myocarditis symptoms occurs within 2 months in 90% of the reported cases and are associated with myocardial eosinophilic infiltrates consistent with drug induced acute hypersensitivity (Type 1, EgE) mediated myocarditis (49).

A preliminary study found the rate of sudden death during Clozapine treatment to be 0.7%, 2.5 times greater than that with other atypical antipsychotic medications (50–52). One factor which may contribute to this finding is that Clozapine decreases heart rate variability more than other atypical antipsychotics (53).

Clinical Vignette

A 70-year-old man had been prescribed pimozide (Orap) 10 mg/day by his neurologist for treatment of a tic disorder. The patient had responded well to this dose with no significant side effects. Six months later, he began to cough frequently and painfully and developed a fever of 101.3°F. His internist prescribed clarithromycin (Biaxin®) 500 mg b.i.d. for 10 days. On day 5, the patient had a syncopal episode and fell. ECG monitor obtained by EMS (emergency medical services) showed a prolonged QTc greater than 606 milliseconds, which progressed to TdP and ventricular fibrillation. He was taken to the hospital after a stable rhythm was restored following emergency medical care, including defibrillation. The patient gradually improved with supportive care and change in antibiotics.

Discussion

Pimozide is a CYP450 isoenzyme 3A4 substrate and clarithromycin is a potent 3A4 inhibitor. The addition of clarithromycin significantly impaired the ability of 3A4 to efficiently metabolize the pimozide. This likely caused the blood level of pimozide to increase significantly for the same dose administered. Pimozide has been shown to increase the QTc interval in a dose-dependent manner. The increased pimozide blood level caused the QTc interval to correspondingly increase. Clarithromycin can also increase the QTc interval. This resulted in a large QTc prolongation, predisposing to TdP, and ventricular fibrillation.

Pharmacokinetic Interactions

The pharmacokinetic interactions and metabolic effects of P450 isoenzyme inhibition is a topic of great importance in view of the prevalence of polypharmacy in the modern world. P450 inhibition can lead to increased plasma levels of an antipsychotic, QTc prolongation, increased vulnerablity to TdP, ventricular arrhythmias, and sudden cardiac death. Harrigan et al. (54) reported on the effect of six antipsychotics on the QTc interval in the absence and presence of metabolic inhibition. This randomized study involved patients with psychotic disorders who had reached a steady state on either haloperidol (Haldol), 15 mg/day ($N = 27$), thioridazine (Mellaril), 300 mg/day ($N = 30$), ziprasidone (Geodon), 160 mg/day ($N = 31$), quetiapine (Seroquel®), 750 mg/day ($N = 27$), olanzapine (Zyprexa®), 20 mg/day ($N = 24$) or risperidone (Risperidol®), 6 to 8 mg/day, increased to 16 mg/day ($N = 25/20$). The mean plasma/serum drug concentrations in nanograms per milliliter after the addition of the metabolic inhibitor was increased for ziprasidone 1.39, risperidone 2.47, olanzapine 1.77, quetiapine 4.03, thioridazine 1.04, and haloperidol 1.94. Haloperidol was inhibited by ketaconazole 400 mg and paroxetine 20 mg to inhibit the pathways of 3A4 and 2D6. Ziprasidone and quetiapine were inhibited by 400 mg of ketoconazole to inhibit the 3A4 pathway. Olanzapine was inhibited with fluvoxamine to inhibit the 1A2 pathway and risperidone and thioridazine were both inhibited by 20 mg of paroxetine inhibiting the 2D6 metabolic pathway. The QTc changes were greatest for thioridazine 30.14 milliseconds and least with olanzapine at 1.7 milliseconds, ziprasidone 15.9 milliseconds, haloperidol 7.1 milliseconds and quetiapine 5.7 milliseconds, respectively. No patient had a QTc interval of greater than 500 milliseconds during this study.

Only 9 of 116 cases of TdP had a QTc interval of less than 500 milliseconds in one study of antipsychotics (55). QT prolongation by itself does not usually cause significant adverse cardiac events. The presence of other factors that lessen the repolarization reserve increases the likelihood of developing a life-threatening arrhythmia.

ANTIDEPRESSANTS

Clinical Vignette

A 21-year-old woman was admitted to the emergency department with confusion and agitation, accompanied by twitching of her upper and lower limbs. She had been diagnosed three years earlier with resistant major depressive disorder. Her primary care physician had tried a variety of medications and combinations to no avail.

Earlier that morning she had an argument on the phone with her boyfriend after which she told him he "would be sorry." After the argument, her boyfriend had gone over to her house to check on her and found her comatose with an empty bottle of amitriptyline beside her.

He immediately called 911, and she was transported by ambulance to the hospital for further treatment. Her vital signs revealed a pulse of 62, blood pressure of 90/55, and temperature of 38°C. She was obtunded and minimally responsive to pain. Secondary to her low level of arousal and instability she was intubated and placed on a ventilator. An arterial blood gas done just before intubation revealed a respiratory acidosis. A computed tomography (CT) scan done of her head was normal. An ECG was done, which showed a pattern consistent with "Brugada syndrome" (right bundle branch block with ST segment elevation in the right precordial leads). Shortly after being placed on telemetry, she developed ventricular fibrillation and her pulse disappeared. Appropriate ACLS (advanced cardiac life support) protocols were followed to restore a normal cardiac rhythm. Despite maximal effort, she was unable to be resuscitated.

Tricyclic Antidepressants

Amitriptyline (Elavil®)
Imipramine (Tofranil®)
Doxepin (Sinequan®)
Clomipramine (Anafranil®)
Desipramine (Norpramin®)
Nortriptyline (Pamelor®) (Tables 3A and 3B)

Tricyclic antidepressants (TCAs) have been used in the treatment of major depressive disorder since the late 1950s. From the mid-1960s, it became apparent that the TCAs in overdose affect cardiac physiology and often resulted in TdP and death.

The cardiovascular side effects of the TCAs are well established and are known to be linked to their capacity to inhibit cardiac and vascular ion channels. Newer antidepressants such as the selective serotonin reuptake inhibitors (SSRIs), and norepinepherine (NE) and DA reuptake inhibitors have been reported to have a more benign cardiovascular profile. This has led to their widespread use as first line treatments for depression. When patients fail to respond to these medicines, often TCAs have to be used. TCAs are also still frequently used in the treatment of chronic pain syndromes such as migraine and prophylaxis. TCAs remain second only to analgesics as the most commonly prescribed drugs implicated in overdose fatalities. This is all the more remarkable considering the decline in their use in the treatment of major depression.

Ion Channel Modulation by TCAs

1. The electrophysiological effects that antidepressants exert on ion channels may well affect the cardiac action potential (cAP), lengthening both depolarization and repolarization phases, widening the QRS complex,

Table 3A Tricyclic Antidepressants

Generic name Trade name	Chemical class (TCAs)	Receptor-effect Class	FDA approved	Major metabolism sites	Enzyme processes inhibited	Usual adult daily dose	Approximate half-life (including active metabolites)
Amitriptyline Elavil®	Tertiary amine tricyclic	NSCA	MDD Prophylaxis of MDD (in unipolar depression) Depressed phase of bipolar disorder[a] Treatment of secondary depression with other mental illnesses, e.g., Schizophrenia and dementia	2C19 2D6 3A4 UGT1A4	2C19[c] 2D6[d]	100–300 mg	16 hr (30) hr
Imipramine Tofranil®	Tertiary amine tricyclic	NSCA	MDD Prophylaxis of MDD (in unipolar depression) Depressed phase of bipolar disorder[a] Eneuresis Treatment of secondary depression with other mental illnesses, e.g. Schizophrenia and Dementia	1A2 2C19 2D6 3A4 UGT1A4 UGT1A3	2C19[d] 2D6[d]	100–300 mg	12 hr (30) hr
Clomipramine Anafranil®	Tertiary amine tricyclic	NSCA	MDD Prophylaxis of MDD Depressed phase of bipolar disorder[a] Eneuresis OCD Treatment of secondary depression illnesses, e.g., with other mental illnesses, e.g., schizophrenia and dementia	2C19 2D6 3A4	2D6[d]	100–250 mg	32 hr (70) hr
Doxepin Sinequan®	Tertiary amine tricyclic	NSCA	MDD Prophylaxis of MDD (in unipolar depression) Depressed phase of bipolar disorder[a] Depression and/or anxiety associated with alcoholism or organic disease Treatment of secondary depression with other mental illnesses, e.g., schizophrenia and dementia	1A2 2D6 3A4 UGT1A4 UGT1A3	None Known	100–300 mg	16 (30) hr

(Continued)

Table 3A Tricyclic Antidepressants (*Continued*)

Generic name Trade name	Chemical class (TCAs)	Receptor-effect Class	FDA approved	Major metabolism sites	Enzyme processes inhibited	Usual adult daily dose	Approximate half-life (including active metabolites)
Nortriptyline Pamelor®	Secondary amine tricyclic	NSCA	MDD Prophylaxis of MDD (in unipolar depression) Depressed phase of bipolar disorder[a] Treatment of secondary depression with other mental illnesses, e.g., schizophrenia and dementia	2D6	2D6[c]	50–150 mg	30 hr
Desipramine Norpramin®	Secondary amine tricyclic	NSCA	MDD Prophylaxis of MDD (in unipolar depression) Depressed phase of bipolar disorder Treatment of secondary depression with other mental illnesses, e.g., schizophrenia and Dementia	2D6	2D6[d]	100–300 mg	30 hr

[a]Use with caution may precipitate manic or hypomanic episode.
[b]Marked inhibition.
[c]Moderate inhibition.
[d]Mild inhibition.

Note: The Arizona Centers for Education and Research on Therapeutics, also known as Arizona CERT or AzCERT, maintains a list and classification of drugs that prolong the QT interval and/or induce torsades de pointes (see Ref. 1).

Abbreviations: NSCA, nonselective cyclic antidepressants; MDD, major depressive disorder; OCD, obsessive compulsive disorder.

Sources: Adapted from Refs. 3, 4, and 5.

Table 3B Tricyclic Antidepressants

Generic name / Trade name	Pharmacological effects on neurotransmitters/receptors responsible for cardiovascular side effects (direct and indirect)						Frequency percentage of adverse cardiovascular reaction to antipsychotics at therapeutic doses				
	NE reuptake blockade — Tachycardia Hypotension	5-HT reuptake blockade — Potentiation of drugs with serotonergic properties risk-ing serotonin syndrome	5HT₂ blockade — Hypotension Weight gain	M1 blockade — Sinus tachycardia QRS changes Potentiation of drugs w/ anticholinergic	H1 blockade — Postural Hypotension Weight gain	α1 blockade — Postural Hypotension Reflex tachycardia	AzCERT class[a] Risk for TdP	Orthostatic hypotension Dizziness	Tachyardia Palpitations	ECG changes	Cardiac arrhythmia ms
Amitriptyline Elavil®	+++	+++	+++	+++	++++	+++	4	>10	>10	>10[b]	>2
Imipramine Tofranil®	+++	+++	+++	+++	+++	+++	4	>30	>10	>10[b]	>2
Clomipramine Anafranil®	+++	++++	+++	+++	+++	+++	4	>10	>10	>10[b]	>2
Doxepin Sinequan®	+++	++	+++	+++	+++++	+++	4	>10	>2	>2[b]	>2
Nortriptyline Pamelor®	++++	++	+++	++	+++	+++	4	>2	>2	>2[b]	>2
Desipramine	++++	++	++	++	++	++	4	>2	>10	>2[b]	>2

[a]The Arizona Centers for Education and Research on Therapeutics, also known as Arizona CERT or AzCERT, maintains a list and classification of drugs that prolong the QT interval and/or induce torsades de pointes (see Ref. 1).

[b]Conduction delays: increased PR, QRS, or QTc interval.

Note: ECG abnormalities usually without cardiac injury.

Sources: Adapted from Refs. 3, 4, and 5.

prolonging the QT interval, or causing Brugada-like electrocardiographic patterns. Lengthening of the depolarization phase can slow conduction through the Purkinje system in the ventricular myocardium. Slowing repolarization can lead to EADs and TdP.

2. Many antidepressants, like many antipsychotics, modulate the cAP by blocking different cardiac ion channels present in ventricular myocytes, including the fast inward I_{Na}, the inward slow I_{Ca} and one or more outward KI_K. Cyclic antidepressants share the same properties as class 1 antiarrhythmics in blocking sodium channels. This causes widening of the QRS complex and as a consequence some degree of QT interval prolongation.

3. The antidepressant-mediated effect on depolarization significantly contributes to the prolongation of the QT interval. Conversely, QT prolongation that is related to I_{Kr} block is solely the result of lengthening of repolarization. This is linked to the greater risk of EADs and TdP. One example of the modulating effect of multiple channel blocks on the repolarization phase is the effect of TCAs on both Na^+ and K^+ channels: the Na^+ channel–blocking effects of these agents may diminish the effect of "I_{Kr} blockade on the prolongation of APD." However, Na^+ channel blockade by antidepressants has been suggested to cause fatal tachyarrhythmias without QT prolongations as a result of a drug-induced, Brugada-like ECG pattern (6).

4. Studies involving the hamster ovary, the human embryonic kidney, rabbit atrial and ventricular myocytes, and rat ventricular myocytes suggest that imipramine and amitriptyline definitively block I_{Na} and also may have blocking properties at both I_{Ca} and I_{Kr}. Thus, all tricyclic compounds may prolong the QT interval in therapeutic doses and will consistently do so when taken in overdose.

The Brugada Syndrome

In addition to QTc prolongation–induced TdP arrhythmia, tricyclic–induced Brugada syndrome has been described as an important cause of sudden death with tricyclic overdose (35,56,57). The Brugada syndrome occurs in about 0.05% to 0.1% of the population (> 3 times the prevalence of the congenital long QT syndrome). This arrhythmic syndrome is characterized by an electrocardiographic pattern of right bundle branch block and ST segment elevation in the right precordial leads and normal QTc interval coupled with sudden death due to primary ventricular tachyarrhythmias (including TdP). Ventricular fibrillation is the most commonly documented terminal arrhythmia (58,59).

QTc Prolongation

Goodnick et al. (60) have published an extensive review of the effects of antidepressants on QT interval in controlled clinical trials. Significant QT and QRS prolongation was reported in depressed patients treated with therapeutic doses

(75 to 180 mg/day) of imipramine for at least three weeks compared with patients treated with placebo, fluoxetine, or bupropion. Imipramine treatment led to a significant QT prolongation that varied between +4 and +20 milliseconds from baseline. Desipramine and clomipramine have also been shown to significantly prolong QT and QRS intervals when used at therapeutic doses (5 mg/kg/ day in children and adolescents) (61). In one study, paroxetine, sertraline, fluvoxamine, fluoxetine, citalopram (SRIs) and venlafaxine (SNRI) did not affect the QT interval or any other ECG parameter when used at therapeutic dose.

All tricyclic compounds that may prolong QT at therapeutic doses have been shown to prolong QT in overdose.

TCA Cardiovascular Toxicity with Overdose

An ingestion of 6.67 mg/kg or more of most TCAs constitutes a moderate to serious exposure, where coma and cardiovascular symptoms are expected. As little as 15 mg/kg may be fatal in a child. Cardiovascular toxicity is the leading cause of death in overdose for tricyclics.

Sinus tachycardia is a common anticholinergic effect. The abrupt blockade of the reuptake of NE also increases the tachycardia. As stated earlier, patients with more serious overdoses may develop conduction disturbances, including prolonged PR interval, QRS widening, QTc prolongation, rightward shift in the axis of the terminal 40 milliseconds of the QRS complex, atrial ventricular block, ventricular dysrrhythmias (TdP, ventricular tachycardia, and fibrillation) and hypotension. QRS duration of 0.16 seconds or longer has been associated with an increased incidence of ventricular dysrrhythmias. Severe cardiac toxicity generally develops within six hours although ECG changes may persist for 48 hours (62).

TCA Cardiovascular Toxicity with Therapeutic Doses

TCAs at therapeutic doses can frequently cause orthostatic hypotension and tachycardia (Table 3B). TCAs cause these problems via their pharmacological effects of blocking $5HT_2$, M_1, H_1, and $\alpha 1$ receptors and their reuptake inhibition of serotonin and NE. These effects are somewhat less pronounced in the secondary amine tricyclics nortriptyline and desipramine than their tertiary amine counterparts amitriptyline and imipramine (Table 3B). The former two compounds are formed from dehydroxylation of the latter two compounds.

In addition, it became apparent in the mid-1960s that tricyclic antidepressant overdose caused more frequent hypotension and tachycardia. This parallels the increased potential for QT prolongation and sudden death that accompanies overdose.

Effects of TCAs on Human Myocardial Contractility

TCAs also appear to have an effect on the contractility of the heart. Strips of atrial tissue obtained during cardiac bypass surgery exposed to increasing concentrations of amitriptyline and desipramine decreased the myocardial contractile force in a dose-dependent manner. These dose-related effects occur at concentrations that have been shown to block fast Na^+ channels in cardiac myocytes (63). This tricyclic dose–related depression of myocardial contractile force is independent of effects on the conduction system. These data suggest another potential manifestation of cardiac toxicity of TCAs, especially when taken in overdose (64).

Selective Serotonin Reuptake Inhibitors

Clinical Vignette

A 75-year-old widower who lived alone had a daughter who lived close to him and checked on him regularly. He had a history of heart failure for which his cardiologist prescribed digoxin and metoprolol. A year after his wife's death, he still appeared to not be his "old self." His daughter noticed that he had become more withdrawn from his friends. He used to meet his friends in the park to play chess, but had not been to the park in over six months. She also noticed that he had very little energy during the day, sometimes not even getting out of bed. She felt that he was sad most of the time and had witnessed several crying episodes. This would have been unheard of for her dad. She was very concerned and took her father to see his family physician. Their family physician diagnosed him with major depressive disorder and prescribed paroxetine. Two days after starting the paroxetine at 20 mg daily he called his family physician indicating he was "not doing so well". He reported feeling "very uneasy on his feet, especially right after standing up". He was frequently lightheaded and had even fallen down once. His pulse was 45 and his blood pressure was 95/55 and he was feeling more lethargic than he had been prior to starting the paroxetine.

The doctor called his pharmacist friend who confirmed the doctor's concern that the patient's symptoms were related to the initiation of the paroxetine. The pharmacist explained that some SSRIs significantly decrease the metabolism of most β-blockers through potent inhibition of the 450 2D6 metabolic pathway.

The family doctor conferred with the patient's cardiologist who recommended a decrease in the patient's metoprolol dose. At a two week follow-up the symptoms of lethargy, lightheadedness and unsteadiness had resolved and the widower's mood was improving.

SSRIs

The success of TCAs in treating depression led to a search for compounds that would have the efficacy of TCAs without the many adverse side effects (particularly the cardiotoxicity in overdose). The answer came in the form of SSRIs. The first member of this new therapeutic class, fluoxetine, was introduced in the United States in 1988. Of the antidepressants, SSRIs appear to be the safest. However, certain SSRIs increase their potential for cardiac toxicity when taken in overdose.

Relative Risk of Sudden Cardiac Death with SSRIs

SSRIs are safer than TCAs, both at therapeutic doses and in overdose. This conclusion was supported by a large cohort study of over 480,000 persons

Table 4A Selective Serotonin Reuptake Inhibitors

Generic name / Trade name	Chemical class (TCAs)	Receptor-effect class	FDA Approved		Major metabolism sites	Enzyme process(es) inhibited	Usual adult daily dose	Approximate half-life (including active metabolites)
Citalopram Celexa®	Phthalane derivative	SSRI	MDD depressed phase of bipolar disorder[a] Prophylaxis of MDD (in unipolar depression)	Treatment of secondary depression with other mental illnesses, e.g., schizophrenia and dementia	2C19 2D6 3A4	2D6[d]	20–60 mg	35 hr
Escitalopram Lexapro- (L-isomer of citalopram)	Phthalane derivative	SSRI	MDD depressed phase of bipolar disorder[a] Prophylaxis of MDD (in unipolar depression)	Treatment of secondary depression with other mental illnesses, e.g., schizophrenia and dementia GAD	2C19 2D6 3A4	2D6[d]	10–20 mg	32 hr
Fluoxetine Prozac® Serafen®	Bicyclic	SSRI	MDD depressed phase of bipolar disorder[a] Bulimia nervosa Obsessive compulsive disorder Prophylaxis of MDD (in unipolar depression)	Treatment of secondary depression with other mental illnesses, e.g., schizophrenia and dementia Bulimia nervosa OCD PDD	2C9 2C19 2D6 3A4	1A2[d] 2B6[c] 2C9[c] **2C19[b]** **2D6[b]** 3A4[c] — —	10–80 mg	50 (240)[f]
Fluvoxamine Luvox®	Monocyclic	SSRI	OCD Prophylaxis of MDD (in unipolar depression)	Treatment of secondary depression with other mental illnesses, e.g., schizophrenia and dementia	1A2 2D6	**1A2[b]** 2B6[c] 2C9[c] **2C19[b]** 2D6[d] 3A4[c]	100–300 mg	18 hr
Paroxetine Paxil® Paxil CR®	Phenyl-piperidine	SSRI	MDD depressed phase of bipolar disorder[a] Prophylaxis of MDD (in unipolar depression) OCD Panic disorder Social anxiety disorder	Treatment of secondary depression with other mental illnesses, e.g., schizophrenia and dementia PTSD PDD GAD	2D6	1A2[d] **2B6[b]** 2C9[d] **2D6[b]** 3A4[c]	20–60 mg 125–75 mg (CR)	22 hr

(Continued)

Table 4A Selective Serotonin Reuptake Inhibitors (*Continued*)

Generic name Trade name	Chemical class (TCAs)	Receptor-effect class	FDA Approved	Major metabolism sites	Enzyme process(es) inhibited		Usual adult daily dose	Approximate half-life (including active metabolites)
Sertaline Zoloft®	Tetrahydro-naphthylmethyl-amine	SSRI	MDD depressed phase of bipolar disorder[a] Prophylaxis of MDD (in unipolar depression) OCD Panic disorder Social anxiety disorder	2B6 2C9 2C19 2D6 3A4	1A2[d] **2B6**[b] **2D6**[b,c,e]	3A4[c] Glucuroni- dation	50–200 mg	24 (66)

[a]The Arizona Centers for Education and Research on Therapeutics, also known as Arizona CERT or AzCERT, maintains a list and classification of drugs that prolong the QT interval and/ or induce torsades de pointes (see Ref. 1).

Abbreviations: SSRI; selective serotonin reuptake inhibitor; MDD, major depressive disorder; OCD, obsessive compulsive disorder; PTSD, posttraumatic stress disorder; GAD, Generalized anxiety disorder; PDD, premenstrual dysphonic disorder.

[a]Use with caution: may precipitate a manic or hypomanic episode.

[b]Marked inhibition (bold) type.

[c]Moderate inhibition.

[d]Mild inhibition.

[e]Sertaline generally exhibits moderate 2D6 inhibition, which becomes marked as the dose approaches 200 mg/day.

[f]Because of the half-life of active metabolite norfluoxetine being >10 days, fluoxetine can have major pharmacokinetic and pharmacodynamic effects with medications started 4 to 8 weeks after it has been discontinued (see Vignette).

Sources: Adapted from Refs. 3, 4, and 5.

Table 4B Selective Serotonin Reuptake Inhibitors

Generic name / Trade name	Pharmacological effects on neurotransmitters/receptors responsible for cardiovascular side effects (direct and indirect)						Frequency percentage of adverse cardiovascular reaction to antipsychotics at therapeutic doses				
	NE reuptake blockade — Tachycardia hypotension	5-HT reuptake blockade — Potentiation of drugs with serotonergic properties risking serotonin syndrome	5HT$_2$ blockade — Hypotension Weight gain	M1 blockade — Sinus tachycardia QRS changes Potentiation of drugs with anticholinergic	H1 blockade — Postural Hypotension Weight Gain	α1 Blockade — Postural Hypotension Reflex tachycardia	AzCERT class Risk for TdP	Orthostatic hypotension	Tachycardia Palpitations	ECG changes	Cardiac arrhythmia ms
Citalopram Celexa®	+	++++	+	+	++	+	4	>2	>2[b]	<2	<%
Escitalppram Lexapro®	+	++++	+	+	+	+	Not listed	>2	>2[b]	<2	<2
Fluoxetine Prozac®	++	++++	++	++	+	+	4	>10	<2[b]	<2	<2[c]
Fluvoxamine Luvox®	++	++++	+	+−	−	+	Not listed	>2	<2[b]	<2	<2
Paroxetine Paxil® Paxil CR®	+++	+++++	+−	++	+−	+	4	>10	<2[b]	<2	<2
Sertraline Zoloft®	++	++++	+	++	+−	++	4	>10	>2[b]	<2	<2

[a]The Arizona Centers for Education and Research on Therapeutics, also known as Arizona CERT or AzCERT, maintains a list and classification of drugs that prolong the QT interval and/or induce torsades de pointes (see Ref. 1).

[b]Bradycardia reported.

[c]Slowing of sinus mode and atrial dysrhythmia.

Sources: Adapted from Refs. 3, 4, and 5.

and nearly 1500 cases of sudden cardiac death occurring in a community setting. The use of SSRIs was not associated with an increased risk of sudden cardiac death. In contrast, the use of TCAs in doses of 100 mg, or higher, of amitriptyline or its equivalent had a 41% increased rate of sudden cardiac death (65).

Comparison of Effect of SSRI with Effect of TCA on Heart Rate Variability

One factor that has been explored in understanding this difference in sudden death is heart rate variability (HRV). A decrease in cardiac vagal tone as suggested by a decrease in HRV has been linked to sudden death in patients with cardiac disease.

Nortriptyline has been shown to have a greater adverse effect (i.e., decrease) on HRV than paroxetine. This is most likely through a stronger vagolytic effect on autonomic function. It is likely that this difference applies to all SSRIs and TCAs (66) (Tables 3B and 4B).

SSRI and Myocardial Infarction

It has been suggested by some research that the SSRIs may have a protective effect on cardiovascular function related to their effect on decreasing platelet aggregation, thereby decreasing the risk of myocardial infarction (67–69). Serotonin is normally released by activated platelets, causing enhanced platelet aggregation and vasoconstriction (70,71). In coronary artery disease both of these can contribute to the pathogenesis of acute MI. SSRIs with high affinity for the serotonin transporter (fluoxetine, paroxetine, sertraline) attenuate platelet activation by depleting serotonin storage (67) and have been shown to decrease platelet activity in patients with coronary artery disease (68). A recent large study among current users of antidepressants with high serotonin transporter affinity had an OR for MI of 0.59 compared with nonusers (56).

The picture, however, is not entirely clear. For instance, a recent study of over 60,000 cases of acute MI and 360,000 matched controls found a substantially increased incidence of acute MI throughout the initial 28 days after an antidepressant prescription and that the increased risk of MI in similar for both TCA and SSRI. More research needs to be done on this topic (57,66).

Cardiovascular Effects of SSRIs at Therapeutic Doses

Syncope, orthostatic hypotension, palpitations, and tachycardia are the cardiovascular symptoms rarely reported during treatment with SSRIs. In addition, QT interval prolongation has also been reported. Up to 6% reduction in mean heart rate is common. On rare occasion, a few of the SSRIs, as noted in Table 4B, have been associated with the occurrence of ventricular fibrillation, ventricular tachycardia, and TdP in postmarketing reports (57,72–77). The chances of developing associated cardiac symptoms increases with overdose.

Pharmacokinetic Interactions

While the SSRIs have low potential for cardiovascular toxicity on their own, it is important to remember the interaction they have with other medications through various enzyme pathways (Tables 4A and 4B). As in the vignette, some SSRIs have the potential to increase the level of many cardiac medications and other QT prolonging medications, which can lead to serious symptoms or events. SSRI levels can also be increased, resulting in an increased risk of cardiovascular toxicity.

Other Antidepressants

SNRIs—Selective Serotonin Norepinephrine Reuptake Inhibitors

Venlafaxine is a phenylethylamine that was introduced in the United States in 1994. It became available in an extended release form in 1998. It was the first noncyclic dual reuptake inhibitor, blocking both serotonin and norepinepherine reuptake (Tables 5A and 5B). Duloxetine hydrochloride (Cymbalta®) is also a member of this class. In 2004, it was approved for the treatment of pain associated with diabetic neuropathy (Tables 5A and 5B).

Cardiovascular Effects at Therapeutic Doses

Venlafaxine (Effexor®) and duloxetine (Cymbalta) can be associated with sustained increases in blood pressure, tachycardia and rarely QTc prolongation. The blood pressure increase is dose related with venlafaxine but may not be with duloxetine. These medications also carry an increased risk of these symptoms as well as worsening prolongation of the QTc, which, in overdose, could lead to fatal arrhythmia.

Pharmacokinetic Considerations

Venlafaxine is a relatively weak, but selective inhibitor of CYP2D6. Therefore, it has relatively few significant drug-drug interactions. Duloxetine (Cymbalta®) is a more potent inhibitor of 2D6 and should be used with caution in 2D6 substrates with a narrow therapeutic index (e.g., type 1C antiarrhythmics, propafenone, flecainide).

NDRI—Norepinephrine Dopamine Reuptake Inhibitors

Bupropion (Wellbutrin®, Wellbutrin SR®, Wellbutrin XL®, Zyban®)

Bupropion is a unicyclic aminoketone that resembles amphetamine. It is structurally unrelated to any other antidepressant available in the United States. Bupropion was released in 1989, when it became clear that its increased seizure

Table 5A Other Antidepressants

Generic name Trade name	Chemical class (TCAs)	Receptor-effect class	FDA approved	Major metabolism sites	Enzyme process(es) inhibited	Approx. half-life hr (including active metabolite)	Usual Adult Dose
Venlafaxine Effexor®	Bicyclic agent Phenylethyl-alanine	SNRI	MDD GAD Social anxiety	2D6	2D6[d]	5 (11)	75–37.5 mg
Duloxetine Cymbalta®	No specific class Chemical designation is (+)-(S)-*N*-methyl-γ-(l-naphthyloxy)-2-thiophenepropylamine hydrochloride	SNRI	MDD GAD Pain due to diabetic peripheral neuropathy	1A2 2D6	2D6[c]	12 hr	60–120 mg
NDRI Bupropion Wellbutrin® Wellbutrin SR® Wellbutrin Xl® Zyban®	Monobicyclic agent aminoketone	NDRI	MDD Prophylaxis of MDD Depressed phase of bipolar disorder[a] Aid in smoking cessation (Zyban)	2B6	2D6[b]	21 hr	150–450 mg
NaSSA Mirtazapine®	Tetracyclic	NaSSA	MDD	1A2 2D6 3A4	None known	20–40 hr	15–45 mg
SARI Trazodone®	Triazolopyridine	SARI	MDD Prophylaxis of MDD Depressed phase of bipolar disorder[a]	3A4 2D6	None known	4–9 hr	150–300 mg

[a]Use with caution, may precipitate a manic or hypomanic episode.
[b]Marked inhibition.
[c]Moderate inhibition.
[d]Mild inhibition.
Abbreviations: SNRI, Selective serotonin norepinephrine reuptake inhibitor; NDRI, norepinephrine dopamine reuptake inhibitor; NaSSA, noradrenergic/specific serotonergic antidepressants; SARI, serotonin-2 antagonists/reuptake inhibitors; MDD, major depressive disorder; GAD, generalized anxiety disorder.

Table 5B Other Antidepressants

| | Pharmacological effects on neurotransmitters/receptors responsible for cardiovascular side effects (direct and indirect) | | | | | | Frequency percentage of adverse cardiovascular reaction to antipsychotics at therapeutic doses | | | | |
| | NE Reuptake blockade | 5-HT Reuptake blockade | 5HT$_2$ blockade | M$_1$ blockade | H$_1$ blockade | α$_1$ blockade | AzCERT[a] Class Risk for TdP | Orthostatic hypotension | Tachycardia Palpitations | ECG changes | Cardiac arrhythmia ms |
Generic name / Trade name	Tachycardia Hypotension	Potentiation Of drugs with serotonergic properties risking serotonin syndrome	Hypotension Weight gain	Sinus Tachycardia QRS changes Potentiation of drugs with anticholinergic agents	Postural hypotension Weight gain	Postural hypotension Reflex Tachycardia					
SNRI[b] Venlafaxine Effexor IR® Effexor XL®	++	++++	+−	−	−	−	**2**	>10[c]	>2[d]	<2[d]	<2
SNRI[b] Duloxetine Cymbalta®	++++	+++++	−	+	+	+	Not listed	>10	>2	—	—
NDRI Bupropion Welbutrin® Zyban®	+	+−	+	+−	+	+	Not listed	>2[b]	>2	<2	<2

(Continued)

Table 5B Other Antidepressants (*Continued*)

	Pharmacological effects on neurotransmitters/receptors responsible for cardiovascular side effects (direct and indirect)						Frequency percentage of adverse cardiovascular reaction to antipsychotics at therapeutic doses				
Generic name / Trade name	NE Reuptake blockade / Tachycardia Hypotension	5-HT Reuptake blockade / Potentiation Of drugs with serotonengic properties risking serotonin syndrome	5HT$_2$ blockade / Hypotension Weight gain	M$_1$ blockade / Sinus Tachycardia QRS changes Potentiation of drugs with anticholinergic agents	H$_1$ blockade / Postural hypotension Weight gain	α_1 blockade / Postural hypotension Reflex Tachycardia	AzCERT Class[a] Risk for TdP	Orthostatic hypotension	Tachycardia Palpitations	ECG changes	Cardiac arrhythmias
NaSSA											
Mirtazapine Remeron®	+	+	++++	++	+++++	++	Not listed	>2	>2	<2	<2
SARI											
Trazodone Desyrel®	+	++	++++	–	++	+++	Not listed	>10[e]	>2	>2	>2[f]

[a]The Arizona Centers for Education and Research on Therapeutics, also known as Arizona CERT or AzCERT, maintains a list and classification of drugs that prolong the QT interval and/or induce torsades de pointes (see Ref. 1).
[b]In clinical practice, hypertension, in some cases severe, requiring acute treatment, has been reported in patients receiving bupropion alone and in patients with and without pre-existing hypertension (PDR).
[c]Small sustained increases in blood pressure in a dose related manner have been observed with Effexor especially at doses greater than 225 mg day.
[d]Increased risk with higher doses.
[e]Less frequent if medication is given after meals.
[f]Patients with preexisting heart disease have a 10% incidence of premature ventricular contractions.
Sources: Adapted from Refs. 3, 4, and 5.

risk was dose related and tended to occur in specific populations. In 1998, bupropion became available in a sustained-release formulation (Wellbutrin SR®) that allows twice a day administration. In 2003, Wellbutrin XL became available in an extended release formulation for once a day dosing.

The neurochemical mechanism of the antidepressant effect of bupropion is not known. Bupropion is a relatively weak inhibitor of the neuronal uptake of NE, serotonin, and DA and does not inhibit monoamine oxidase. (Tables 5A and 5B)

Cardiovascular Effects at Therapeutic Doses

Treatment-related emergent hypertension has been reported in 2% to 4% of patients in treatment trials with bupropion. Other cardiovascular symptoms are quite infrequent (Table 5B). In a retrospective review of over 7000 bupropion overdoses, cardiovascular disturbances were extremely uncommon (78). Deaths following overdoses of bupropion with no concurrent drugs are rare (79). Tachycardia is common in overdose (i.e., up to 45%). However, hypotension is rare, with reports of no significant cardiac symptoms in doses up to 4500 mg.

Pharmacokinetic Interactions

Bupropion is a potent 2D6 inhibitor. Therefore, combining with drugs that are metabolized primarily by 2D6 (e.g. metoprolol, flecainide, paroxetine, etc.) should be done with caution.

NaSSA—Noradrenergic/Specific Serotonergic Antidepressants

Mirtazapine (Remeron®)

Mirtazapine (Remeron®) released in 1996 is chemically related to mianserin, an antidepressant long used in Europe. Mirtazapine is not a specific reuptake blocker of any monoamine neurotransmitter. It is an antagonist of central pre-synaptic α_2 adrenergic receptors resulting in increased norepinephrine release. The increased noradrenergic tone results in a rapid increase in synaptic serotonin levels by mobilizing serotonin release secondary to stimulation of α_1 adrenergic receptors on serotonin cell bodies.

Cardiovascular Effects

Tachycardia, hypertension, and hypotension have been reported following thera-peutic use. In premarketing studies, the mean QTc change was +1.6 milliseconds for mirtazapine and an increase in heart rate of 3.4 bpm. There have been no fatalities reported with mirtazapine alone despite reported overdoses of 50 times the normal daily dose.

SARI—Serotonin-2 Antagonists/Reuptake Inhibitors

$5HT_2$ Receptor Antagonists

Trazodone (Desyrel®)
Nefazodone (Serzone®)

Trazodone was synthesized in Italy in the mid-1960s and introduced in the United States in 1981. Due to excessive sedation, postural hypotension and ataxia, trazodone was rarely tolerated at the recommended therapeutic doses of 400 mg to 600 mg. Nefazodone (Serzone®) was synthesized in the 1980s with the intent of improving the side-effect profile of trazodone. It was introduced in the United States in 1995 (80).

In late 2003, the manufacturer withdrew Serzone® from markets in the United States and Canada following reports of hepatotoxicity. Nefazodone is still available generically.

The principal effect of both trazodone and nefazodone appears to be antagonism of the postsynaptic $5HT_2A$ and $5HT_2C$ receptors. This antagonism causes a paradoxical downregulation of $5HT_2$ sites. These are linked to other receptors including the $5HT_1A$ receptor, which is thought to be important in depression.

In addition, nefazodone and trazodone likely stimulate the $5HT_1A$ site and block the reuptake of serotonin to a modest degree in comparison to the SSRIs. In addition, a major metabolite of both nefazodone and trazodone is a potent direct agonist of serotonin, mostly at the $5HT_2C$ receptor (81).

Cardiovascular Effects

The most common cardiovascular side effect during trazodone therapy is postural hypotension, which may be accompanied by syncope. In clinical trials, the cardiovascular side effects of trazodone reported in 1% or more of patients included hypertension, hypotension, syncope, bradycardia, or palpitations. In healthy volunteers, trazodone 150 mg administered in a single dose was found to significantly prolong the QTc interval (82). Trazodone has been associated with the initiation of ventricular tachycardia on as little as 50 mg daily.

Bradycardia and first-degree heart block are the most frequent cardiovascular findings in overdose. Sporadic reports of hypotension, nonspecific ST-T–wave changes, QT prolongation, ventricular premature depolarization, right bundle branch block, T-wave inversion, delayed intraventricular conduction, first-degree AV block, and TdP have been noted. In one case series of trazodone overdose, 77% of the patients developed QTc interval prolongation and 32% developed dysrrhythmias including TdP. All of the patients with dysrrhythmias had prolonged QTc intervals (82).

Pharmacokinetic Effects

Trazodone is primarily metabolized by CYP3A4 and CYP2D6 pathways. Its active metabolite via 3A4 metabolism, m-chlorphenylpiperazine (m-CPP), is anxiogenic and is further metabolized by 2D6. The concentration of m-CPP may be increased in 2D6 "poor metabolizers" and by the concomitant use of potent inhibitors. Trazodone metabolism is also altered by 3A4 inhibitors and inducers. Trazodone itself is not known to inhibit any CYP enzymes.

Monoamine Oxidase Inhibitors

Clinical Vignette

A 65-yr-old college professor was brought to the emergency room (ER) by his wife of 40 years. She reported that she and her husband were at a party with friends, when her husband began complaining of a horrible headache. She stated that, on the way to the hospital, he was complaining of blurry vision and his heart "pounding out of his chest" before he passed out. Her husband's blood pressure was 230/110 and heart rate was 100. The ER physician asked the woman if her husband was taking any medicines. She told him that her husband had suffered for many years from severe depression which had not responded to multiple trials of traditionally utilized antidepressants. She added that 6 months ago he had been started on the new MAOI Selegeline patch. Initially then dose was 6 mg patch daily. After two months the dose was increased to 9 mg daily. Then 2 months ago the patch was increased to 12 mg and the professor's depression lifted substantially for the first time in many years.

The patient's wife asserted that her husband had not had to follow any diet restrictions on the 6 mg patch and had begrudgingly loosely followed the dietary restrictions on Tyramine containing foods as the dose had been increased. Since he had previously had no difficulty despite some "cheating" on the restrictions, he decided on his birthday to have some red wine and aged cheese despite the restrictions not to do so.

The doctor administered phentolamine to the patient and was able to restore the professor's blood pressure to within normal range. The patient remained neurologically infact and after an overnight stay on the observation unit was discharged home.

He proclaimed a new resolve to stick to the Tyramine restricted diet.

MAOIs

In the early 1950s, investigators noted that their tuberculosis patients showed improvement in their mood when treated with iproniazid, a monoamine oxidase inhibitor (MAOI). Iproniazid proved ineffective for tuberculosis, but its impact on patients' moods led to some of the earliest double-blind studies in psycho-pharmacology. These studies demonstrated that the MAOIs were effective antidepressants. The observations that the MAOIs were antidepressants that degraded NE and serotonin became cornerstones of the so-called biogenic amine theory of depression (83).

The first-generation MAOIs, isocarboxazid (Marplan®), phenelzine (Nardil®) and trancypromine (Parnate®) have few direct effects on neurotransmitter uptake or receptor blockade. Instead, they inhibit MAO in various organs. They exert their greatest effects on monoamine oxidase A (MAOA), for

Table 6 Monoamine Oxidase Inhibitors

Generic Name Trade Name	Chemical classification	FDA approved	Usual adult daily dose	Approximate half-life	Orthostatic hypotension dizziness	Tachycardia	ECG changes	Cardiac Arrhythmia
Isocarboxid Marplan®	Irreversible MAOI	Refractory depression[a] Atypical depression[a] Phobic anxiety states Social phobia	30–50 mg	2.5	>10%	—	>2%	>2%
Phenelzine Nardil®	Irreversible MAOI	Refractory depression[a] Atypical depression[a] Phobic anxiety States Social phobia	45–90 mg	1.5–4	>10%	>10%[b]	<2%[c]	<2%
Trancypromine Parnate®	Irreversible MAOI	Refractory depression[a] Atypical depression[a] Phobic anxiety States Social phobia	20–60 mg	2.4	>10%	>10%[b]	>2%[c]	<2%
Selegeline Transdermal patch EMSAM®	Irreversible MAOI	MDD	6–12 mg	24-hr transdermal patch	—[d]		—	

[a]Atypical depression—patients manifesting hypochondriasis, somatic anxiety, irritability, and often hypersomnia and increased appetite with weight gain along with other symptoms of depression.
[b]Bradycardia also reported.
[c]Shortened QT interval reported.
[d]Hypertension reported between 1% and 1.0%.
Abbreviations: MAOI, monoamine oxidase inhibitor; ECG, electrochardiogram; MDD, major depressive disorder.

which NE and serotonin are primary substrates. They exert less of an effect on monoamine oxidase B (MAOB), which acts primarily on other amines (e.g., phenylethylamine and dopamine). In addition, MAO is found in the gut mucosa and is responsible for degrading various amines that can act as false transmitters and produce hypertensive crises.

Clinical Indications

Our present MAOIs are indicated for refractory depression or atypical depression (patients showing hypochrondriasis, somatic anxiety irritability, frequently increased appetite and hypersomnia; rather than insomnia and decreased appetite). In addition, they are FDA approved for phobic anxiety states or social phobia. MAOIs have been limited in their use because of the proclivity to cause hypertensive crises when combined with tyramine-containing foods and multiple medications as in the vignette. For example, hypertensive crises may occur in patients receiving MAOIs with other MAOIs, meperidine (Demerol®), tricyclic antidepressants, sympathomimetics (including amphetamines, over-the-counter cold-, hayfever-, or weight-reducing preparations containing vasoconstrictors (guanethidine, methyldopa, reserpine, dopamine, levodopa, and tryptophan). MAO in the intestinal tract degrades tyramine. When MAO is inhibited by MAOIs, the individual is at risk for absorbing large amounts of tyramine and probably other substances (e.g., phenylethylamine), which can act as false transmitters or indirect agonists and elevate blood pressure. Various foods that are high in tyramine are prohibited when one is taking an MAOI. The current MAOIs irreversibly bind MAO to such a degree that it takes approximately two weeks after the MAOI is stopped for the enzyme to regenerate. During this time, tyramine and drug interactions may occur. Thus, it is important to inform patients that they should maintain their dietary and drug restrictions for two weeks after the MAOI is discontinued. This should be done by gradual taper.

Adverse Cardiovascular Effects at Therapeutic Doses

Isocarboxazid, phewelzine and trancypromine have a greater than 10% incidence of hypotension and dizziness in clinical trials (Table 6). Isocarboxazid does not appear to affect the heart rate to any significant degree. Both phewelzine and trancypromine have a greater than 10% incidence of tachycardia, although bradycardia has also been reported.

Mild overdose or the early phase of severe toxicity may manifest with hypertension, tachycardia, flushing, and palpitations. Profound hypotension, bradycardia, cardiovascular collapse, and asystolic arrest may be noted following overdose of MAOIs alone. Ingestion of greater than 2 to 3 mg/kg of an MAOI should be considered potentially life-threatening and 4 to 6 mg/kg or greater is consistent with reported fatalities (84).

Caution needs to be exercised not only in combining MAOIs with other medications (e.g., pseudoephedrine-containing decongestants), but also when switching from antidepressants to an MAOI. Switching from a nonselective cyclic antidepressant (e.g., SSRI, NDRI, SNRI, or NaSSA) to an irreversible MAOI (e.g., isocarboxazid, phewelzine or trancypromine) requires a wash-out period of five half-lives before starting the MAOIs. This is to insure that the patient will not experience a significant and potentially fatal serotonin syndrome. Symptoms of a serotonin syndrome include tremor, diaphoresis, rigidity, myoclonus, autonomic disregulation, potentially progressing to hyperthermia, rhabdomyolysis, coma, and death.

Selegeline Transdermal Patch (EMSAM®)

In 2006, a transdermal patch of selegilene (EMSAM) was introduced for treatment of major depression. At the 6 mg-dose, there is no restriction on tyramine-containing foods. At 9-mg and 12-mg doses, dietary restrictions are recommended. Selegeline transdermal patch 6 mg/24 hours for 10 days coadministered with pseudoephedrine (60 mg, 3 times daily) failed to show any significant changes in blood pressure. However, EMSAM coadministered with phenylpropanolamine (PPA; 25 mg every 4 hours × 6 doses) did demonstrate a higher incidence of significant blood pressure elevations compared with EMSAM or PPA alone. This suggests a possible pharmacodynamic interaction. Present recommendations are to avoid the concomitant use of sympathomimetic agents with EMSAM.

MOOD STABILIZERS

Clinical Vignette

A 19-year-old college student presented to the ER with complaints of nausea, vomiting, and diarrhea for four days. He reported that for the last day he had been unable to keep any fluids down. His other symptoms included cough, rhinorhea, and subjective fever. He had gotten very weak and stated that he felt slightly disoriented. His medical history was only significant for bipolar disorder type I. He had been treated with lithium for the past three years without incident. On exam, the patient had very dry oral mucosa and poor skin turgor. His pulse rate was 50, blood pressure 100/70, and temperature was 37.9 C. Nasopharyngeal swab was positive for influenza A. The patient was admitted with the diagnosis of dehydration secondary to influenza. Supportive treatment with IV fluids was started. On admission, the internist on call noticed that the patient's pulse was averaging around 50 bpm. This is inappropriately slow in response to dehydration. He noticed that the patient was on lithium and immediately ordered a lithium level and an ECG. The ECG revealed sinus bradycardia with a junctional escape rhythm of 45b bpm. The lithium level was 1.8 mEq/L (normal therapeutic range 0.8–1.2 mEq/L). Lithium was held and the patient was monitored on telemetry. Over the next four days, the patient's heart rate gradually returned to normal. A repeat lithium level was 0.90. An exercise stress test was performed, before discharge, to eliminate the possibility of underlying or residual sinus node dysfunction. During the stress test, the patient had appropriate sinus node response, achieving 80% of his maximal predicted heart rate. He was discharged to home with a 48-hour Holter monitor that revealed no further bradycardia. He was also educated about the possibility of lithium toxicity as a result of dehydration.

Lithium carbonate (Lithobid®)

Lithium is an element of the alkalai-metal group with the atomic number 3. Lithium is indicated for the treatment of manic episodes and in maintenance therapy to prevent or diminish the intensity of subsequent manic episodes in patients with bipolar disorder. Clinically, it is often used as an adjunctive agent in patients with partially remitted depression.

Lithium was reported to have therapeutic efficacy in the treatment of mania as early as 1949. However, it was not until the mid-1970s that compelling evidence from clinical trial data definitively documented these effects. Identifying the optimal therapeutic dosage range through serum level monitoring was the main prerequisite that allowed this advance in psychiatric treatment. Lithium was the first psychiatric drug to utilize blood level monitoring. Lithium appears to

1. modulate the balance between excitory and inhibitory effects of various neurotransmitters such as Serotonin (5HT), nonepinephrine (NE), glutamate, GABA(γ-aminobutyric acid) and dopamine.
2. affect neural plasticity through its effects on glycogen synthetase kinase-3β cyclic AMP dependent kinase and protein kinase C, and
3. adjust signaling activity via effects on second messenger activity (85).

Cardiovascular Toxicity with Therapeutic Doses

Lithium is generally safe at therapeutic levels from a cardiovascular standpoint. However, lithium has had the following adverse cardiovascular effects reported: edema, new onset congestive heart failure, heart block, hypertension, myocariditis, and sinus node dysfunction. An estimated 28% to 40% of patients may experience first-degree AV block or other cardiac conduction abnormalities while receiving lithium. The changes are relatively benign, require no treatment, and do not require discontinuation of lithium therapy (86).

Little correlation exists between serum lithium levels and severity of intoxication in acute lithium overdoses. Lithium levels as high to 3 to 6 mEq/L have been noted in asymptomatic patients. The generally accepted therapeutic level is 0.6 to 1.2 mEq/L. Toxic levels are usually noted as (*i*) mild to moderate—1.5 to 2.5 mEq/L, (*ii*) severe—2.5 to 3.0 mEq/L, and (*iii*) levels greater than 3 to 4 mEq/L may lead to serious morbidity and possibly mortality, especially in patients on chronic lithium therapy who have comorbidities. Mortality from lithium toxicity as a single-agent overdose is rare. Patients surviving a dose as high as 84,000 mg have been reported.

The cardiovascular effects that may develop following severe, usually chronic intoxication include T-wave changes, bundle branch block, bradycardia, junctional rhythm, and hypotension. Chronic lithium intoxicated patients with serum levels of 1.5 mEq/L or greater show a significantly greater incidence of cardiac deterioration than acutely intoxicated individuals (87). Acutely intoxicated patients do not exhibit T-wave abnormalities. However, 50% of the chronically intoxicated patients exhibit these changes (88). The pathophysiology of this occurrence is unclear (87). Commonly occurring ECG abnormalities with chronic lithium poisoning are U-waves, intraventricular conduction defect, prolongation of the QTc interval, and T-wave flattening or inversion.

Carbamazepine (Tegretol®)

Carbamazepine is an anticonvulsant and specific analgesic for trigeminal neuralgia. In the early 1970s, Japanese researchers reported that it was effective in many bipolar patients who were refractory to lithium. Since that time, multiple controlled studies have documented the utility of carbamezapine in the treatment of acute mania and in maintenance therapy. Because of its pharmacokinetic interactions and its side effects (e.g., risk of aplastic anemia, agranulocytosis, hyponatremia), it is somewhat cumbersome to use.

Adverse Cardiovascular Effects

Cardiovascular effects, although rare, have been reported to include hypertension, hypotension, syncope and collapse, edema, and aggravation of coronary artery disease. In addition, isolated cases of cardiac dysrrhythmias, Stoke-Adams attacks, and congestive heart failure have been reported.

In carbamazepine poisoning, sinus tachycardia is common. Cardiac conduction defects (prolonged PR, QRS, and QTc intervals) have also been noted. Hypotension, myocardial depression, sinus bradycardia, and sinus dysrrhythmia may occur in severe overdose. Cardiovascular effects are inconsistent and are usually not clinically significant (89,90).

Lamotrigine (Lamictal®)

Lamotrigine (Lamictal®) is an antiepileptic drug of the phenyltriazine class chemically unrelated to existing antiepileptic drugs and is approved for the maintenance treatment of bipolar I disorder.

Adverse Cardiovascular Effects

Lamotrigine (Lamictal®) has been shown to be generally safe from a cardiac perspective. Pre-marketing studies have shown a minor incidence of increased

PR interval that was not clinically significant following therapeutic Lamotrigine doses (91).

Overdoses involving up to 15 g of Lamictal have been reported, some of which have been fatal (5). On the other hand, no ECG abnormalities were reported in an overdose involving greater than 4000 mg of Lamotrigine and a plasma-Lamotrigine concentration of 52 μg/mL. In nearly 500 cases of lamotrigine overdose, tachycardia was present in 21 cases; but conduction disturbances occurred in only two cases (92).

Valproic Acid (Depakene®)

Divalproex Sodium (Depakote®)

Divalproex sodium (Depakote®) is the most frequently used preparation due to less of a tendency to cause gastrointestinal side effects.

Adverse Cardiovascular Effects

Valproic acid has not demonstrated cardiac toxicity at therapeutic doses given orally. The manufacturer reports that tachycardia, hypertension, palpitations, hypotension, postural hypotension, and edema have occurred with valproic acid intravenous therapy. Refractory hypotension, tachycardia, QTc prolongation, and cardiac arrest may develop after severe overdose of valproic acid. The QTc prolongation is likely related to diminished K^+ currents in the cardiomyocytes (93). Severe toxicity has been associated with ingestion of 19 to 45 gms in adults. The majority of adverse outcomes following valproic acid overdoses have occurred at peak drug levels more than 450 μg/ml.

Topiramate (Topamax®)

Topiramate is a sulfamate-substituted monosaccharide antiepileptic medication that is also approved for prophylaxis of migraine headaches. Although it is not FDA approved for mood disorders, it is frequently used as adjunctive therapy.

Adverse Cardiovascular Effects

Hypotension, hypertension, postural hypotension, arrhythmias, palpitations, atrioventricular block, bundle branch block, and angina pectoris have been rarely described with the administration of topiramate at therapeutic levels. Topamax is generally free of serious cardiovascular adverse events. The toxic dose of topiramate has not been established in humans. Doses up to 1600 mg daily were tolerated in clinical trials. In a series of 567 patients with topiramate overdose, only one patient developed a conduction disturbance (94).

SUMMARY/CONCLUSION

Advances in psychopharmacology have dramatically transformed the management of mental disorders. The documented success of antipsychotics, antidepressants, and mood-stabilizing agents has resulted in a proliferation of highly effective therapies for previously untreatable conditions. This therapeutic success has also been accompanied by the sobering recognition of the potential harm these agents can have in selected individuals for a variety of possible reasons. Some of these adverse cardiovascular effects occur at therapeutic doses. Others occur as a result of overdose. It is incumbent upon the responsible health care provider to be familiar with the potential for adverse cardiovascular consequences of pharmacological treatment of this vulnerable population.

REFERENCES

1. AzCert—The Arizona Centers for Education and Research on Therapeutics, also known as Arizona CERT or AzCert, maintains a list and classification of drugs that prolong the QT interval and/or induce torsades de pointes.
2. Cozza KL, Armstrong SC, Oesterheld JR. Concise Guide to Drug Interaction Principles for Medical Practice: Cytochrome P450s, UGTs, P-Glycoproteins, 2nd ed. chap. 19, Psychiatry. Alington, VA: American Psychiatric Publishing, Inc., 2003: 345–382.
3. Bezchlibnyk-Butler KZ, Jeffries JJ. Clinical Handbook of Psychotropic Drugs. Cambridge, MA: Hogrefe and Huber, 2006:2–65, 77–123, 161–191.
4. Goodman and Gillman. Chap. 17: Drug therapy of depression and anxiety disorders; chap. 18 Pharmacotherapy of psychosis and mania. In: L. L. Brunton, Lazo JS, Parker KL, eds. The Pharmacological Basis of Therapeutics, 11th ed. New York: McGraw-Hill, Medical Publishing Division, 2006:429–460, 461–500.
5. Physicians' Desk Reference. Antidepressant agents; antipsychotic agents; biopolar agents. In: Phisicians' Desk Reference 2007, 61 ed. Thomson PDR 2007.
6. Davidson M. Risk of cardiovascular disease and sudden death in schizophrenia. J Clin Psychiatry 2002; 63(suppl 9):5–11.
7. FDA Psychopharmacologic Drugs Advisory Committee. Briefing Document for Zeldox Capsules (ziprasidone HCl). July 19 2000. Available at: http://www.fda.gov/ohrms/dockets/ac/00/backgrd/3619b1a.pdf.
8. Titier K, Girodet PO, Verdoux H, et al. Atypical antipsychotics: from potassium channels to torsade de pointes and sudden death. Drug Saf 2005; 28(1):35–51.
9. Montanez A, Ruskin JN, Hebert PR, et al. Prolonged QTc interval and risks of total and cardiovascular mortality and sudden death in the general population: a review and qualitative overview of the prospective cohort studies. Arch Intern Med 2004; 164(9):943–948.
10. Haverkamp W, Breithardt G, Camm AJ, et al. The potential for QT prolongation and proarrhythmia by non-antiarrhythmic drugs: clinical and regulatory implications. Report on a policy conference of the European Society of Cardiology. Eur Heart J 2000; 21(15):1216–1231.
11. Glassman AH, Bigger JT, Jr. Antipsychotic drugs: prolonged QTc interval, torsade de pointes, and sudden death. Am J Psychiatry 2001; 158(11):1774–1782.

12. Buckley NA, Sanders P. Cardiovascular adverse effects of antipsychotic drugs. Drug Saf 2000; 23(3):215–228.
13. Malik M, Camm AJ. Evaluation of drug-induced QT interval prolongation: implications for drug approval and labelling. Drug Saf 2001; 24(5):323–351.
14. Roden DM. Taking the "idio" out of "idiosyncratic": predicting torsades de pointes. Pacing Clin Electrophysiol 1998; 21(5):1029–1034.
15. Committee for Proprietary Medicinal Products. Points to consider: The assessment of the potential for QT interval prolongation by non-cardiovascular medicinal products. December 1997. Available at: http://www.emea.eu.int/pdfs/human/swp/098696en.pdf.
16. Justo D, Prokhorov V, Heller K, et al. Torsade de pointes induced by psychotropic drugs and the prevalence of its risk factors. Acta Psychiatr Scand 2005; 111(3):171–176.
17. Rouleau F, Asfar P, Boulet S, et al. Transient ST segment elevation in right precordial leads induced by psychotropic drugs: relationship to the Brugada syndrome. J Cardiovasc Electrophysiol 2001; 12(1):61–65.
18. Henderson RA, Lane S, Henry JS. Life-threatening ventricular arrhythmia (torsade de pointes) after haloperidol overdose. Hum Exp Toxicol 1991; 10:59–62.
19. Frassati D, Tabib A, Lanchaux B, et al. Hidden cardiac lesions and psychotropic drugs as a possible cause of sudden death in psychiatric patients: a report of 14 cases and review of the literature. Can J Psychiatry 2004; 49(2):100–105.
20. Hall BF, Lockwood TD. Toxic cardiomyopathy. The effect of antipsychotic antidepressant drugs and calcium on myocardial protein degradation and structural integrity. Toxicology Appl Pharmacology 1986; 86:308–324.
21. Testai L, Bianucci AM, Massarelli I, et al. Torsadogenic cardiotoxicity of antipsychotic drugs: a structural feature, potentially involved in the interaction with cardiac HERG potassium channels. Curr Med Chem 2004; 11(20):2691–2706.
22. Reilly JG, Ayis SA, Ferrier IN, et al. QTc-interval abnormalities and psychotropic drug therapy in psychiatric patients. Lancet 2000; 355(9209):1048–1052.
23. Kongsamut S, Kang J, Chen XL, et al. A comparison of the receptor binding and HERG channel affinities for a series of antipsychotic drugs. Eur J Pharmacol 2002; 450(1):37–41.
24. Adamantidis MM, Kerram P, Dupuis BA. In vitro electrophysiological detection of iatrogenic arrhythmogenicity. Fundam Clin Pharmacol 1994; 8(5):391–407.
25. Drici MD, Wang WX, Liu XK, et al. Prolongation of QT interval in isolated feline hearts by antipsychotic drugs. J Clin Psychopharmacol 1998; 18(6):477–481.
26. Gluais P, Bastide M, Caron J, et al. Risperidone prolongs cardiac action potential through reduction of K+ currents in rabbit myocytes. Eur J Pharmacol 2002; 444(3):123–132.
27. Kitayama H, Kiuchi K, Nejima J, et al. Long-term treatment with antipsychotic drugs in conventional doses prolonged QTc dispersion, but did not increase ventricular tachyarrhythmias in patients with schizophrenia in the absence of cardiac disease. Eur J Clin Pharmacol 1999; 55(4):259–262.
28. Mehtonen OP, Aranko K, Malkonen L. A survey of sudden death asociated with the use of antipsychotic or antidepressant drugs: 49 cases in Finland. Acta Psychiatr Scan 1991; 84:58–64.
29. Leestma JE, Koenig KL. Sudden death and phenothiazines. Arch Gen Psychiatry 1968; 18:137–148.

30. Kelly HG, Fay JE, Laverty SG. Thioridazine hydrochloride (Mellaril); its effect on the electrocadiogram and a report on two fatalities with electrocardiographic abnormalities. Can Med Assoc J 1963; 89:645–654.

31. Hulisz DT, Dasa SL, Black LD, et al., Complete heart block and torsade de pointes associated with thioridazine poisoning. Pharmacotherapy 1994; 14(2):239–245.

32. Flugelman MY, Tal A, Pollack S, et al. Psychotropic drugs and long QT syndromes: case reports. J Clin Psychiatry 1985; 46(7):290–291.

33. Kiriike N, Maeda Y, Nishiwaki S, et al. Iatrogenic torsade de pointes induced by thioridazine. Biol Psychiatry 1987; 22(1):99–103.

34. Fulop G, Phillips RA, Shapiro AK, et al. ECG changes during haloperidol and pimozide treatment of Tourette's disorder. Am J Psychiatry 1987; 144(5):673–675.

35. Committee on Safety of Medicines-Medicines Control Agency. Cardiac arrhythmias with pimozide (Orap). Current Problems in Pharmacovigilance 1995; 21:1.

36. Lischke V, Behne M, Doelken P, et al. Droperidol causes a dose-dependent prolongation of the QT interval. Anesth Analg 1994; 79(5):983–986.

37. Sharma ND, Rosman HS, Padhi ID. Torsade de pointes associated with intravenous haloperidolin critically ill patients. Am J Cardiol 1998; 81: 238–240.

38. Drolet B, Zhang S, Deschenes D, et al. Droperidol lengthens cardiac repolarization due to block of the rapid component of the delayed rectified potassium current. J Cardiovasc Electrophysiol 1999; 10:1597–1604.

39. Fayer SA. Torsades de pointes ventricular tachyarrhythmia associated with haloperidol. J Clin Psychopharmacol 1986; 6(6):375–376.

40. Kriwisky M, Perry GY, Tarchitsky D, et al. Haloperidol-induced torsades de pointes. Chest 1990; 98(2):482–484.

41. Hunt N, Stern TA. The association between intravenous haloperidol and torsades de pointes: three cases and a literature review. Psychosomatics 1995; 36:541–549.

42. Nasrallah HA, White T, Nasrallah AT. Lower mortality in geriatric patients receiving risperidone and olanzapine versus haloperidol. Am J Geriatri Psychiatry 2004; 12(4): 437–439.

43. Liperoti R, Gambassi G, Lapane KL, et al. Conventional and atypical antipsychotics and the risk of hospitalization for ventricular arrhythmias or cardiac arrest. Arch Intern Med, 2005; 165(6):696–701.

44. Newcomer JW, Haupt DW. The metabolic effects of antipsychotic medications. Can J Psychiatry 2006; 51(8):480–491.

45. Newcomer JW. Insulin resistance and metabolic risk during antipsychotic treatment. Presented at the American Psychiatric Association symposium Insulin Resistance and Metabolic Syndrome in Neuropsychiatry; Atlanta, GA; May 23, 2005.

46. Drieling T, Biedermann NC, Schärer LO, et al. [Psychotropic drug-induced change of weight: a review]. Fortschr Neurol Psychiatr 2007; 75(2):65–80.

47. Merrill DB, William G. Adverse cardiac effects associated with clozapine. J Clin Psychopharmacology 2005; 25(1):32–41.

48. Canada NP. Association of Clozaril (clozapine) with cardiovascular toxicity [Dear Healthcare professional letter). 2002.

49. Killian JG, Kerr K, Lawrence C, et al. Myocarditis and cardiomyopathy associated with clozapine. Lancet 1999; 354(9193):1841–1845.

50. Modai I, Hirschmann S, Rava A, et al. Sudden death in patients receiving clozapine treatment: a preliminary investigation. J Clin Psychopharmacol 2000; 20(3): 325–327.

51. Tie H, Walker BD, Singleton CB, et al. Clozapine and sudden death. J Clin Psychopharmacol 2001; 21(6):630–632.
52. Warner B, Hoffmann P. Investigation of the potential of clozapine to cause torsade de pointes. Adverse Drug React Toxicol Rev 2002; 21(4):189–203.
53. Cohen H, Loewenthal U, Matar M, et al., Association of autonomic dysfunction and clozapine. Heart rate variability and risk for sudden death in patients with schizophrenia on long-term psychotropic medication. Br J Psychiatry 2001; 179:167–171.
54. Harrigan EP, Miceli JJ, Anziano R, et al. A randomized evaluation of the effects of six antipsychotic agents on QTc, in the absence and presence of metabolic inhibition. J Clin Psychopharmacol 2004; 24(1):62–69.
55. Bednar MM, Harrigan EP, Anziano RJ, et al. The QT Interval. Prog Cardiovasc Dis 2001; 43(5 part 2):1–45.
56. Golino P, Piscione F, Willerson JT, et al. Divergent effects of serotonin on coronary-artery dimensions and blood flow in patients with coronary atherosclerosis and control patients. N Engl J Med 1991. 324(10):641–648.
57. Borys DJ, Setzer SC, Ling LJ, et al. Acute fluoxetine overdose: a report of 234 cases. Am J Emerg Med 1992; 10(2):115–120.
58. Naccarelli GV, Antzelevitch C. The Brugada syndrome: clinical, genetic, cellular, and molecular abnormalities. Am J Med 2001; 110:573–581.
59. Vieweg WV, Wood MA. Tricyclic antidepressants, QT interval prolongation, and torsade de pointes. Psychosomatics 2004; 45(5):371–377.
60. Goodnick PJ, Jerry J, Parra F. Psychotropic drugs and the ECG: focus on the QTc interval. Expert Opin Pharmacother 2002. 3(5):479–498.
61. Leonard HL, Meyer MC, Swedo SE, et al. Electrocardiographic changes during the desipramine and clomipramine treatment in children and adolescents. J Am Acad Child Adolesc Psychiatry 1995; 34(11):1460–1468.
62. Boehnert MT, Lovejoy FH, Jr. Value of the QRS duration versus the serum drug level in predicting seizures and ventricular arrhythmias after an acute overdose of tricyclic antidepressants. N Engl J Med 1985; 313(8):474–479.
63. Heard K, Cain BS, Dart RC, et al. Tricyclic antidepressants directly depress human myocardial mechanical function independent of effects on the conduction system. Acad Emerg Med 2001; 8(12):1122–1127.
64. Bailey B, Buckley NA, Amre DK. A meta-analysis of prognostic indicators to predict seizures, arrhythmias or death after tricyclic antidepressant overdose. J Toxicol Clin Toxicol 2004; 42(6):877–888.
65. Ray WA, Meredith S, Thapa PB, et al. Cyclic antidepressants and the risk of sudden cardiac death. Clin Pharmacol Ther 2004; 75(3):234–241.
66. Tata LJ, West J, Smith C, et al. General population based study of the impact of tricyclic and selective serotonin reuptake inhibitor antidepressants on the risk of acute myocardial infarction. Heart 2005; 91(4):465–471.
67. Poole R. Is it healthy to be chaotic? Science 1989; 243:604–607.
68. Xiong GL, West J, Smith C, et al. Prognosis of patients taking selective serotonin reuptake inhibitors before coronary artery bypass grafting. Am J Cardiol 2006; 98(1):42–47.
69. Hergovich N. Paroxetine decreases platelets in serotonin storage and platelet function in human beings. Clin Pharmacol Ther 2000; 68:435–442.
70. Serebruany VL. Effective selective serotonin reuptake inhibitors on platelets in patients with coronary arter disease. Am J Cardiol 2001; 87:1398–1400.

71. Sauer WH, Berlin JA, Kimmel SE. Selective serotonin reuptake inhibitors and myocardial infarction. Circulation 2001; 104(16):1894–1898.

72. Wernicke JF. The side effect profile and safety of fluoxetine. J Clin Psychiatry 1985; 46:29–67.

73. Stark P, Hardison CD. A review of multicenter controlled studies of fluoxetine vs. imipramine and placebo in outpatients with major depressive disorder. J Clin Psychiatry 1985; 46(3 pt 2):53–58.

74. Amital D, Amital H, Gross R, et al. Sinus bradycardia due to fluvoxamine overdose. Br J Psychiatry 1994; 165(4):553–554.

75. Goeringer KE, Raymon L, Christian GD, et al. Postmortem forensic toxicology of selective serotonin reuptake inhibitors: a review of pharmacology and report of 168 cases. J Forensic Sci 2000; 45(3):633–648.

76. Sauer WH, Berlin JA, Kimmel SE. Effect of antidepressants and their relative affinity for the serotonin transporter on the risk of myocardial infarction. Circulation 2003; 108(1):32–36.

77. Segura LJ, Bravo B. Postmortem citalopram concentrations: alone or along with other compounds. J Forensic Sci 2004; 49(4):814–819.

78. Cymbalta® delayed-release oral capsules, duloxetine HCl delayed-release oral capsules. Product information. Indianapolis, IN: Eli Lilly and Company; 2007.

79. Harris CR, Gualtieri J, Stark G. Fatal bupropion overdose. J Toxicol Clin Toxicol 1997; 35(3):321–324.

80. Belson MG, Kelley TR. Bupropion exposures: clinical manifestations and medical outcome. J Emerg Med, 2002; 23(3):223–230.

81. Schatzberg AF, Cole JO, DeBattista C, eds. Manual of Clinical Psychopharmacology. 5th ed. Washington, DC: American Psychiatric Publishing Inc., 2005:65.

82. Burgess CD, Hames TK, George CF. The electrocardiographic and anticholinergic effects of trazodone and imipramine in man. Eur J Clin Pharmacol 1982; 23: 417–421.

83. Schatzberg AF, Cole JO, DeBattista C, eds. Manual of Clinical Psychopharmacology. 5th ed. Washington, DC: American Psychiatric Publishing Inc., 2005:36.

84. Monoamine Oxidase Inhibitors. In: POISINDEX® System [Internet database]. Greenwood Village, Colo: Thomson Micromedex. Updated periodically. Accessed June 5, 2008.

85. Schatzberg AF, Cole JO, DeBattista C, eds. Manual of Clinical Psychopharmacology. 5th ed. Washington, DC: American Psychiatric Publishing Inc., 2005.

86. Martin CA, Plaseik MT. First degree AV block in patients on lithium carbonate. Can J Psychiatry 1985; 30:114–116.

87. Michaeli J, Ben-Ishay D, Kidron R, et al. Severe hypertension and lithium intoxication. JAMA 1984; 251:1680 (letter).

88. Shannon MW, Eisen T, Linakis J. Clinical features of acute versus chronic lithium intoxication. Vet Hum Toxicol 1989; 31:370 (abstr 164).

89. Larsen G, Caravati M. Electrocardiographic effects of carbamazepine toxicity. Vet Hum Toxicol 1991(33):367 (abstr).

90. Salzman MB, Valderrama E, Sood SK. Carbamazepine and fatal eosinophilic myocarditis. N Engl J Med 1997; 336(12):878–879.

91. Matsuo F, Bergen D, Faught E, et al. Placebo-controlled study of the efficacy and safety of lamotrigine in patients with partial seizures. U.S. Lamotrigine Protocol 0.5 Clinical Trial Group. Neurology 1993; 43(11):2284–2291.

92. Lofton AL, Klein-Schwartz W. Evaluation of lamotrigine toxicity reported to poison centers. Ann Pharmacother 2004; 38:1811–1815.
93. Spiller HA, Krenzelok EP, Klein-Schwartz W, et al. Multicenter case series of valproic acid ingestion: serum concentrations and toxicity. J Toxicol Clin Toxicol 2000; 38(7):755–760.
94. Lofton AL, Klein-Schwartz W. Evaluation of toxicity of topiramate exposures reported to poison centers. Hum Exp Toxicol 2005; 24(11):591–595.

10

Adverse Effects of Drugs on Electrophysiological Properties of the Heart

Cynthia A. Carnes

College of Pharmacy, and Davis Heart and Lung Research Institute, The Ohio State University, Columbus, Ohio, U.S.A.

Gary Gintant

Department of Integrative Pharmacology, Global Pharmaceutical Research and Development, Volwiler Society, Abbott Laboratories, Abbott Park, Illinois, U.S.A.

Robert Hamlin

Veterinary Biosciences, Davis Heart and Lung Research Institute, The Ohio State University, Columbus, Ohio, U.S.A.

INTRODUCTION

The heart possesses at least (*i*) three electrophysiological properties (chronotropy or automaticity, dromotropy or conductivity, bathmotropy or irritability) (1,2); (*ii*) 9 tissues or electrophysiological phenotypes (atrial myocardium, ventricular myocardium [epicardial, midmyocardial ("M"), and endocardial tissues]), His-Purkinje fibers, sinoatrial (SA) node, atrioventricular (AV) node, atrio-AV nodal junctional fibers, and internodal pathways]; (*iii*) 15 or more voltage- or ligand-gated ion channels, pumps, and exchangers (3); and (*iv*) 6 or more relatively large signaling molecules [ryanodine, sarco/endoplasmic reticulum Ca^{++} ATPase

(SERCA), phospholambam, protein kinase A and C, calcineurin, sarcoplasmic calcium buffers] that may be potential targets for therapeutic or toxic effects of drugs. Because of the potential subtlety of toxic effects [e.g., small changes in heart rate, minor lengthening of corrected QT (QTc)], and because they may not be manifested for years (e.g., doxorubicin, mercury, arsenic), or may require high doses or concomitant provocateurs (e.g., hypertrophy, diabetes, heart failure, metabolites, electrolyte disturbances), it is sometimes difficult to ascertain the potential for toxicity. Acute toxic cardiovascular effects (as with strychnine or supratherapeutic concentrations of dofetilide) may be easily identified, but subtle effects [as with rofecoxib (4)] of arsenic, mercury, lead, phentermine-fenfluramine (5), 5-hydroxy-tryptamine $_{2B}$ (5-HT$_{2B}$) agonists may be difficult to identify, yet result in far greater morbidity and mortality. Notably, a leading cause of recent removals of drugs from the market is toxicity due to electrophysiological effects on the heart, specifically delayed repolarization, and the ventricular arrhythmia, torsades de pointes (TdP) (6). This chapter will review proarrhythmic electrophysiological actions, provide examples of how such effects are manifest, and discuss methods of identifying potential toxic signals (7–14).

NORMAL CARDIAC ELECTROPHYSIOLOGY

Overview

Each normal heart beat begins with a wave of depolarization, originating from the SA node in the right atria, which travels over internodal pathways to the AV node and through the atria, then through the AV node and rapidly down the His-Purkinje system, and finally slowly through the ventricles (15–18). The electrocardiogram (ECG) (Fig. 1) (a recording of voltages from the body surface) demonstrates when the atria (P wave) and ventricles (QRS complex) are depolarized, when the atria (Ta wave) and ventricles (ST-T complex) are repolarized, and the time between the onsets of depolarization of the atria and of the ventricles (PQ interval). Cardiac electrograms (voltages recorded from within the heart or on its surface) demonstrate electrical activity at localized, precise cardiac locations. These can be recorded either with catheters, electrodes designed to measure monophasic action potentials (MAPs), or plunge electrodes placed within the ventricular wall. More typically, electrograms (such as those from the specialized conduction system within the ventricle) are used to define spread of conduction through this region.

General Electrophysiological Properties of the Heart (19)

Chronotropy

Chronotrophy [chronos (time); automaticity, rhythmicity] refers to the intrinsic ability of tissues of the heart to discharge spontaneously. Chronotropy determines heart rate (a vital sign, because our predecessors recognized its importance

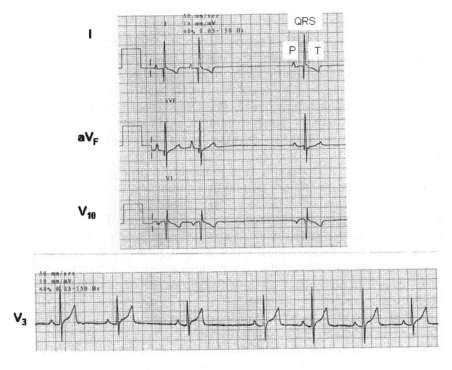

Figure 1 ECG showing component deflections with a description of their origins. Example of four leads from a dog that characterize the electrocardiographic properties. Any of the leads can be used for measurements of heart rate and durations of all important intervals. The P wave corresponds to atrial depolarization, the QRS complex corresponds to ventricular depolarization, and the T wave corresponds to ventricular repolarization. *Abbreviation*: ECG, electrocardiogram.

in clinical medicine), which is usually expressed as beats/min or may also be expressed as the interbeat interval (measured in milliseconds). Heart rate is one of three primary determinants of myocardial oxygen consumption; thus, a drug that accelerates heart rate may place the heart at an energetic imbalance (i.e., increases myocardial oxygen consumption and decreases myocardial oxygen delivery).

A "hierarchy of pacemakers" exists in the heart (15,20–23) defined by differences in intrinsic rates of discharge (automaticity); in dogs, the typical rates of discharge (beats per minute) are SA node, (100); internodal pathways, 70; junctional tissue between atria and AV node, 40–60; and His-Purkinje tissue (20–50). The region with the most rapid diastolic depolarization, the SA node, is the "usual" or dominant pacemaker, thus determining heart rate; after SA nodal discharge, the depolarization of the rest of the heart activates potential (latent) pacemakers, resetting their cycles and effectively suppressing their automaticity. Note that under normal conditions, atrial and ventricular working myocardium lack automaticity.

Dromotropy

Dromotrophy (Greek, "running") refers to the ability of a structure to propagate a wave of depolarization (24). Each tissue comprising the heart propagates a wave of depolarization at a different velocity[a], depending on its anatomic and physiological properties and the direction of propagation (isotropy) through the fibers. In general, propagation is more rapid in the direction parallel to the long axis of the fiber, and in fibers with greater amplitudes of the action potential upstroke (defined as the voltage difference between the resting potential and the action potential overshoot).

Action potentials originating from within the SA node preferentially propagate to the right atrium over exit pathways comprising transitional (T) fibers, and then traverse the atria at a velocity of approximately 1 m/sec. This wave of depolarization produces the P wave recorded on the surface ECG and initiates atrial contraction. The wave is preferentially and more rapidly conducted to the AV node (25) over three modified ridges of myocardium serving as internodal conducting pathways. These pathways have been described as "functional," and likely result from nonuniform anisotropic alignment of the myocardial cellular bundles within the atrial myocardium.

Next, the cardiac impulse is conducted between the atrial and ventricular chambers through a specialized structure known as the AV node. AV conduction is primarily reflected in the duration of the PQ (PR) interval on the ECG. Conduction through the head of the AV node is extremely slow (0.025 m/sec), providing time for atrial depolarization and contraction (to eject a small quantity of blood[b] into the ventricles before ventricular contraction). The AV node can be separated into three physiological sections, namely, the atrial-nodal (AN), nodal (N), and nodal-His (NH) bundle; the NH region is the most distal of the nodal regions. Slowed conduction through the node is primarily the result of slowed conduction through the N region, where conduction is dependent on the weak influx of Ca^{++} ions through L-type calcium channels (Cav1.2). Velocity of conduction over the AV node is modulated by the same factors that determine the rate of discharge of the SA node; whatever increases heart rate usually accelerates AV conduction; whatever decreases heart rate slows AV conduction. Thus, parasympathetic (vagal) stimulation slows conduction, and sympathetic stimulation and increasing temperature speed conduction. These actions would be expected on the basis of the dense sympathetic and parasympathetic innervation of the nodes. Vagomimetics (e.g., edrophonium, digitalis), β-adrenergic blockers (e.g., esmolol, atenolol), and Ca^{++} channel blockers (e.g., verapamil,

---

[a] It is interesting, however, that cells comprising the same tissues are relatively uniform in size and that velocities of propagation for identical tissues are similar across the animal kingdom.

[b] Atrial contraction normally contributes approximately 15% (5% at slow heart rates and 35% at high heart rates) of the blood the ventricle is destined to eject; however, atrial contraction sets the positions of the AV valves and minimizes regurgitation through them. Thus, drugs that alter AV conduction may impact on ventricular stroke volume without altering the force of ventricular contraction.

diltiazem) retard AV conduction and may lead to decremental conduction and block. Adenosine dramatically decreases the rate of slow diastolic depolarization in the SA node (decreases heart rate) and slows conduction through the AV node by activation of the acetylcholine-activated K channel (I_{KACh}) that contributes to the reduced excitability of the node.

Next, the wave of excitation is conducted at a velocity of 2 to 5 m/sec over the His-Purkinje system, expediting an orderly sequence of rapid activation of the terminal arborizations of Purkinje fibers on the endocardial surface of the ventricles. In primates and carnivores, the Purkinje fiber-ventricular muscle transitional zones are located as a subendocardial reticulum (26,27). From the endpoints of the Purkinje fibers, the propagating wave of depolarization conducts rather slowly through the ventricular myocardium (conduction of 0.4 m/sec). Velocity of conduction through ventricular myocardium depends on the rate of rise (phase 0) of the action potential, as determined by the availability and activation of the Na^+ channels (which are modulated by resting membrane potential). Thus, hyperkalemia and ischemia slow ventricular conduction by depolarizing the ventricular myocardium and reducing the fast inward sodium current. Drugs that reduce (or block) the fast inward sodium current (class I antiarrhythmic drugs, such as quinidine, or the specific Na channel blocker tetrodotoxin) slow conduction by reducing the net inward depolarizing current necessary for rapid ventricular propagation.

Dromotropy may be measured in vitro; however, it is often inferred by measuring intervals on the ECG, which is described in detail below.

Bathmotropy

Bathmotropy (from *bathmos*, "threshold") refers to the ease with which a cell may be stimulated or excited (excitability). For a cell to reach threshold and fire an action potential, net inward current must predominate. For working atrial and ventricular myocardium, the action potential upstroke is due to a net depolarizing current provided by I_{Na}, the rapid inward sodium current. One must also consider the properties of the cardiac syncytium when considering bathmotropy, as the threshold must be exceeded over a critical length (liminal length) before impulse propagation occurs. This quantity of depolarized tissue provides sufficient net inward current (source current) to depolarize adjacent tissues (the sink) to beyond the threshold potential to initiate and sustain propagation. In general, bathmotropy may be increased by reducing the resting membrane potential (thus bringing the resting potential closer to the threshold potential), and supernormal bathmotropy may lead to arrhythmia. When bathmotrophy is supernormal, there is an increased susceptibility to any oscillations in the resting potential, which can initiate extrasystoles and proarrhythmia. Notably, in diseases where bathmotrophy is enhanced (e.g., postmyocardial infarction, heart failure, or electrolyte imbalances), there is an increased risk of drug-induced arrhythmias (e.g., digitalis-induced arrhythmias).

Refractoriness

Refractoriness refers to periods when the heart, tissue, or myocyte is not able to be electrically stimulated, requires a more intense stimulus to initiate a response, or responds at a reduced level. After each cardiac depolarization, there is a period of time when the heart is refractory to stimulation, this is termed the absolute refractory period and occurs toward the end of each action potential. The relative refractory period immediately follows, during which time greater stimulus intensity (or duration) is needed to elicit an active response (as compared with stimulation long after repolarization has ended). In general, decreased refractoriness in atria is associated with potential proarrhythmia. In general, for action potentials initiated with fast upstrokes (fast responses due to massive inrush of sodium ions carried as fast inward sodium current), refractoriness is approximated by the action potential duration, and the duration may be used as a surrogate for the refractory periods. However, this surrogate for refractoriness may be unreliable during ischemia, alterations in extracellular (K^+), or in the presence of drugs that delay reactivation of depolarizing ionic channels (i.e., I_{Na} in atrial or ventricular myocardium, or I_{Ca} in nodal tissues). Refractoriness is measured using standardized techniques as described below.

Electrogenesis of the Cardiac Action Potential

Voltage-Dependent Ion Channels

Electrical activity of all excitable tissue is determined by net flux of ions crossing the cardiac membrane through ion channels or carried by ionic pumps, transporters, or exchangers. Functionally, ion channels can be considered as structures consisting of a conducting pore coupled to a selectivity filter (that determines the type of ions that may pass) coupled to a voltage-dependent gating mechanism (that controls when the channel is in either conducting or non-conducting states). In the case of voltage-sensitive channels, gating is controlled by the transmembrane potential; an example would be the fast inward sodium channel responsible for the upstroke of working atrial and ventricular fibers, where channels transiently open when the membrane is depolarizing, leading to the voltage- and time-dependent activation and inactivation. Ion channels may also be modulated by neurotransmitters and hormones, providing for modulation of electrical activity in response to changing physiological conditions (e.g., calcium current increases in response to activation of a G-protein-coupled receptor) (28), resulting in increased inotropy of ventricular tissues, but decreased current in response to muscarinic stimulation. In the case of ligand-gated channels, channel-ligand interactions are necessary to control channel gating; the acetylcholine-activated K channel I_{KAch} present in atrial and nodal tissues is an example.

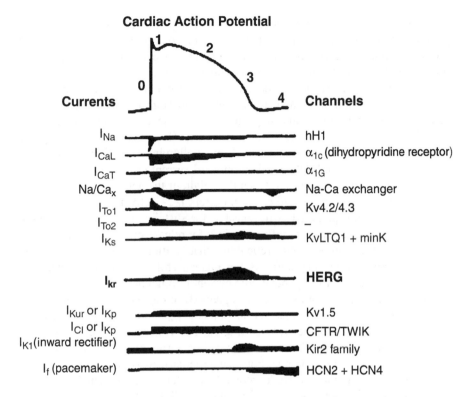

Figure 2 Ionic currents and channels involved in the electrogenesis of a ventricular myocyte. The upper trace illustrates a generalized cardiac ventricular action potential, with the different phases labeled; phase 0 is termed the upstroke, phase 1 is termed early repolarization, phase 2 is termed the plateau, and phase 3 is termed terminal repolarization. Any slow depolarization arising after terminal repolarization from the resting (or diastolic) membrane potential is termed phase 4 depolarization. The lower traces display individual ionic currents contributing to the action potential. Currents are indicated on left, and corresponding channels on right. The time course of individual currents is depicted by the filled shapes, with inward (depolarizing) current shown as downward shapes, and outward (repolarizing current) shown as upward shapes. See text for further discussion. Adapted from Ref. 108.

Components of the Cardiac Action Potential (29,19)

In order to appreciate the adverse effects of drugs on cardiac electrophysiology, it is necessary to understand the electrogenesis of the cardiac action potential (Fig. 2). Note that only cells possessing the property of normal automaticity (e.g., SA-nodal cells, cells of internodal pathways, cells at the atrial-AV nodal junction, and those of the His-Purkinje conduction system in the ventricles) would display phase 4 depolarization, as normal atrial and ventricular myocardium do not demonstrate automaticity.

On the basis of their voltage and time dependence, different currents predominate during each phase of the action potential (Fig. 2). The fast inward sodium current is responsible for the rapid upstroke of the action potential (phase 0). This current rapidly activates and inactivates (within a few milliseconds), providing sufficient depolarizing current to ensure rapid, nondecremental conduction of the cardiac impulse through the working atrial and ventricular myocardium. Rapid depolarization of the cardiac cell triggers the sequential activation of other cardiac channels (K^+, Ca^{++}), generating the remainder of the action potential waveform. Following the initial rapid depolarization, an early (but brief) transient outward current (I_{to}) rapidly activates to ensure phase 1 repolarization and to set the height of the action potential plateau (also known as phase 2). Inward calcium current $I_{Ca,L}$ activated during phases 1 and 2 of the action potential is responsible for sustaining the action potential plateau, providing the calcium influx required for release of intracellular calcium stores from the sarcoplasmic reticulum that initiates cardiac contraction (excitation-contraction coupling). As the plateau shifts toward more negative values, outward (repolarizing) potassium current through hERG (I_{Kr}) increases to trigger terminal repolarization (known as phase 3) of the action potential. During slower stimulation (with longer action potentials), another potassium current known as I_{Ks} also contributes repolarizing current. During (and following) final repolarization, I_{K1} is rapidly activated, ensuring terminal repolarization and a stable resting membrane potential. Following repolarization, the sodium/calcium exchanger may continue to extrude intracellular calcium accumulated during the action potential in exchange for extracellular sodium (driven by the electrochemical gradients of sodium and calcium), generating a net inward (depolarizing) current. In addition, the activity of the sodium-potassium adenosine triphosphatase-activated (Na-K-ATPase) pump increases, generating a net outward current as it transports accumulated intracellular sodium out of the cell (at the expense of ATP) to maintain ionic homeostasis.

Unlike atrial and ventricular working fibers, SA nodal fibers do not display a stable resting membrane potential (30). Instead the SA node demonstrates slow depolarization commencing at the end of the action potential. This slow depolarization typically arises from a maximum diastolic potential (of approximately -60 mV) to a threshold value of approximately -40 mV to initiate an action potential upstroke that propagates from the node to surrounding transitional cells and working atrial myocardium. Thus, pacemaker activity in the SA node reflects the integrated response of multiple ionic channels generating net inward current to sustain depolarization leading to threshold and firing of the action potential. The I_F channel (also referred to as the "funny channel"), a cation-selective inward current activated by hyperpolarization and intracellular cAMP, plays a major role in regulating normal automaticity in the sinus node (31). β-receptor stimulation accelerates, and vagal stimulation slows, cardiac rate by increasing and decreasing I_F, respectively, at diastolic potentials via changes in cAMP levels. Current through T-type calcium channels (which activates at more negative membrane potentials than L-type calcium channels) likely also plays a role in determining the rate of diastolic depolarization in the SA node of some species. Near threshold potentials, this inward current diminishes and is replaced by inward calcium current carried through L-type calcium channels. Finally, repolarization of the sinus node action potential is promoted by two K^+ currents (I_{Kr} and I_{Ks}), whose contributions may vary with species (32). More recent studies have also implicated oscillations in internal calcium as contributing to diastolic depolarization (33,34). The reader is referred to a more detailed description later in this chapter (sect. "Normal Automaticity").

Electrical Heterogeneity of the Ventricular Wall

It has long been appreciated that differences in the action potential configuration exist across the ventricular wall (Fig. 3). For example, differences in the action potential duration from epicardial and endocardial regions of the ventricle have been implicated in the genesis of the QT interval of the ECG (35). More recently, transmural differences across the entire ventricular wall (encompassing epicardial, midmyocardial, and endocardial regions) have been characterized (20,32). These differences arise (at least in part) from differences in the expression of

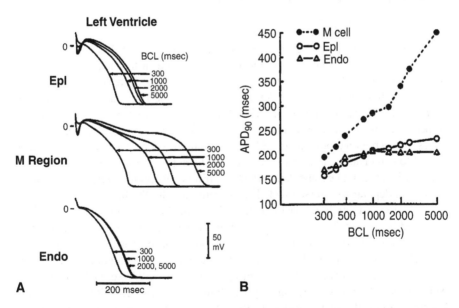

Figure 3 Transmural differences in action potential duration in vitro across the canine left ventricular free wall. (**A**) Note prominent "spike and dome" configuration of epicardium and cells from midmyocardial (M cell) regions, compared with higher plateau and absence of "notch" shape in endocardial cells. (**B**) Also note substantial differences in rate dependence of the action potential of epicardial (EPI), deep subepicardial (M cells), and endocardial (Endo) cells in canine left ventricle on extreme slowing of stimulation. Adapted from Ref. 109.

sarcolemmal ion channels transmurally, between apex and base, and between left ventricle and right ventricle. Ventricular epicardium typically displays prominent phase 1 repolarization followed by a relatively positive phase 2 (termed a "spike and dome" configuration), reflecting a greater contribution of the transient outward current than in the endocardium. During excessively slow rates, action potentials from the midmyocardial region of ventricle demonstrate significant prolongation compared with either epi- or endocardium. This characteristic of these cells (termed "M cells") likely results from a smaller I_{Ks} and residual or slow sodium current. Finally, the endocardial action potential is characterized with a plateau voltage that is typically less positive than the epicardium, and an action potential duration longer than the epicardium. Differences in the configurations of the action potential and differences in the time order of repolarization of the varying regions of the ventricular wall are responsible for genesis of the ST-T on the ECG. In various in vitro models, drugs that delay ventricular repolarization have been shown to exaggerate transmural differences in repolarization, thereby increasing spatial dispersion of repolarization (36), an effect considered to be proarrhythmic (below).

Normal and Abnormal Cardiac Electrogenesis

Normal Automaticity

As described above (sect. "Components of the Cardiac Action Potential"), the SA node of the heart normally is the most automatic site in the heart and therefore normally serves as the dominant pacemaker (37), a property termed normal automaticity. While cells within the AV node and Purkinje fibers are also capable of normal automacity, their rate of firing (40–60 beats/min and 20–40 beats/min, respectively) is typically lower than that of the SA node. When an electrical impulse arises from a region other than the SA node to initiate a depolarization, that impulse is said to originate from an ectopic focus. If the ectopic discharge follows a long pause, it is termed an escape depolarization; if it occurs prematurely, it is termed a premature depolarization (see sect."Electrocardiography Studies").

 Action potentials of pacemaker cells in the SA and AV nodes are characterized by a slow diastolic depolarization (phase 4 depolarization) that leads to threshold and the firing of slow response-type action potentials (Fig. 4). Nodal cell action potentials are characterized by calcium current–dependent upstrokes with slow rates of upstroke depolarization (typically <50 V/sec) compared with working atrial and ventricular myocardium (typically 100–200 V/sec) and Purkinje fibers (typically 400–600 V/sec), where fast inward sodium current causes depolarization. Figure 4 illustrates the numerous ionic channels and exchangers postulated to play a role in phase 4 depolarization in the sinus node. On repolarization, deactivation of the repolarizing current (I_{Kr}) occurs, along with activation of a hyperpolarization-activated cyclic nucleotide (HCN) gate depolarizing nonselective cation current (I_f), which contributes to the initial

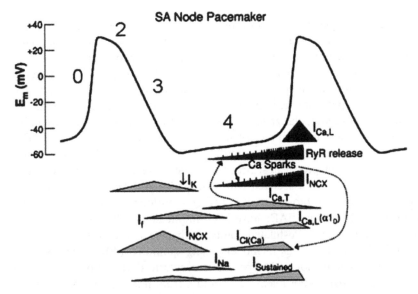

Figure 4 Currents contributing to normal automaticity in sinus node. Phases indicated phase 0, 3, 4 predominate. Note the lack of a stable resting potential, and that the maximum diastolic potential is typically in the range of –50 to –60 mV. Adapted from Ref. 33.

phase of diastolic depolarization. Subsequently, intracellular calcium release (termed "sparks") from ryanodine release channels within the sarcoplasmic reticulum of SA-nodal cells, which may elicit a depolarizing sodium-calcium exchange current (33). In addition, inward calcium current carried first by I_{CaT} and subsequently by I_{CaL} channels leads to further depolarization, and on reaching threshold, the firing of the next action potential takes place. This integrated response provides potential redundancies for diastolic depolarization and guarantees a continuing rhythm despite perturbations of any one current. Drugs may affect heart rate by directly or indirectly modulating ion channels. For example, ivabradine slows sinus rate by selectively blocking the I_F current in sinus node (38). Interestingly, heart rate slowing in vitro with blockade of I_F appears to be self-limiting, possibly due to redundancy in the mechanisms responsible for ensuring diastolic depolarization. In contrast, catecholamines (NE) increase rate by enhancing cAMP levels, which can modulate multiple processes (including $I_{Ca,L}$, I_f, and Ca release from sarcoplasmic reticulum) to increase sinus rate.

Abnormal Automaticity—Triggered Activity, Early and Delayed Afterdepolarizations

A cardiac arrhythmia is defined as any abnormality in the rate, regularity, or site of origin of the cardiac impulse or a disturbance in the conduction of that impulse such that the normal sequence of activation is altered. This section addresses abnormalities in the site of origin of the cardiac impulse. Under certain conditions, cells typically not automatic may generate extra beats following stimulation. Such activity, termed triggered activity, is said to arise or result from a prior "triggering" event [hence the term "triggered activity" (39)]. Triggered activity results from afterdepolarizations that arise either during or after the preceeding action potential; activity occurring prior to the end of repolarization are termed early afterdepolarizations (EADs), while those occurring after full repolarization (during diastole) are termed delayed afterdepolarizations (DADs) (Fig. 5). Under certain conditions, afterdepolarizations may initiate premature electrical activity that propagates throughout the ventricles to generate extrasystoles. EADs are often associated with drug-induced delayed cardiac repolarization (action potential prolongation or QT/QTc prolongation on the ECG) and are bradycardia dependent. EADs have been implicated in the initiation of TdP arrhythmias (see below). Postulated ionic mechanisms responsible for EADs include K^+ channel block [as in models using quinidine (40)], enhanced late sodium current, reactivation of L-type calcium current during prolonged action potential plateau (10), and/or release of calcium from intracellular sarcoplasmic reticulum stores leading to inward current via Na/Ca exchange [see views of Sipido (41)].

In contrast, DADs are typically associated with rapid heart rates and are attributed to "calcium overload" of cardiac cells, such as occurs with inhibition of Na^+-K^+ ATPase with cardiac glycosides or β-adrenergic stimulation (42). DADs are thought to occur as a result of spontaneous calcium release from the sarcoplasmic reticulum, as occurs during calcium overload, resulting in subsequent activation of a transient inward current via the forward mode Na/Ca exchanger. It should be noted that EADs and DADs need not be considered in strict isolation, as it is also possible to generate EADs and DADs in the same preparation in vitro. Notably, both EADs and DADs can give rise to ectopic beats that can initiate proarrhythmia [e.g., extrasystoles during the T wave ("R on T phenomena") linked to the initiation of ventricular fibrillation].

Reentry

Reentry is thought to be the most common mechanism of cardiac arrhythmias. Reentrant arrhythmias require an underlying substrate, namely, dispersion of both conduction velocities and refractory periods within a region of the heart. The simplest way to picture reentry is illustrated in Figure 5c.

METHODS TO STUDY DRUG EFFECTS ON CARDIAC ELECTROPHYSIOLOGY

It is instructive to consider methods used to study drug effects on cardiac electrophysiology on the basis of the level of complexity and integration of the biological systems under study (36,43–46). Studies of individual ion currents

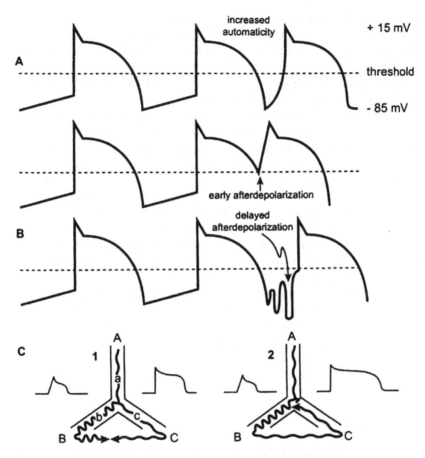

Figure 5 Mechanisms for initiation of arrhythmias. Panel A: Increased automaticity results from a net influx of positive charge, causing phase 4 (diastolic) depolarization. Panel B: Two forms of triggered activity (EAD and DAD). With triggered activity, the previous depolarization triggers abnormal depolarizations so that they reach threshold either during phase 3 of the triggering action potential (early), or after the triggering cell has repolarized fully (delayed). Panel C: Initiation and propagation of reentry. Note that while pathway A exhibits slowed conduction, it has a normal refractory period. Contrast pathway B exhibits normal conduction, but a longer refractory period (longer action potential). When a properly timed premature impulse propagates into both bifurcations, the premature impulse may block in pathway B (because of longer refractory period), while slowly conducting through pathway A (slowed conduction). By the time the impulse exits pathway A, pathway B is no longer refractory and is reexcited in a retrograde manner. At this point, the circuit can repeatedly reexcite itself, to maintain a "reentrant" rapid arrhythmia. *Abbreviations*: EAD, early afterdepolarization; DAD, delayed afterdepolarizations.

represent the simplest preparations to study, ideally reflecting the activity of a single channel type. The next higher level of complexity and systems integration consist of the cardiac cell, with multiple ion channels contributing ionic currents to define the cardiac action potential. Small cardiac tissue preparations (Purkinje fibers, papillary muscles) represent a more complex system, in which myocytes of the same type typically "synchronize" activity, possibly with the involvement of other cell types (e.g., embedded nervous tissues). Larger cardiac preparations (including transmural slices and cardiac "wedge" preparations) provide for integration of multiple cardiac electrophysiological phenotypes. The highest levels of integration are represented by whole hearts studied either in vitro (Langendorff preparations) or in vivo in an intact organism, the latter including the influence of neuronal and hormonal interactions and potential drug metabolites. The selection of species and tissues are critical considerations when conducting repolarization studies as a surrogate marker of proarrhythmia (47,48). For example, hERG plays a minimal, if any, role in determining repolarization of the rat ventricle. Thus, repolarization studies using rat ventricular myocytes or tissues would likely not be useful in characterizing hERG blockade as a marker for proarrhythmia. Repolarization is sexually dimorphic in humans and other mammals, with females having longer QT intervals after puberty. Female sex also increases the risk of hERG blockade–induced proarrhythmia. The use of cardiac tissue derived from female animals may provide increased sensitivity for detecting drug-induced repolarization defects (47,49,50). Some representative studies employing each of these systems will be described below.

Ion Current Studies

Cardiac ionic currents are typically studied either in native myocytes or in expression systems, where the channel of interest is heterologously expressed in a cell culture system (Fig. 6). For a successful study in heterologous expression systems, the amplitude of the current under study must be larger than (or easily identified or "isolated" from) background currents. For studies of individual currents in native myocytes, the current of interest must be isolated by suppression of other ion currents present using pharmacological and/or biophysical methods. The obvious advantage of studying native currents is the fact that the channel and all associated subunits (that may influence channel gating or drug-channel interactions) are present; this may not be the case in heterologous expression systems. However, interpretations of studies are simpler (and throughput generally faster) using heterologous versus native systems.

Following due consideration of experimental conditions, IC_{50} values for hERG block are compared with anticipated free therapeutic (or Cmax) plasma concentrations to predict the potential for delayed repolarization. In general, a safety margin of ≥ 30 (Cmax/IC_{50}, where Cmax is the maximal expected concentration and IC_{50} is the concentration resulting in half-maximal block of

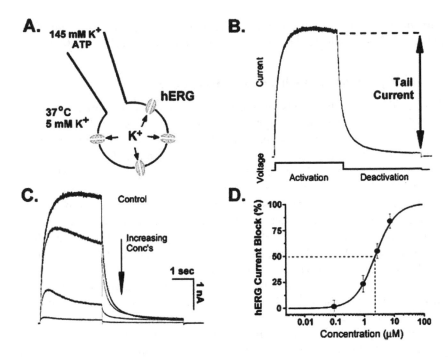

Figure 6 hERG ionic current study. An example of a study evaluating drug blocks of hERG current is illustrated. Panel A represents a cell expressing the hERG channel attached to a patch pipette containing 145 mM K^+ and ATP (to support channel activity). The outward current (activated by depolarization) is carried by K^+ ions flowing out of the cell through hERG channels. Panel B illustrates the growth of outward current during a depolarizing voltage clamp pulse. The activating (depolarizing) voltage clamp pulse elicits voltage-dependent activation of the channel, resulting in an increasing outward current (upward deflection). On repolarization, the channel deactivates, as reflected in the declining outward current trace (labeled "Tail Current"). Changes in the amplitude of the outward tail current are typically measured to assess current block. Panel C illustrates the concentration-dependent effects of a drug that preferentially blocks open (conducting) hERG channels. During each depolarizing pulse to a constant voltage, outward current in the presence of drug is progressively reduced, consistent with greater drug block later during the voltage clamp pulse. With the application of each depolarizing pulse, current levels during the depolarizing pulse are progressively reduced, demonstrating concentration dependence of current block. This effect is also reflected in the reduction of the tail current amplitudes elicited on repolarization. Concentration-dependent block is graphically summarized in Panel D, which characterizes block potency using a Hill function to characterize with an IC_{50} value (in this particular example, 2.3 mM). *Abbreviation*: ATP, adenosine 5'-triphosphate. Adapted from Ref. 110.

hERG) is considered by some as a minimal value to target to ensure cardiac safety with respect to delayed repolarization (51). It should be noted that based primarily on regulatory concerns, hERG studies have been the main focus of ion current studies used to assess the electrophysiological effects of drugs on the heart; however, other cardiac currents (including I_{Na}, $I_{Ca,L}$, I_{K1}, I_{Ks}) are often studied to further evaluate the safety of drugs on cardiac electrical activity.

In Vitro Repolarization: Cellular and Tissue Studies

These studies evaluate effects on cardiac depolarization/repolarization using isolated myocytes or tissues. Preparations can range (in order of complexity) from single isolated myocytes, to papillary muscles and Purkinje fibers, to slices or "wedges" of ventricular tissues (Figs. 7, 8). Action potentials can be recorded using either conventional whole-cell patch or perforated patch techniques (isolated cells) or sharp microelectrodes (isolated cells or tissues). Regarding repolarization (action potential) studies from single myocytes, conventional whole-cell patch techniques alter the intracellular milieu of cells under study, possibly affecting ion channel behavior (but provide the ability to introduce compounds intracellularly). Perturbations of the intracellular milieu are mini-mized using perforated patch techniques (at the expense of slightly higher access resistance). Microelectrode (52) (or sharp electrode) techniques provide for minimal changes to the intracellular milieu but are often difficult to achieve without physically damaging myocytes. Beat-to-beat variability may be greater for isolated myocytes compared with tissues, as tissues form a functional syn-cytium with electrical coupling between cells, providing more stable beat-to-beat recordings. Repolarization studies using cardiac tissues provide the ability to

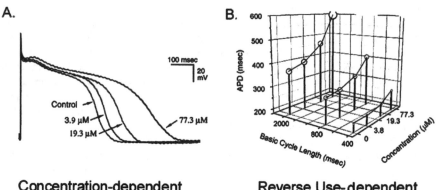

A.

B.

Concentration-dependent Prolongation

Reverse Use-dependent Prolongation

Figure 7 Repolarization studies with grepafloxacin. Panel **A**: concentration-dependent prolongation of canine Purkinje fiber repolarization. Panel **B**: reverse use–dependent prolongation. For any given concentration, prolongation is greater at the slower stimu-lation rate [2000 milliseconds basic cycle length (30 beats/min)] compared with faster stimulation rates (800 and 400 milliseconds basic cycle lengths, corresponding to 75 and 150 beats/min, respectively). Hence, prolongation is greater with lesser "use" or activity (hence the phrase reverse use–dependence). Adapted from Ref. 44.

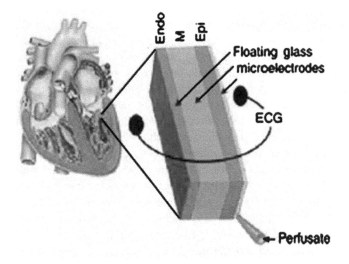

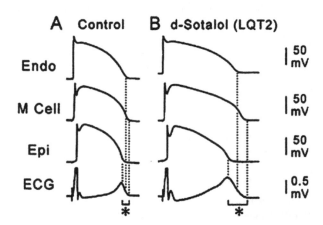

Figure 8 Wedge preparation for studying cellular electrophysiology in vitro. (*Top*) A left ventricular wedge of tissue is isolated for in vitro electrophysiologic study. The tissue is perfused to maintain viability. Recordings can be made from the endocardial (endo), mid-myocardial (M), and epicardial (Epi) region, and a pseudo-ECG (ECG) can be simultaneously recorded. (*Bottom*) Recordings from a left ventricular wedge preparation (**A**) before and (**B**) after treatment with d-sotalol, an IKr (hERG) blocker. Note that repolarization (end of the action potential) varies across the ventricle, thus providing dispersion of repolarization that is exaggerated by sotalol (see Fig. 5 for the role of nonuniform repolarization to reentrant arrhythmias). *Abbreviation*: ECG, electrocardiogram. Adapted from Refs. 111,112.

assess electrophysiological changes from nearly all regions of the heart. Most tissues have been well characterized in the literature (providing for easy comparisons of drug-free "controls" when critically comparing data sets). In addition, one might expect less variability between preparations with tissues, as minimal interventions are necessary when preparing tissues for study (as compared with, e.g., the multistep dissaggregation methods necessary to isolate myocytes). Purkinje tissues, from such animals as rabbits and canines, allow for easy harvest. Purkinje fibers also possess less contractile elements (53) compared with ventricular muscle and thus tend to provide more stable recordings from a mechanical perspective, allowing for maintained impalements throughout an experiment (useful for direct comparisons of pre- and postdrug recordings). Papillary muscles (such as that of guinea pigs), which are smaller in diameter than those from larger species to minimize the growth of an anoxic core, are also easily dissected for either electrophysiological or contractility studies. Both tissue preparations have been well characterized and widely used for electrophysiological studies of drugs (44,54). Sinus node preparations from the rabbit and guinea pig have also been well characterized; in general, sinus node studies from dogs are not performed because of an overlaying endocardial muscle layer preventing microelectrode access.

As the action potential represents the integrated response of multiple ion channels, pumps, and exchangers, a drug's effect on repolarization may reflect its actions on multiple ionic currents (Fig. 2) (Table 1). Thus, repolarization

Table 1 Potential Manifestations of Electrophysiologic Adverse Effects

Drug	Cellular effect	Potential ECG effect
Sodium channel block	Block I_{Na}, slow conduction in working myocardium	P wave prolongation PR prolongation QRS prolongation
L-type calcium channel block	Action potential triangulation Negative inotropy Negative chronotropy Slowed AV-node conduction	Bradycardia PR prolongation
I_{Kr}/hERG channel block	Delayed repolarization Early afterdepolarizations	QT/QTc prolongation Proarrhythmia
I_{Ks} channel block	Delayed repolarization in the presence of β-adrenergic stimulation	QT prolongation Proarrhythmia
I_{K1} channel block	Depolarization of resting potential	Abnormal automaticity
I_F channel block	Slowing of normal (and potentially abnormal) phase 4 depolarization	Slowing of sinus rate
Cardiac glycosides	Delayed afterdepolarizations Calcium overload	Many forms of proarrhythmia are possible at toxic concentrations
Increased I_{KACh} (adenosine)		Transient AV node block

Abbreviations: AV, atrioventricular.

studies may be considered as assaying across multiple ionic currents simultaneously. Since the activity of specific channels dominate during different phases of the ventricular action potential, it is possible to deduce drug effects on various ionic currents on the basis of changes in the action potential configuration. For example, drugs that inhibit the fast sodium current (responsible for the action potential upstroke of fast response-type action potentials) would be expected to reduce the maximum rate of rise of the upstroke (Vmax); this effect may also be accompanied by a reduction in the amplitude or overshoot of the action potential upstroke. The local anesthetic effects of most drugs that decrease fast inward sodium current are exaggerated at slower heart rates. This rate-dependent modulation has been termed reverse use dependence. Drugs that inhibit the initial transient outward current (responsible for phase 1 repolarization and establishing an initial plateau voltage) would act to slow repolarization and likely generate a more positive plateau. Calcium channel–blocking drugs (by reducing inward calcium current) would be expected to reduce the height of the plateau and elicit a more triangulated action potential configuration. Drugs that block I_{Kr} current would be expected to prolong the action potential by delaying the transition to phase 3 terminal repolarization. Finally, drugs that block the inward rectifier current I_{K1} responsible for final repolarization and setting the resting membrane potential would act to extend (or shoulder) the terminal phase of repolarization and elicit depolarization of the resting membrane potential. With sufficient block of I_{K1}, tissue would depolarize, leading to reduced (and eventual) loss of excitability. Because of the complex nature of interactions between membrane voltage and currents, it can be difficult to reliably deduce the precise mechanisms resulting in abnormalities, particularly during the plateau and repolarization phases. Therefore, assignment of mechanisms to any repolarization effects should be followed up with studies of the suspected ionic currents. Finally, it is not surprising that some drugs affect the heart by affecting multiple cardiac currents. For example, the antiarrhythmic drug verapamil was developed on the basis of its ability to block the L-type cardiac calcium channel. However, it was later shown to be a potent I_{Kr}/hERG channel blocker as well (55). Despite the often-cited association between hERG block and the rare but potentially lethal arrhythmia TdP (56), verapamil is not associated clinically with TdP. This apparent discrepancy is readily explained by the "multiple channel blockade" by verapamil; that is, that block of the cardiac calcium channel mitigates the deleterious effects of delayed repolarization expected from hERG block alone. This "protective" effect of the calcium channel block in the presence of hERG block has also been demonstrated in vitro with nifedipine reversing the action potential duration–prolonging effects of dofetilide (57). These examples illustrate the importance of considering a drug's effect on the ensemble of currents responsible for the action potential when evaluating cardiac toxicity.

While it is important to understand cellular electrophysiological effects on any individual cell or tissue type, it is also important to consider differences in drug effects across different regions of the heart. This may be done using simultaneous, multiple impalements from different cardiac regions. Preparations used in such studies of ventricular myocardium include (*i*) superfused sliced papillary muscle (52), (*ii*) superfused thin slices of ventricular muscle (typically produced using a dermatome), or (*iii*) perfused "wedges" of ventricular myocardium (Fig. 8) (36,58–60). The last preparation typically provides for simultaneous action potential recordings from the cut/exposed edges of epicardial, midmyocardial, and endocardial regions using microelectrodes (held in place via wire supports and described as "floating microelectrodes"). This approach provides for comparisons of differences in electrophysiological actions in three regions (e.g., increased "dispersion" of repolarization, a mechanism linked to proarrhythmia), information that cannot be obtained in any other manner. However, it should be recognized that this technique is challenging in practice, practiced by few laboratories, and considered a low throughput approach. Drugs that prolong repolarization typically have greater effects on Purkinje and "M" cells than epicardial or endocardial muscle (61,62), providing for improved sensitivity to detect repolarization delays with smaller sample sizes.

In Vitro Repolarization: Whole Heart Studies

Whole heart studies can be conducted either in vitro or in vivo. Langendorff preparations (in vitro), in which excised hearts are retrogradely perfused through the aortic root, remain a means by which true arrhythmias can be recorded (63). Classic (traditional) ECGs represent the sum of electrical activity as recorded from body surface. However, ECGs can also be recorded from electrodes placed around isolated hearts in superfusate-filled recording chambers (volume-conducted ECGs). Differential recordings from two electrodes placed directly on the cardiac surface can be used to record ECG-like signals (pseudo ECGs).

It is also possible to record action-potential-like traces from either endo-or epicardial surfaces of Langendorff-perfused hearts. Using two catheter-mounted electrodes, one in contact with either the epicardial or endocardial surface, a MAP is obtained. While smaller in amplitude than true transmembrane recordings and typically less stable, such recordings faithfully reflect the time course of repolarization of tissues under and surrounding the recording electrode (64). MAP recordings have proven useful in correlating changes in repolarization with ECG changes in in vivo experiments. More recently, MAP recordings have been used to evaluate beat-to-beat instability associated with QT-prolonging drugs and proarrhythmia such as TdP (46,65,66). MAP recordings from epicardial cells have been compared with optical recordings obtained using voltage-sensitive dyes verifying the time course of electrical activity [reviewed in (67)]. Voltage-sensitive dye studies can be used to record action potentials from a portion of the whole heart. This technique is limited to the epicardial surface and is technically demanding.

A primary advantage of whole heart in vitro (Langendorff) preparations for ECG studies is the exquisite control of experimental conditions (68,69).

Specifically, one can control heart rate and/or rhythm (with either atrial or ventricular pacing), ionic conditions, and drug concentrations (the latter providing for exposures that may not be attainable in vivo because of extracardiac effects). Indeed, it is possible to test for proarrhythmic effects of drugs in vitro by evaluating their effects on hearts exposed to known proarrhythmic risk factors (e.g., hypokalemia). It is also possible to generate diseased hearts (e.g., heart failure) that are then isolated and studied ex vivo in the presence of drugs and/or additional proarrhythmic risk factors. Obviously, one difference in this approach, compared with in vivo studies, is the loss of neurohumoral influences that may modulate drug effects.

Electrocardiography Studies

Electrocardiography is the study of minute voltages measured on the body surface by waves of depolarization and repolarization (70,71). It involves the heart as a generator of voltage, the body as a conductor of the voltages to the body surface, leads that conduct the voltages from the body surface to the electrocardiograph, and the electrocardiograph or voltmeter, which detects, amplifies, and records the voltages as ECGs. Although ECGs may be quantified and interpreted by evermore sophisticated digital computational methods (72), the most important link in electrocardiography is still the well-trained human interpreter who may make observations (e.g., subtle changes in configurations of ST-T or PQ segment, appearance of high-frequency components to QRS). However, evolving detection algorithms and processing techniques are quickly changing the way ECGs are read and analyzed.

As mentioned previously, the ECG comprises a series of deflections and intervals between them. The P wave is produced by atrial depolarization, the QRS by ventricular depolarization, the Ta wave (if present) by atrial repolarization, the ST-T complex by ventricular repolarization. In some recordings, U waves (waves on terminal part or immediately following the T wave) may be present, thought to arise from either repolarization of Purkinje fibers or "M" fibers in the middle region of the ventricular free wall. The end of the QRS or the beginning of the ST-T is termed the J point. Frequently, the end of the QRS complex contains a relatively low amplitude, slowly inscribed deflection termed the J wave, which is actually produced by early ventricular repolarization (mediated by K^+ conductance through I_{TO} channels). The PQ interval is the time between onsets of atrial and ventricular depolarization. Most animal ECGs do not possess an ST segment, which in normal humans is a relatively flat line between the end of the QRS complex and the beginning of the T wave. The absence of a flat ST segment in many (smaller) animals with more rapid heart rates is explained by the observation that ventricular repolarization begins even before ventricular depolarization is completed, thus the ST segment and T wave fuse. This is particularly true in mice and rats in whom ventricular repolarization begins well within the time course for ventricular depolarization such that the peak of the T wave sometimes actually occurs in the descending limb of the QRS complex.

The electrocardiograph measures the potential difference (electromotive force, or voltage) between two regions. Typically, electrodes are attached to all four limbs and often to points on the thorax, and there are standardized pairs of electrodes used for each ECG lead. For example: lead I (voltage between left and right arms), II (voltage between left leg and right arm), III (voltage between left leg and left arm), aVR (voltage at the right arm paired against a near 0 voltage), aVL (voltage at the left arm paired against a near 0 voltage), aVF (voltage at the left leg paired against a near 0 voltage), and the V leads (voltage from specific points on the thorax paired against a near 0 voltage). Leads I, II, III, aVR, aVL, and aVF consitute the so-called limb leads, and the V leads are termed unipolar thoracic leads. Although 12 leads are typically used to diagnose disease in humans, electrocardiography is used in toxicology or safety pharmacology to determine, principally, heart rate and rhythm; durations of P, PQ, QRS, and QT; and whether the J point may be displaced. Because studies in toxicology and safety pharmacology are usually rather short in duration and because chamber size is rarely an endpoint of importance, measuring amplitudes of deflections in leads in which atrial or ventricular enlargement may be identified is seldom useful. Thus, 1 to 3 leads appear(s) to be sufficient to identify changes of toxicological significance.

Configurations and durations of component deflections and intervals on the ECG are species dependent, and to include specifics for each species is beyond the scope of this chapter. However, since the heart of a mouse is tiny— and all pathways are comparably smaller—when compared to the heart of a dog, then intervals/durations (P, PQ, QRS) depending on the length of those pathways will be proportionally shorter, despite myocyte size, which appears to be similar across species (73). ECG identification of drug toxicity may be done using standard ECGs (Table 1) (Fig. 1). A useful ECG display (Fig. 1) may include three orthogonal leads (I, aV_F, V_{10}) and a unipolar lead placed on the thorax close to the left ventricle (V_3). Lead V_3 is termed a proximity lead because of its closeness to the greatest mass of the left ventricle, and it is most useful for detecting myocardial injury (i.e., J-point deviation) and for exhibiting T waves whose terminations are clearly defined (for easy measurement of the end of the QT interval [QT_{END}]. Respirations (Fig. 9) produce large fluctuations in heart rate (HR), termed respiratory sinus arrhythmia (RSA) (74,75). This is the normal rhythm for a quiet, healthy dog. All animals manifest an RSA but usually to a lesser degree than in dogs.

Chronotropy refers to changes in heart rate. In studies on toxicology or safety pharmacology, HR is an extremely important parameter—the measure of the chronotropic state that reflects sympathetic and parasympathetic tone. It is usually measured as the number of beats/6 sec $\times$ 10 (the number of 6-seconds periods in 1 minute). However, it can be observed that because of the pronounced RSA, HR may vary according to precisely where in the tracing it is

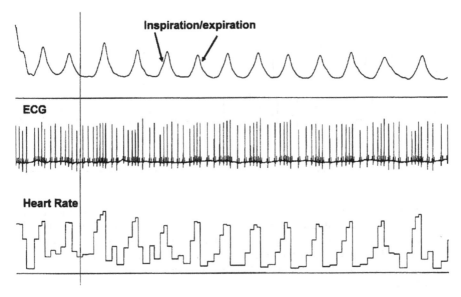

Figure 9 Respiratory sinus arrhythmia recorded in a dog. This occurs most commonly at rest or during sleep. During respiratory sinus arrhythmia, heart rate accelerates during inspiration and slows during expiration. Tracings (*top to bottom*) by respiratory motion, ECG, heart rate. *Abbreviation*: ECG, electrocardiogram.

measured. Heart rate may also be calculated based on the interval between consecutive beats expressed in milliseconds. In fact with RSA, the HR is never the single number obtained by integrating over time, rather it jumps from fast to slow according to the phase of respiration. For example, a continuously recorded ECG from a dog during a period of sleep (Fig. 9) may show periods when the heart rate is 15 beats/min as well as occasional P waves not followed by QRS complexes (2nd degree AV block), both of which are consistent with high parasympathetic tone. In the same animal during excitement, the HR may reach 180 beats/min. Thus, the enormous variability for even normal dogs makes identifying a potential toxic chronotropic effect difficult. Nonetheless, there is no better modality than an ECG for identifying an effect of a drug or test article on chronotropy. Typically, one reports changes relative to baseline or compared with an animal receiving vehicle at the same time. Representative ECGs from a dog are shown to demonstrate the chronotropic effects of the I_F ("funny" current) blocker zatebradine (Fig. 10) (7) and the parasympatholytic atropine (76). Because heart rate is a prime determinant of cardiac output, coronary blood flow, and myocardial oxygen demand, even a small but prolonged change may translate into a significant liability, albeit not an instant liability (refer to Ref. 74 for more information on heart-rate modulation of cardiac function).

Dromotropy refers to changes in conduction through the heart. ECGs are also useful for identifying negative dromotropy through the atria (by lengthening

HR/minute

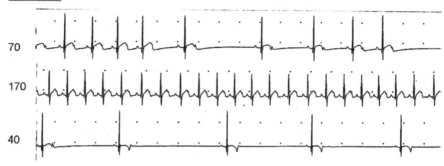

Figure 10 ECG from healthy, quiet dog (*top*), after receiving a parasympatholytic dose of atropine (*middle*) and after receiving a "funny" (I_F) channel blocker, zatebradine (*bottom trace*). Toxic effects of drugs manifested by changing heart rate are evaluated best by electrocardiography. The rhythms are RSA (*top*), sinus tachycardia (*middle*), and sinus bradycardia (*bottom*). *Abbreviations*: ECG, electrocardiogram; RSA, respiratory sinus arrhythmia.

of the P wave), through the AV transmission system (by lengthening of the PQ interval), and through ventricular myocardium (by lengthening of QRS duration). Notice that ECG (Fig. 11), in response to quinidine, demonstrates prolongation of the QRS complex (because of blocking of I_{Na}), as well as prolongation of the QT interval (because of blocking of I_{Kr}), and abolition of the J wave (because of blocking of I_{TO}) (77,78). Prolongation of the PQ interval (without an invasively measured His bundle electrogram) is not necessarily a satisfactory method for identifying an I_{Na} effect, since the PQ is determined by the velocity of conduction from SA to AV nodes (I_{Na} determined) as well as conduction through the AV node ($I_{Ca,L}$ dependent).

The ECG is the best method for identifying the toxic potential for a drug or test article to increase ectopic activity. Such activity may arise from atria or ventricles and may be categorized as normal (arising from normally automatic fibers) or abnormal (such as arising from EADs or DADs), depending on the conditions (as reviewed above). Normal ectopic activity may occur (Fig. 12, top) after a long pause in SA nodal discharge (escape depolarizations, which can arise from a normally automatic tissue such as the AV node or Purkinje fibers). In contrast, it may arise from an abnormally automatic focus or it may occur (Fig. 12, bottom) earlier than anticipated (premature depolarization). If there is more severely increased irritability, bursts (so-called paroxysms) of premature depolarizations (Fig. 13) may occur, or if there is an escape rhythm, a sequence of ectopic depolarizations may occur after a pause in the sinus rhythm and at a slow rate (Figs. 13B and 14). Escape rhythms occur commonly in response to catecholamines or to amphetamine and are thought to result from either increased normal automaticity or DADs. Typically, they occur when sympathetic drive is elevated

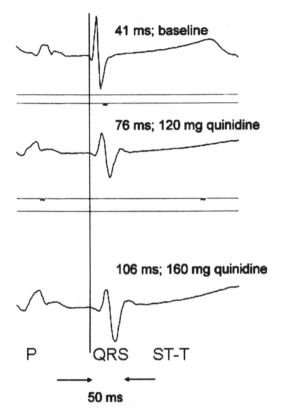

41 ms; baseline

76 ms; 120 mg quinidine

106 ms; 160 mg quinidine

P   QRS   ST-T

50 ms

Figure 11   Effects of quinidine on the ECG in a pig. The ECG is shown before (*top*) and after (*middle, bottom*) two doses of quinidine. The ECG demonstrates QRS prolongation due to slowing of myocardial conduction velocity (negative dromotropism), secondary to the I_{Na}-blocking property of quinidine (41 to 76 to 106 ms). Note that the I_{Kr}-blocking property of quinidine also results in prolongation of the QT interval. ECGs were recorded at high paper speed. The vertical line indicates the onset of the QRS. *Abbreviation*: ECG, electrocardiogram.

(a β_1-adrenergic effect) and when there is simultaneous elevation of parasympathetic activity because of a reflex initiated by elevation of blood pressure (an α_1-adrenergic effect). In leads II or aV$_F$, QRS complexes of ectopic depolarizations arising from the left ventricle are usually predominantly negative (Fig.14), and when arising from the right ventricle, they are predominantly positive (Fig. 13B).

    Cardiac glycosides (such as digoxin and digitoxin) and thiobarbiturates (thiamylal sodium and thiopental sodium) can produce ventricular bigeminy (Fig. 15) characterized by a beat of sinus origin alternating with a ventricular ectopic depolarization. Most commonly, this arrhythmia is caused by DADs triggered by the preceding sinus beat. Bigeminy due to thiobarbiturates is usually

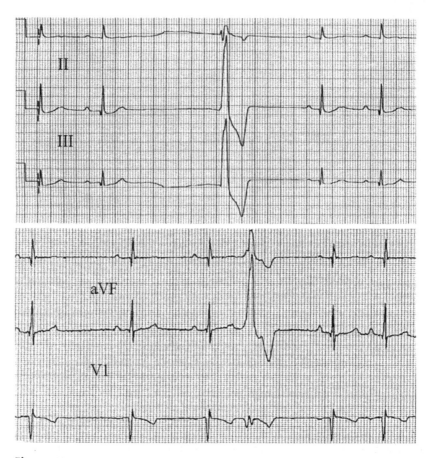

Figure 12 Two discrete forms of ventricular ectopic depolarization in the dog. ECG leads I, II, and III (*top trace*) and I, aVF, V10 (*bottom trace*) showing two forms of ectopic depolarizations originating from specialized conduction tissue of the right ventricle. Note that the QRS complexes of the premature depolarizations are predominantly positive in a lead in which it is normally positive, indicating a right ventricular origin. The ectopic depolarization at the type occurring after a long pause in sinus discharge, and is termed an "escape beat" and is shown in the top panel. In contrast, the ectopic depolarization in the bottom trace occurs prematurely and is termed a "premature beat". *Abbreviation*: ECG, electrocardiogram.

benign and terminates when the anesthetic is eliminated; bigeminy due to digitalis may lead to ventricular fibrillation but may be terminated almost instantly with diphenylhydantoin (an interesting laboratory experiment).

Many drugs from divergent therapeutic classes and with highly divergent chemical structures (e.g., antibiotics, antihistamines, antipsychotics, prokinetics) may slow ventricular repolarization (i.e., lengthen the QT interval or QTc), particularly in persons with hereditary defects in the hERG (I_{KR}) channel. In rare

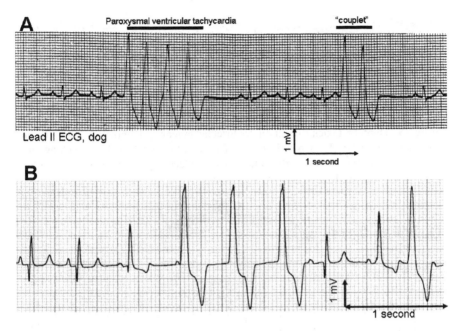

Figure 13 Catecholamine-induced cardiac arrhythmias. (**A**) Ventricular arrhythmia resulting from catecholamine toxicity. Lead II ECG showing short bursts of right ventricular premature depolarizations. (**B**) Cardiac arrhythmia resulting from norepinephrine. Norepinephrine elevates both sympathetic and parasympathetic efferent activity. This rhythm is typical of one produced by a sympathomimetic that both vasoconstricts (elevating systemic arterial pressure) and elicits increased parasympathetic activity. *Abbreviation*: ECG, electrocardiogram.

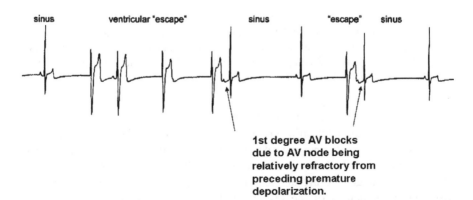

Figure 14 Another form of catecholamine toxicity induced by a β-2 adrenergic agonist. The ECG (lead AVF) illustrates a short paroxysm of escape ventricular tachycardia resulting from increased automaticity. *Abbreviations*: ECG, electrocardiogram; AVF, augmented unipolar lead obtained from the foot.

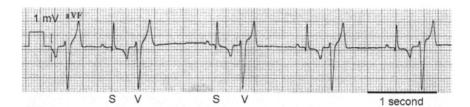

S   V   S   V   1 second

Figure 15 Digitalis toxicity results in ventricular bigeminy [alternating sinus (S) and premature ventricular (V) depolarizations]. This is attributed to DADs resulting from digitalis toxicity. This form of arrhythmia is also produced by thiobarbiturate anesthesia. *Abbreviation*: DADs, delayed afterdepolarizations.

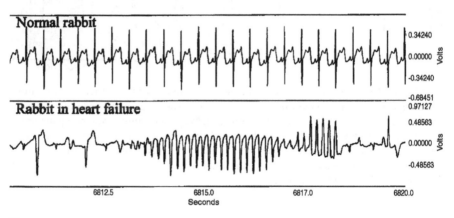

Figure 16 Example of ECGs from a normal rabbit and from a rabbit with heart failure after exposure to a torsadogen (dofetilide). In the heart failure example, this results in a rapid, polymorphic ventricular tachycardia—torsade de pointes. Notice the "twisting" (torsade) of polarity of QRS complexes around the baseline. In this example TdeP ends spontaneously. *Abbreviation*: ECG, electrocardiogram.

instances, excessive delays in ventricular repolarization may lead to a polymorphic ventricular tachycardia termed "torsades de pointes" (meaning "twisting of the points," Fig. 16) that may deteriorate into ventricular fibrillation. It has been estimated that TdP may occur in only 1 in 10,000 to 1 in 1,000,000 persons receiving torsadogenic drugs and lead to sudden death in approximately 20% of instances. Lengthening of the QT interval (or QTc interval after appropriate correction for heart rate changes) is a well-known phenomenon and is a recognized surrogate marker for TdP proarrhythmia (79–82). It has been suggested that no drug is considered safe unless it is first tested to determine if it lengthens QTc, particularly in a dose-dependent and reverse use–dependent manner (i.e., in

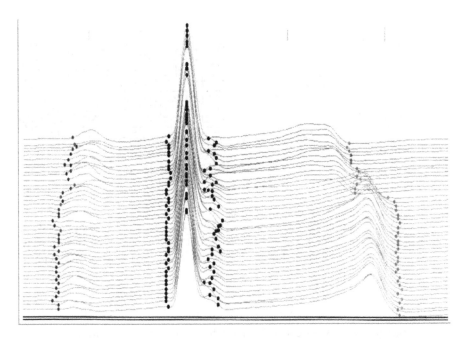

Figure 17 ECGs from dog given sotalol orally. Recordings are "stacked-up" from the baseline (*top trace*) to the ECG obtained four hours postdosing. Fiduciary points mark (from *left to right*) beginning of P, beginning of QRS, end of QRS, and end of T. Notice lengthening of QT, slight lengthening of PQ, but little change in QRS durations. This demonstrates a clear QT liability. This display technique permits easy detection of time-dependent changes in characteristic ECG waveforms. *Abbreviation*: ECG, electrocardiogram.

the presence of a slowed heart rate). It has been postulated that a ventricular premature depolarization is the initiating event for TdP; this depolarization may arise either from an EAD (likely carried by reactivated L-type calcium current) on a substrate of excessive dispersion of repolarization within the ventricle. This arrhythmia is likely perpetuated due to reentry within the ventricle.

In toxicological or safety pharmacology studies, it is important to obtain an ECG using a lead (Fig. 1) from which QT_{END} may be measured with the greatest accuracy and precision. To monitor the progression of QT prolongation, it is often convenient to "stack-up" serial ECGs (Fig. 17) using waterfall plots, with QRS complexes aligned. This allows detection of any progression in the duration of the QT interval. However, as slowing of heart rate itself can cause QT interval prolongation, this confounding factor must be considered when evaluating such plots. Drug-induced changes in autonomic tone may also affect the QT interval absent direct drug effects on net cardiac repolarizing current and should be considered in the absence of evidence of direct effects on cardiac membrane currents.

Another potential toxic manifestation of drugs is the production of myocardial injury. Injury may be produced by a direct cytotoxic effect (e.g., as with

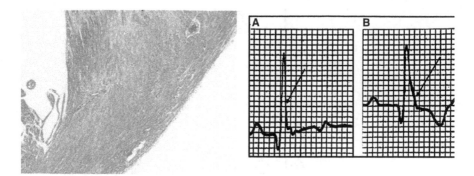

Figure 18 Myocardial necrosis (*left*) produced by abnormal energetics (ratio of myocardial oxygen consumption to oxygen delivery). This form of scarring results in abnormal fracturing of the wave of depolarization as it traverses the fibrotic myocardium. This is manifested as a "sloppy" descent of the R wave (*arrows*) in the QRS complex.

the anthracycline, doxorubicin administered long term), or by altering myocardial energetics (as with excessive catecholamines that alter the relationship between myocardial oxygen consumption and blood flow). Animals whose hearts are driven rapidly and forcefully for prolonged periods may develop, first, acute injury manifested by J-point deviation and then, cell death with replacement of myocardium by fibrous tissue over longer periods of time (Fig. 18). Because fibrosis causes fractionation of otherwise smooth waves of depolarization traversing the myocardium and because myocardial disease in general may produce erratic waves of depolarization, quite commonly the QRS complexes from subjects with myocardial injury have high-frequency components manifested as beads, slurs, or notches, or may have a prolonged descent to R waves. During acute myocardial injury with a sufficient volume of injured myocardium, the J point (ST segment) of the ECG is usually deviated (elevated or depressed) from the baseline. This occurs whenever the myocardium is injured, whether by ischemia or otherwise. When heart rate and/or myocardial contractility increases, myocardial oxygen demand increases, and in the absence of adequate coronary flow reserve, regions of ischemia develop. Since the subendocardium of the left ventricle consumes more oxygen than any other region of the heart, ischemia is most likely to develop there. Subendocardial ischemia of the left ventricular free wall often produces J-point depression (Fig. 19A) in leads (e.g., II, III, aV_F, V_3) "facing" the left ventricular free wall. When the stress leading to ischemia terminates, the J-point returns toward normal. For example, in response to coronary vasoconstriction produced by arginine vasopressin, the myocardium becomes ischemic and J-point depression may occur (Fig. 19B). Unfortunately there are no limits for what deviations are normal in animal models.

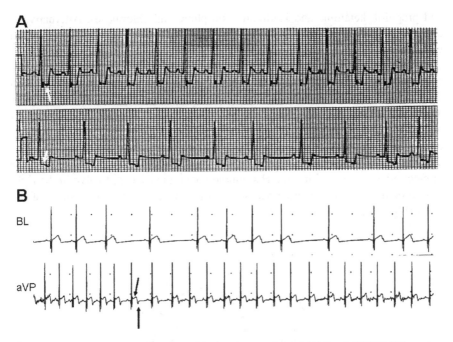

Figure 19 J point changes because of ischemia or necrosis. (**A**) Lead II ECG (25 mm/sec paper speed) from a dog receiving 2-ug/kg norepinephrine. Top trace 30 seconds post-dose, bottom trace 10 minutes postdose. J-point depressions (*white arrows*) indicate subendocardial injury (ischemia) worse when heart rate is elevated because of imbalance between myocardial oxygen delivery and uptake (increased drastically because of increased contractility and rate). (**B**) Lead II ECG before (*top*) and after (*bottom*) exposure to a high concentration of arginine vasopressin. Notice the increase in heart rate and the J-point elevation (*arrow from top*) and terminal T-wave inversion (*arrow from bottom*). These patterns indicate subepicardial ischemia of the left ventricular free wall. *Abbreviation*: ECG, electrocardiogram.

Invasive Electrophysiological Studies

For clinical diagnosis and to explore potential toxic effects of test articles, it is often useful to record voltages directly from the surface of the heart (15). Such recordings are termed cardiac electrograms. Electrograms are frequently recorded during studies involving programmed electrical stimulation (PES) (see below). These studies may determine if a disease process or a drug possesses the potential to produce arrhythmias (most often arrhythmias resulting from reentry), but also permits measurements of refractory periods of atrial and ventricular myocardium or the atrioventricular conduction system (15,51,83,84). Cardiac electrography and PES are often performed in humans in an unsedated state, but when performed on animals, they are usually anesthetized lightly (e.g., midazolam and propofol, ketamine and isoflurane, morphine and chloralose). Alternatively, animals may be preinstrumented with pacing and recording electrodes placed under anesthesia and then studied while conscious.

Since many drug-induced arrhythmias do not occur spontaneously, invasive electrophysiological studies provide a means to evaluate the presence of a drug-induced proarrhythmic substrate—which would provide the opportunity for an adverse electrophysiological event to initiate an arrhythmia. Instrumentation for these studies is performed by guiding catheters containing the electrodes by either fluoroscopy or echocardiography. Individual electrodes affixed to a cardiac catheter contact the ventricular and/or atrial endocardial surface, and a pair of electrodes contacts either the His bundle above the tricuspid valve in the right atrium or the left main bundle accessed easily through a Valsalva sinus of the aorta (Fig. 20).

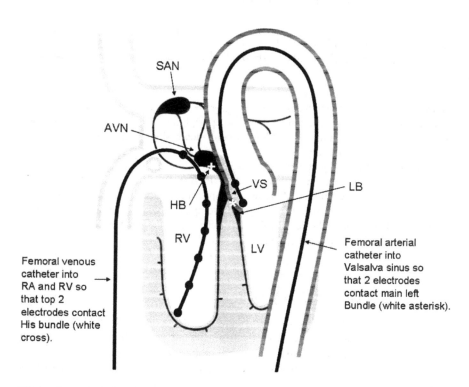

Figure 20 Schematic diagram of the heart into which two cardiac catheters containing multiple electrodes have been introduced. Electrodes on the catheter from the femoral artery touch the left main bundle in a VS. Electrodes on the catheter from the femoral vein touch the HB located just above the tricuspid valve in the right atrium. Positions of the SAN and AVN are identified. *Abbreviations*: VS, Valsalva sinus; HB, His bundle; SAN, sinoatrial node; AVN, atrioventricular node.

Sinus Node Function

Electrophysiological testing may evaluate how drugs affect function of the SA node and the pathway between the SA node and the right atrium. Sinus node recovery time (Fig. 21) and SA conduction time [from SA node to right atrium, sinus node conduction time (SNCT), Fig. 22] may be measured by pacing the sinus node in the right atrium at the junction of the cranial vena cava. The right atrium is paced for approximately 1 minute at a rate significantly more rapid than the rate of SA nodal discharge to overdrive the sinus pacemaker. The shortest time between the last paced beat and the first spontaneous sinus beat measures the sinus node recovery time. The corrected sinus node recovery time (cSNRT) is the SNRT minus the P-P interval proceeding the pacing epoch. This is the time required for the slow diastolic depolarization in the sinus node to reach the threshold value at which more rapid depolarization and excitation develop. For healthy dogs, the SNRT is <850 milliseconds, but it is modulated by anesthesia (if used), temperature, autonomic

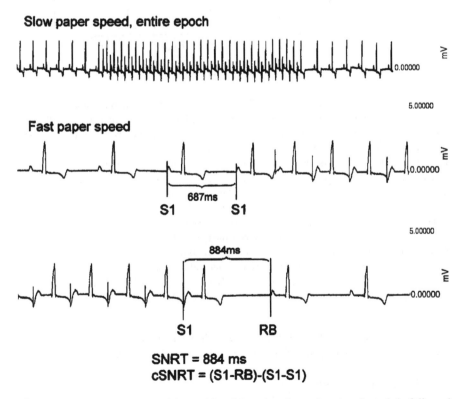

Slow paper speed, entire epoch

Fast paper speed

687ms

S1   S1

884ms

S1   RB

SNRT = 884 ms
cSNRT = (S1-RB)-(S1-S1)

Figure 21 SNRT is measured by rapid atrial pacing that, when terminated, is followed by a sinus nodal discharge. The duration between cessation of pacing and the 1st sinus discharge (RB, Recovery Beat) is the SNRT; the SNRT minus the normal interbeat interval is the (cSNRT). Drugs that affect automaticity often lengthen the SNRT. *Abbreviations*: SNRT, sinus node recovery time; cSNRT, corrected sinus node recovery time.

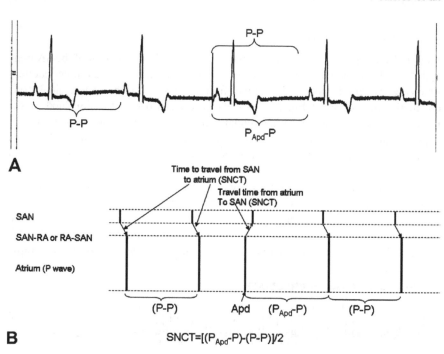

A

B   SNCT=[(P$_{Apd}$-P)-(P-P)]/2

Figure 22 Determination of the SNCT. (**A**) A "late" atrial premature depolarization is introduced by pacing the right atrium near the SA node. The SNCT is calculated as half of the interval between the paced beat and the next beat of sinus origin minus the normal interbeat interval. (see Fig. 21 for further explanation.) (**B**) A modified Lewis diagram (after the great British cardiologist, Sir Thomas Lewis) shows a short vertical line representing SA nodal discharge, a short oblique line representing conduction from the SA node to the right atrium, and a longer vertical line representing atrial depolarization. The interval between the pre-mature atrial depolarization and the next atrial depolarization of sinus origin is the time required for the impulse to enter the SA node over the pathway, the time required to reset the SA node so it will discharge normally, and the time required for the impulse to travel from SA node into the right atrium. Thus, the duration required to for the impulse to travel into and out of the SA node from the right atrium is equal to interval between the paced beat and the next sinus beat minus the normal interbeat interval. But the SNCT (either into or out of the SA node) would be half of that. *Abbreviations*: SA, sinoatrial; SNCT, sinus node conduction time.

balance, and of course chronotropic effects of drugs, all of which are determined by the activity of underlying ion channels (e.g., I_F, $I_{Ca,L}$, I_{CaT}, I_{Kr}).

Refractory Periods

Effects of drugs or test articles on the refractory period are extremely important predictors of the likelihood of toxicity manifested as arrhythmia. Refractory periods of atria, AV node, and ventricles may be measured using intracardiac catheters. To estimate the effective (absolute) refractory period of the ventricle, the ventricle is paced at a fixed rate above the sinus rate, for eight so-called

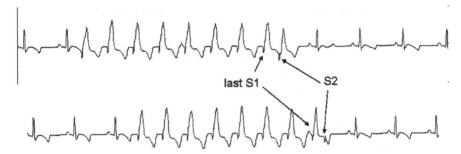

Figure 23 Determination of the ventricular effective refractory period. The right ventricle is paced with eight rapid, conditioning stimuli (S1's), followed by an S2 that occurs early (*top*) but is propagated through the ventricle, that is, a QRS complex follows S2. However, when S2 was introduced still earlier it fell in the effective refractory period of the ventricle and was not propagated (*bottom*), that is, no QRS followed the pacing spike. The shortest S1-S2 that was not propagated determines the duration of the effective refractory period. Note the wide appearance of the QRS, which results from ventricular pacing, in comparison with the narrow QRS occurring in sinus rhythm (first 2 beats) where the ventricle is activated via the rapidly conducting His-Purkinje system.

conditioning stimuli (S1), followed by a premature stimulus (S2); S2 comes progressively earlier (typically 5-milliseconds decrements) with each cycle. When S2 falls in the effective refractory period (Fig. 23), it will not be conducted, that is, it will not produce/elicit a QRS complex. However, if it falls beyond the effective refractory period, it will propagate and elicit a ventricular (QRS) response (Fig. 23). Thus, the shortest interval between the last S1 and S2 that is not conducted is the effective refractory period. Analagous methods may be used to determine the refractoriness of the atria or AV node.

AV Node Function

Refractory periods of the AV conduction system may be estimated in an analogous manner, Figs. 24, 25). The refractory period of the AV node depends on autonomic activity, health of the AV node, and heart rate; the faster the heart rate, the shorter the refractory periods. Many drugs or test articles affect the refractoriness of the AV node, and those that prolong it may have clinical utility for slowing ventricular response (e.g., calcium channel blockers, digitalis) but also may produce adverse effects by producing high degree AV blocks (Fig. 26) or desynchronizing the timing of activation between atria and ventricles. This is of particular concern when there is underlying pathology in the AV node (e.g., fibrosis, which may be increased with advanced age).

Potentially valuable information about drug toxicity on propagation over the AV conduction system may be obtained by pacing protocols and by His bundle electrography (Fig. 20). The His bundle electrogram consists of voltages recorded from two electrodes placed in juxtaposition to the His bundle located in the right atrium just above the tricuspid valve or juxtaposed to the left main

AV conduction time (S2-QRS) with shortening of S1-S2

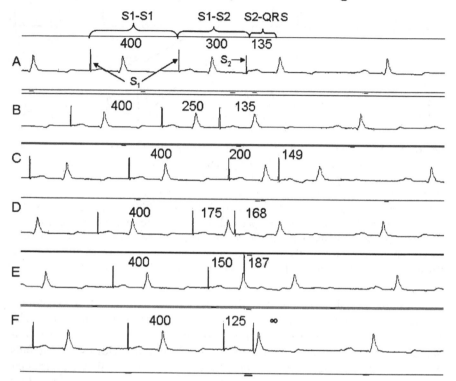

Figure 24   Assessment of AV node conduction. With a basic S1-S1 (conditioning) cycle length of 400 ms (between *arrows*), an S2 is inserted earlier and after the S1. Notice that the PQ intervals for S2s in A and B are 135 ms, but that the PQ interval lengthens (C, D, E) as the S1-S2 becomes shorter and shorter, until there is no PQ following the S2 that followed the S1 by only 125 ms. The right atrium is paced with eight conditioning stimuli and a ninth stimulus is imposed progressively earlier after the eight conditioning stimulus. If the ninth stimulus is conducted through the AV transmission system so that the PQ interval is normal [Fig. 24 (A,B), and Fig. 25, abscissal points 250–300 ms], the conduction is unimpaired. If the impulse is conducted but at a lower velocity (i.e., taking more time to activate the ventricles, manifested as prolongation of the PQ interval), the impulse reached the AV node in its relative refractory period [Fig. 24 (C–E), and Fig. 25, abscissal points 225 through 150 ms]. If the impulse was not conducted at all (i.e., no QRS complex followed the P wave), then the impulse reached the AV node in its effective (absolute) refractory period [Fig. 24 (F) and Fig. 28, abscissal point 125 ms]. *Abbreviation*: AV, atrioventricular.

bundle approached from a Valsalva sinus. The His bundle electrogram consists of three sets of spikes. The first set, termed the "A," is produced by the wave of depolarization traversing the right atrium. The second set, termed the "H," is produced by the wave of depolarization traveling down the His bundle. The third

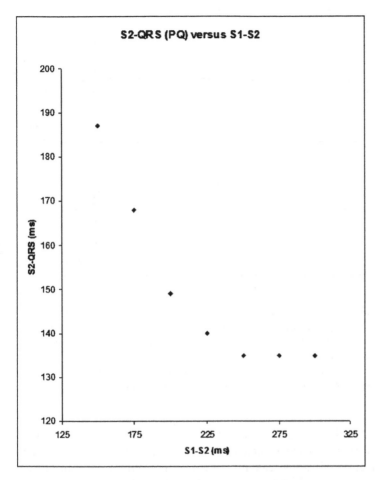

Figure 25 AV node refractory period. A plot of PQ interval (S2-S1) versus the S1-S2 (a measure of the prematurity of S2). Notice that as S2-S1 shortens initially, S1-S2 remains constant because the AV node is fully recovered, that is, out of the relative refractory period. But when S1-S2 shortens more and more, S2-S1 lengthens more and more because the AV node is in its relative refractory period. But after the S1-S2 becomes still shorter, no S2-S1 exists, because the S2 entered the AV node in its effective refractory period. *Abbreviation*: AV, atrioventricular.

set, termed the "V," is produced by the waves of depolarization traversing the ventricle. The A-V interval approximates the PQ interval on the ECG. The A-V interval comprises the A-H (normally ~ 80% of the A-V or PQ), and the H-V (normally ~ 20% of the A-V or PQ). The A-H is the time required for the wave of depolarization to travel from the atrium, through the AV node, and down the short portion of the His bundle immediately inferior to the AV node. Since the vast majority of the A-H is spent traversing the head of the AV node, the A-H is

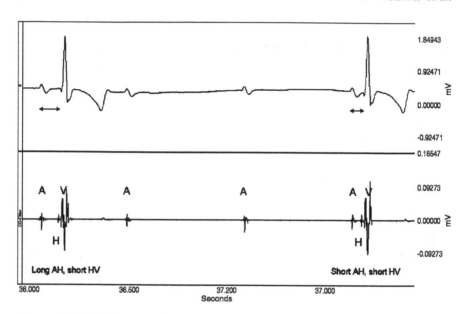

Figure 26 ECG demonstrating periods of second degree AV block (some P waves not followed by QRS complexes, but all QRS complexes are preceded by P waves with a "reasonably" constant PQ interval) after treatment with methacholine. The His bundle electrogram (*bottom trace*) shows the A-H-V for conducted beats, but only the A for nonconducted beats. Thus, this block is confirmed to be within the AV node and not in the His-Purkinje system. *Abbreviations*: EEG, electrocardiogram; AV, atrioventricular.

considered to primarily reflect velocity of propagation through the AV node. Since propagation through this portion of the AV node is dependent on depolarizing current through L-type calcium channels, A-H lengthening most likely reflects a reduction of L-type calcium current. Diltiazem, a calcium channel blocker, is a drug, which prolongs AV conduction; therefore it (Fig. 27) lengthens the PQ interval when compared with baseline. For example, it may be important to determine if drug-induced prolongation of AV conduction—observed by lengthening of the PQ interval—occurs because of retarded conduction through the superior (head of the AV node) or inferior portion (including the His bundle) of the AV transmission system. Propagation in the former is affected by autonomic control and drugs that usually affect $I_{Ca,L}$ (or less often I_{Na}), whereas the latter is affected by drugs that reduce fast inward sodium current (I_{Na}) or more seriously by fibrosis, inflammation, or neoplasia.

Atrial and Ventricular Function

In addition to evaluating refractory periods in the atria and ventricles, as described above, conduction can also be measured. In the atria, this can be done using multiple recording electrodes within a chamber, (e.g., high-right to low-right atrium) to measure conduction time before and after application of a test article.

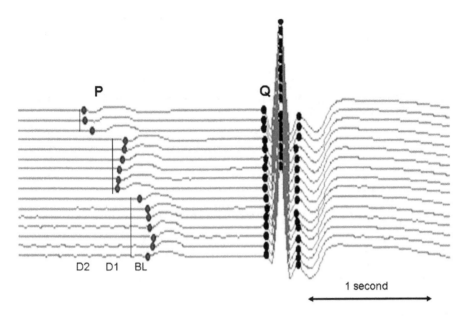

Figure 27 Drug-induced slowing of AV node conduction. ECG (*stacked*) recorded from a pig treated with sequential doses of diltiazem. ECGs are from baseline (BL) (starting at the bottom) and after 0.25 mg/kg of diltiazem (D1) and after 0.5 mg/kg of diltiazem (D2), administered intravenously. Fiduciary points mark (*from left to right*) beginning of P, beginning of QRS, end of QRS, and end of T. Note the dose-dependent prolongation of the PQ interval. *Abbreviations*: EEG, electrocardiogram; AV, atrioventricular.

Conduction within the specialized conduction system of the ventricles can be assessed by the H-V interval (Fig. 28) The H-V interval is the time required to travel from the His bundle to the first portion of the ventricle depolarized, that portion usually being the apical third of the interventricular septum. The H-V is determined by the velocity of propagation over His-Purkinje system and is modulated by fast inward sodium current. Thus, lengthening of the H-V interval most likely reflects a reduction of fast inward sodium current.

Methods to Provoke Arrhythmias: Programmed Electrical Stimulation (15,84,85)

The predilection to develop ventricular arrhythmia by reentry may be predicted by searching for repetitive spontaneous ventricular responses following ventricular pacing. PES is used to elicit reentrant arrhythmias; the ventricle is paced with eight conditioning stimuli (S1) and then with one (S2), two, (S3), or three (S4) extrastimuli; with each extrastimuli occurring within 15 milliseconds of the effective refractory period of the preceding paced beat (Fig. 29). Typically, a bipolar stimulating electrode is placed in contact with the subendocardium of the right ventricle, most often at the apex but occasionally at the outflow tract of the

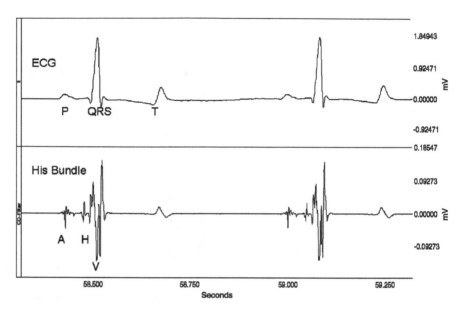

Figure 28 An ECG (*top trace*) and an electrogram from the main left bundle (*bottom trace*) showing normal P, QRS, and T waves on the ECG, and corresponding A, H, and V waves in the electrogram. Notice that AH is normally four to five times the duration of HV, indicating that 85% to 90% of the duration of the PQ interval is spent by the wave of depolarization traveling from SA node to AV node and through the head of the AV node to the left main bundle, with only 10% to 15% of the time spent traveling over the His-Purkinje system to the first portion of the ventricle depolarized (the apical third of the interventricular septum). *Abbreviations*: EEG, electrocardiogram; AV, atrioventricular; AH, atrium-His; HV, His-ventricle.

right ventricle. Stimulation is usually a square wave of twice the mid-diastolic threshold and 2 milliseconds in duration. Note that in a normal heart, the pacemaker is suppressed after the extrastimuli, such that there should be a brief period of cardiac arrest, followed by reinitiation of sinus rhythm. If a substrate for a reentrant arrhythmia is present, the paced beats are immediately followed by rapid ventricular premature depolarizations or a ventricular tachycardia (Fig. 30 bottom) Should an irreversible hemodynamically unstable arrhythmia (ventricular fibrillation or sustained ventricular tachycardia) develop, the subject may be externally countershocked with a DC current of 50 to 150 J and will almost always recover (if the countershock is delivered soon after onset of the arrhythmia). This form of PES is the best method of determining if a drug or test article possesses a tendency to produce ventricular arrhythmias by a reentrant mechanism. As mentioned previously, a tendency to develop arrhythmia by increased automaticity may be predicted by seeking the arrhythmic dose of epinephrine (Fig. 14) or alternatively by the use of sustained (e.g., 30 sec)

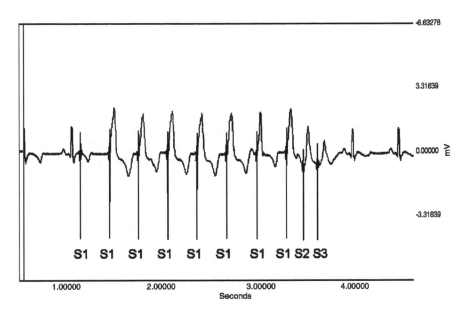

Figure 29 Lead II ECGs showing eight conditioning S1 stimuli followed by premature S2 and S3 extrastimuli. Either ventricle is paced rapidly with eight conditioning stimuli (S1s) followed by an S2 and an S3 that occur prematurely. In hearts not prone to develop reentrant arrhythmias, the heart returns to a sinus rhythm after the S3. *Abbreviation*: EEG, electrocardiogram.

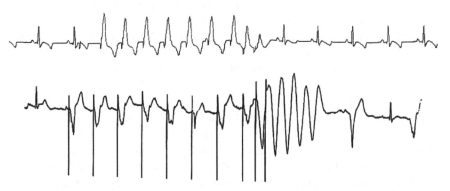

Figure 30 Induction of ventricular arrhythmia. In hearts prone to develop reentrant arrhythmias, the use of ventricular pacing with extrastimuli may induce ectopic activity, termed "repetitive ventricular responses" (RVR). These may evolve into hemodynamically unstable ventricular tachycardia or ventricular fibrillation, thus a defibrillator should be on hand when this provocative test is used to assess arrhythmic potential.

high-rate ventricular pacing. For example, torsadogenic risk (enhanced risk of TdP arrhythmia) may be identified by challenging rabbits in heart failure (Fig. 16) with the test article in question and assessing the presence of this arrhythmia.

ANIMAL MODELS

Electrocardiography and invasive electrophysiological studies remain mainstays for identifying, in vivo, toxicity or potentially toxic effects of drugs on electrophysiological properties of the heart. However, many issues have evolved surrounding in vivo studies utilizing electrocardiography, probably the most contentious of which are animal models (species/strains, age, gender, awake/anesthetized, spontaneous diseases, and what agents) and the use of provocateurs [e.g., programmed stimulation (85), arrhythmic dose of epinephrine (86,87), and sudden change in posture].

Animal models to detect or to predict toxicity to electrophysiological function of the hearts should fulfill all demands imposed on animal models in general. They should possess high sensitivity and specificity for predicting toxicity in man; their preparation should be facile and with a high yield; they should be as inexpensive as possible to purchase and to house, and they should employ neither endangered species nor species dangerous to investigators; they should be docile and large enough for instrumentation and for adequate sampling; they should possess polymorphisms that render them responsive to potential toxicity; they should not be selected because they always have been, or because others have or do. Finally, surrogates for man may be selected because they conserve more genetic similarity to man; however, there is little to no evidence that general genetic similarity translates to more accurate prediction when comparing results from a species to man. Merely possessing similar genes is no assurance that they translate to phenotypical similarity that might make a particular subhuman animal a better or lesser surrogate for predicting toxicity in man.

Most studies have been conducted on dogs (as larger animals) and on rats, mice, rabbits, or guinea pigs (as smaller animals). Nonhuman primates are selected for some test articles principally because they demonstrate metabolism of those test articles most resembling predicted metabolism in humans. Dogs may be eliminated as subjects for some test articles because of their emetic sensitivity or because they may lack the pathways to produce active metabolites that manifest toxicity (e.g., N-acetylprocainamide, a metabolite of the antiarrhythmic drug procainamide). Rats are excluded from studies of potential toxins whose toxicity is mediated via the hERG (I_{Kr}) channel, since they effectively lack functional I_{Kr} current. Rabbits are excluded from studies of potential toxins whose toxicity is mediated via cholinergic receptors (76). Guinea pigs and some rabbits are excluded from studies of potential toxins whose toxicity is mediated via I_{TO} channels because they lack that channel. Birds are excluded from studies in which toxicity may be manifested by effects on ventricular transverse tubules, since they lack these tubules.

Polymorphisms in receptors may restrict use of infrahuman mammals (88) as surrogates for man; however, these restrictions may not be more limiting than searching for toxicity in man because of polymorphisms in man that translate to obvious differences in phenotype. It is not surprising that all humans do not respond identically to either toxic or therapeutic properties of drugs or that humans do not respond identically to infrahuman mammals. Therefore, there is an argument that conducting toxicological studies on animals with vast and varying genetic differences may optimize the chances of identifying a potential toxic effect in man—at least in some individuals. Most toxicological research is conducted using subjects (species and strains) with the greatest possible genetic similarity. This, most often, reduces variability in parameters being interrogated and decreases the number of subjects necessary to achieve satisfactory statistical power. If the genetic strain happens to possess the phenotype that exhibits toxicity, then the selection of genetically similar individuals is justified. However, if the genetic strain happens not to possess the phenotype, then the sensitivity of a study for predicting toxicity in man, using that strain, will be 0. Unless the specific target, when affected by the test article, is known and unless it is known whether or not the target exists in a specific species or strain, the species/strain selected may be useless.

Once the species/strain is selected, the parameters to be interrogated should be selected and the variance of the parameters evaluated/estimated to determine the number of subjects required to achieve the desired statistical power.[c] The variance of the parameters is affected by multiple parameters, and the initial assessment should include variability arising from conscious versus anesthetized preparations, or the need for restraint. If the animal is to be studied awake or heavily sedated or narcotized, which chemical restraints are least likely to obfuscate the results? There is little point evaluating chronotropy in an untrained monkey restrained in a chair, since the heart rate will be nearly fixed at close to 240 beats/min, and no test article is likely to drive it faster (or possibly even reduce the rate). An animal restrained with all general anesthetics except morphine-chloralose or dial-urethane may have ventricular irritability increased (as with low concentration of halothane[d]), or decreased (as with high concentrations of halothane). A distinct advantage, however, to volatile anesthetics is the ability to maintain relatively constant tissue concentrations. A well-calibrated vaporizer set to deliver 2% isoflurane should sustain a relatively constant tissue concentration of anesthetic. This is nearly impossible with anesthetics given parenterally, since (*i*) tissue concentrations are almost never measured and will change depending on rates of infusion, metabolism, and excretion and (*ii*) there is typically a long time between when a blood sample is drawn, the anesthetic

---

[c] This variance, the alpha level, and the differences sought are all required to calculate power, and most Laboratory Animal Care and Use Committee (ILACUC) and sponsors of research require, a priori, estimates of power.

[d] In addition, most volatile anesthetics are power-negative inotropes.

concentration is measured, and remedial action may be taken. Obviously, variability of tissue concentrations of anesthetics with their own cardiovascular effects may impact on identifying potential toxicities of test articles (89).

For example, the ganglioplegic property of barbiturates will produce an initial cardioacceleration, then cardiodeceleration as arterial blood pH and body temperature fall (though temperature may be controlled by externally applied heat). Thiobarbiturates frequently produce ventricular bigeminy and block many cardiac ion currents at higher concentrations) (90,91). Xylazine is an α-2 agonist, which produces pronounced early cardiodeceleration and may favor production of escape rhythms; acepromazine is an α-1 antagonist, which may block arrhythmias mediated by stimulation of α-1 adrenergic receptors. Opiates are powerfully vagomimetic; these may favor development of escape ventricular ectopy or may suppress enhanced irritability. Morphine chloralose is an anesthetic combination, which is thought to maintain autonomic activity identical with that of a naturally sleeping animal. However, as it must be given in rather large volumes and produces hemodilution, it should be prepared in lactated Ringer's solution (to preserve normalcy of serum electrolytes). The potential effects of reductions in protein and erythrocyte concentrations—but not amounts—should be considered when using chloralose. In general, if a study is designed to determine pharmacokinetics, the type of anesthesia is less important than if the study is designed to determine cardiovascular, respiratory, or autonomic effects.

Why would chemical restraint ever be used? It removes pain, the removal of which is of value for both humane reasons and to prevent sympathoadrenal surges. It allows for a stable preparation insensitive to psychological influences. It allows for more extensive instrumentation. In general, parameter variability is reduced under chemical restraint. A question as of yet unanswered is: How often does chemical restraint obfuscate identifying a toxic potential for a test article to be used in man?

DISEASE MODELS: (92–94)

Drugs are not given to healthy persons, and it is well known that persons with diseases may not always respond to drugs as healthy persons might. For example, persons with ventricular hypertrophy, heart failure, and electrolyte imbalance are more prone to develop TdP than are persons in good health. A logical question is "why search for toxicity in a preparation different from the target species to which a drug may be given?" For example, if simvastatin is given to patients with hypercholesterolemia, why not search for toxicity in animal models with hypercholesterolemia? We know full well that at different stages of clinical trials, males and females, young and old, and persons of varying ethnic origins may be included in the study population. The more varied the individuals, the more extrapolatable should be the results to the general population[e].

---

[e]A corollary to that statement is the better controlled the study, the less extrapolatable should the results be to the general population.

With the availability of animal models with iatrogenic diseases manifested commonly in man (e.g., streptozotocin-induced diabetes, coronary ligation–induced heart failure, aortic-banded-induced left ventricular hypertrophy), would use of those surrogate preparations uncover toxic liabilities not demonstrable when studying normal surrogates? What would be the extra costs in dollars and animal life to conduct them? Which disease models should be used? Would the models, in fact, improve sensitivity without reducing specificity even more? Would regulatory agencies accept, expect, or demand such studies? Do more persons manifest morbidity and mortality from toxic drugs or from efficacious drugs being denied because they were thought to be toxic? Is the price paid for studying genetic similarity (where the cost of these studies is reduced because of less variability in parameters measured) offset by the reduced generalizability to a broad population?

TORSADES DE POINTES

Sudden cardiac death occurs in approximately 300,000 persons in the United States each year, and approximately 15,000 of those deaths are thought to be due to the polymorphic ventricular tachycardia termed "torsades de pointes," which evolves into ventricular fibrillation approximately 20% of the time. Although many drugs used for treating heart disease (e.g., quinidine, ibutilide, sotalol) (40,95,96) may produce TdP at high concentrations or in the presence of multiple risk factors, often the culprit drug (termed a torsadogen) is used for a non-life-threatening disease (e.g., colds, allergy, anxiety, depression). Thus, drug-induced death from TdP is particularly devastating (unexpected), and regulatory agencies and the pharmaceutical industry are greatly concerned about the risk of TdP (97,98). In fact, a common cause for removal of a drug from the marketplace is torsadogenicity (99–101).

TdP is thought to occur most often in people taking rather high doses of torsadogenic or/and in those who may have inadvertently increased drug exposure by blocking metabolism of torsadogenic agents (e.g., by ingestion of grapefruit juice, erythromycin, ketoconazole). TdP is linked with polymorphisms/mutations in ion channels responsible for affecting ventricular repolarization (congenital long QT syndromes) and in cases where drugs may affect ventricular repolarization (acquired long QT syndrome, Fig. 31). Such ion channels include the delayed rectifier current that plays a prominent role in defining ventricular repolarization in humans and higher mammals (I_{Kr}) as well as toxins that inhibit sodium channel closure (e.g., ATXII) (102,103) to augment depolarizing current to delay repolarization. Drugs linked with TdP are found in almost every therapeutic class (e.g., antihistamines, antipsychotics, prokinetics, antibiotics). The initiating electrocardiogaphic pattern of acquired long TdP consists of a rather slow heart rate, a long QT, a long interbeat interval (not always present) (104) followed by a short interbeat interval, due to a closely coupled premature ventricular depolarization occurring on the T wave of the

Delayed Repolarization: Links to Torsade

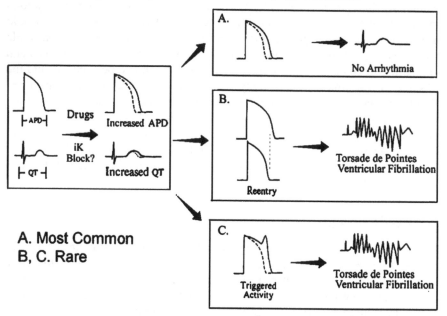

Figure 31 Drug-induced delayed repolarization and potential mechanisms of torsades de pointes. Delayed repolarization typically leads to delayed repolarization with no further consequences (right panel **A**). Two postulated mechanisms responsible for torsades de pointes arrhythmia are illustrated in lower panels. A drug that promotes greater dispersion of repolarization in different regions of the heart (e.g., greater prolongation in mid-myocardium vs. endocardium) could set the stage for block and reentry, leading to proarrhythmia (panel **B**). It has also been postulated that drug-induced prolongation could lead to EADs and triggered activity, resulting in torsades de pointes (panel **C**). To complicate matters further, both B and C could occur simultaneously to promote proarrhythmia. Adapted from Ref. 113. *Abbreviation*: EADs, early afterdepolarizations.

previous beat of sinus origin, and a rapid polymorphic ventricular tachycardia with QRS complexes changing polarity. It appears that the long interbeat interval preceding TdP "triggers" abnormal function of specific ion channels determining ventricular repolarization, such that when a beat is initiated with a short interbeat interval, the channel physiology sustains the depolarized membrane at a potential that permits abnormal calcium influx that triggers EADs. Although long QT is a putative marker for TdP, it is actually a marker for the abnormal repolarization and calcium cycling that are the proximate causes of the arrhythmia.

Although TdP is rare, regulatory agencies are concerned greatly with this arrhythmia and impose enormous demands on the pharmaceutical industry to minimize the likelihood of marketing a potentially torsadogenic agent. The reader is referred to recent reviews (99,101,105).

A FINAL NOTE ABOUT ADDRESSING ELECTROPHYSIOLOGICAL HAZARD RISK ASSESSMENTS—PHARMACEUTICAL AND REGULATORY CONCERNS

As mentioned previously, drug regulatory agencies and the pharmaceutical industry are interested in identifying toxic or potential toxic effects of drugs on electrophysiological properties of the heart (97,98). Drugs may exert toxicity by functionally affecting ion channels specific for depolarization (e.g., I_{Na}) and/or repolarization (e.g., I_{Kr}) (56,106). For example, blockade of I_{Na}, as with quinidine, may slow conduction through atria (prolonging the P wave), through the ventricles (prolonging the QRS complex), or across the AV conduction system (prolonging the PQ interval). Of course, reduced calcium conductance may also prolong the PQ interval and may decrease rate of discharge of SA node. These effects may translate to impaired force of contraction because of decreased synchrony of contraction within the ventricles or between the atria and the ventricles, and/or because of decreased availability of calcium to initiate excitation-contraction coupling. These effects may be observed with high concentrations of drugs or with rapidly escalating concentrations. Drugs (e.g., dofetilide, cisapride) that block hERG (I_{Kr}) or that retard closure of sodium channels (veratridine, ATXII) delay repolarization, typically produce prolongation of the QT interval on the ECG.

Some drugs have been linked to the rare but potentially lethal arrhythmia TdP, forcing warnings on product labels and/or their removal from the market. In fact, as mentioned above, QT liability is a common cause for drug removal from the market. This has led to the expectation by regulatory agencies that effects of all drugs on hERG physiology will be studied (98). While liability to block hERG has high sensitivity (with the exception of arsenic trioxide and pentamidine, which inhibit trafficking of hERG channels to the cell surface membrane), many drugs that block hERG do not possess, or possess minimially, torsadogenic liability (verapamil, pentobarbital, amiodarone), either because they possess multichannel effects or because they may decrease heterogenicity of ventricular repolarization. Drugs that block cardiac calcium current may lead to triangulation of the action potential (the action potential becomes less "rectangular," repolarizing more gradually) and possibly negative inotropy (reduced contractility). While the safety/utility of triangulation is still debated (8,107), negative inotropic effects are to be avoided. Controversy regarding I_{K1} block may be related to the extent of block, with smaller levels of I_{K1} block leading to minimal changes in excitability (and possibly some prolongation of terminal repolarization), while greater levels of I_{K1} block leading to slowed (or blocked) conduction and eventual inexcitability. It has been suggested that the proximate cause of TdP is not reduced repolarizing current per se but delayed repolarization affecting internal calcium cycling (41). This concept is consistent with the recognition that delayed repolarization and QT interval prolongation is a surrogate marker of proarrhythmia. Adaptive preclinical studies melding in vitro studies [including ion currents and repolarization (action potential duration) studies] with in vivo studies (including thorough ECG analysis) that are properly and statistically powered will provide the best understanding of potential risks of cardiac toxicity with novel drug candidates.

REFERENCES

1. Barr RC. Genesis of the electrocardiogram. In: Macfarlane PW, Lawrie TDV, eds. Comprehensive Electrocardiology: Theory and Practice in Health and Disease. Vol 1. New York: Perganmon Press, 1989:129–151.
2. Scher AM, Spach MS. Cardiac depolarization and repolarization and the elctrocardiogram. In: Berne RM, Sperelakis N, Geiger SR, eds. Handbook of Physiology, Section 2: The cardiovascular system. Bethesda: American Physiological Society, 1979:357–392.
3. Bers DM. Excitation-Contraction Coupling and Cardiac Contractile Force. Dordrect, The Netherlands: Kluwer Academic Publishers, 2001.
4. Topol EJ. Failing the public health–rofecoxib, Merck, and the FDA. N Engl J Med 2004; 351:1707–1709.
5. Connolly HM, Crary JL, McGoon MD, et al. Valvular heart disease associated with fenfluramine-phentermine. N Engl J Med 1997; 337:581–588.
6. Connolly SJ, Dorian P, Roberts RS, et al. Comparison of beta-blockers, amiodarone plus beta-blockers, or sotalol for prevention of shocks from implantable cardioverter defibrillators: the OPTIC Study: a randomized trial. JAMA 2006; 295:165–171.
7. Furukawa Y, Xue YX, Chiba S, et al. Effects of zatebradine on ouabain-, two-stage coronary ligation- and epinephrine-induced ventricular tachyarrhythmias. Eur J Pharmacol 1996; 300:203–210.
8. Hondeghem LM. TRIad: foundation for proarrhythmia (triangulation, reverse use dependence and instability). Novartis Found Symp 2005; 266:235–244.
9. Hondeghem LM, Snyders DJ. Class III antiarrhythmic agents have a lot of potential but a long way to go. Reduced effectiveness and dangers of reverse use dependence. Circulation 1990; 81:686–690.
10. January CT, Riddle JM. Early afterdepolarizations: mechanism of induction and block. A role for L-type Ca2+ current. Circ Res 1989; 64:977–990.
11. Jiao Z, De Jesus VR, Iravanian S, et al. A possible mechanism of halocarbon-induced cardiac sensitization arrhythmias. J Mol Cell Cardiol 2006; 41:698–705.
12. Miyamoto S, Zhu B, Teramatsu T, et al. QT-prolonging class I drug, disopyramide, does not aggravate but suppresses adrenaline-induced arrhythmias. Comparison with cibenzoline and pilsicainide. Eur J Pharmacol 2000; 400:263–269.
13. Ranger S, Nattel S. Determinants and mechanisms of flecainide-induced promotion of ventricular tachycardia in anesthetized dogs. Circulation 1995; 92:1300–1311.
14. Rosen MR, Legato MJ. Repolarization: physiological and structural determinants, and pathophysiological changes. Eur Heart J 1985; 6(suppl D):3–14.
15. Fogoros RN. Electrophysiologic Testing. Malden, MA: Blackwell Science, Inc, 1999.
16. Hamlin RL, Smith CR. Anatomical and physiological basis for interpretation of the electrocardiogram. Am J Vet Res 1960; 21:701–709.
17. Horan LG, Flowers NC. Electrocardiography and vectorcardiography. In Heart Disease, ed. E. Braunwald, 198-Philadelphia: WB Saunders, 1980.

18. Tilley LP. Essentials of Canine and Feline Electrocardiography. Philadelphia: Lea & Febiger, 1992.
19. Zipes DP, Jalife J. Cardiac electrophysiology: From cell to bedside. Philadelphia: WB Saunders, 2004.
20. Antzelevitch C, Dumaine R. Electrical heterogeneity in the heart: Physiological, pharmacological and clinical implications. In: Fozzard H, Solaro RJ, ed. Handbook of Electrophysiology: The Heart. New York: Oxford University Press, 2002: 654–692.
21. Boyett MR, Honjo H, Kodama I. The sinoatrial node, a heterogeneous pacemaker structure. Cardiovasc Res 2000; 47:658–687.
22. Irisawa H, Brown HF, Giles W. Cardiac pacemaking in the sinoatrial node. Physiol Rev 1993; 73:197–227.
23. Opthof T. Embryological development of pacemaker hierarchy and membrane currents related to the function of the adult sinus node: implications for autonomic modulation of biopacemakers. Med Biol Eng Comput 2007; 45:119–132.
24. Kleber AG, Rudy Y. Basic mechanisms of cardiac impulse propagation and associated arrhythmias. Physiol Rev 2004; 84:431–488.
25. Mazgalev TN, Ho SY, Anderson RH. Anatomic-electrophysiological correlations concerning the pathways for atrioventricular conduction. Circulation 2001; 103: 2660–2667.
26. Hamlin RL, Robinson FR, Smith CR. Electrocardiogram and vectorcardiogram of Macaca mulatta in various postures. Am J Physiol 1961; 201:1083–1089.
27. Hamlin RL, Smith CR, Redding RW. Time-order of ventricular activation for premature beats in sheep and dogs. Am J Physiol 1960; 198:315–321.
28. Kang M, Chung KY, Walker JW. G-protein coupled receptor signaling in myocardium: not for the faint of heart. Physiology (Bethesda) 2007; 22:174–184.
29. Carmeliet E. Cardiac ionic currents and acute ischemia: from channels to arrhythmias. Physiol Rev 1999; 79:917–1017.
30. Satoh H. Sino-atrial nodal cells of mammalian hearts: ionic currents and gene expression of pacemaker ionic channels. J Smooth Muscle Res 2003; 39:175–193.
31. Mangoni ME, Marger L, Nargeot J. If current inhibition: cellular basis and physiology. Adv Cardiol 2006; 43:17–30.
32. Nerbonne JM, Kass RS. Molecular physiology of cardiac repolarization. Physiol Rev 2005; 85:1205–1253.
33. Bers DM. The beat goes on: diastolic noise that just won't quit. Circ Res 2006; 99:921–923.
34. Lakatta EG, Maltsev VA, Bogdanov KY, et al. Cyclic variation of intracellular calcium: a critical factor for cardiac pacemaker cell dominance. Circ Res 2003; 92: e45–e50.
35. Noble D, Cohen I. The interpretation of the T wave of the electrocardiogram. Cardiovasc Res 1978; 12:13–27.
36. Antzelevitch C, Shimizu W, Yan GX, et al. Cellular basis for QT dispersion. J Electrocardiol 1998; 30(suppl):168–175.
37. Brown HF. Electrophysiology of the sinoatrial node. Physiol Rev 1982; 62:505–530.
38. Savelieva I, Camm AJ. Novel If current inhibitor ivabradine: safety considerations. Adv Cardiol 2006; 43:79–96.
39. Moak JP, Rosen MR. Induction and termination of triggered activity by pacing in isolated canine Purkinje fibers. Circulation 1984; 69:149–162.

40. Roden DM, Thompson KA, Hoffman BF, et al. Clinical features and basic mechanisms of quinidine-induced arrhythmias. J Am Coll Cardiol 1986; 8:73A–78A.
41. Sipido KR. Calcium overload, spontaneous calcium release, and ventricular arrhythmias. Heart Rhythm 2006; 3:977–979.
42. Rosen MR. Cellular electrophysiology of digitalis toxicity. J Am Coll Cardiol 1985; 5:22A–34A.
43. Anyukhovsky EP, Sosunov EA, Rosen MR. Regional differences in electrophysiological properties of epicardium, midmyocardium, and endocardium. In vitro and in vivo correlations. Circulation 1996; 94:1981–1988.
44. Gintant GA, Limberis JT, McDermott JS, et al. The canine Purkinje fiber: an in vitro model system for acquired long QT syndrome and drug-induced arrhythmogenesis. J Cardiovasc Pharmacol 2001; 37:607–618.
45. Hamlin RL, Cruze CA, Mittelstadt SW, et al. Sensitivity and specificity of isolated perfused guinea pig heart to test for drug-induced lengthening of QTc. J Pharmacol Toxicol Methods 2004; 49:15–23.
46. Hondeghem LM, Hoffmann P. Blinded test in isolated female rabbit heart reliably identifies action potential duration prolongation and proarrhythmic drugs: importance of triangulation, reverse use dependence, and instability. J Cardiovasc Pharmacol 2003; 41:14–24.
47. Cheng J. Evidences of the gender-related differences in cardiac repolarization and the underlying mechanisms in different animal species and human. Fundam Clin Pharmacol 2006; 20:1–8.
48. Lu HR, Marien R, Saels A, et al. Species plays an important role in drug-induced prolongation of action potential duration and early afterdepolarizations in isolated Purkinje fibers. J Cardiovasc Electrophysiol 2001; 12:93–102.
49. Lu HR, Remeysen P, Somers K, et al. Female gender is a risk factor for drug-induced long QT and cardiac arrhythmias in an in vivo rabbit model. J Cardiovasc Electrophysiol 2001; 12:538–545.
50. Pham TV, Rosen MR. Sex, hormones, and repolarization. Cardiovasc Res 2002; 53:740–751.
51. Redfern WS, Carlsson L, Davis AS, et al. Relationships between preclinical cardiac electrophysiology, clinical QT interval prolongation and torsade de pointes for a broad range of drugs: evidence for a provisional safety margin in drug development. Cardiovasc Res 2003; 58:32–45.
52. Solberg LE, Singer DH, Ten Eick RE, et al. Glass microelectrode studies on intramural papillary muscle cells. Description of preparation and studies on normal dog papillary muscle. Circ Res 1974; 34:783–797.
53. Carnes CA, Geisbuhler TP, Reiser PJ. Age-dependent changes in contraction and regional myocardial myosin heavy chain isoform expression in rats. J Appl Physiol 2004; 97:446–453.
54. Hayashi S, Kii Y, Tabo M, et al. QT PRODACT: a multi-site study of in vitro action potential assays on 21 compounds in isolated guinea-pig papillary muscles. J Pharmacol Sci 2005; 99:423–437.
55. Zhang S, Zhou Z, Gong Q, et al. Mechanism of block and identification of the verapamil binding domain to HERG potassium channels. Circ Res 1999; 84:989–998.
56. Roden DM. Taking the "idio" out of "idiosyncratic": predicting torsades de pointes. Pacing Clin Electrophysiol 1998; 21:1029–1034.

57. Martin RL, McDermott JS, Salmen HJ, et al. The utility of hERG and repolarization assays in evaluating delayed cardiac repolarization: influence of multi-channel block. J Cardiovasc Pharmacol 2004; 43:369–379.
58. Yan GX, Antzelevitch C. Cellular basis for the electrocardiographic J wave. Circulation 1996; 93:372–379.
59. Yan GX, Antzelevitch C. Cellular basis for the normal T wave and the electrocardiographic manifestations of the long-QT syndrome. Circulation 1998; 98:1928–1936.
60. Yan GX, Shimizu W, Antzelevitch C. Characteristics and distribution of M cells in arterially perfused canine left ventricular wedge preparations. Circulation 1998; 98:1921–1927.
61. Sicouri S, Moro S, Elizari MV. d-Sotalol Induces Marked Action Potential Prolongation and Early Afterdepolarizations in M but Not Empirical or Endocardial Cells of the Canine Ventricle. J Cardiovasc Pharmacol Ther 1997; 2:27–38.
62. Strauss HC, Bigger JT Jr., Hoffman BF. Electrophysiologial and beta-receptor blocking effects of MJ 1999 on dog and rabbit cardiac tissue. Circ Res 1970; 26:661–678.
63. Skrzypiec-Spring M, Grotthus B, Szelag A, et al. Isolated heart perfusion according to Langendorff—still viable in the new millennium. J Pharmacol Toxicol Methods 2007; 55:113–126.
64. Franz MR. Current status of monophasic action potential recording: theories, measurements and interpretations. Cardiovasc Res 1999; 41:25–40.
65. Fossa AA, Wisialowski T, Magnano A, et al. Dynamic beat-to-beat modeling of the QT-RR interval relationship: analysis of QT prolongation during alterations of autonomic state versus human ether a-go-go-related gene inhibition. J Pharmacol Exp Ther 2005; 312:1–11.
66. Thomsen MB, Verduyn SC, Stengl M, et al. Increased short-term variability of repolarization predicts d-sotalol-induced torsades de pointes in dogs. Circulation 2004; 110:2453–2459.
67. Efimov IR, Nikolski VP, Salama G. Optical imaging of the heart. Circ Res 2004; 95:21–33.
68. Hamlin RL, Cruze CA, Mittelstadt SW, et al. Sensitivity and specificity of isolated perfused guinea pig heart to test for drug-induced lengthening of QTc. J Pharmacol Toxicol Methods 2004; 49:15–23.
69. Valentin JP, Hoffmann P, De Clerck F, et al. Review of the predictive value of the Langendorff heart model (Screenit system) in assessing the proarrhythmic potential of drugs. J Pharmacol Toxicol Methods 2004; 49:171–181.
70. Bayley RH. Biophysical Prinicples of Electrocardiography. New York: Paul B. Hoeber, Inc, 1958.
71. Hamlin RL, Burton RR, Leverett SD, et al. Ventricular activation process in minipigs. J Electrocardiol 1975; 8:113–116.
72. Stein IM, Ferriero T. Letter: Computer analysis of ECG's. N Engl J Med 1976; 294:1128–1129.
73. Loughrey CM, Smith GL, MacEachern KE. Comparison of Ca2+ release and uptake characteristics of the sarcoplasmic reticulum in isolated horse and rabbit cardiomyocytes. Am J Physiol Heart Circ Physiol 2004; 287:H1149–H1159.
74. Hamlin RL, Nakayama T, Nakayama H, et al. Effects of changing heart rate on electrophysiological and hemodynamic function in the dog. Life Sci 2003; 72: 1919–1930.

75. Hamlin RL, Smith CR, Smetzer DL. Sinus arrhythmia in the dog. Am J Physiol 1966; 210:321–328.

76. Olson ME, Vizzutti D, Morck DW, et al. The parasympatholytic effects of atropine sulfate and glycopyrrolate in rats and rabbits. Can J Vet Res 1994; 58:254–258.

77. Thompson KA, Blair IA, Woosley RL, et al. Comparative in vitro electrophysiology of quinidine, its major metabolites and dihydroquinidine. J Pharmacol Exp Ther 1987; 241:84–90.

78. Yamamoto K, Tamura T, Imai R, et al. Acute canine model for drug-induced Torsades de Pointes in drug safety evaluation-influences of anesthesia and validation with quinidine and astemizole. Toxicol Sci 2001; 60:165–176.

79. Aytemir K, Maarouf N, Gallagher MM, et al. Comparison of formulae for heart rate correction of QT interval in exercise electrocardiograms. Pacing Clin Electrophysiol 1999; 22:1397–1401.

80. Funck-Brentano C, Jaillon P. Rate-corrected QT interval: techniques and limitations. Am J Cardiol 1993; 72:17B–22B.

81. Hnatkova K, Malik M. "Optimum" formulae for heart rate correction of the QT interval. Pacing Clin Electrophysiol 1999; 22:1683–1687.

82. Malik M. Problems of heart rate correction in assessment of drug-induced QT interval prolongation. J Cardiovasc Electrophysiol 2001; 12:411–420.

83. Billman GE, Hamlin RL. The effects of mibefradil, a novel calcium channel antagonist on ventricular arrhythmias induced by myocardial ischemia and programmed electrical stimulation. J Pharmacol Exp Ther 1996; 277:1517–1526.

84. Rahimtoola SH, Zipes DP, Akhtar M, et al. Consensus statement of the Conference on the State of the Art of Electrophysiologic Testing in the Diagnosis and Treatment of Patients with Cardiac Arrhythmias. Circulation 1987; 75:III3–III11.

85. Brugada P, Green M, Abdollah H, et al. Significance of ventricular arrhythmias initiated by programmed ventricular stimulation: the importance of the type of ventricular arrhythmia induced and the number of premature stimuli required. Circulation 1984; 69:87–92.

86. Mullin LS, Azar A, Reinhardt CF, et al. Halogenated hydrocarbon-induced cardiac arrhythmias associated with release of endogenous epinephrine. Am Ind Hyg Assoc J 1972; 33:389–396.

87. Navarro R, Weiskopf RB, Moore MA, et al. Humans anesthetized with sevoflurane or isoflurane have similar arrhythmic response to epinephrine. Anesthesiology 1994; 80:545–549.

88. Wymore RS, Gintant GA, Wymore RT, et al. Tissue and species distribution of mRNA for the IKr-like K+ channel, erg. Circ Res 1997; 80:261–268.

89. Chaves AA, Dech SJ, Nakayama T, et al. Age and anesthetic effects on murine electrocardiography. Life Sci 2003; 72:2401–2412.

90. Carnes CA, Muir WW, III, Van Wagoner DR. Effect of intravenous anesthetics on inward rectifier potassium current in rat and human ventricular myocytes. Anesthesiology 1997; 87:327–334.

91. Nattel S, Wang ZG, Matthews C. Direct electrophysiological actions of pentobarbital at concentrations achieved during general anesthesia. Am J Physiol 1990; 259:H1743–H1751.

92. Billman GE. A Comprehensive Review and Analysis of 25 Years of Data From an in vivo Canine Model of Sudden Cardiac Death: Implications for Future Antiarrhythmic Drug Development. Pharmacol Ther 2006; 808–835.

93. Hamlin RL. Animal models of ventricular arrhythmias. Pharmacol Ther 2007; 113: 276–295.
94. Janse MJ, Opthof T, Kleber AG. Animal models of cardiac arrhythmias. Cardiovasc Res 1998; 39:165–177.
95. Cubeddu LX. QT prolongation and fatal arrhythmias: a review of clinical implications and effects of drugs. Am J Ther 2003; 10:452–457.
96. MacNeil DJ, Davies RO, Deitchman D. Clinical safety profile of sotalol in the treatment of arrhythmias. Am J Cardiol 1993; 72:44A–50A.
97. Anonymous ICHS7A Safety pharmacology studies for human pharmaceuticals Washington, DC: U.S. Food and Drug Administration, 2001.
98. Anonymous ICHS7B safety pharmacology studies for assessing the potential for delayed ventricular repolarization (QT interval prolongation) by human pharmaceuticals. Washington, DC: U.S. Food and Drug Administration, 2002.
99. Roden DM. Drug-induced prolongation of the QT interval. N Engl J Med 2004; 350:1013–1022.
100. Roden DM, Temple R. The US Food and Drug Administration Cardiorenal Advisory Panel and the drug approval process. Circulation 2005; 111:1697–1702.
101. Shah RR. Drug-induced QT interval prolongation–regulatory guidance and perspectives on hERG channel studies. Novartis Found Symp 2005; 266:251–280.
102. Moss AJ, Zareba W, Benhorin J, et al. ECG T-wave patterns in genetically distinct forms of the hereditary long QT syndrome. Circulation 1995; 92:2929–2934.
103. Roden DM. Long QT syndrome: reduced repolarization reserve and the genetic link. J Intern Med 2006; 259:59–69.
104. Gbadebo TD, Trimble RW, Khoo MS, et al. Calmodulin inhibitor W-7 unmasks a novel electrocardiographic parameter that predicts initiation of torsade de pointes. Circulation 2002; 105:770–774.
105. Kannankeril PJ, Roden DM. Drug-induced long QT and torsade de pointes: recent advances. Curr Opin Cardiol 2007; 22:39–43.
106. Eckhardt LL, Rajamani S, January CT. Protein trafficking abnormalities: a new mechanism in drug-induced long QT syndrome. Br J Pharmacol 2005; 145:3–4.
107. Hondeghem LM. Relative contributions of TRIaD and QT to proarrhythmia. J Cardiovasc Electrophysiol 2007; 18:655–657.
108. 1991. The Sicilian gambit. A new approach to the classification of antiarrhythmic drugs based on their actions on arrhythmogenic mechanisms. Task Force of the Working Group on Arrhythmias of the European Society of Cardiology. Circulation 84:1831–1851.
109. Sicouri S, Antzelevitch C. A subpopulation of cells with unique electrophysiological properties in the deep subepicardium of the canine ventricle. The M cell. Circ Res 1991; 68:1729–1741.
110. Gintant GA, Su Z, Martin RL, et al. Utility of hERG assays as surrogate markers of delayed cardiac repolarization and QT safety. Toxicol Pathol 2006; 34:81–90.
111. Carlsson L. In vitro and in vivo models for testing arrhythmogenesis in drugs. J Intern Med 2006; 259:70–80.
112. Shimizu W, Antzelevitch C. Sodium channel block with mexiletine is effective in reducing dispersion of repolarization and preventing torsade des pointes in LQT2 and LQT3 models of the long-QT syndrome. Circulation 1997; 96:2038–2047.
113. Ebert SN, Liu XK, Woosley RL. Female gender as a risk factor for drug-induced cardiac arrhythmias: evaluation of clinical and experimental evidence. J Womens Health 1998; 7:547–557.

11

Cardiovascular Effects of Steroidal Agents

Russell B. Melchert

Department of Pharmaceutical Sciences, University of Arkansas for Medical Sciences, College of Pharmacy, Little Rock, Arkansas, U.S.A.

Scott M. Belcher

Department of Pharmacology and Cell Biophysics, University of Cincinnati College of Medicine, Cincinnati, Ohio, U.S.A.

Richard H. Kennedy

Department of Physiology, Loyola University Medical Center, Stritch School of Medicine, Maywood, Illinois, U.S.A.

INTRODUCTION

Overview

The steroidal agents are a group of compounds with remarkable diversity in target tissues and actions. Steroidal agents include androgens, estrogens, progestins, glucocorticoids, mineralocorticoids, cholesterol, bile acids, cardiac glycosides, and other compounds. Receptors for steroids are found throughout the cardiovascular system of nearly every species examined. Not surprisingly, the cardiovascular system is the target of many steroid actions through either indirect effects or direct effects mediated by direct interaction of the steroids with vascular or cardiac cells. In addition, continued identification of rapid signaling mechanisms of steroid action raise questions as to the diversity of cardiovascular tissues that may be susceptible to steroid-mediated effects. Similarly, increased awareness and identification of environmental or novel synthetic compounds acting through steroid receptors underscores the importance of understanding the cardiovascular effects of steroidal agents, especially with regard to toxicological implications. Finally, the extensive hepatic metabolism of these agents coupled with the great diversity in target tissues leaves the steroids susceptible to a wide variety of drug, chemical, or physiological interactions. This chapter is not intended to undermine the importance of steroid function in other classical target tissues; rather, the focus of this chapter will be on the known effects of steroidal agents on the vasculature and the heart, with special emphasis on identification of future areas for steroid research. Where possible, emphasis will be placed on human studies, providing mechanistic information regarding the cardiovascular effects of steroidal agents. However, contributions from animal models have made a tremendous impact on defining the mechanisms of action of steroidal agents on the cardiovascular system, and these studies are included where necessary and possible.

Review of Steroidal Agents

Steroidal agents include both naturally occurring and synthetic derivatives of compounds structurally based on the cyclopentanoperhydrophenanthrene ring illustrated in Table 1. A thorough review of the chemical structures of steroidal agents can be found in the first reference (1). This group of compounds includes classical sex steroid hormones (androgens, estrogens, progestins), mineralocorticoids, glucocorticoids, cholesterol and bile acids, and the cardiotonic steroids known as cardiac glycosides. All of these classes of steroidal agents may influence cardiovascular function through either systemic neurohumoral effects or through direct interactions with myocardial and vascular tissue.

Androgens and Anabolic Steroids

Androgens and synthetic derivatives of androgens are more appropriately known as androgenic-anabolic steroids (AASs). The AASs are divided into two structural classes: (*i*) nonalkylated AASs (e.g., testosterone and ester derivatives of testosterone, 19-nortestosterone or nandrolone, and 17-β-ester derivatives of nandrolone, boldenone, dehydroepiandrosterone, and androstenedione) and (*ii*) 17-α-alkylated AASs (e.g., fluoxymesterone, methandrostenolone, methenolone, methyltestosterone, oxandrolone, oxymetholone, and stanozolol) (2,3). The essential difference between these two classes of AASs is the ability of the 17-α-alkylated compounds to resist first-pass metabolism by the liver and to reach significant blood concentrations following oral administration (4,5). Incidentally, the structural modification to improve oral bioavailability has resulted in AASs that are associated with increased prevalence of hepatotoxicity (6). Whether this structural modification results in significant differences in the cardiovascular effects of AASs is not entirely known, but some literature

Table 1 The Steroid Nucleus and Classification of Steroidal Agents

The steroid nuceus: cyclopentanoperhydrophenanthrene ring

I. Androgens and anabolic steroids
  A. Nonalkylated AASs
    androstenedione
    boldenone
    dehydroepiandrosterone
    dihydrotestosterone
    nandrolone (19-nortestosterone)
    testosterone (and ester formulations)
    trenbolone
  B. 17-α-Alkylated AASs
    danazol
    fluoxymesterone
    desoxymethyltestosterone
    methandrostenolone
    methenolone
    methyltestosterone
    oxandrolone
    oxymetholone
    stanozolol

II. Estrogens
  A. Endogenous estrogens
    17-β-estradiol
    estrone
    estriol
  B. Synthetic estrogens
    diethylstilbesterol (nonsteroidal)
    equilin
    17-β-estradiol (ester formulations)
    ethinyl estradiol
    mestranol
    quinestrol

III. Progestins
  A. Progesterone-like progestins
    hydroxyprogesterone
    medroxyprogesterone
    progesterone
  B. 19-Nortestosterone-like progestins
    desogestrel
    norethindrone
    norethynodrel
    norgestimate
    norgestrel

IV. Mineralocorticoids
  aldosterone

V. Glucocorticoids
  A. Endogenous glucocorticoids
    corticosterone
    cortisone
    hydrocortisone (cortisol)
  B. Synthetic glucocorticoids
    alclometasone
    amcinonide
    beclomethasone
    betamethasone
    clobetasol
    desonide
    desoximetasone
    dexamethasone
    diflorasone
    fludrocortisone
    flunisolide
    fluocinolone
    fluocinonide
    fluorometholone
    flurandrenolide
    halcinonide
    medrysone
    methylprednisolone
    mometasone
    paramethasone
    prednisolone
    prednisone
    triamcinolone

VI. Cholesterol and bile acids
  cholesterol
  cholic acid
  chenodeoxycholic acid
  deoxycholic acid
  lithocholic acid
  ursodeoxycholic acid

VII. Cardiac glycosides
  digoxin
  digitoxin
  ouabain

Abbreviation: AASs, androgenic-anabolic steroids.

suggests that there is, in fact, a clear structure-activity relationship for effects of AASs on lipid metabolism, as discussed below.

Historically, the AASs have been used clinically to treat anemia, breast cancer, hereditary angioneurotic edema, endometriosis, and osteoporosis (5–7). Because improved treatments for those conditions have been developed, the most appropriate clinical use of AASs is currently replacement therapy for hypogonadal males or perhaps to treat chronic wasting syndromes associated with cancer or other diseases. Many of the AASs have been removed from the United States market (e.g., methandrostenolone). Nonetheless, AASs continue to be used illicitly in attempts to improve athletic performance or physical appearance (8). Importantly, self-administration of AASs for these illicit purposes often follows regimens that incorporate doses of AASs that are 10 to 200 times the normal therapeutic doses of these agents (9). Therefore, when discussing the adverse cardiovascular effects of AASs, it is critical to include observations from individuals using these high-dose regimens.

Estrogens

Estrogen, 17-β-estradiol, estrone, and estriol are the primary naturally occurring estrogens in animals and humans. Synthetic derivatives of estrogen include esterified versions (e.g., estradiol valerate and estradiol cypionate) and ethinyl estradiol, mestranol, quinestrol, and equilin (10). In addition, synthetic nonsteroidal estrogens have been made, including diethylstilbesterol, and many other synthetic chemicals have estrogenic activity such as the pesticides DDT (dichlorodiphenyltrichloroethane, 1,1,1-trichloro-2,2-bis[*p*-chlorophenyl]ethane) and methoxychlor, the monomer of polycarbonate plastics bisphenol A, and other industrial chemicals such as polychlorinated biphenyls (10,11). Recent attention has focused on the naturally occurring environmental estrogens or phytoestrogens (found in soy-based foods) such as flavones and isoflavones (e.g., genistein) and coumestan derivatives (12,13). Together, the synthetic chemicals and naturally occurring substances that serve as estrogen receptor (ER) agonists fall into the general classification of endocrine disruptors. Thus, discussion of the cardiovascular effects of estrogenic compounds applies to a wide variety of steroidal and nonsteroidal agents that are either naturally occurring or man made.

Estrogens and synthetic derivatives of estradiol have been used for 50 years as oral contraceptive drugs or as hormone replacement therapy (HRT) for ovariectomized (OVXed) or postmenopausal women to reduce the occurrence of osteoporosis. In addition, HRT has been used to reduce the risk of cardiovascular disease in postmenopausal women, although current literature raises concern regarding this use, especially in light of a possible increased risk of thromboembolic complications (14–16). Despite the many years of clinical use, a clear understanding of the cardiovascular effects of exogenous estrogens has been slow to develop. Initial reports were based on high-dose estrogen administration for oral contraception; however, current practice involves a dramatic reduction in total estrogen doses for oral contraception (10,17). Thus, ironically, discussion of the cardiovascular effects of estrogens must include observations from individuals using lower-dose regimens of estrogens, which is in direct opposition to examining cardiovascular effects of high-dose androgens.

Progestins

The primary progestational hormone synthesized and secreted by the ovaries and adrenal glands is progesterone. Like the androgens, progestins can be grouped into two major chemical classes: (*i*) compounds with high first-pass metabolism by the liver that must be administered by injection (e.g., hydroxyprogesterone caproate and progesterone), and (*ii*) compounds with an ethinyl group at the 17 position or methyl group at the 6 position, which reduce first-pass metabolism and allow oral administration (e.g., desogestrel, medroxyprogesterone, norethindrone, norethynodrel, norgestrel, and norgestimate) (10). Importantly, however, these compounds may also be grouped according to structural similarity to either progesterone (hydroxyprogesterone and medroxyprogesterone) or 19-*nortestosterone* (desogestrel, norethindrone, norethynodrel, norgestimate, and norgestrel). This classification is clinically important as those compounds with structural similarity to 19-nortestosterone retain significant androgenic activity (10,18).

The primary clinical uses of progestins are for contraception or HRT, and for such purposes progestins are more frequently combined with estrogens than used alone (19). Antagonists of the progesterone receptor (e.g., mifepristone or RU486) have been developed and used as abortifacient agents.

Mineralocorticoids

Aldosterone is the primary mineralocorticoid, and it is synthesized and secreted by the adrenal glands. Natural mineralocorticoids are not used for therapeutic purposes, but natural and synthetic corticosteroid-derived agents with mineralocorticoid activity can have profound impact on the cardiovascular system (20). The mineralocorticoid receptor also has at least limited affinity for many steroidal agents including androgens, estrogens, progestins, and glucocorticoids. Therefore, cardiovascular effects associated with mineralocorticoid activity must be considered for many steroidal agents. In addition, structural modifications of mineralocorticoids have produced some therapeutically useful agents that act as antagonists of mineralocorticoid receptors (e.g., spironolactone, eplerenone). Studies have suggested that these antagonists may be useful in limiting the adverse cardiac remodeling observed after myocardial infarction (21).

Glucocorticoids

Cortisol, or hydrocortisone, and corticosterone are the predominant glucocorticoids synthesized and secreted by the adrenal glands. In addition to hydrocortisone, there are presently over 20 different synthetic glucocorticoids used clinically in the United States. Among the numerous glucocorticoids are alclometasone, amcinonide, beclomethasone, betamethasone, clobetasol, desonide, desoximetasone, dexamethasone, diflorasone, fludrocortisone, flunisolide, fluocinolone, fluocinonide, fluorometholone, flurandrenolide, halcinonide, medrysone, methylprednisolone, mometasone, paramethasone, prednisolone, prednisone, and triamcinolone (22). Many of these drugs are used topically, but several are used systemically for replacement therapy in patients with adrenal insufficiency, and for the treatment of various inflammatory conditions. In addition, glucocorticoids are most often used in regimens of short duration (1 week or less); however, a significant population of patients with chronic inflammatory conditions exists throughout the world, and many of these patients undergo long-term glucocorticoid therapy. The glucocorticoids have long been known to exert significant effects on cardiovascular function (23). Moreover, cardiovascular morbidity and mortality is increased in patients with Cushing's syndrome (24). Therefore, a clear understanding of the mechanisms responsible for the adverse cardiovascular effects of glucocorticoids is needed.

Cholesterol and Bile Acids

Cholesterol and bile acids are steroidal agents, and as with the aforementioned compounds, the bile acids are synthesized in the body from cholesterol. The cardiovascular effects of cholesterol will not be included in this chapter because of numerous previous reviews; however, the effects of other steroidal agents on lipoprotein-cholesterol metabolism will be considered here. The primary bile acids in the body are cholic acid, chenodeoxycholic acid, deoxycholic acid, lithocholic acid, and ursodeoxycholic acid (25). These agents are rarely used therapeutically with the exception of ursodeoxycholic acid, which receives occasional use for dissolution of gallstones (25). Because the bile acids are primarily found in the intestinal tract and are largely confined to this region via enterohepatic recirculation, potential cardiovascular effects of these agents will not be considered in this chapter.

Cardiac Glycosides

The cardiac glycosides also represent a group of steroidal agents with profound effects on the cardiovascular system. Indeed, these steroidal agents were likely the first identified to have direct actions upon myocardial tissue. Other than to point out that cardiac glycosides share in the cyclopentanoperhydrophenanthrene ring of the steroidal agents listed above, this chapter will not review the cardiovascular effects of these drugs. For a more complete review of the cardiovascular toxicities of cardiac glycosides, see the chapter titled "Adverse Effects of Drugs on Cardiac Electrophysiology, Rhythm, and Ion Flux" in this text.

Mechanisms of Steroid Action

Steroidal agents exert their effects through a variety of mechanisms. These mechanisms can be classified into "genomic" (meaning, nuclear hormone

Table 2 Characteristics of Steroid Mechanisms of Action

Genomic mechanisms	Rapid signaling mechanisms
1. receptor mediated	1. receptor- or nonreceptor mediated
2. slowly developing (>1–2 hr)	2. rapidly developing (< 1–2 hr)
3. interaction with steroid response element	3. no direct interaction with steroid response element
4. altered gene transcription	4. no effect on gene transcription or indirect and delayed effects on gene transcription
5. response inhibited by actinomycin D	5. immediate response unaffected by actinomycin D
6. response inhibited by cycloheximide	6. immediate response unaffected by cycloheximide

receptor–mediated mechanisms) or "nongenomic" (meaning, rapid signaling mechanisms). The major characteristics of these mechanisms are discussed below and summarized in Table 2.

The Nuclear Hormone Receptor Mechanism

The founding principles for the mechanism for steroid action are now well over 30 years old and sufficiently well established to commonly be called the "classic" or "classical" mechanism. The classic mechanisms of steroid action are based on intracellular protein receptors specific for androgens, estrogens, progestins, mineralocorticoids, glucocorticoids, etc., which function as ligand-activated transcription factors. The steroid hormone receptors belong to the large superfamily of human nuclear hormone receptors that include receptors for a variety of other ligands (e.g., thyroid hormone, retinoic acid, vitamin D). Many of the nuclear hormone receptors, including the estrogen, glucocorticoid, peroxisome proliferator-activated, progesterone, and retinoic acid receptors, are expressed from multiple genes, and/or from multiple transcripts that give rise to functional receptor isoforms with unique ligand-binding and transcriptional properties. Furthermore, several genes encoding proteins closely related to receptors of the nuclear hormone receptors (orphan receptors) have been discovered, for which ligands have not yet been identified. The role of the orphan receptors in the cardiovascular actions of steroids is not known but could add to the complexity of steroid action on cardiovascular physiology.

The "classical" steroid hormone mechanism is diagrammatically outlined in Figure 1. The steroid hormone receptors are localized to the intracellular compartment. To varying degrees, circulating steroids are tightly bound by specific serum proteins, with only the unbound or "free-fraction" available to act as ligands at the steroid receptors. The biologically active free steroids first cross the plasma membrane and are then bound by steroid receptors located either in the cytosol or nucleus to form a hormone or receptor complex. In the inactive or unoccupied state, steroid receptors are frequently associated with multiprotein

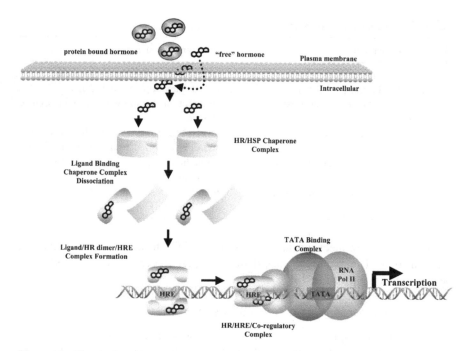

Figure 1 Classical nuclear hormone mechanism of action.

complexes containing chaperone protein [e.g., the 90 kD heat shock protein (HSP)]. Steroid binding results in dissociation of the receptor from the chaperone protein complex and proteolytic modification of the receptor (26–29). The ligand-steroid receptor complex translocates to the nucleus (if cytosolic), and forms a ligand/receptor/DNA ternary complex by binding as a dimer at a specific promoter hormone response element (HRE), and mediates either up- or down-regulation of target-gene transcription (20,27). The specific response to receptor activation is governed by formation of protein-protein interactions between the active receptor or HRE complex and coregulatory factors, which trigger chromatin remodeling and the formation of higher order complexes that interact with the basal transcription or RNA polymerase II machinery. In addition to cell specific expression of receptors and coregulators, the complexity of the steroid-mediated transcriptional response is further increased by the ability of most steroid receptors to form and function as a receptor-ligand-HRE complex via receptor homodimerization or heterodimerization at their respective response elements (30,31).

The general features of the classical mechanism of nuclear receptor action can adequately explain many of the effects of steroids on gene transcription. However, it is important to point out that clear demonstration of expression and function of some nuclear receptors in specific cardiac cell populations remains controversial. The unclear role of ERs in cardiac myocytes stands as the prime example of this ongoing debate. Of course, long-held exceptions to the classical model include the mechanism of actions for the anesthetic effects of progesterone at the GABA receptor, and the cardiac glycosides, which inhibit the sodium/potassium ATPase. Moreover, the question of how steroidal agents regulate highly integrated effects such as proliferation, cellular hypertrophy, metabolism, biosynthesis and metabolism, and secretion has been difficult to understand with explanations imparted solely by effects of nuclear hormone receptors on steroid responsive transcription.

Rapid Signaling Mechanisms

Along with an increasing number of transmembrane receptors and enzymes with activities directly modified by steroids, steroids also directly regulate a variety of intracellular signaling cascades. These signaling effects can be observed with a rapid onset (minutes to seconds) that is independent of de novo changes in gene expression. In the most well-characterized examples of rapid steroid signaling action, the rapid signaling effects are initiated via steroid-selective receptor-like systems. The increased understanding of the signaling actions of steroids has raised some questions as to the primary mode of action of steroidal agents (32). Examples of the rapid signaling mechanisms of steroid action are found in a variety of tissues, with most studies related to actions of gonadal steroid hormone in reproductive tissues and are not related directly to cardiovascular function or health.

Cardiovascular-relevant evidence for rapid actions of steroids include studies of Koenig and colleagues (33), who demonstrated that nanomolar concentrations of testosterone induce rapid increases in ornithine decarboxylase activity and polyamine concentrations and acute stimulation of calcium fluxes and calcium-mediated membrane transport systems in rat ventricular myocytes exposed for less than one minute. The authors suggested that the effects were consistent with androgen receptor–mediated events (33). However, questions arose as to whether androgen receptor–mediated alterations in gene transcription could have accounted for the aforementioned effects of testosterone because of the swift nature of the responses. The authors hypothesized that testosterone effects on ornithine decarboxylase were, at least in part, mediated by posttranslational modification of the enzyme by androgen receptor–mediated phosphorylation or dephosphorylation (33). More recently, these studies have been extended to demonstrate that increased ornithine decarboxylase activity and polyamine concentrations in cardiac myocytes might contribute to positive inotropic effects of dihydrotestosterone (34). Furthermore, polyamines may affect cardiac ion homeostasis, as spermidine and putrescine are known modulators of potassium current (35). Thus, nontranscriptional regulation of potassium currents by testosterone may contribute to gender differences in QTc interval (36). Finally, it is probable that testosterone and other androgens exert at least some of their effects on ventricular myocytes by rapid androgen receptor–mediated mechanisms.

Additional support for rapid androgenic mechanisms comes from studies of prostate cells. Farnsworth demonstrated that androgens bind to sodium/ potassium ATPase in prostatic plasma membranes and can activate the ATPase to regulate metabolic activity (37). In addition, evidence strongly suggests the coexistence of non-DNA binding androgen receptors in endoplasmic reticulum (microsomal fractions) of rat ventral prostate tissue that was not simply due to contamination of the fractions (38). Therefore, it is reasonable to speculate that androgens may also affect cardiac myocyte function through interactions with sodium/potassium ATPase or other enzyme targets in both receptor- and nonreceptor-mediated fashion. Indeed, more recent studies have also demonstrated that epiandrosterone (a metabolite of dehydroepiandrosterone) can block L-type calcium channel activity in ventricular myocytes in a manner similar to that of dihydropyridines (39). In contrast, testosterone was shown to rapidly increase intracellular calcium in rat cardiac myocytes, perhaps through a plasma membrane receptor associated with a pertussin toxin-sensitive G protein pathway (40). Overall, more research is need to clearly delineate the rapid signaling mechanisms associated with androgen action in the heart.

Of most relevance to the vascular system is the well-established rapid estrogen signaling mechanism operating in vascular endothelium (41). Rapid estrogen signaling in human vascular endothelium rapidly increases the generation of nitric oxide (NO) by kinase-mediated activation of eNOS (Fig. 2). A transcriptional variant of estrogen receptor alpha (ERα46) acts as a membrane-associated receptor in a caveolin 1–associated multiprotein signaling complex

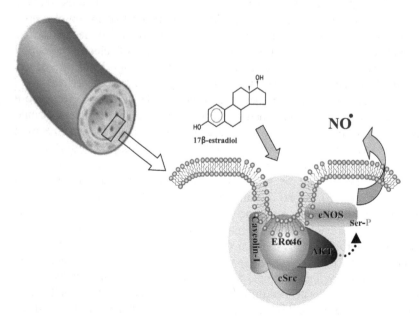

Figure 2 Proposed model for membrane-initiated vascular responses to estradiol.

located in specialized subdomains of the plasma membrane. Estrogen binding at ERα46 stimulates c-SRC activity leading to PI3K activity and Akt activation. Serine phosphorylation of eNOS by Akt stimulates nitric oxide synthase (NOS) enzymatic activity, resulting in increased NO generation. The vasoregulatory actions of E2-mediated NO generation may play an important role in homeostasis of cardiovascular function.

Further support for rapid modes of steroid action that could apply to the cardiovascular system comes from initial research into alternative mechanisms of estrogen action in hormone responsive cancers. Using MCF-7 (Michigan Cancer Foundation) breast cancer cells, Migliaccio and colleagues demonstrated that estradiol, coupled to the ER, elicited tyrosine kinase activation of the p21ras signaling pathway, resulting in activation of extracellular signal–regulated kinases [ERK 1/2, part of the mitogen-activated protein kinase (MAPK) family] and culminating in stimulation of MCF-7 cell growth (42). Furthermore, estradiol has been shown to enhance cardiac fibroblast proliferation through a rapid signaling mechanism. Lee and Eghbali-Webb found that estrogen stimulated cardiac fibroblast DNA synthesis through activation of ERK 1/2, and these effects were blocked by the ER antagonist tamoxifen or by the MAPK inhibitor PD98059 (43). Numerous demonstrations of subpopulation of ERs similar to the nuclear hormone receptors have been identified as localized to, or associated with, the plasma membrane in various cell types. Therefore, evidence suggests that at least part of the mechanism of action of estrogens in most cells involves binding to membrane-associated ERs and stimulation of MAPK pathways. Given the similarities of the steroid superfamily of receptors, it is reasonable to speculate that other steroidal agents also act in a rapid cell-specific fashion on the cardiovascular system through membrane-localized steroid receptors.

In summary, literature suggests that steroidal agents act in part by steroid nuclear receptor–mediated alterations in gene transcription (i.e., classic mechanisms) and in part by steroid receptor– or nonreceptor–mediated rapid signaling mechanisms. Many of the direct signaling actions of steroids impact growth or death signaling pathways such as the MAPKs and the regulation of calcium homeostasis. These rapid signaling effects may be especially important in the failing heart or following myocardial infarction. Whether multiple mechanisms for specific steroids are active in individual cells of the cardiovascular system and to what degree they are integrated into normal or pathophysiological responses of cells and tissues comprising the cardiovascular system are not known.

VASCULAR EFFECTS OF STEROIDAL AGENTS

Indirect Effects of Steroidal Agents on the Vasculature: Lipid Metabolism

The causative relationship between hypercholesterolemia and atherosclerosis is no longer regarded as a controversial theory, as the mechanisms responsible for low-density lipoprotein cholesterol–induced atherosclerosis are increasingly

understood. The major atherogenic carriers of cholesterol are low-density lipoprotein (LDL) and β-very low-density lipoprotein (β-VLDL), yet high-density
lipoprotein (HDL) is almost universally regarded as nonatherogenic, if not
antiatherogenic (44,45). Furthermore, evidence suggests that LDL-C, low-density
lipoprotein cholesterol, initiates atherosclerotic plaque development when it is
oxidized to a form that initiates injury and inflammation (45). Conclusions
regarding atherogenic lipoproteins were reached following years of clinical
research into risk factors for atherosclerosis and observations of patients with
familial hypercholesterolemia. On the basis of these conclusions, current clinical
practice includes monitoring serum LDL-C and HDL-C and attempts to decrease
elevated LDL-C while increasing HDL-C.

Endogenous Sex Steroids and Risk of Coronary Artery Disease

Endogenous androgens, estrogens, and progestins have long received attention as
possible mediators of gender differences in the risk of coronary artery disease.
Now well accepted is the approximate twofold increased risk of coronary artery
disease in men compared with premenopausal women (46). The clinical literature from which numerous inconclusive and/or disparate results have been
obtained is extensive (46). Thus, the purpose of the following review is not to
revisit the entire clinical literature with regard to mortality rates and risk of
coronary artery disease as they relate to levels of endogenous sex steroids.
Rather, the purpose is to consider the effects of exogenous androgens, estrogens,
and progestins on lipid metabolism (Table 3), as these data likely have significant pharmacological and toxicological relevance with regard to the increasing
identification of heretofore-unknown androgenic, estrogenic, and progestogenic
compounds to which humans are exposed. It is, nonetheless, worthwhile to
consider some of the conclusions reached by Kalin and Zumoff (46) regarding
endogenous levels of androgens, estrogens, and progestins. First, although both

Table 3 Potential Effects of Exogenous Steroids on Lipoprotein Metabolism

Steroid class	HTGL	TC	LDL-C	HDL-C
Androgens and anabolic steroids				
Nonalkylated	↑	↑	↑	↓
17-α-Alkylated	↑↑	↑↑	↑↑	↓↓
Estrogens	↓	↓	↓	?
Progestins	↑	↑	↑	↓
Mineralocorticoids	—	—	—	—
Glucocorticoids	?	↑	↑	↑ or ↓

Abbreviations: HTGL, hepatic triglyceride lipase; TC, total serum cholesterol; LDL-C, low-density
lipoprotein cholesterol; HDL-C, high-density lipoprotein cholesterol; ↑, increased; ↓, decreased;
↑↑, larger increase; ↓↓, larger decrease; —, no significant effect; ?, unknown effects. Supporting
references are found throughout the text.

are usually normal prior to myocardial infarction, endogenous estradiol levels are elevated and testosterone levels are decreased for up to one year in men who survive myocardial infarction. Second, progesterone is normal prior to but elevated for short periods (less than 1 year) following myocardial infarction, and this alteration may be stress related. Third, pregnancy (high levels of endogenous estrogens and progestins) appears to provide protection against coronary artery disease. Fourth, men with cirrhosis of the liver have high endogenous estrogen levels and low endogenous testosterone levels, and this appears to be associated with a decreased risk of coronary artery disease. And fifth, women with elevated endogenous testosterone appear to have an increased risk of coronary artery disease. In summary, these clinical studies support the hypothesis that estrogens provide protection from coronary artery disease, whereas androgens may increase the risk of coronary artery disease. The observed effects of exogenous androgens, estrogens, and progestins on lipid metabolism also support this hypothesis.

Androgens and Anabolic Steroids

The AASs have long been known to alter lipid metabolism in humans and animals, and the effects of AASs on lipid metabolism have been reviewed previously (3,47–49). Net effects of AASs on lipid metabolism are generally observed to include significant elevations in LDL-C and significant reductions in HDL-C. However, as discussed below, effects of individual AASs on lipid metabolism may vary significantly, and a structure-activity relationship appears to explain, at least partially, this variability.

While alterations in lipid metabolism that include significantly elevated LDL and reduced HDL have long been associated with atherosclerosis, and the AASs are known to affect lipid metabolism in such a manner, experimental evidence supporting the hypothesis that AASs promote atherosclerosis is lacking (47). Nonetheless, potential causes for differences in death rates from coronary artery disease have included androgen-induced alterations in lipid metabolism (46), and suggestion has been made to include women with signs of androgen excess as being at a greater risk of coronary artery disease (50). Also of note, the reduction of serum HDL induced by AASs in humans is of greater magnitude than alterations produced by any other pharmacological agent or nonpharmacological factor including smoking and obesity (47). Therefore, understanding the mechanisms responsible for AAS-induced reductions in serum HDL is of utmost importance.

The exact mechanisms for AAS-induced alterations in lipid metabolism are largely unknown; however, the genomic mechanisms could largely account for these effects. In support of this theory, evidence suggests that AASs upregulate or induce hepatic triglyceride lipase (HTGL), which catabolizes HDL, yet AASs have little effect on lipoprotein lipase, which liberates fatty acids from triglycerides and converts VLDL and chylomicrons into atherogenic β-VLDL. For example, subjects given 7.5 mg/day of oxandrolone for three weeks had significantly higher activities of postheparin plasma HTGL activity compared with control subjects, but no differences in lipoprotein lipase were observed (51). Similarly, subjects given 6 mg/day of stanozolol had significantly increased activity of HTGL but unaltered lipoprotein lipase compared with their pre-treatment levels, and the elevated HTGL activity appeared to correlate with reduced serum HDL levels in these subjects (52). Furthermore, increases in HTGL induced by stanozolol were subsequently found to precede decreases in serum HDL (53). Nearly identical results on HDL and HTGL have been reported in men who were self-administering high doses of AASs (54,55). However, these studies were hampered by a general lack of ability to control diet, dose and purity of the AAS, and other factors (3).

A structure-activity relationship for the effects of AASs on lipid metabolism appears to exist, and this relationship is most likely unrelated to the relative androgenic potencies of the AASs. In a crossover study in weightlifters given 6 mg/day oral stanozolol or 200 mg/wk intramuscular testosterone enanthate for six weeks, HDL-C was reduced by 33% during stanozolol administration and 9% during testosterone administration (56). Stanozolol increased HTGL activity by 123%, while testosterone only increased HTGL activity by 25%. Interestingly, LDL-C was increased by 29% in the stanozolol-treated group, whereas LDL-C decreased by 16% in the testosterone-treated group (56). A subsequent study found similar results (57). Eighteen subjects were divided into three groups and for 12 weeks given either 280 mg/wk testosterone enanthate, 280 mg/wk testosterone enanthate plus 250 mg testolactone (aromatase inhibitor) orally four times daily, or 20 mg methyltestosterone orally twice daily (57). Subjects treated with methyltestosterone or testosterone enanthate plus testolactone had significant decreases in HDL-C, while subjects treated with testosterone enanthate alone had no significant changes in HDL-C. Reductions in HDL-C were preceded by increases in HTGL in subjects treated with methyltestosterone or testosterone enanthate plus testolactone, but subjects treated with testosterone enanthate alone had no significant changes in HTGL (57). To further clarify the effects of the aromatase inhibitor testolactone, a subsequent study recruited 14 male weightlifters, and in a randomized crossover design, administered to them 200 mg/wk testosterone enanthate, 250 mg testolactone orally four times daily, or a combination of testosterone enanthate and testolactone (58). Serum testosterone levels increased during all three treatments; however, serum estradiol was unchanged during treatment with testolactone or testosterone enanthate plus testolactone, and serum estradiol increased by 47% when subjects received testosterone enanthate alone. These results strongly suggested that testolactone inhibited testosterone aromatization to estradiol (58). While testolactone had minimal effects on lipid metabolism, testosterone decreased HDL-C, and testosterone plus testolactone appeared to further decrease HDL, but the changes were not significantly different. There was, however, a significant difference when comparing effects of the regimens on HTGL; testosterone enanthate increased HTGL by 21%, while testosterone enanthate plus testolactone increased HTGL by 38% (58).

In summary, many clinical studies demonstrate that AASs alter lipid metabolism in humans, and the alterations most frequently include elevated LDL-C and decreased HDL-C. A structure-activity relationship has been established, which suggests that 17-α-alkylated AASs have a greater effect on lipid metabolism through induction of HTGL and subsequent reduction of plasma HDL-C. When an aromatizable androgen is administered (e.g., testosterone), the effects on HTGL and HDL are not as profound, and evidence suggests that the conversion of testosterone to estradiol may impart a slight protective effect.

Estrogens and Progestins

The effects of estrogens on lipid metabolism are nearly opposite to those of androgens. Estrogens dose-dependently increase HDL-C and commonly produce reductions in total and LDL-C, although higher doses or higher potencies of estrogens produce a different pattern of altered lipid metabolism where LDL and VLDL may be increased (59). In direct contrast to estrogens, the effects of synthetic progestins, particularly those with structural similarity to 19-nortestosterone, on lipid metabolism are nearly identical to those of androgens. These sex hormone–mediated alterations in lipid metabolism may at least partially explain gender differences in coronary artery disease.

From the numerous clinical studies evaluating exogenous estrogens and progestins, Kalin and Zumoff (46) concluded that (*i*) postmenopausal estrogen replacement therapy may protect against coronary artery disease; (*ii*) oral contraceptives using high-dose synthetic estrogens likely increase the risk of coronary thrombosis, but not coronary atherosclerosis; and (*iii*) oral contraceptives using synthetic progestins with androgenic activity may increase the risk of myocardial infarction. A more recent study suggests that the currently used, low-dose estrogen and progestin oral contraceptives do not increase the risk of myocardial infarction (17). Nonetheless, studies have continued to raise concern that HRT can increase the risk of coronary heart disease, especially thromboembolic events (14–16). Although the magnitude of this increased risk may depend on the doses of individual agents, duration of therapy, preexisting disease, and other factors, many physicians are advising women to avoid this therapy unless required by postmenopausal symptoms.

In terms of lipid metabolism alone, many of the effects of estrogens are generally regarded as protective in terms of atherosclerosis, while commonly used combined estrogen and progestin HRT may result in no net beneficial effects because the estrogen effects may be diminished by those of progestins (18,19). For example, in a cross-sectional study of 693 postmenopausal French women over two years, 27 received transdermal unopposed (no progestin) estradiol, 165 received transdermal estradiol plus a progestin, and 501 women received no HRT (60). Women receiving HRT had lower serum total cholesterol, triglycerides, apolipoprotein B, and LDL-C and VLDL-C. However, no significant differences in HDL-C were found, and the results suggested that women administered combined HRT (86% of treated women) may have had beneficial effects of estradiol reduced by progestins (60). Interestingly, the effects of estrogens on lipid metabolism may be more profound in those individuals who have hyperlipidemias prior to HRT. For example, in women with normal blood cholesterol levels, estrogen therapy via oral or transdermal administration reduced total and LDL-C by up to 10%; whereas, in women with hyper-cholesterolemia, estrogen therapy via oral or transdermal administration reduced total and LDL-C levels by up to 20% (59).

As with androgens, the mechanisms responsible for estrogen- and/or progestin-induced alterations in lipid metabolism are largely unknown; however, the mechanisms involved for estrogens may include steps that are in direct opposition of those observed with androgens. Genomic mechanisms are likely responsible for estrogen- or progestin-induced alterations in lipid metabolism. Estrogens are thought to inhibit HTGL expression or activity, thus promoting HDL levels (59,61) and antagonizing the actions of androgens. Conceivably, the estrogen-estrogen receptor complex could act as a regulatory factor that interferes with or reduces HTGL expression. Similar to androgens, estrogens have not been clearly demonstrated to affect lipoprotein lipase (59). Because many of the progestins have significant androgenic activity (18,46), it should come as no surprise that at least one mechanism for progestin-induced alterations in lipid metabolism includes upregulation and/or activation of HTGL (61). Furthermore, the human androgen receptor shares 82% amino acid homology of the two zinc finger structural motifs and 75% and 56% amino acid homology of two other important regions (likely hormone binding domains) with that of human progesterone receptors, and the HREs for androgen and progesterone receptors are very similar, if not identical (27,62).

An additional mechanism regarding potential beneficial effects of estrogens on lipid metabolism deserves mention. That is, experimental evidence suggests that estrogens may serve as antioxidants, thus behaving similarly to α-tocopherol. Specifically, estrogen was shown to inhibit the oxidation of LDL induced by copper or by exposure to endothelial cells (63). However, these in vitro experiments required extremely high concentrations of estradiol (1.25–2.5 μM). Presumably the rigorous in vitro conditions led to requirements for high estradiol concentrations, and in vivo radical production may be much lower than that produced in vitro, so that conceivably this antioxidant mechanism could function in the intact vasculature (63).

In summary, exogenous estrogens produce alterations in lipid metabolism that are opposite to those elicited by androgens, so total and LDL-C is frequently reduced, while HDL-C is elevated. Exogenous progestins, in contrast, appear to produce alterations in lipid metabolism that are very similar to those induced by androgens. The primary target leading to sex steroid–altered lipid metabolism appears to be HTGL, and it is likely that sex steroid receptors regulate HTGL expression. Future research into the mechanisms responsible for sex steroid–induced alterations in lipid metabolism should include clear identification of the molecular targets of the receptors and delineation of transcriptional activity of the receptors at the gene-encoding HTGL.

Glucocorticoids

In contrast to androgens, estrogens, and progestins, the effects of glucocorticoids on lipid metabolism are less clear. Even though individuals with Cushing's syndrome frequently have elevated serum levels of all lipids and lipoproteins, including LDL-C and HDL-C, difficulties have prevented sound conclusions regarding effects of exogenous glucocorticoids on lipid metabolism (64). Nonetheless, treatment with glucocorticoids frequently results in elevated total, LDL-C, and HDL-C—a lipid profile somewhat different from that induced by androgens, estrogens, and progestins.

Clinical studies evaluating the effects of exogenous glucocorticoid therapy on lipid metabolism have been frequently conducted in heart or kidney transplant recipients; however, not many of these studies have been published. In 92 patients who received heart transplants, 52% were above the sex- and age-adjusted 75th percentile, and 35% were above the 90th percentile for total cholesterol, with similar elevations observed in LDL-C and HDL-C (65). Prednisone exposure was the strongest predictor of both total and LDL-C levels independent of other clinical variables (65). In 500 renal transplant recipients, hypercholesterolemia occurred in 82% of the patients, and there was a strong correlation between prednisone doses and cholesterol levels, which were significantly reduced when prednisone doses were decreased (66). It is important to note that examination of transplant patients to draw firm conclusions regarding glucocorticoid-induced alterations in lipid metabolism is difficult because of concomitant immunosuppressant therapy, often with cyclosporine, which may independently alter lipid metabolism. However, some studies in patients with various inflammatory conditions provide some support for the observed glucocorticoid-induced lipid alterations in transplant recipients.

When 46 female patients with systemic lupus erythematosus (SLE) were compared with 30 matched control subjects, SLE patients receiving prednisone (32 of the 46 patients) had significantly elevated total and LDL-C compared with SLE patients not receiving prednisone and control subjects (67). In addition, cholesterol levels correlated with daily prednisone dosage in treated patients with SLE (67). In contrast, a study involving 23 patients with rheumatic disease who received prednisone for one month showed that total and HDL-C were significantly increased, but LDL-C was unchanged (68). Interestingly, women may be more susceptible to glucocorticoid-induced alterations in lipid metabolism. For example, in patients receiving long-term (>3 years) glucocorticoid treatment for connective tissue disorders and asthma, women, but not men, had significantly elevated total cholesterol and decreased HDL-C (69). Even though many studies have focused on chronic therapy, effects of glucocorticoids on lipid metabolism can surface fairly rapidly. For example, six male and six female subjects given prednisone showed significant increases in total and HDL-C within 48 hours after initiation of treatment; LDL-C did not increase significantly (70). Overall, available clinical literature suggests that chronic exogenous glucocorticoid therapy frequently results in elevated total, LDL-C, and HDL-C; however, these changes are inconsistent when comparing all reports. Further studies are required to clarify glucocorticoid effects.

As with androgens, estrogens, and progestins, mechanisms for glucocorticoid-induced alterations in lipid metabolism are largely unknown. The mechanism could partially be explained by changes in LDL receptor expression (71), which are most likely mediated by a genomic mechanism. More detailed information regarding the mechanism(s) could be provided by future animal studies because at least one animal study suggested that glucocorticoids slow the catabolism of LDL-C. Cynomolgus monkeys given prednisone developed increased total cholesterol, including elevated LDL-C and depressed HDL-C, and there was a decrease in the fractional catabolic rate of LDL (72). Thus, definitive mechanistic studies of glucocorticoid-induced alterations in lipid metabolism are lacking, yet clarification of cellular or molecular mechanisms will be important as new agonists and antagonists of glucocorticoid receptors are identified.

In summary, a major systemic influence of steroidal agents on cardiovascular function is steroid-induced hyperlipidemias. Androgens, progestins, and glucocorticoids appear to be the primary steroidal agents that may alter lipid metabolism in such a manner as to favor development of atherosclerosis. The most likely target of these steroidal compounds appears to be HTGL. In contrast to androgens, progestins, and glucocorticoids, available evidence suggests that estrogens impart a protective effect against undesirable lipid profiles. If all estrogenic agonists elicit this type of response, then concerns regarding altered lipid metabolism secondary to environmental or industrial chemical estrogens may be unjustified. Nonetheless, as new agonists and antagonists of steroidal receptors are identified, a clear understanding of the mechanisms responsible for steroid-mediated changes in lipid metabolism will become increasingly important. This importance may be best exemplified by examples listed above, where particular members of a class of steroidal agents (e.g., androgens) display quite different effects on lipid metabolism. Although it is useful to discuss all steroidal agents as classes, a caveat regarding compound-specific differences is in order.

Other indirect hemodynamic actions of steroidal agents, including effects on blood pressure, circulating electrolytes and volume, autonomic function, thrombogenesis, and hematopoiesis will not be discussed in detail in this chapter. Although these indirect effects may be quite important, results of numerous human investigations have been inconclusive, only limited information is available, or the actions are well defined with reviews or chapters being available to describe the effects (e.g., effects of mineralocorticoids on electrolytes, volume, and blood pressure). The remainder of the chapter will focus on direct effects of steroidal agents on the vasculature and heart.

Direct Effects of Steroidal Agents on the Vasculature

Increasing evidence suggests that steroidal agents may exert cardiovascular effects through direct actions on smooth muscle and/or endothelial cells lining the vasculature (20). In addition, significant evidence demonstrates the presence of steroid receptors in the vasculature (Table 4). Thus, the vasculature is a target for direct steroid actions, and major effects are summarized in Table 5. Even with this evidence, however, results are limited in that few human studies have been conducted, and confounding factors in these studies, such as hypercholesterolemia and hypertension, are difficult to eliminate. Further evidence for direct steroid-mediated alterations in vascular tone stems largely from whole animal and in vitro experiments. Overall, these experiments certainly provide strong support for consideration of the vasculature as a target for direct steroid action.

Androgens and Anabolic Steroids

Autoradiographic evidence for the presence of androgen receptors in the vasculature was found in 1981 when McGill and Sheridan reported finding specific tritiated dihydrotestosterone binding in vascular smooth muscle and endothelial cells from male and female baboons (73). These experiments provided the foundation for identification of the vasculature as a target for direct androgen action. Evidence for direct AAS effects on the vasculature comes mostly from animal studies. However, conflicting results preclude definitive conclusion as to whether AAS promote vascular constriction or dilation, and, of course, regional vascular variability in response may be significant.

Animal models have provided evidence that AAS alter vascular reactivity. First, one week treatment of male and female rats with testosterone was found to increase maximum tension and potency for the vasoconstrictive response to

Table 4 Evidence for Vascular Steroid Receptors in Various Species: Location, Isoforms, and Methods Employed for Detection

	Species	Location	Isoforms	Methods
Androgen receptors	baboon	VSMC and EC	?	RB
Estrogen receptors	rats, monkeys, humans	VSMC and EC	α and β	IB, RNaseP, RT-PCR
Progesterone receptors	rats, rabbits, humans	VSMC	?	IH, RT-PCR
Mineralocorticoid and glucocorticoid receptors	rats, rabbits, humans	VSMC and EC	Type I and II	RB, SRE

Abbreviations: VSMC, vascular smooth muscle cells; EC, endothelial cells; ?, unknown; SRE, binding or activation of steroid response elements; IB, immunoblotting; IH, immunohistochemistry; RB, radioligand binding; RT-PCR, reverse transcription-polymerase chain reaction; RNaseP, ribonuclease protection assay. Supporting references are found throughout the text.

Table 5 Potential Direct Effects of Exogenous Steroids on the Vasculature

Steroid class	Types of studies	Endothelium-dependent effects	Endothelium-independent effects	Possible net effects on reactivity
Androgens and anabolic steroids	animal	↓ NO signaling	?	vasoconstriction in vivo and vasodilation in vitro
Estrogens	human and animal	↑ NO signaling, ↑ NOS	↓ Ca^{++} influx or ↑ Ca^{++} efflux	vasodilation in vivo and in vitro
Progestins	animal	↓ NO signaling?	↓ Ca^{++} influx	?
Mineralocorticoids	human and animal	?	↑ Na^+ influx ↑ Na^+ channels ↑ Ca^{++} influx	vasoconstriction
Glucocorticoids	human and animal	↓ NO signaling, ↓ protacyclin	↑ ACE ↑ AT receptors ↓ Na^+ influx ↑ Ca^{++} influx	vasoconstriction

Abbreviations: NO, nitric oxide signaling; NOS, nitric oxide synthase; ACE, angiotensin converting enzyme; AT, angiotensin II; ?, unknown effects. Supporting references are found throughout the text.

prostaglandin $F_{2\alpha}$ ($PGF_{2\alpha}$) in female, but not male, aortic rings with intact endothelium (74). This suggested that the female has a greater capacity than the male for AAS-induced changes in vascular smooth muscle contraction (74). Subsequently, Ferrer and colleagues examined the effects of chronic (4 to 12 weeks) nandrolone administration in male rabbits on vasodilator responses of isolated aorta (75). Nandrolone treatment was not associated with any significant changes in blood pressure throughout the treatment period (75). In thoracic aorta, endothelium-dependent relaxation induced by acetylcholine and the calcium ionophore, A23187, was abolished in nandrolone-treated rabbits; however, similar results were not observed in mesenteric and femoral arteries (75). Furthermore, acetylcholine- or sodium nitroprusside–induced increases in cyclic GMP were abolished by nandrolone treatment, and the authors concluded that nandrolone reduced NO-mediated relaxation in thoracic aorta by inhibition of guanylate cyclase, while endothelial NO production (surmised from bioassay data) was unaltered (75). Further evidence for direct effects of androgens on endothelium-dependent relaxation was obtained by Farhat and colleagues (76). They administered testosterone to pigs for two weeks, then assessed vascular reactivity in segments of left anterior descending (LAD) coronary artery. In vessels obtained from male and female pigs, testosterone treatment significantly increased the maximum response of intact vessels to potassium chloride (KCl) and

$PGF_{2\alpha}$. Interestingly, endothelial denudation significantly decreased the testosterone effects on vascular responses to KCl and $PGF_{2\alpha}$ in segments obtained from male but not female pigs, while there was no significant sex difference in the response of LAD segments from placebo-treated pigs to KCl and $PGF_{2\alpha}$ (76).

At least one case report stemming from a human study exists in the literature that may confirm the observed effects of AASs on vascular reactivity found in animal models (77). Seven men were recruited for measurement of forearm blood flow responses to brachial artery infusion of methacholine (MC) and sodium nitroprusside (SNP). The investigators found one man to have vasodilatory responses to MC and SNP that were 71% and 51% (respectively) lower in the second measurement session compared with the first (77). It was later serendipitously discovered that this individual had been self-administering high-dose testosterone, which he initiated following the first blood flow measurement. The authors concluded that AAS use may induce changes in NO-mediated vasodilatory responses that appear to lie distal to the endothelium, perhaps in the vascular smooth muscle (77). This supposition was supported by the observed effects of nandrolone on rabbit aorta discussed previously (75).

Opposite actions of AASs on vascular reactivity were reported when aortic or coronary artery rings were obtained and acutely exposed to AAS in vitro. For example, testosterone elicited an endothelium-independent relaxation of isolated rabbit coronary artery and aortic rings, and coronary artery rings were more sensitive to testosterone-induced relaxation than aortic rings (78). Results were similar in preparations isolated from male and nonpregnant female rabbits. Further, testosterone-induced relaxation of coronary artery rings was inhibited by barium chloride, a potassium channel inhibitor. The authors concluded that altered potassium conductance was at least partially involved in the mechanism of testosterone-induced relaxation, but it is important to note that the concentration of testosterone required for relaxation in these experiments was 1 μM or higher (78). Similarly, Costarella and colleagues demonstrated that testosterone produced direct relaxation of rat thoracic aorta when administered to aortic rings in vitro (79). Supraphysiological concentrations (>25 μM) of testosterone relaxed phenylephrine-precontracted endothelium-intact aortic rings, and pretreatment of endothelium-denuded rings with 50 μM testosterone reduced the sensitivity to phenylephrine (79). From these experiments, the authors concluded that testosterone has a direct vasodilating effect, involving endothelium-dependent and endothelium-independent mechanisms (79). Somewhat in contrast to this acute vasodilatory effect, studies by Ceballos and colleagues showed that concentrations of testsoterone as low as 0.1 nM acted acutely to antagonize the vasodilator effect of adenosine in isolated rat heart, possibly via increased synthesis and release of thromboxane A_2 (80). More recent evidence supports vasodilatory properties of AAS including dilation of coronary and pulmonary arteries. For example, testosterone was demonstrated to produce vasodilation in the pulmonary vasculature most likely through rapid signaling mechanisms involving inhibition of calcium channels (81). In addition, dehydroepiandrosterone induced acute vasodilation of porcine coronary arteries in in vitro experiments using isolated coronary artery rings and in vivo experiments where coronary flow increased significantly (82).

In summary, the literature suggests that long-term treatment with AASs may promote vasoconstriction through mechanisms involving NO, perhaps at the level of inhibiting NO signaling through downregulation of guanylyl cyclase. However, when AASs are administered in supraphysiological concentrations to in vitro preparations, a net relaxing effect is observed. In contrast, lower concentrations may act acutely to antagonize vasodilators such as adenosine. At this point, it is tempting to speculate that the former effects result from genomic mechanisms of AAS action; whereas, the rapid effects of AAS result from nongenomic mechanisms (20), but further research is required to delineate the mechanisms and clarify discrepancies.

Estrogens

In contrast to androgens, a considerable amount of work, including human and animal studies, has been completed in attempts to understand the direct effects of estrogens on the vasculature. Impetus for this work stems from epidemiological data suggesting that the "atheroprotective" effects of estrogens are not entirely explained by beneficial effects on lipid metabolism, and that additional direct effects of estrogens on the vascular wall likely contribute to this phenomenon (20,83,84). Functional ERs have been identified in human vascular smooth muscle cells from mammary artery and saphenous vein (85,86) and in human endothelial cells isolated from aorta and umbilical vein (87). Recent investigations have demonstrated that both forms of ERs (classic ERα and recently identified β) are expressed in coronary artery and cultured aortic smooth muscle from cynomolgus monkeys (88), and that ERβ is increased in male rat aortic smooth muscle and endothelial cells as early as two days and persists up to two weeks following balloon injury (89). These data suggest that estrogen receptor beta (ERβ) may participate in vascular remodeling following injury.

Human studies support the hypothesis that estrogens exert beneficial effects on the vasculature. In a human study in the early 1990s, 11 women (mean age 58 ± 8 years) with angina, coronary artery disease, and clinical evidence of estrogen deficiency were recruited, randomly assigned to two groups, 1 mg 17-β-estradiol sublingual or placebo, and then subjected to exercise testing on two separate days (90). Nitrates other than sublingual nitroglycerine were withdrawn two days before the study, whereas calcium channel blockers and β-adrenoceptor blocking agents were withdrawn four and five days (respectively) prior to the study. As for sublingual nitroglycerine, subjects were withdrawn from therapy at least six hours prior to exercise testing. Interestingly, sublingual estradiol delayed the onset of signs of myocardial ischemia on the electrocardiogram and increased exercise tolerance in a manner similar to that of sublingual nitroglycerin as demonstrated in other studies (90). These results suggested that estradiol exerts direct acute coronary vasodilating effects in menopausal women. Subsequent human studies support this observation. For example, flow-mediated, endothelium-dependent brachial artery vasodilation was greater in postmenopausal subjects given 17-β-estradiol for nine weeks compared with those given placebo (91). Similar findings on brachial artery blood flow were reported in a study where postmenopausal women were given infusions of 17-β-estradiol (92), suggesting that both long-term and acute administration of estradiol promotes vasodilation. In an investigation using angiography and Doppler analysis of coronary flow velocity, intracoronary infusion of 17-β-estradiol prevented epicardial coronary artery constriction induced by acetylcholine and potentiated the vasodilator coronary microvascular response to acetylcholine (93). The effect of estradiol on coronary dynamics was similar in women regardless of angiographically apparent left coronoary artery atherosclerosis. The authors concluded that physiological levels of 17-β-estradiol acutely potentiated endothelium-dependent vasodilation of both large coronary arteries and coronary microvascular resistance arteries of postmenopausal women (93). Interestingly, a subsequent and similar coronary blood flow investigation that included men confirmed previous findings in postmenopausal women but found no evidence that 17-β-estradiol modulates acetylcholine-induced coronary artery responses in men (94). Overall, these data strongly suggest that estradiol exerts prominent vasodilating effects in the coronary vasculature of postmenopausal women.

In vitro and whole animal studies also support the hypothesis that estrogens exert beneficial effects on the vasculature and provide some evidence as to possible mechanisms of action. Given the observed endothelium-dependent effects of estrogens in human studies, numerous whole animal and/or in vitro experiments have focused on estrogen modulation of NO as a potential mechanism. From these studies, sufficient evidence exists to conclude that exogenous estrogens induce NOS and increase NO release, thus promoting endothelium-dependent vasodilation in a variety of species and vascular beds, possibly via both transcriptional mechanisms and via ERα with activation of PI3K/Akt and phosphorylation of eNOS (95) and that endogenous estrogens may be responsible for gender differences in vascular responsiveness via NO-mediated mechanisms (96–101). Importantly, the observed effects of estrogens on NO-mediated vasodilation are accompanied by improvements in myocardial function in dogs, as indicated by reductions in both myocardial infarct size and the occurrence of ischemia- and reperfusion-induced ventricular arrhythmias (102). In addition to effects on NO, Dubey and colleagues reported that metabolites of estradiol with little affinity for ERs inhibit endothelin-1 production in endothelial cells, possibly via inhibition of MAPK activity (103). Furthermore, it has been demonstrated that estrogen (*i*) decreases endothelium-mediated prostaglandin H synthase–dependent vasoconstriction and the sensitivity of the thromboxane A_2/PGH_2 receptor (104,105) and (*ii*) acts via a receptor-dependent, PI3K/Akt-mediated pathway to enhance production of vasodilator epoxyeicosatrienoic acids (106). Studies in rat heart suggest that the coronary vasodilation elicited by acute estrogen treatment involves prostaglandin release and K_{ATP} channel activation in addition to calcium channel blockade (107). Conversely, it was reported that estrogen treatment of OVXed rats suppresses isoprenaline-induced relaxation of aortic rings via mechanisms involving cytochrome P450 metabolites (108). It is interesting to note that estrogen augments, rather than attenuates, vasoconstrictor responsiveness in vessels isolated from ERβ-deficient mice (109).

Several studies have demonstrated calcium channel blocking effects of estrogens in vascular smooth muscle that could account for the observed vaso-dilation (110). These acute exposure studies include electrophysiological experiments (111,112), fluorescent measurements of intracellular calcium (113), or contraction measurements in response to the calcium channel agonist BayK 8644 (114). In general, these studies are hampered by the high concentrations (often in excess of 1 μM) of estrogen required to demonstrate or to suggest calcium channel blocking effects. It is plausible that nonspecific membrane flu-idity alterations induced by intercalation of estrogen into the lipid bilayer con-tributed to the observed effects in these studies (20). Nonetheless, sufficient evidence to rule out the possibility that estrogens act acutely as calcium channel antagonists does not exist. In addition, studies in porcine coronary artery smooth muscle cells suggested that estradiol acts acutely via ERs to diminish the intra-cellular calcium response to endothelin-1 by increasing calcium efflux (115). Also, with respect to chronic actions studies in isolated aortic smooth muscle cells from rats indicate that ovariectomy (OVX) increases phenylephrine- and depolarization-induced cell contraction and intracellular calcium, suggesting that physiological levels of estrogen (or progesterone) alter calcium entry processes (116).

Lower concentrations of estrogens (<400 nM) have also been demonstrated to exert antiproliferative effects on rat carotid artery segments (117) and on porcine LAD coronary artery segments (118). Interestingly, preincubation of rat, but not porcine, vascular segments with the partial ER agonist tamoxifen inhibited the effects of estradiol, suggesting that ERs may mediate the observed anti-proliferative effects of estrogen on vascular smooth muscle cells. Mechanisms for estrogen-induced inhibition of vascular smooth muscle proliferation might also include insulin-like growth factor I (IGF-I) receptors because estrogen-treated rabbits displayed reduced IGF-I receptor mRNA in their coronary arteries (119). Also, Hong and colleagues, using cultured rat aortic smooth muscle cells, showed that estradiol preincubation inhibits angiotensin II–induced cell proliferation and endothelin-1 expression at least in part by decreasing reactive oxygen species (ROS) formation and activation of the ERK pathway (120). Some precautions regarding experimental models are in order for future studies. For example, in primary rabbit vascular smooth muscle cell cultures, 17-β-estradiol (10 nM) delayed cell cycle reentry, thus prolonging the quiescent phase prior to rapid proliferation in vitro; however, when secondary or tertiary cultures were exam-ined, 17-β-estradiol actually promoted proliferation (121). This study of rabbit vascular smooth muscle cells is extremely important, as future studies must consider the phenotypic state of the cells prior to examining effects of estrogens.

A final possible mechanism for estrogen's beneficial effects on vasculature involves the potential antioxidant activity of the hormone. As discussed previously, 17-β-estradiol was found to inhibit in vitro copper-induced oxidation of LDL, but the concentrations required for antioxidant activity were extremely high, in excess of 1 μM (63). Furthermore, estradiol was found to protect DNA from hydroperoxide-induced damage, but again high concentrations (18 μM) were required (122). Perhaps the most convincing data for antioxidant effects of estradiol are found in a study by Kim and colleagues (123). Thirty-nine male dogs were given either 100 μg/kg 17-β-estradiol subcutaneously or an equal volume of vehicle for two weeks prior to instigation of cardiac ischemia/reperfusion injury. The investigators found a decreased incidence of ventricular arrhythmias in estradiol-treated compared with vehicle-treated dogs, and n-pentane in exhaled air (an index of lipid peroxidation) was lower in estradiol-treated animals (123). Moreover, artery segments from estradiol-treated dogs generated less superoxide anion after hypoxia/reoxygenation than those obtained from vehicle-treated dogs (123). In addition, later studies in rat aortic vascular smooth muscle cells showed that physiological to pharmacological concentrations of estradiol metabolites such as methoxyestradiol can act acutely via nonreceptor mechanisms to serve as antioxidants and diminish oxidant damage and associated cell proliferation and migration (124). Thus, available in vitro data still leave some concern that the concentrations of estrogens required for acute antioxidant effects are too high to assume similar effects occur in vivo; however, at least one in vivo study suggests that with chronic administration estrogens may indeed act to enhance antioxidant mechanisms.

In summary, apart from altered lipid metabolism, four mechanisms have been proposed to explain the beneficial vascular effects of estrogens: (*i*) estrogen-mediated vasodilation through upregulation and/or activation of NOS (i.e., endothelium-dependent vasodilation); (*ii*) estrogen-mediated vasodilation through effects on calcium influx or efflux (i.e., endothelium-independent vasodilation); (*iii*) estrogen modulation of vascular smooth muscle and/or endothelial cell proliferation; and (*iv*) antioxidant effects of estrogen providing protection from endothelial damage. Whether any or all of these actions are necessary to produce the observed beneficial vascular effects of estrogens is currently unknown. In addition, further research is required to determine if these observed actions are receptor mediated and/or if they involve genomic and/or nongenomic mechanisms.

Progestins

As with androgens, little is known about the direct effects of progestins on the vasculature. Progesterone receptors are most likely expressed throughout the vasculature, including the coronary vasculature; however, evidence for expression of these receptors is limited. Not surprisingly, progesterone receptors are expressed in arterial vessels of the reproductive tract in rabbits and humans, more specifically in uterine arteries (125). In addition, Perrot-Applanat and colleagues (126) found immunocytochemical evidence of progesterone receptor expression in varicose saphenous veins from men, and pre- and postmenopausal women, and progesterone receptors have also been detected in human and rat aortic smooth muscle cells (127). As discussed below, the vasculature serves as a target for direct progestin action, and it is plausible that both genomic and nongenomic, progesterone receptor–mediated mechanisms could account for progestin actions. In support of the nongenomic mechanism, a full-length cDNA clone for a membrane-bound progesterone receptor has been constructed from porcine vascular smooth muscle cells (128).

The effects of progesterone on vascular reactivity are not entirely clear, as the limited animal and in vitro studies provide some conflicting information. In rabbit coronary artery rings, high concentrations of progesterone (>1 µM) induced significant relaxation in potassium-, $PGF_{2\alpha}$-, or BayK 8644-precontracted arteries, with no differences in progesterone-induced relaxation being observed in endothelium-intact and -denuded preparations isolated from male and female rabbits (129). The authors concluded that progesterone elicited an endothelium-independent relaxation by altering calcium influx, but again high concentrations of progesterone were required. Progesterone-induced inhibition of calcium current in smooth muscle was later found using human intestinal cells in electrophysiological experiments (130). Furthermore, at least one study provided evidence that while estradiol induced NOS activity in tissues from guinea pigs, progesterone treatment did not (98). These findings further support an endothelium-independent effect of progesterone on vascular reactivity. Yet, other evidence suggests that while progesterone minimally alters endothelium-dependent vascular reactivity, it may antagonize estrogen-induced vasodilation. Miller and Vanhoutte examined OVXed dogs treated with estrogen, progesterone, or estrogen plus progesterone (131). Estrogen-treated dogs had similar coronary vasodilatory responses as described in other studies, but when progesterone was added, the vasodilatory response of estrogen was inhibited (131). As with estrogens, studies also suggest that progesterone may inhibit arterial smooth muscle proliferation (127). Overall, acute and chronic mechanisms and effects of progesterone on vascular reactivity are not well understood, and further research is indicated. Furthermore, it is quite possible that the different classes of progestins may have strikingly different effects on the vasculature, where, e.g., progestins chemically related to 19-nortestosterone may antagonize the beneficial vasodilation produced by estrogens.

Glucocorticoids and Mineralocorticoids

Adrenal steroids (glucocorticoids and mineralocorticoids) increase blood pressure in humans, and this response is not entirely explained by renal mechanisms such as increased sodium and water retention (132). Thus, examination of direct effects of adrenal steroids on the vasculature has been the subject of several investigations. Functional receptors for both glucocorticoids and mineralocorticoids were found in rabbit aorta and femoral and carotid arteries (133,134). More recently, evidence for membrane-bound mineralocorticoid receptors was found in membrane preparations from human mononuclear leukocytes (135) and porcine kidney and liver (136,137). Despite identification of classical adrenal steroid receptors in vascular cells, whether membrane-bound glucocorticoid or mineralocorticoid receptors are expressed in vascular cells is not known.

Few human and whole animal studies have been conducted to examine direct effects of glucocorticoids or mineralocorticoids on the vasculature; thus, most of the evidence for direct effects was generated with in vitro models. Nonetheless, some evidence has been published, suggesting direct glucocorticoid alterations in vascular reactivity. Six human subjects were placed on a restricted nitrate diet and treated with 80 mg/day cortisol (138). Cortisol significantly increased systolic and mean arterial blood pressure, and there was an associated reduction in plasma nitrate or nitrite after 3, 4, and 5 days of cortisol treatment. The authors concluded that the results supported a role for NO in cortisol-induced hypertension in humans (138). Indeed, glucocorticoid-induced hypertension may involve endothelium-mediated vasoconstriction and/or reduced vasodilation, but whether reduced NO production is involved is unknown. For example, direct glucocorticoid-altered vascular reactivity may involve inhibition of prostacyclin synthesis. In human endothelial cell cultures, dexamethasone (0.01–100 nM) reduced histamine-, bradykinin-, and calcium ionophore A23187–induced prostaglandin I_2 (prostacyclin) and prostaglandin E_2 formation within four hours of exposure (139). Furthermore, a glucocorticoid receptor antagonist (cortisol-21-mesylate) and cycloheximide blocked the effects of dexamethasone on prostaglandin synthesis (139). The hypothesis that glucocorticoid-induced hypertension involves reductions in endothelial prostacyclin production (140) is certainly worthwhile, but subsequent data suggest that other mechanisms also participate in the hypertensive response.

Additional mechanisms for direct glucocorticoid actions in the vasculature include alterations in the cellular renin-angiotensin system. For example, dexamethasone (100 nM) increased angiotensin converting enzyme (ACE) mRNA and activity in rat aortic smooth muscle cell cultures (141). Interestingly, glucocorticoids have also been shown to increase angiotensin II type 1A receptors in vascular smooth muscle cells (142), and this effect was shown to participate in dexamethasone-induced hypertension in rats (143). Furthermore, a glucocorticoid response element for the rat angiotensin II type 1A receptor was later reported (144). Overall, glucocorticoids may increase angiotensin II production in vascular smooth muscle and enhance angiotensin II responsiveness by upregulating angiotensin II receptors.

Glucocorticoids may also affect vascular reactivity by altering electrolyte transport across the vascular smooth muscle cell plasma membrane. For example, in rabbit aortic smooth muscle cell cultures, dexamethasone (100 nM) increased sodium influx within 48 hours of exposure (145). This effect was completely blocked by the glucocorticoid antagonist RU486 and significantly reduced by progesterone (145). Actinomycin D and cycloheximide (protein synthesis inhibitors) also blocked the enhanced sodium influx, suggesting a genomic mechanism for dexamethasone (145). Calcium influx may also participate in direct glucocorticoid actions on vascular smooth muscle. When rabbits were given silastic implants containing dexamethasone, blood pressure was elevated compared with sham-treated controls (146). Interestingly, when the treated rabbits' aortas were excised, aortic rings from the dexamethasone-treated animals exhibited calcium influx at a rate twice that of rings from sham-treated animals (146). Thus, glucocorticoids could alter vascular smooth muscle contractions by enhancing sodium and/or calcium influx. The channels or transporters involved have not been fully elucidated.

Regarding mineralocorticoids, aldosterone rapidly increases vascular resistance in man. Wehling and colleagues recruited 17 subjects with suspected coronary artery disease, and enrolled them in a double-blind, placebo-controlled, randomized parallel trial (147). During cardiac catheterization, intravenous administration of 1 mg aldosterone rapidly (within 10 minutes) increased systemic vascular resistance and cardiac output compared with placebo (147). Results of this human experiment provide strong evidence for nongenomic, direct actions of mineralocorticoids on the vasculature.

Regarding the mechanisms of mineralocorticoid-induced alterations in vascular reactivity, the most likely explanation is that aldosterone mediates electrolyte transport across vascular smooth muscle cell plasma membranes. At least part of this mechanism is similar to that of glucocorticoids. Aldosterone was shown to stimulate sodium influx in vascular smooth muscle cells, and both genomic and nongenomic mechanisms may account for this effect. Support for a genomic mechanism stems from data demonstrating that physiological concentrations of aldosterone (5 nM) required 7 to 10 days to increase sodium influx in rabbit aortic smooth muscle cell cultures, and rabbits treated for four weeks with 2 mg/day aldosterone had increased sodium channel density in aortic smooth muscle membranes (148). In contrast, aldosterone (1 nM) stimulated sodium influx after only four minutes of exposure in rat vascular smooth muscle cells (149). This effect appeared to be mediated by aldosterone stimulation of the sodium/hydrogen exchanger via a nongenomic mechanism (149).

Other mechanisms may also participate in aldosterone-mediated vascular reactivity. For example, aldosterone stimulates calcium influx in rat aortic vascular smooth muscle cells (150) and in porcine endothelial cells (151). The calcium effect of aldosterone in vascular smooth muscle cells may be mediated by phospholipase C (PLC), as aldosterone was shown to increase inositol 1,4,5-trisphosphate (IP_3) levels within 30 seconds of exposure in rat vascular smooth muscle cells, and inhibitors of PLC blocked this effect (149). Furthermore, the involvement of PLC would be expected to increase diacylglycerol (DAG) and activate protein kinase C (PKC). Indeed, increased levels of DAG were observed in rat vascular smooth muscle cells exposed to 1 nM aldosterone for 30 seconds, and increased translocation of PKCα from cytosolic to particulate fractions (indicating activation) was observed within five minutes of aldosterone exposure (152). Somewhat in contrast, studies in porcine coronary artery vascular smooth muscle cells showed that physiological concentrations of aldosterone increased intracellular cAMP levels (153), an action often associated with vasodilation. Whether the observed signaling mechanisms of aldosterone in vascular smooth muscle and/or endothelial cells are mediated by membrane-associated mineralocorticoid receptors is not known, although the reported effect on cAMP levels was not antagonized by mineralocorticoid receptor inhibitors.

In summary, glucocorticoids and mineralocorticoids induce hypertension, and at least part of this effect is likely produced by direct glucocorticoid- or mineralocorticoid-induced increases in vascular resistance. Mechanisms for adrenal steroid–induced alterations in vascular reactivity are beginning to be understood. Further research is required to determine whether genomic and/or nongenomic, receptor-mediated mechanisms are responsible for increased vascular smooth muscle contractility. Further research is also required to understand the effects of adrenal steroids on endothelial cells and whether glucocorticoids or mineralocorticoids might alter the NO system.

CARDIAC EFFECTS OF STEROIDAL AGENTS

Steroid Receptors and Steroids in the Heart

Androgen Receptors and Androgens

Significant evidence demonstrates that steroid receptors are expressed in cardiac tissue (Table 6) and that the heart is a target organ for direct steroid action (Table 7). Over 20 years ago, autoradiographic evidence for androgen receptor

Table 6 Evidence for Cardiac Steroid Receptors in Various Species: Location, Isoforms, and Methods Employed for Detection

	Species	Location	Isoforms	Methods
Androgen receptors	rats, dogs, monkeys, baboons, humans	atria and ventricles	A form	AR, IB, RB, RT-PCR
Estrogen receptors	rats, rabbits	atria and ventricles	α and β	AR, IH, RNaseP, RT-PCR
Progesterone receptors	rats	?	?	IB
Mineralocorticoid receptors	rats, guinea pigs	atria and ventricles	Type I	AR, RB
Glucocorticoid receptors	rats	ventricles	Type II	AR, RB

Abbreviations: AR, autoradiography; IB, immunoblotting; IH, immunohistochemistry; RB, radioligand binding; RT-PCR, reverse transcription-polymerase chain reaction; RNaseP, ribonuclease protection assay; ?, unknown. Supporting references are found throughout the text.

Table 7 Potential Direct Effects of Exogenous Steroids on the Heart

Steroid class	Cardiac myocytes	Cardiac fibroblasts
Androgens and anabolic steroids	hypertrophic growth, ↑ ornithine decarboxylase, ↑ pyruvate kinase, ↑ lactate, dehydrogenase, altered ion homeostasis	↑ collagen synthesis
Estrogens	↑ L-type Ca^{++} channels, ↓ L-type Ca^{++} current, ↑ Na^+/K^+ ATPase, prolonged QT interval	↑ or ↓ proliferation
Mineralocorticoids	hypertrophic growth with high glucose, ↑ Cl^-/HCO_3^- exchanger, ↑ Na^+/H^+ antiporter, ↑ Na^+/K^+ ATPase	↑ collagen synthesis
Glucocorticoids	hypertrophic growth, ↑ angiotensinogen, ↑ AT receptors	↑ collagen synthesis

Abbreviations: AT, angiotensin II. Supporting references are found throughout the text.

expression was found in rat heart muscle (154). Two years later, McGill and colleagues reported evidence for androgen receptor expression in atrial and ventricular cardiac myocytes from female rhesus monkeys and baboons (155). More recently, full-length androgen receptors (A form; 110 kD) were identified in human fetal heart tissue by immunoblotting; whereas, truncated androgen receptors (B form; 87 kD) were not detectable (156). Most recently, mRNA transcripts for androgen receptors were detected by reverse transcription-polymerase chain reaction (RT-PCR) in cardiac myocytes isolated from male and female adult rats, pooled cardiac myocytes isolated from male and female neonatal rats, and heart tissue obtained from male and female adult rats, male and female adult dogs, male and female neonatal humans, and male and female adult humans (157). Thus, androgen receptors are most likely expressed in the hearts of nearly every mammalian species regardless of age or sex—an "equal opportunity" receptor.

Interestingly, the rat heart accumulates testosterone to levels that are greater than those observed in more classical androgen target tissue. For example, in uncastrated adult male rats, radioimmunoassay revealed cardiac tissue testosterone levels that were four-fold higher than skeletal muscle and two-fold higher than prostate tissue, possibly because of the low levels of 5-α reductase in the heart (154). Similar findings were reported in humans, where men were found to have higher postmortem cardiac testosterone concentrations than striated muscle, and the cardiac hormone profile suggested low levels of 5-α reductase activity (158). Interestingly, steroid production in the heart may vary in the disease process. For example, steroid-metabolizing enzymes and testosterone are elevated in the hypertrophic heart, clearly indicating a role for heart-specific steroid metabolism during cardiac hypertrophy (159). Clearly, the heart is a target organ for androgens, but the physiological and/or pathophysiological roles of cardiac androgen receptors are unknown. In addition, the heart contains the metabolic capacity to produce and metabolize steroidal hormones, and these processes may be altered during disease. Thus, further research is required to delineate cause-effect relationships of these observations.

ERs and Estrogens

Evidence for cardiac ERs was obtained shortly before evidence for androgen receptors when Stumpf and colleagues found tritiated estradiol binding in the nuclei of atrial myocytes by autoradiography (160). Since then, two forms of the ER have been identified (α and β), and both forms appear to be expressed in heart tissue. For example, in adult male rats, ERβ was found by immunohistochemistry (161), and in hearts from adult male and female mice, mRNA transcripts for ERα and ERβ were found by ribonuclease protection assay (162). In addition, functional ERs were found in both male and female neonatal rat cardiac myocytes and cardiac fibroblasts, and 17-β-estradiol treatment (1 nM for 24 hours) increased ERα and ERβ and progesterone receptor expression in cardiac myocytes (163). Also of note is the possibility that ER expression in the heart changes following injury. For example, ERα was upregulated (as determined by immunohistochemistry and RT-PCR) in cholesterol-fed rabbits that received cardiac-aorta transplants (164). Furthermore, androstendione and testosterone were found to stimulate ERα and ERβ expression and activate an estrogen-responsive reporter plasmid in neonatal rat cardiac myocytes, perhaps through cardiac aromatase conversion of these precursors to estrogen (165). These results provide evidence for androgen- and estrogen-mediated upregulation of ERs and suggest local cardiac production of estrogens. Therefore, it is clear that the heart is also a target organ for estrogens, but the physiological and/ or pathophysiological roles of cardiac ERs are not known.

Other Steroid Receptors

As for other steroid receptors in the heart, less information is available. Progesterone receptors are expressed in the hearts of male and female neonatal rats, and expression of progesterone receptors may be induced by estrogen (163). In atrial and ventricular cytosols from adult male and female rats, radioligand evidence for aldosterone binding to type I mineralocorticoid receptors was found, and in a manner similar to that of classical aldosterone target tissue, aldosterone and corticosterone had similar binding affinities (1–2 nM), whereas dexamethasone had a much lower affinity (166). In these experiments, relative levels of type I mineralocorticoid receptors were higher in atria than ventricles, and relative levels of type II (classic glucocorticoid) receptors were higher in ventricles than atria (166). Type I mineralocorticoid receptors were also found in guinea pig heart, and cortisol and aldosterone appeared to have equivalent affinity for this receptor (167).

Most interestingly, there is evidence for local cardiac production of both aldosterone and corticosterone. Rat hearts were found to express the terminal synthetic enzymes for aldosterone (aldosterone synthase) and corticosterone (11-β-hydroxylase), aldosterone and corticosterone were found in rat heart tissue, and rat hearts responded to angiotensin II or adrenocorticotrophin by increasing aldosterone or corticosterone synthesis, respectively (168). Importantly, cardiac aldosterone concentrations in these rats were estimated to be 16 nM, which would be approximately 17-fold higher than aldosterone concentrations in the plasma (168).

Regarding progestins, progesterone may also bind to mineralocorticoid receptors. However, in contrast to other guinea pig tissues such as kidney and colon where progesterone and aldosterone appeared to have equal affinity for mineralocorticoid receptors, progesterone demonstrated 10- to 100-fold less affinity than aldosterone for guinea pig heart mineralocorticoid receptors (169). Also worthy of note is that other members of the steroid receptor superfamily are also found in the heart. For example, autoradiography and immunocytochemistry techniques demonstrated the presence of receptors for 1,25-dihydroxyvitamin D_3 in the right atrium of male and female mice (170). Overall, progesterone, mineralocorticoid, and glucocorticoid receptors appear to be expressed in the heart of a variety of species, and agonists for these receptors may exhibit binding to all three types of receptors, thus challenging researchers with complex signaling and control mechanisms. As with androgen and ERs, whether subpopulations of progesterone, mineralocorticoid, or glucocorticoid receptors are plasma membrane associated is not known.

In summary, it appears that the heart is a target organ for steroidal agents. At present, however, studies are just beginning to identify the physiological and pathophysiological roles for these cardiac steroid receptors. In addition, the role of plasma membrane–bound steroid receptors in the heart is currently being elucidated. A wide range of future research regarding cardiac steroid receptors and mechanisms of action thus lies nearly untouched.

Direct Effects of Steroids on the Heart

Androgens and Anabolic Steroids

Evidence for a direct pathological effect of androgens on cardiac tissue was first described by Behrendt and Boffin in 1977 (171); about the same time that evidence for cardiac androgen receptors was reported. Adult female wistar rats were given weekly intramuscular injections of 1.65 mg/kg methandrostenolone for three weeks. Using transmission electron microscopy, hearts from rats treated with methandrostenolone had swollen and elongated mitochondria, and myofibrils demonstrated either disintegrated, widened and twisted Z-bands or complete dissolution of the sarcomeric units. The authors concluded that methandrostenolone administration induced myocardial lesions that were similar to those observed during early heart failure (171). These results suggested that in vivo administration of AASs may induce myocardial necrosis and/or apoptosis.

Indeed, in vitro studies demonstrated that several AASs induce cell death of cultured neonatal rat cardiac myocytes (172,173) or apoptosis of skeletal myocytes (174); however, the concentrations of AASs required to induce cardiac myocyte death or skeletal myocyte apoptosis were in the micromolar range. More recently, stanozolol and testosterone, also at high concentrations (0.1–100 µM), induced dose-dependent apoptotic cell death of rat ventricular myocytes (175). Alternatively, AAS may produce necrosis and/or apoptosis in the heart though indirect actions. For example, castration of male rats or treatment with flutamide (antiandrogen) improved myocardial function following ischemia-reperfusion injury, effects that were possibly attributable to proinflammatory (e.g., increased expression of TNF-α, IL-1β, and IL-6) and/or proapoptotic properties of testosterone (176). Therefore, whether AASs may induce myocardial necrosis and/or apoptosis in humans self-administering enormous doses of AASs seems possible but is currently unknown and requires further research.

Increasing evidence suggests that androgens may induce hypertrophic growth of cardiac myocytes through an androgen receptor–mediated mechanism. First, however, it is important to note that men have larger hearts than women, even after correction for body weight and height, and despite similar numbers of myocytes (177). However, left ventricular (LV) mass is only slightly lower in girls than boys prior to puberty (177). Thus, gender differences in cardiac size may be related to sex steroids, and endogenous testosterone–induced cardiac hypertrophy may indeed be a normal physiological response. Furthermore, even if endogenous testosterone were found to be responsible for increased cardiac size in men, the clinical significance in terms of adverse cardiovascular outcomes following administration of exogenous androgens would not be clear. The increased cardiac size in men may represent a normal physiological variation without adverse consequences. For example, in a study of 436 black patients (163 male, 273 female) with no angiographic evidence of coronary artery disease, 52% of the men and 44% of the women had left ventricular hypertrophy (LVH), and a two-fold greater relative risk of cardiac death was found among women with LVH than men with LVH (178). Thus, endogenous androgen–induced cardiac hypertrophy as a sole cause of gender differences in cardiac size has not been proven, and its relationship to cardiovascular disease is questionable.

Exogenous androgens, on the other hand, may impart an increased risk of pathological cardiac hypertrophy in those who self-administer supra-physiological doses. Several human studies demonstrate increased LV mass in AAS users compared with nonusers; however, an important disclaimer to all these studies is the inherent inability to control specific AAS(s) used, dose, or purity. Urhausen and colleagues used one- and two-dimensional echocardiography and found increased LV posterior wall and septum thickness and increased LV wall thickness to LV internal diameter ratios in 21 AAS using body builders compared with 7 nonusing control body builders (179). Importantly, there was an impairment of diastolic function in the body builders using AASs (179). Similar results were reported by De Piccoli and colleagues when they found echocardiographic evidence for increased ventricular septal thickness, increased LV mass, increased end-diastolic volume indices, and increased isovolumetric relaxation time in 14 body builders self-administering AAS compared with 14 body builders not using AASs and 14 sedentary individuals (180). The investigators also found that cardiac structural modifications persisted in individuals who withdrew from AASs for approximately nine weeks (180). Sachtleben and colleagues reported similar findings regarding altered cardiac structure in AAS-using body builders, but they observed no AAS-associated changes in myocardial shortening fraction (181). Finally, at least one study similar to those previously discussed, found no association between AAS use in weight lifters and LVH or clinically detectable systolic or diastolic dysfunction (182). Although some controversy exists, an association between high-dose AAS use and LVH in humans is likely, given the results of animal experiments.

Animal studies have demonstrated similar anabolic effects of androgens on the heart. First, and as with humans, animal hearts are known to exhibit sexual dimorphism. For example, male A/J mice, and Sprague-Dawley, Wistar, and Fischer 344 rats have slightly larger ventricles (not corrected for body weight) than their female counterparts (183–186), and orchiectomized rats were found to have reduced heart weight compared with normal, sham-operated control males (187). Koenig and colleagues found that male mice also had substantially higher specific activities of lysosomal hydrolases and mitochondrial cytochrome C oxidase than female mice, and that these gender differences were abolished by orchiectomy (185). Cardiac contractile properties may also exhibit sexual dimorphism. For example, papillary muscle from male rats exhibited markedly different contractile properties from age-matched female rats in that the time course of isometric contraction was decreased and the velocity of shortening during isotonic contractions was increased in tissue from males (184). Wang and colleagues found that cardiac muscle isolated from female rats was more sensitive to extracellular calcium when compared with tissue from age-matched males (188). Adult female rat hearts had greater steady state mRNA levels for contractile proteins [α- and β-myosin heavy chain (MHC) and sarcomeric actin] and structural proteins (collagen type I, cytoskeletal actin, and connexin 43) when compared with their age-matched male counterparts (186), although Morris and colleagues (189) reported that OVX in adult rats does not affect myosin iso-enzyme distribution. Interestingly, studies in neonatal rat ventricular myocytes showed that testosterone (1 μM) treatment for 8 to 24 hours increases β_1-adrenoceptor, L-type calcium channel, androgen receptor, and Na/Ca exchanger mRNA levels (190). Clearly, there are sex- and sex steroid–mediated differences in cardiac structure and function, and these differences may confound studies examining effects of exogenous sex steroids.

As in human studies, administration of exogenous androgens to animals was found to elicit hypertrophic cardiac growth. Initial studies of the effects of exogenous androgens on cardiac ultrastructural morphology demonstrated that methandrostenolone administration (1.65 mg/kg intramuscularly once weekly) to female rats for 13 weeks resulted in an increase of intermediate-sized filaments in muscle cells of the left ventricle (191). Several subsequent studies have demonstrated anabolic effects of androgens on the hearts of castrated animals. For example, testosterone (but not estrogen or progesterone) administration for five to six weeks to castrated male rats was found to induce significant right ventricular hypertrophy (RVH) (192). Testosterone administration to orchiectomized mice induced a marked anabolic effect as demonstrated by increased ventricular wet weight, and increases in total protein and RNA, while total DNA remained constant (185). Furthermore, testosterone administration partially restored the reduced heart weight (193) and the reduced V_1 MHC isoenzyme levels in orchiectomized rats (194). These effects of androgens may be mediated in part via myocardial ACE expression as ventricular ACE mRNA and protein are more abundant in male than female mouse ventricle, with the levels of this enzyme in male myocardium being significantly decreased by androgen deprivation (195). In addition, data suggest that androgen receptor activation may enhance the responsiveness to angiotensin II. Ikeda and colleagues reported that the heart-to-body weight ratio and the concentric hypertrophy and ERK 1/2 and ERK 5 activation elicited by angiotensin II is diminished in androgen receptor knockout (ARKO) as compared with wild-type male mice (196). Conversely, angiotensin II produced a greater cardiac fibrosis with greater expression of collagens type I and II as well as TGF-β1 in the ARKO mice. Interestingly, short-term (2 weeks) testosterone administration to rats restored the reduced α MHC levels that were observed in OVXed rats (197), and dihydrotestosterone was shown to cause a concentric cardiac remodeling in OVXed rats, possibly via increased IGF-1 (198). Finally, testosterone administration to young male rats (30-day-old) also restored castration-induced reductions in cardiac protein synthesis (199).

Hearts from other species also respond to androgens in an anabolic manner. In dogs, administration of methandienone (1.5 mg/kg/day orally for 6 weeks) resulted in a significantly increased heart weight that was associated with reduced cardiac responses to inotropic load, and the pressure-volume diagram revealed that the left ventricles of treated animals worked on larger ventricular volumes (200). Interestingly, exogenous testosterone and methyltestosterone increased rainbow trout heart growth to levels that were approximately 1.7 times that of control fish (201).

Overall, androgens appear to increase heart weight by producing increases in RNA and protein synthesis. The mechanisms involved in this effect may involve ACE, IGF-1, and ERKs; however, further research is required to delineate the exact mechanisms. However, exposure of neonatal rat cardiac myocyte cultures to dihydrotestosterone and testosterone was found to increase protein synthesis to levels comparable to that of angiotensin II, and the effects of dihydrotestosterone and testosterone were blocked by the androgen antagonist cyproterone acetate (157). Although high concentrations (1 μM) of androgens were used in these in vitro experiments, when combined with data from ARKO mice (196), these results suggest that androgen-induced cardiac hypertrophy is mediated through androgen receptors and that cultured cardiac myocytes may be a useful model for determining mechanisms of androgen-induced hypertrophy.

Because there are gender differences in coronary artery disease and myocardial infarction, studies have also examined effects of androgens on cardiac ischemia/reperfusion injury and postinfarction remodeling with somewhat conflicting results. Experiments in rat ventricular myocytes showed that testosterone acts acutely to decrease the rate of cardiomyocyte death elicited by a model of ischemia, possibly via activation of mitochondrial K_{ATP} channels (202), whereas studies in hearts isolated from adult female and castrated male rats demonstrated that acute treatment with testosterone decreased functional recovery and increased MAPKs and caspase-3 activation following ischemia/reperfusion (203). Cavasin and colleagues showed in mice that chronic testosterone exposure promotes myocardial inflammation, thus diminishing early healing and remodeling and enhancing cardiac rupture within one week of acute infarction (204). In contrast, studies in rats showed that chronic testosterone treatment led to an increased LVH with diminished LV end-diastolic pressure and wall stress (205); infarct size and mortality were not affected. These conflicting results may be mediated by differences in species, doses, duration of exposure, experimental models, etc. Continued studies are required to better delineate the actions of physiological or pharmacological doses of androgens on ischemia/reperfusion injury and recovery as well as the underlying mechanisms.

A variety of other effects including alterations in specific enzyme systems, ion fluxes, and structural matrices may occur in cardiac myocytes exposed to androgens. For example, Koenig and colleagues demonstrated that exposure of rat ventricular cubes and acutely isolated ventricular myocytes to testosterone (10 nM) resulted in increased ornithine decarboxylase activity and subsequent polyamine levels, and increased endocytosis, hexose transport, and amino acid transport (33). All of these testosterone effects were blocked by the specific ornithine decarboxylase inhibitor α-difluoromethylornithine. More recently, these studies have been extended to demonstrate that increased ornithine decarboxylase activity and polyamine concentrations in cardiac myocytes might contribute to positive inotropic effects of dihydrotestosterone (34). Furthermore, polyamines may affect cardiac ion homeostasis, as spermidine and putrescine are known modulators of potassium current (35). In castrated male rats, testsosterone administration increased the activity of pyruvate kinase (206). In addition, total levels of lactate dehydrogenase were decreased in the hearts of guinea pigs exposed to methandrostenolone in combination with inclined treadmill running (207).

As for acute androgen-induced alterations in cardiac ion homeostasis and contractility, testosterone (10 nM) produced rapid (<30 seconds) stimulation of calcium influx and efflux in rat ventricular cubes and isolated myocytes (33), suggesting that androgens may exert effects in cardiac myocytes via nongenomic mechanisms. Studies by Velasco and colleagues (208) also showed that dihydrotestosterone increases contractility and intracellular cAMP levels in isolated rat left atrium, although at relatively high concentrations (10–100 μM). In contrast, an in vitro study using neonatal rat cardiac myocyte cultures found no immediate (<13 minutes) changes in intracellular calcium concentrations when fura-2-loaded myocytes were exposed to high concentrations (100 μM) of testosterone (173).

Other investigators have reported effects of chronic androgen exposure on cardiac electrical properties and/or ion channels. For example, dihydrotestosterone downregulated mRNA for two cardiac potassium channels and prolonged the QT interval in OVXed rabbits (209). Somewhat in contrast, repolarization was found to be slower and longer in castrated when compared with normal men (210), and castration of male mice prolonged the QT interval of the ECG, increased action potential duration in ventricular myocytes, and decreased the expression of Kv1.5 and its associated current density in these cells (211). Testosterone replacement reversed these effects (212).

As for cardiac structural matrices, Takala and colleagues reported that methandienone (1.5 mg/kg/day) in combination with endurance exercise in dogs increased collagen concentration in the right ventricular (RV) wall (213). Furthermore, sialic acid in the glycocalyx (participates in maintaining normal electrical activity) was increased in castrated rats receiving testosterone replacement (214).

In summary, endogenous androgens are likely to be at least partially responsible for gender-related differences in cardiac size and function. Exogenous androgens, particularly in the high doses used for illicit purposes, may induce cardiac hypertrophy. It is logical to speculate that many of these effects are mediated by genomic mechanisms. However, a variety of acute effects of androgens on cardiac tissue have been found, and the rapidity of these effects suggest that androgens may alter cardiac function through nongenomic mechanisms. Future research is required to clarify the signaling pathways of androgens in the heart.

Estrogens and Progestins

Although compelling evidence suggests that androgens are at least partially responsible for gender differences in cardiac size and function, these sex differences could, of course, also be a result of direct effects of estrogens and/or progestins on the heart. Most likely, however, is the possibility that gender differences in cardiac size and function are produced by exposure to variable concentrations of all sex steroids and secondary to the alterations in hemodynamics produced by the sex steroids. In short, and as with androgens, the direct effects of estrogens and progestins on the heart are currently being elucidated.

Currently, there is great interest in studying the potential direct effects of estrogens and progestins on cardiac structure and function. This interest stems largely from the fact that sex differences in cardiovascular mortality are not entirely explained by protective effects of estrogens on lipid metabolism and from identification of hormone receptors in the heart. For example, it has been reported that medroxyprogesterone treatment of postmenopausal women increases LV mass and circulating IGF-1 (215). In addition, several clinical studies have indicated that the LVH and wall thickening resulting from systemic hypertension is greater in women when compared with men (216–218). In fact, some investigators have reported that hypertensive hypertrophic cardiomyopathy is seen in women but rarely in men (219).

Gender-related differences in cardiac contractile function have also been observed in hypertensive patients. As estimated by echocardiographically measured ejection fraction, both hypertensive and normotensive women have been found to display greater LV systolic function when compared with men (220,221). This difference in systolic function is paralleled by gender-associated differences in LV geometry (222), which is known to influence ejection fraction and fractional shortening (223). Concentric hypertrophy is more prevalent in hypertensive women, whereas eccentric hypertrophy is more prevalent in men (218,224). Similarly, a study by Aurigemma and Gaasch identified gender differences in both LV structure and function in older patients with pressure-overload hypertrophy; female hearts had smaller chamber dimensions, greater wall thickness, lower stress, and, as a result, a higher ejection fraction than male hearts (225). Thus, clinical data suggest that when presented with pressure overload female hearts are better able to retain systolic function via maintained wall thickness, while male hearts are more prone to progress to eccentric hypertrophy and transition into failure.

Animal models also show a sexual dimorphism in cardiac structure and function following pressure overload. Male spontaneously hypertensive rats (SHR), spontaneously hypertensive heart failure rats (SHHF), and Dahl salt-sensitive rats show accelerated progression to heart failure when compared with females (222,226–228). Similarly, aortic banding in Wistar rats resulted in depressed cardiac reserve (229) and earlier transition to heart failure in males (230). Female rats exhibited greater LV systolic pressure and lower LV diastolic pressure than male rats after aortic banding, and with increasing hypertrophy, female rats showed less cardiac dysfunction than males (230). Although some reports have suggested that the degree of hypertrophy does not correlate with the degree of hypertension in animal models (231,232), Wallen and colleagues found a correlation between blood pressure and heart-to-body weight ratio in both male and female SHR and WKY rats, with females having greater ratios in both strains (233). In contrast to clinical data reported by Krumholz and colleagues (224), Toth and coworkers reported that female Dahl salt-sensitive hypertensive rats exhibit an eccentric hypertrophy, whereas males exhibit a concentric hypertrophy (228). Interestingly, Pelzer's group showed that long-term administration of estradiol or an ERα selective agonist to OVXed SHR rats attenuated cardiac hypertrophy and increased cardiac contractile function (234). The disparity among these reports may reflect differences in timing and/or duration of estrogen exposure, age, species, and duration or extent of the pressure overload.

Although clinical studies regarding postinfarction cardiac remodeling in early to middle adulthood are limited somewhat by the occurrence of heart attacks in females, gender differences and the role of sex hormones in ischemic damage and postinfarction cardiac remodeling are being examined in animal models. Work by Booth and colleagues in anesthetized rabbits showed that estrogens act acutely via ERα-dependent mechanisms to protect the heart from ischemia/reperfusion injury, thereby decreasing infarct size (235). A study in hearts isolated from intact, OVXed and estradiol-treated/ OVXed rats indicated that the damage caused by global ischemia/reperfusion is more severe in the OVXed group, indicating that estrogen also elicits chronic effects that are cardioprotective (236); a subsequent study in hearts isolated from male ERα knockout and wild-type mice suggested that ERα plays a role in this cardioprotective mechanism (237).

Experiments examining postinfarction remodeling have produced somewhat inconsistent results. Work in castrated and hormone (estradiol or testosterone)-treated male and female mice showed that estrogen diminishes, while testosterone promotes, the remodeling and deterioration of contractile function observed 4 to 12 weeks after coronary ligation; infarct sizes were not significantly different among the groups (238). In contrast, experiments in intact, OVXed and OVXed/E2-treated female rats showed no difference among the three groups in LV function or in ACE message levels three weeks after coronary artery ligation (239). Experiments in ERβ knockout and wild-type female mice showed increased mortality and heart failure in the knockout mice eight weeks after coronary occlusion (240), suggesting that estrogen acts through ERβ to improve the remodeling process. Interestingly, another study of coronary artery ligation in intact, OVXed and estradiol-treated/OVXed rats suggested that estrogen is detrimental during the early postinfarction period, causing an increased infarct size and a trend toward increased mortality, but is subsequently associated with normalized wall tension and limited LV dilatation (241). Further disparity is observed in a study by van Eickels and colleagues who found that estradiol treatment of OVXed mice decreases both the infarct size caused by left coronary artery ligation and early cardiomyocyte apoptosis; however, after six weeks, LV mass and mortality were greater in the estradiol group (242). An antiapoptotic action of estradiol was also demonstrated in neonatal rat ventricular myocytes treated with staurosporine and found to correlate with reduced activity of caspase-3 and NF-κB transcription factors (243). Thus, in general, most studies suggest that estrogen elicits cardioprotective effects, both in terms of initial infarct damage and subsequent remodeling; however, continued work is required to identify the causes of the somewhat contradictory results.

Numerous studies have begun to examine possible mechanisms by which estrogen may act upon the heart to affect cardiac hypertrophy. Some data suggest that estrogen activates antihypertrophic pathways or inhibits hypertrophic pathways. For example, studies in neonatal rat ventricular myocytes showed that the observed antihypertrophic action of estradiol was ER dependent and mediated by cGMP, possibly as a result of ANF release (244) or by direct interaction of estradiol with membrane-bound guanylate cyclase (245). Nuedling and coworkers (246) reported that estradiol stimulates expression of both iNOS and eNOS in neonatal and adult cardiomyocytes, and Dash and colleagues (247) showed that estrogen can increase MAP kinase phosphatase (MKP-1), an inhibitor of p38 MAPK, and thereby antagonize norepinephrine-induced hypertrophy. Work in hearts isolated from OVXed and E2-treated OVXed rats showed that functional recovery after global ischemia was better and coronary TNFα levels were reduced in hearts from E2-treated animals; when perfused in vitro, a TNFα inhibitor improved function and reduced apoptosis and necrosis in OVXed hearts but did not have a significant effect on OVXed/E2-treated hearts (248).

In contrast, other data suggest that estrogens activate hypertrophic-signaling paths. For example, experiments by de Jager and colleagues (249) in neonatal rat cardiomyocytes suggested that estradiol acts through ERs, ERK 1/2 activation, and serum response elements (SREs) to increase expression of early growth response gene-1 (Egr-1), a factor that is enhanced by several known cardiac hypertrophic stimuli. Other studies in isolated cardiomyocytes, as well as in castrated and estradiol-treated female SHR rats, demonstrated that estrogens diminish the expression of the B subtype, but not the A subtype, endothelin receptor (250).

It is possible that the cardioprotective actions of estrogen observed by some investigators are mediated in part by effects on oxidant damage, HSPs, or ion homeostasis. Studies in intact, OVXed and OVXed and E2-treated rats, as well as H9c2 cells, showed that estrogen diminishes basal- and iron-stimulated lipid peroxidation in the myocardium (251). Urata and colleagues (252) reported that estradiol protects ERβ expressing H9c2 cells from H_2O_2-induced apoptosis via an ER-dependent increase in glutaredoxin (GRX) and λ-glutamylcysteine synthetase, a rate limiting enzyme in GSH synthesis, while others (253) showed that estradiol treatment of adult rat cardiomyocytes protects the cells against hypoxic insult by a mechanism involving increased HSP72 and NFκB activation. Similarly, experiments examining trauma-hemorrhage in rats suggested that treatment with an ERβ agonist prevented the resulting decrease in cardiac function by maintaining or even enhancing levels of HSP 32, 60, 70, and 90 (254). In contrast, Shinohara and colleagues reported that estrogen inhibits HSP 72 expression (255). With respect to possible mechanisms involving ion homeostasis, ischemia/reperfusion studies in hearts isolated from OVXed rats showed that pre- and postischemia perfusion with estradiol improves recovery of ventricular function and limits changes in intracellular pH, sodium, and calcium levels during reperfusion, possibly due in part to release of NO (256). Experiments in H9c2 cells showed that 24-hour pretreatment with estradiol increased K_{ATP} channel formation and pinacidil-stimulated current density, and protected the cells from intracellular calcium loading in response to hypoxia-reoxygenation (257). Similarly, coronary perfusion with estrogen prior to coronary angioplasty was shown to limit myocardial ischemic insult as monitored by ECG, chest pain and lactate levels in humans, with the protective effect of estrogen being limited by glibenclamide, a K_{ATP} channel inhibitor (258).

In addition, work has shown that estrogens can affect the function of cardiac fibroblasts. Cardiac fibroblasts comprise approximately 90% of the nonmuscle cells of the heart and are involved in maintaining the functional and structural integrity of the myocardium (43,259). Clearly, there are gender-related differences in the rate of cardiac fibroblast proliferation, and 17-β-estradiol affects cardiac fibroblast proliferation; however, it is not clear whether 17-β-estradiol increases or decreases this proliferative process, for example, cardiac fibroblasts isolated from adult female rats had over three-fold higher rates of tritiated thymidine incorporation when compared with cardiac fibroblasts from adult male rats (186). This gender difference was even more striking in cells isolated from neonatal rats, as cardiac fibroblasts from female rats had over nine-fold higher amounts of tritiated thymidine incorporation when compared with fibroblasts from males (186). Subsequently, 17-β-estradiol (1 nM; 24-hour exposure) was shown to increase proliferation of neonatal cardiac fibroblasts by 10%, as indicated by bromodeoxyuridine incorporation; whereas, the metabolites of estradiol, estrone and 2-hydroxyestrone (both used at 1 nM for 24 hours), were shown to increase cardiac fibroblast proliferation by approximately 30% and 50%, respectively (260). Similarly, 17-β-estradiol (10–20 nM; 12-hour exposure) was shown to increase proliferation of cardiac fibroblasts isolated from adult female rats as determined by tritiated thymidine incorporation (43). 17-α-Estradiol (inactive estrogen) had no effect on proliferation, and tamoxifen blocked the 17-β-estradiol-induced proliferation (43). Furthermore, 17-β-estradiol rapidly (<10 minutes) increased MAPK activity in these cells, an effect that was blocked by tamoxifen and the MAPK pathway inhibitor PD98059 (43). Importantly, PD98059 also blocked 17-β-estradiol-induced increases in tritiated thymidine incorporation, suggesting that estrogen-induced proliferation of cardiac fibroblasts was produced by ER activation of the MAPK pathway (43). In contrast, other investigators showed that 17-β-estradiol (1 nM) and progesterone (10 nM), but not 17-α-estradiol, inhibit fetal calf serum–induced proliferation of cardiac fibroblasts isolated from both male and female adult rats (259). The estrogen metabolite 2-hydroxyestradiol was more potent than 17-β-estradiol at inhibiting cardiac fibroblast proliferation in these experiments (259). Also important, progesterone was shown to enhance the antiproliferative effects of estradiol in these experiments, and the phytoestrogens biochanin A and daidzein also inhibited fetal calf serum–induced cardiac fibroblast proliferation (259). Overall, data suggest that estrogens and progestins modulate cardiac fibroblast proliferation, but results are seemingly contradictory with some demonstrating an increase and others showing a decrease in proliferation. Further research is definitely needed.

As with androgens, estrogens appear to exert a variety of other direct effects on the heart, and these effects primarily involve alterations in membrane ion pumps or channels. For example, endogenous sex hormone–related differences appear to exist in the expression of proteins involved in calcium homeostasis. Binding studies with tritiated nitrendipine demonstrated that OVXed, SHRs had decreased numbers of nitrendipine binding sites, and replacement of estradiol returned those numbers to nearly control values (261). Other experiments by these investigators suggested that L-type calcium channel numbers were not affect by testosterone (261). Studies in cardiomyocytes isolated from estrogen-treated, OVXed rabbits suggested that estrogen may also result in epicardial-endocardial transmural differences in calcium channel density (262). Other research suggests that estradiol may act acutely to interfere with calcium current. High concentrations (micromolar range) of 17-β-estradiol inhibited L-type calcium current in male rat ventricular myocytes (263), in isolated adult guinea pig ventricular myocytes (260), in isolated adult guinea pig ventricular myocytes exposed to endothelin-1 (264), and in isolated rat and human ventricular myocytes (265). However, Meyer and colleagues demonstrated that ventricular L-type calcium current stimulated by isoproterenol was much more susceptible to inhibition of 17-β-estradiol, and the inhibitory effect could be seen at 1 nM estradiol (265). Combined with previous investigations, these results suggest that estrogens may inhibit L-type calcium current in vivo at physiological concentrations. In contrast, Buitrago and coworkers reported that physiological concentrations of estradiol enhance calcium influx in isolated rat ventricle via receptor-mediated increases in cAMP (266).

Other ion channels or pumps may also be affected by estrogens. For example, OVXed dogs treated with estradiol had increased sodium/potassium ATPase activity in cardiac sarcolemmal membranes compared with untreated OVXed dogs, and the experiments suggested that estradiol allosterically stimulated potassium activation of the enzyme (267). The authors suggested that this estradiol-mediated upregulation of sodium/potassium ATPase may impart a protective effect against ischemic insult by improving the maintenance of cation homeostasis in cardiac myocytes (267). Experiments by Ren and colleagues in rat ventricular myocytes demonstrated that OVX decreases contractile function, calcium responsiveness, Akt activation, and the SERCA2a-to-PLB ratio, all of which were restored by estradiol replacement (268).

Also worthy of note, however, is the possibility that some estrogen-induced alterations in ion homeostasis are deleterious in terms of cardiac rhythm. For example, women have longer QT intervals and increased risk of Torsade de pointes ventricular tachycardia after exposure to antiarrhythmic agents such as quinidine (209). Prolonged QT intervals (209) and extended action potential duration of papillary muscle (269) have been observed in OVXed rabbits treated with estradiol. In addition, experiments in guinea pig ventricular myocytes showed that 17-β-estradiol acts acutely to prolong action potential duration, primarily by inhibiting the rapidly and slowly activating components of the delayed outward K^+ current (I_K) (270). Thus, results suggest that estrogens may modulate potassium currents via changes in expression as well as acute actions. In addition, studies in canine Purkinje fibers and isolated canine LV cells have suggested that gender differences in the adrenergic responsiveness of the slow delayed rectifier K^+ current (I_{Ks}) (271) and in transmural distribution of repolarizing currents (272) may play a role in the increased susceptibility to arrhythmias in female heart.

In summary, the heart is a target organ for estrogens and progestins; however, little is known about the direct effects of progestins on the heart. Available studies indicate that both cardiac myocytes and fibroblasts may be susceptible to endogenous and exogenous estrogens. Further research is needed to clarify the growth-inhibiting or growth-enhancing effects of estrogens and progestins, as these studies may very well reveal important roles of sex steroids in cardiac remodeling. More research is also needed to understand the effects of estrogens and progestins on cardiac ion channels and pumps, especially to determine whether these effects involve altered expression of ion homeostatic proteins or nongenomic or direct interference of the channels and/or pumps by estrogens. Finally, since available data suggest that estrogens may affect cardiac myocytes and fibroblasts by both genomic and nongenomic mechanisms, a wide avenue of research is open to clarifying the mechanisms whereby estrogens and progestins directly affect the heart.

Mineralocorticoids and Glucocorticoids

Given the presence of mineralocorticoid and glucocorticoid receptors as well as local aldosterone and corticosterone synthesis in the heart, there is little doubt that cardiac tissue is a target for mineralocorticoids and glucocorticoids. It is, however, interesting to note that aldosterone synthesis in the heart may only occur, or may be enhanced, under pathological conditions. Work by Kayes-Wandover and White (273) suggested that corticosterone and deoxycorticosterone, but not cortisol or aldosterone, are synthesized in normal adult human heart, while Nakamura and colleagues (274) reported that aldosterone is produced by failing, but not normal adult heart, and Tsybouleva and coworkers (275) found that myocardial aldosterone and aldosterone synthase mRNA levels are increased significantly in humans with hypertrophic cardiomyopathy.

Available evidence suggests that aldosterone stimulates cardiac fibrosis (276,277). Rats receiving a chronic infusion of aldosterone responded with a significant rise in cardiac interstitial collagen in both the hypertrophied left ventricles and nonhypertrophied right ventricles (278). Similarly, Robert and colleagues demonstrated that rats treated with aldosterone and increased salt intake for two months developed arterial hypertension, moderate LVH, and numerous foci of proliferating nonmuscle cells with bilateral fibrosis (279). The investigators found that hypertrophy and increased atrial natriuretic peptide mRNA levels were restricted to the left ventricle, and because fibrosis was found in both ventricles, they suggested that fibrosis was independent of hemodynamic factors. Direct actions of aldosterone on fibroblasts were verified by Brilla and colleagues who found significantly increased collagen synthesis in adult rat cardiac fibroblast cultures exposed to aldosterone (280).

Other studies have suggested that aldosterone can also act directly on cardiomyocytes to cause hypertrophy. Sato and Funder observed hypertrophic growth in neonatal rat cardiac myocyte cultures exposed to aldosterone (10 nM) with high glucose (30 mM), but not in cells exposed to aldosterone alone, high glucose alone, or dexamethasone (10 nM) with or without high glucose (281). In addition, Tsybouleva and coworkers showed that aldosterone enhances hypertrophic markers in rat cardiac myocytes via a protein kinase D (PKD)-dependent mechanism and increased collagen and TGF-β expression in rat cardiac fibroblasts via a PI3K-p100delta mechanism (275). These direct effects on myocytes and fibroblasts were antagonized by the mineralocorticoid receptor antagonist spironolactone. Spironolactone also antagonized the interstial fibrosis, myocyte disarray, and diastolic dysfunction observed in a cardiac troponin T (cTnT)-Q92 trangenic mouse model of human hypertrophic cardiomyopathy.

Other direct cardiac effects of mineralocorticoids also deserve attention. For example, exposure of neonatal rat cardiac myocyte cultures to aldosterone for 24 hours resulted in increased chloride/bicarbonate exchanger six days following exposure and increased sodium/hydrogen antiporter nine days following exposure (282). Furthermore, physiological concentrations of aldosterone (nM range) induced rapid increases in mRNA for sodium/potassium ATPase in both neonatal and adult rat cardiac myocyte cultures, with increases in sodium/potassium ATPase protein and transport activity also being observed in the adult cells (283). In addition, aldosterone may have acute, nongenomic effects on the heart. Chai and colleagues reported that pathological concentrations of aldosterone elicit a negative inotropic response in isolated human trabeculae and potentiate the vasoconstriction elicited by angiotensin II in isolated human coronary arteries (284). These actions were found to be associated with PKC and ERK 1/2 activation, respectively, but were not blocked by mineralocorticoid receptor antagonists.

With respect to glucocorticoids, in contrast to the study by Sato and Funder (281), other investigators reported that dexamethasone administration to neonatal rats produces cardiac hypertrophy as indicated by increased heart-to-body weight ratio, elevated total cardiac protein content, elevated actin content, increased total protein-to-total DNA ratio (285), increased α-MHC and decreased β-MHC expression (286). Uninephrectomized rats treated with corticosterone and increased salt intake developed increased cardiac interstitial collagen in both ventricles compared with control animals, although the effect was modest compared with the increased cardiac fibrosis observed in aldosterone-treated animals (277). Regarding a potential mechanism of these effects, hearts from adult rats pretreated with dexamethasone had increased angiotensinogen mRNA (287). Furthermore, in rats subjected to unilateral renal artery clips and later given subcutaneous dexamethasone, mRNAs for angiotensin II type 1a and 1b receptors were both significantly increased (288). Finally, glucocorticoid-induced hypertrophic growth may be short lived and/or reversed over time. Czerwinski and colleagues found that female rats given hydrocortisone developed peak cardiac enlargement after seven days of treatment, but the enlargement returned nearly to control levels by 15 days of continued treatment (289). In addition, deVries and coworkers reported that treatment of rat pups on days 1 through 3 resulted in decreases in heart weight, early degeneration of cardiomyocytes, and myocyte hypertrophy at 45 weeks of age (290).

In summary, both mineralocorticoids and glucocorticoids appear to induce cardiac fibrosis and possibly hypertrophic growth. Thus, both cardiac fibroblasts and cardiac myocytes may be targets for mineralocorticoids and glucocorticoids. In addition, the presence of local cardiac mineralocorticoid and glucocorticoid systems also strongly suggests that these hormones have direct effects on the heart and may play both physiological and pathological roles in cardiac structure and function. Whether mineralocorticoids and glucocorticoids induce their direct actions in cardiac tissue through genomic or nongenomic mechanisms or both is currently not known.

FURTHER CONSIDERATIONS REGARDING STEROIDAL AGENTS AND CARDIOVASCULAR FUNCTION

Until the actions of single steroidal agents on the cardiovascular system are better understood, it is unlikely that the more common situation of simultaneous exposure of the heart and vasculature to combinations of steroidal agents will be fully appreciated. For example, under physiological conditions multiple endogenous steroids are present in the circulation at any given moment. Even in the case of exogenous steroid administration, rarely is one steroidal agent administered as demonstrated by illicit AAS use, where numerous androgens are used concomitantly in high doses, and by HRT or oral contraceptives where estrogens are frequently coprescribed with progestins. Furthermore, little is known regarding the effects of multiple steroidal agents on circulating transport proteins, and thus whether concomitant administration of multiple steroidal agents affects the free fraction of circulating steroid. Thus, the effects of steroid-steroid interactions in the cardiovascular system will be difficult to study and to understand, but future research must bear this consideration.

Similarly, an ever-increasing body of literature continues to describe potential drug-exogenous steroid interactions. For example, because most steroidal agents undergo significant hepatic metabolism, the administration of any other chemical entity that may modify hepatic metabolism most certainly subjects an individual to drug-steroid interactions. In addition, there is emerging information regarding other drug-steroid interactions with significant implications regarding cardiovascular function. As a case in point, cocaine and nandrolone (19-nortestosterone) administered concomitantly to SHRs resulted in heart weights that were greater than those in rats that received either agent alone (291). Myocardial inflammatory and fibrotic changes were also more evident in rats treated with nandrolone alone or cocaine plus nandrolone than in rats that received vehicle or cocaine alone (291).

Additionally, future research should consider the possibility that physiological adaptations may interact with steroidal agents. In pointing to a specific example, recall that exogenous self-administration of high doses of AASs may increase the risk of cardiac hypertrophy. Many users of illicit AAs are weight trainers and/or body builders, and weight lifters have long been known to exhibit increased LV mass, LV wall thickness, and intraventricular septal wall thickness together with decreased LV systolic internal dimensions (292,293). Thus, the possibility of interactions between physiological adaptations to exercise training and exogenous androgens should be considered.

Finally, increasing evidence suggests that cytokines and/or growth factors may interact with steroidal agents. For example, it is now known that interleukin-6 can stimulate the androgen receptor in the absence of androgen (294). Furthermore, epidermal growth factor may activate ERs independently of estrogen ligand (295). Thus, any physiological or pathophysiological condition that alters cytokine and/or growth factor release may impart interactions with endogenous steroids and/or induce cardiovascular effects similar to steroidal agents, but independent of cognate ligand.

In summary, the above interactions represent several issues that require continued research. In addition, it is highly likely that future research will identify even further confounding interactions with steroidal agents. However, as in any area, the need to understand the mechanisms of action of the sex steroids and their direct effects on organ systems remains a primary goal in this field. Interactions can be best understood once the cellular mechanisms of the individual agents and/or conditions are elucidated.

CONCLUSIONS: CARDIOVASCULAR TOXICOLOGY AND STEROIDAL AGENTS

In considering the toxicological implications of the information presented here, it is imperative to first point out that limitations prevent complete discussion of every reported cardiovascular consequence of steroidal agents. Therefore, the chapter focused on the effects of steroidal agents on lipid metabolism and direct actions of steroidal agents on the vasculature and heart. As such, the chapter should teach that any exogenous agent that may interact with steroid receptors and/or endogenous steroid ligands should be considered as a potential disrupter of normal cardiovascular function. The focus of the chapter was somewhat narrow in that only the major steroidal agents were discussed. Now, however, it is important to realize that continued research into pharmacological and toxicological modulators of steroid receptor signaling is identifying an increasing number of ligands for steroid receptors as well as an increasing number of receptor isoforms. Examples include pharmaceutical interest in nonsteroidal agonists and antagonists of steroid receptors and their subtypes, and toxicological interest in endocrine disrupters, including naturally occurring and industrial chemicals that serve as agonists and/or antagonists of steroid receptors. Possibilities for future research into cardiovascular effects of steroidal agents appear to be infinite in number.

REFERENCES

1. Brueggemeier RW, Miller DD, Witiak DT. Cholesterol, adrenocorticoids, and sex hormones. In: Foye WO, Lemke TL, Williams DA, eds. Principles of Medicinal Chemistry. 4th ed. Baltimore, MD: Williams & Wilkins, 1995:444–497.
2. Kopera, H. The history of anabolic steroids and a review of the clinical experience with anabolic steroids. Acta Endocrinol 1985; 110(suppl 271):11–18.
3. Melchert RB, Welder AA. Cardiovascular effects of androgenic-anabolic steroids. Med Sci Sports Exerc 1995; 27:1252–1262.
4. Barbosa J, Seal US, Doe RP. Effects of anabolic steroids on haptoglobulin, orosomucoid, plasminogen, fibrinogen, transferrin, ceruloplasmin, α_1-antitrypsin, β-glucoronidase and total serum protein. J Clin Endocrinol 1971; 33:388–398.
5. Rahwan RG. The pharmacology of androgens and anabolic steroids. Am J Pharm Ed 1988; 52:167–177.
6. Haupt HA, Rovere GD. Anabolic steroids: a review of the literature. Am J Sports Med 1984; 12:469–484.
7. Council on Scientific Affairs. Medical and nonmedical uses of anabolic-androgenic steroids. J. Am Med Assoc 1990; 264:1923–2927.
8. Yesalis CE, Barsukiewicz CK, Kopstein AN, et al. Trends in anabolic-androgenic steroid use among adolescents. Arch Pediatr Adol Med 1997; 151:1197–1206.
9. Narducci WA, Wagner JC, Hendrickson TP, et al. Anabolic steroids – A review of the clinical toxicology and diagnostic screening. Clin Toxicol 1990;. 28:287–310.
10. Williams CL, Stancel GM. Estrogens and progestins. In: Hardman JG, Limbird LE, Molinoff PB, et al. eds. Goodman & Gilman's The Pharmacological Basis of Therapeutics. 9th ed.. New York, NY: McGraw-Hill, 1995:1411–1440.
11. Cummings AM. Methoxychlor as a model for environmental estrogens. Crit Rev Toxicol 1997; 27:367–379.
12. Santell RC, Chang YC, Nair MG, et al. Dietary genistein exerts estrogenic effects upon the uterus, mammary gland and the hypothalamic/pituitary axis in rats. J Nutr 1997; 127:263–269.
13. Sheehan DM. Herbal medicines, phytoestrogens and toxicity: risk:benefit considerations. Proc Soc Exp Biol Med 1998; 217:379–385.
14. Blakely JA. The heart and estrogen/progestin replacement study revisited. Arch Intern Med 2000; 160:2897–2900.
15. Mosca L. The role of hormone replacement therapy in the prevention of postmenopausal heart disease. Arch Intern Med 2000; 160:2263–2272.
16. Prentice RL, Langer R, Stefanick ML, et al. Combined postmenopausal hormone therapy and cardiovascular disease: toward resolving the discrepancy between observational studies and the women's health initiative clinical trial. Am J Epidemiol 2005; 162:404–414.

17. Sidney S, Siscovick DS, Petitti DB, et al. Myocardial infarction and use of low-dose oral contraceptives: a pooled analysis of 2 US studies. Circulation 1998; 98: 1058–1063.

18. Hirvonen E, Malkonen M, Manninen V. Effects of different progestogens on lipoproteins during postmenopausal replacement therapy. New Eng J Med 1981; 304 560–563.

19. Sorensen KE, Dorup I, Hermann AP, et al. Combined hormone replacement therapy does not protect women against the age-related decline in endothelium-dependent vasomotor function. Circulation 1998; 97:1234–1238.

20. Christ M, Wehling M. Cardiovascular steroid actions: swift swallows or sluggish snails? Cardiovasc Res 1998; 40:34–44.

21. Cohn JN, Colucci W. Cardiovascular effects of aldosterone and post-acute myocardial Infarction pathophysiology. Am J Cardiol 2006; 97(suppl):4F–12F.

22. Schimmer BP, Parker KL; Adrenocorticotropic hormone; adrenocorticol steroids and their synthetic analogs; synthesis and actions of adrenocortical hormonesi. In: Hardman JG, Limbird LE, Molinoff PB, et al., eds. Goodman & Gilman's The Pharmacological Basis of Therapeutics. 9th ed. New York, NY: McGraw-Hill, 1995:1459–1485.

23. Page IH, McCubbin JW. Cardiovascular reactivity. Circ Res 1954; 2:395–408.

24. Ross EJ, Linch DC. Cushing's syndrome – killing disease. Discriminatory value of signs and symptoms aiding early diagnosis. Lancet 1982; 2:646–649.

25. Brunton LL. Agents affecting gastrointestinal water flux and motility; emesis and antiemetics; bile acids and pancreatic enzymes. In: Hardman JG, Limbird LE, Molinoff PB, et al., eds. Goodman & Gilman's The Pharmacological Basis of Therapeutics. 9th ed. New York, NY: McGraw-Hill, 1995:917–936.

26. Alarid ET. Lives and times of nuclear receptors. Mol Endocrinol 2006; 20:1972–1981.

27. Carson-Jurica MA, Schrader WT, O'Malley BW. Steroid receptor family: structure and functions. Endocr Rev 1990; 11:201–220.

28. Veldscholte J, Berrevoets CA, Zegers ND, et al. Hormone-induced dissociation of the androgen receptor-heat-shock protein complex: use of a new monoclonal antibody to distinguish transformed from nontransformed receptors. Biochemistry 1992; 31:7422–7430.

29. Wahli W, Martinez E. Superfamily of steroid nuclear receptors: positive and negative regulators of gene expression. FASEB J 1991; 5:2243–2249.

30. O'Malley BW. Steroid hormone receptors as transactivators of gene expression. Breast Cancer Res Treat 1991; 18:67–71.

31. Jain S, Pulikuri S, Zhu Y, et al. Differential expression of the peroxisome proliferator-activated receptor γ (PPARγ) and its coactivators steroid receptor coactivator-1 and PPAR-binding protein PBP in the brown fat, urinary bladder, colon, and breast of the mouse. Am J Pathol 1998; 153:349–354.

32. Wehling M. Looking beyond the dogma of genomic steroid action: insights and facts of the 1990s. J Mol Med 1995; 73:439–447.

33. Koenig H, Fan CC, Goldstone AD, et al. Polyamines mediate androgenic stimulation of calcium fluxes and membrant transport in rat heart myocytes. Circ Res 1989; 64:415–426.

34. Bordallo C, Rubin JM, Varona AB, et al. Increases in ornithine decarboxylase activity in the positive inotropism induced by androgens in isolated left atrium of the rat. Eur J Pharmacol 2001; 422:101–107.

35. Carnes CA, Dech SJ. Effects of dihydrotestosterone on cardiac inward rectifier K (+) current. Int J Androl 2002; 25:210–214.
36. Bai CX, Kurokawa J, Tamagawa M, et al. Nontranscriptional regulation of cardiac repolarization currents by testosterone. Circulation 2005; 112:1701–1710.
37. Farnsworth WE. The prostate plasma membrane as an androgen receptor Memb Biochem 1990; 9:141–162.
38. Steinsapir J, Muldoon TG. Role of microsomal receptors in steroid hormone action. Steroids 1991; 56:66–71.
39. Gupte SA, Tateyama M, Okada T, et al. Epiandrosterone, a metabolite of testosterone precursor, blocks L-type calcium channels of ventricular myocytes and inhibits myocardial contractility; J Mol Cell Cardiol 2002; 34:679–688.
40. Vicencio JM, Ibarra C, Estrada M, et al. Testosterone induces an intracellular calcium increase by a nongenomic mechanism in cultured rat cardiac myocytes. Endocrinology 2006; 147:1386–1395.
41. Moriarty K, Kim KH, Bender JR. Estrogen receptor-mediated rapid signaling. Endocrinology 2006; 147:5557–5563.
42. Migliaccio A, Di Domenico M, Castoria G, et al. Tyrosine kinase/p21ras/MAP-kinase pathway activation by estradiol-receptor complex in MCF-7 cells. EMBO J 1996; 15:1292–1300.
43. Lee HW, Eghbali-Webb M. Estrogen enhances proliferative capacity of cardiac fibroblasts by estrogen receptor- and mitogen-activated protein kinase-dependent pathways. J Mol Cell Cardiol 1998; 30:1359–1368.
44. Grundy SM. Cholesterol and coronary heart disease. Future directions. J Am Med Assoc 1990; 264:3053–3059.
45. Steinberg D, Witztum JL. Lipoproteins and atherogenesis. Current concepts. J Am Med Assoc 1990; 264:3047–3052.
46. Kalin MF, Zumoff B. Sex hormones and coronary disease: a review of the clinical studies. Steroids 1990; 55:330–352.
47. Glazer G. Atherogenic effects of anabolic steroids on serum lipid levels Arch Intern Med 1991; 151:1925–1933.
48. Rockhold RW. Cardiovascular toxicity of anabolic steroids. Ann Rev Pharmacol Toxicol 1993; 33:497–520.
49. Sullivan ML, Martinez CM, Gennis P, et al. The cardiac toxicity of anabolic steroids Prog Cardiovasc Dis 1998; 41:1–15.
50. Wild RA, Grubb B, Hartz A, et al. Fert. Steril 1990; 54:255–259.
51. Ehnholm C, Huttunen JK, Kinnunen PJ, et al. Effect of oxandrolone treatment on the activity of lipoprotein lipase, hepatic lipase and phospholipase A_1 of human postheparin plasma. New Eng J Med 1975; 292:1314–1317.
52. Haffner SM, Kushwaha RS, Foster DM, et al. Studies on the metabolic mechanism of reduced high density lipoproteins during anabolic steroid therapy. Metabolism 1983; 32:413–420.
53. Applebaum-Bowden D, Haffner SM, Hazzard WR. The dyslipoproteinemia of anabolic steroid therapy: increase in hepatic triglyceride lipase activity precedes the decrease in high density lipoprotein$_2$ cholesterol. Metabolism 1987; 36:949–952.
54. Kantor MA, Bianchini A, Bernier D, et al. Androgens reduce HDL_2-cholesterol and increase hepatic triglyceride lipase activity. Med Sci Sports Exerc 1985; 17:462–465.
55. Lenders JWM, Demacker PNM, Vos JA, et al. Deleterious effects of anabolic steroids on serum lipoproteins, blood pressure, and liver function in amateur body builders. Int J Sports Med 1988; 9:19–23.

56. Thompson PD, Cullinane EM, Sady SP, et al. Contrasting effects of testosterone and stanozolol on serum lipoprotein levels. J Am Med Assoc 1989; 261:1165–1168.

57. Friedl KE, Hannan CJ, Jones RE, et al. High-density lipoprotein cholesterol is not decreased if an aromatizable androgen is administered. Metabolism 1990; 39:69–74.

58. Zmuda JM, Fahrenbach MC, Younkin BT, et al. The effect of testosterone aromatization on high-density lipoprotein cholesterol level and postheparin lipolytic activity. Metabolism 1993; 42:446–450.

59. Samsioe G. Cardiovascular disease in postmenopausal women. Maturitas 1998; 30:11–18.

60. Bongard V, Ferrieres J, Ruidavets JB, et al. Transdermal estrogen replacement therapy and plasma lipids in 693 French women. Maturitas 1998; 30:265–72.

61. Nabulsi AA, Folsom AR, White A, et al. Association of hormone-replacement therapy with various cardiovascular risk factors in postmenopausal women. New Eng J Med 1993; 328:1069–1075.

62. Distelhorst CW. Steroid hormone receptors. J Lab Clin Med 1993; 122:241–244.

63. White CR, Darley-Usmar V, Oparil S. Gender and cardiovascular disease. Recent insights. Trends Cardiovasc Med 1997; 7:94–100.

64. Henkin Y, Como JA, Oberman A. Secondary dyslipidemia. Inadvertant effects of drugs in clinical practice. J Am Med Assoc 1992; 267:961–968.

65. Becker DM, Chamberlain B, Swank R, et al. Relationship between corticosteroid exposure and plasma lipid levels in heart transplant recipients. Am J Med 1988; 85:632–638.

66. Vathsala A, Weinberg RB, Schoenberg L, et al. Lipid abnormalities in cyclosporine-prednisone-treated renal transplant recipients. Transplantation 1989; 48:37–43.

67. Ettinger WH, Goldberg AP, Applebaum-Bowden D, et al. Dyslipoproteinemia in systemic lupus erythematosus. Effect of corticosteroids. Am J Med 1987; 83:503–508.

68. Ettinger WH, Klinefelter HF, Kwiterovitch PO. Effect of short-term, low-dose corticosteroids on plasma lipoprotein lipids. Atherosclerosis 1987; 63:167–172.

69. Jefferys DB, Lessof MH, Mattock MB. Corticosteroid treatment, serum lipids, and coronary artery disease. Postgrad Med J 1980; 56:491–493.

70. Zimmerman J, Fainaru M, Eisenberg S. The effects of prednisone therapy on plasma lipoprotein and apolipoproteins: a prospective study. Metab Clin Exp 1984; 33: 521–526.

71. Markell MS, Friedman EA. Hyperlipidemia after organ transplantation. Am J Med 1989; 87:61N–67N.

72. Ettinger WH, Dysko RC, Clarkson TB. Prednisone increases low density lipoprotein in cynomolgus monkeys fed saturated fat and cholesterol. Arteriosclerosis 1989; 9:848–855.

73. McGill HC, Sheridan PJ. Nuclear uptake of sex steroid hormones in the cardiovascular system of the baboon. Circ Res 1981; 48:238–244.

74. Maddox YT, Falcon JG, Ridinger M, et al. Endothelium-dependent gender differences in the response of the rat aorta. J Pharmacol Exp Therap 1987; 240:392–395.

75. Ferrer M, Encabo A, Marin J, et al. Chronic treatment with the anabolic steroid, nandrolone, inhibits vasodilator repsonses in rabbit aorta. Eur J Pharmacol 1994; 252:233–241.

76. Farhat MY, Wolfe R, Vargas R, et al. Effect of testosterone treatment on vasoconstrictor response of left anterior descending coronary artery in male and female pigs. J Cardiovasc Pharmacol 1995; 25:495–500.

77. Green DJ, Cable NT, Rankin JM, et al. Anabolic steroids and vascular responses. Lancet 1993; 342:863.

78. Yue P, Kanu C, Beale C, et al. Testosterone relaxes rabbit coronary arteries and aorta. Circulation 1995; 91:1154–1160.

79. Costarella CE, Stallone JN, Rutecki GW, et al. Testosterone causes direct relaxation of rat thoracic aorta. J Pharmacol Exp Therap 1996; 277:34–39.

80. Ceballos G, Figueroa L, Rubio I, et al. Acute and nongenomic effects of testosterone on isolated and perfused rat heart. J Cardiovasc Pharmacol 1999; 33:691–697.

81. Jones RD, English KM, Pugh PJ, et al. Pulmonary vasodilatory action of testosterone: evidence of a calcium antagonistic action. J Cardiovasc Pharmacol 2002; 39:814–823.

82. Hutchison SJ, Browne AE, Ko E, et al. Dehydroepiandrosterone sulfate induces acute vasodilation of porcine coronary arteries in vitro and in vivo. J Cardiovasc Pharmacol 2005; 46:325–332.

83. Farhat MY, Lavigne MC, Ramwell PW. The vascular protective effects of estrogen. FASEB J 1996; 10:615–624.

84. Selzman CH, Whitehill TA, Shames BD, et al. The biology of estrogen-mediated repair of cardiovascular injury. Ann Thorac Surg 1998; 65:868–874.

85. Karas RH, Baur WE, van Eickles M, et al. Human vascular smooth muscle cells express an estrogen receptor isoform. FEBS Lett 1995; 377:103–108.

86. Karas RH, Patterson BL, Mendelsohn ME. Human vascular smooth muscle cells contain functional estrogen receptor. Circulation 1994; 89:1943–1950.

87. Venkov CD, Rankin AB, Vaughan DE. Identification of authentic estrogen receptor in cultured endothelial cells: a potential mechanism for steroid hormone regulation of endothelial function. Circulation 1996; 94:727–733.

88. Register TC, Adams MR. Coronary artery and cultured aortic smooth muscle cells express mRNA for both the classical estrogen receptor and the newly described estrogen receptor beta. J Steroid Biochem Mol Biol 1998; 64:187–191.

89. Lindner V, Kim SK, Karas RH, et al. Increased expression of estrogen receptor-β mRNA in male blood vessels after vascular injury. Circ Res 1998; 83:224–229.

90. Rosano GMC, Sarrel PM, Poole-Wilson PA, et al. Beneficial effect of oestrogen on exercise-induced myocardial ischemia in women with coronary artery disease. Lancet 1993; 342:133–136.

91. Lieberman EH, Gerhard MD, Uehata A, et al. Estrogen improves endothelium-dependent, flow-mediated vasodilation in postmenopausal women. Ann Int Med 1994; 121:936–941.

92. Gilligan DM, Badar DM, Panza JA, et al. Acute vascular effects of estrogen in postmenopausal women. Circulation 1994; 90:786–791.

93. Gilligan DM, Quyyumi AA, Cannon RO, et al. Effects of physiological levels of estrogen on coronary vasomotor function in postmenopausal women. Circulation 1994; 892545–2551.

94. Collins P, Rosano GMC, Sarrel PM, et al. 17 beta-estradiol attenuates acetylcholine-induced coronary arterial constriction in women but not men with coronary artery disease. Circulation 1995; 92:24–30.

95. Simoncini T, Fornari L, Mannella P, et al. Novel non-transcriptional mechanisms for estrogen receptor signaling in the cardiovascular system Interaction of estrogen receptor α with phosphatidylinositol 3-OH kinase. Steroids 2002; 67:935–939.

96. Stallone JN. Role of endothelium in sexual dimorphism in vasopressin-induced contraction of rat aorta. Am J Physiol 1993; 265:H2073–H2080.

97. Collins P, Shay J, Jiang C et al. Nitric oxide accounts for dose-dependent estrogen-mediated coronary relaxation after acute estrogen withdrawal. Circulation 1994; 90:1964–1968.

98. Weiner CP, Lizasoain I, Baylis SA, et al. Induction of calcium-dependent nitric oxide synthase by sex hormones. Proc Nat Acad Sci U S A 1994;, 91:5212–5216.

99. Gorodeski GI, Yang T, Levy MN, et al. Effects of estrogen in vivo on coronary vascular resistance in perfused rabbit hearts. Am J Physiol 1995; 269:R1333–R1338.

100. Sanchez A, Gomez MJ, Dorantes AL, et al. The effect of ovariectomy on depressed contractions to phenylephrine and KCl and increased relaxation to acetylcholine in isolated aortic rings of female compared to male rabbits. Br J Pharmacol 1996; 118:2017–2022.

101. Node K, Kitakaze M, Kosaka H, et al. Roles of NO and Ca^{2+}-activated K^+ channels in coronary vasodilation induced by 17β-estradiol in ischemic heart failure. FASEB J 1997; 11:793–799.

102. Node K, Kitakaze M, Kosaka H, et al. Amelioration of ischemia- and reperfusion-induced myocardial injury by 17β-estradiol. Role of nitric oxide and calcium-activated potassium channels. Circulation 1997; 96:1953–1963.

103. Dubey RK, Jackson EK, Keller PJ, et al. Estradiol Metabolites Inhibit Endothelin synthesis by an estrogen receptor-independent mechanism. Hypertension 2000; 37:640–644.

104. Davidge ST, Zhang Y. Estrogen replacement suppresses a prostaglandin H synthase-dependent vasoconstrictor in rat mesenteric arteries. Circ Res 1998; 83:388–395.

105. Zhang L, Kosaka H. Sex-specific acute effect of estrogen on endothelium-derived contracting factor in the renal artery of hypertensive Dahl rats. J Hypertension 2002; 20:237–246.

106. Huang A, Sun D, Wu A, et al. Estrogen elicits cytochrome P450-mediated flow-induced dilation of arterioles in NO deficiency Role of PI3K-Akt phosphorylation in genomic regulation. Circ Res 2004; 94:245–252.

107. Hügel S, Neubauer S, Zan Lie S, et al. Multiple mechanisms are involved in the acute vasodilatory effect of 17β-estradiol in the isolated perfused rat heart. J Cardiovasc Pharmacol 1999; 33:852–858.

108. Yamaguchi K, Honda H, Tamura K, et al. Possible mechanisms for the suppressing action of 17-β-estradiol on β-adrenoceptor-mediated vasorelaxation in rat aorta. Eur J Pharmacol 2001; 427:61–67.

109. Zhu Y, Bian Z, Lu P, et al. Abnormal vascular function and hypertension in mice deficient estrogen receptor β. Science 2002; 295:505–508.

110. Collins P, Rosano GMC, Jiang C, et al. Cardiovascular protection by oestrogen—a calcium antagonist effect? Lancet 1993; 341:1264–1265.

111. Kitazawa T, Hamada E, Kitazawa K, et al. Non-genomic mechanism of 17β-oestradiol-induced inhibition of contraction in mammalian vascular smooth muscle. J Physiol 1997; 499:497–511.

112. Zhang F, Ram JL, Standley PR, et al. 17 β-estradiol attenuates voltage-dependent Ca^{2+} currents in A7r5 vascular smooth muscle cell line. Am J Physiol 1994; 266: C975–C980.

113. Han S-Z, Haraki H, Ouchi Y, et al. 17 beta-estradiol inhibits Ca^{2+} influx and Ca^{2+} release induced by thromboxane A_2 in porcine coronary artery. Circulation 1995; 91:2619–2626.
114. Cohen ML, Susemichel AD. Effect of 17β-estradiol and the nonsteroidal benzo-thiophene, LY117018 on in vitro rat aortic responses to norepinephrine, serotonin, U46619, and BAYK 8644. Drug Devel Res 1996; 37:97–104.
115. Prakash YS, Togaibayeva AA, Kannan MS, et al. Estrogen increase Ca^{2+} efflux from female porcine coronary arterial smooth muscle. Am J Physiol Heart Circ Physiol 1999; 276:H926–H934.
116. Murphy JG, Khalil RA. Gender-specific reduction in contractility and $[Ca^{2+}]_i$ in vascular smooth muscle cells of female rat. Am J Physiol Cell Physiol 2000; 278: C834–C844.
117. Vargas R, Hewes B, Rego A, et al. Estradiol effect on rate of proliferation of rat carotid segments: effect of gender and tamoxifen. J Cardiovasc Pharmacol 1996; 27:495–499.
118. Vargas R, Wroblewska B, Rego A, et al. Oestradiol inhibits smooth muscle cell proliferation of pig coronary artery. Br J Pharmacol 1993; 109:612–617.
119. Lou H, Ramwell PW, Foegh ML. Estradiol 17-β represses insulin-like growth factor I receptor expression in smooth muscle cells from rabbit cardiac recipients. Transplantation 1998; 66:419–426.
120. Hong HJ, Liu JC, Chan P, et al. 17beta-extradiol downregulates angiotensin-II-induced endothelin-1 gene expression in rat aortic smooth muscle cells. J. Biomed. Sci 2004; 11:27–36.
121. Song J, Wan Y, Rolfe BE, et al. Effect of estrogen on vascular smooth muscle cells is dependent upon cellular phenotype. Atherosclerosis 1998; 140:97–104.
122. Tang M, Subbiah MT. Estrogens protect against hydrogen peroxide and arachidonic acid induced DNA damage. Biochim Biophys Acta 1996; 1299:155–159.
123. Kim YD, Chen B, Beauregard J, et al. 17Beta-estradiol prevents dysfunction of canine coronary endothelium and myocardium and reperfusion arrhythmias after brief ischemia/reperfusion. Circulation 1996; 94:2901–2908.
124. Dubey RK, Atyurina YY, Tyurin VA, et al. Estrogen and tamoxifen metabolites protect smooth muscle cell membrane phospholipids against peroxidation and inhibit cell growth. Circ Res 1999; 84:229–239.
125. Perrot-Applanat M, Groyer-Picard MT, Garcia E, et al. Immunocytochemical demonstration of estrogen and progesterone receptors in muscle cells of uterine arteries in rabbits and humans. Endocrinology 1988; 123:1511–1519.
126. Perrot-Applanat M, Cohen-Solal K, Milgrom E, et al. Progesterone receptor expression in human saphenous veins. Circulation 1995; 92:2975–2983.
127. Lee WS, Harder JA, Yoshizumi M, et al. Progesterone inhibits arterial smooth muscle cell proliferation. Nature Med 1997; 3:1005–1008.
128. Falkenstein E, Meyer C, Eisen C, et al. Full-length cDNA sequence of a proges-terone membrane-binding protein from porcine vascular smooth muscle cells. Biochem Biophys Res Commun 1996; 229:86–89.
129. Jiang CW, Sarrel PM, Lindsay DC, et al. Progesterone induces endothlium-inde-pendent relaxation of rabbit coronary artery in vitro. Eur J Pharmacol 1992; 211:163–167.
130. Bielefeldt K, Waite L, Abboud FM, et al. Nongenomic effects of progesterone on human intestinal smooth muscle cells. Am J Physiol 1996; 271:G370–G376.

131. Miller VM, Vanhoutte PM. Progesterone and modulation of endothelium-dependent responses in canine coronary arteries. Am J Physiol 1991; 261:R1022–R1027.

132. Whitworth JA, Scoggins BA. A 'hypertensinogenic' class of steroid hormone activity in man? Clin Exp Pharmacol Physiol 1990; 17:163–166.

133. Kornel L, Kanamarlapudi N, Ramsay C, et al. Arterial steroid receptors and their putative role in the mechanism of hypertension. J Steroid Biochem 1983; 19:333–344.

134. Kornel L, Kanamarlapudi N, Ramsay C, et al. Studies on arterial mineralocorticoid and glucocorticoid receptors: evidence for the translocation of steroid-cytoplasmic receptor complexes to cell nuclei. Clin Physiol Biochem 1984; 2:14–31.

135. Wehling M, Christ M, Theisen K. Membrane receptors for aldosterone: a novel pathway for mineralocorticoid action. Am J Physiol 1992; 263:E974–E979.

136. Christ M, Sippel K, Eisen C, et al. Non-classical receptors for aldosterone in plasma membranes from pig kidneys. Mol Cell Endocrinol 1994; 99:R31–R34.

137. Meyer C, Christ M, Wehling M. Characterization and solubilization of novel aldosterone-binding proteins in porcine liver microsomes. Eur J Biochem 1995; 229:736–740.

138. Kelly JJ, Tam SH, Williamson PM, et al. The nitric oxide system and cortisol-induced hypertension in humans. Clin Exp Pharmacol Physiol 1998; 25:945–946.

139. Lewis CD, Campbell WB, Johnson AR. Inhibition of prostaglandin synthesis by glucocorticoids in human endothelial cells. Endocrinology 1986; 119:62–69.

140. Axelrod L. Inhibition of prostacyclin production mediates permissive effects of glucocorticoids on vascular tone. Perturbations of this mechanism contribute to pathogenesis of Cushing's syndrome and Addison's disease. Lancet 1983; 1 (8330):904–906.

141. Fishel RS, Eisenberg S, Shai S-Y, et al. Glucocorticoids induce angiotensin-converting enzyme expression in vascular smooth muscle. Hypertension 1995; 25:343–349.

142. Sato A, Suzuki H, Murakami M, et al. Glucocorticoid increases angiotensin II type 1 receptor and its gene expression. Hypertension 1994; 23:25–30.

143. Sato A, Suzuki H, Nakazato Y, et al. Increased expression of vascular angiotensin II type 1A receptor gene in glucocorticoid-induced hypertension. J Hypertension 1994; 12:511–516.

144. Guo D-F, Uno S, Ishihata A, et al. Identification of a cis-acting glucocorticoid responsive element in the rat angiotensin II type 1A promoter. Circ Res 1995; 77:249–257.

145. Kornel L, Manisundaram B, Nelson WA. Glucocorticoids regulate Na^+ transport in vascular smooth muscle through the glucocorticoid receptor-mediated mechanism. Am J Hyperten 1993; 6:736–744.

146. Kornel L, Prancan AV, Kanamarlapudi N, et al. Study on the mechanisms of glucocorticoid-induced hypertension: glucocorticoids increase transmembrane Ca^{2+} influx in vascular smooth muscle in vivo. Endocrine Res 1995; 21:203–210.

147. Wehling M, Spes CH, Win N, et al. Rapid cardiovascular action of aldosterone in man. J Clin Endocrinol Metab 1998; 83:3517–3522.

148. Kornel L, Smoszna-Konaszewska B. Aldosterone (ALDO) increases trans-membrane influx of Na^+ in vascular smooth muscle (VSM) cells through increased synthesis of Na^+ channels. Steroids 1995; 60:114–119.

149. Christ M, Douwes K, Eisen C, et al. Rapid effects of aldosterone on sodium transport in vascular smooth muscle cells. Hypertension 1995; 25:117–123.

150. Wehling M, Neylon CB, Fullerton M, et al. Nongenomic effects of aldosterone on intracellular Ca^{2+} in vascular smooth muscle cells. Circ Res 1995; 76:973–979.
151. Schneider M, Ulsenheimer A, Christ M, et al. Nongenomic effects of aldosterone on intracellular calcium in porcine endothelial cells. Am J Physiol 1997; 272: E616–E620.
152. Christ M, Meyer C, Sippel K, et al. Rapid aldosterone signaling in vascular smooth muscle cells: involvement of phospholipase C, diacylglycerol, and protein kinase C alpha. Biochem Biophys Res Comm 1995; 213:123–129.
153. Christ M, Günther A, Heck M, et al. Aldosterone not estradiol, is the physiological agonist for rapid increases in cAMP in vascular smooth muscle cells. Circulation 1999; 99:1485–1491.
154. Krieg M, Smith K, Bartsch W. Demonstration of a specific androgen receptor in rat heart muscle: relationship between binding, metabolism, and tissue levels of androgens. Endocrinology 1978; 103:1686–1694.
155. McGill HC, Anselmo VC, Buchanan JM, et al. The heart is a target organ for androgen. Science 1980; 207:775–777.
156. Wilson CM, McPhaul MJ. A and B forms of the androgen receptor are expressed in a variety of human tissues. Mol Cell Endocrinol 1996; 120:51–57.
157. Marsh JD, Lehmann MH, Ritchie RH, et al. Androgen receptors mediate hypertrophy in cardiac myocytes. Circulation 1998; 98:256–261.
158. Deslypere JP, Vermeulen A. Influence of age on steroid concentrations in skin and striated muscle in women and in cardiac muscle and lung tissue in men. J Clin Endocrinol Metab 1986; 61:648–653.
159. Thum T, Borlak J. Testosterone, cytochrome P450, and cardiac hypertrophy. FASEB J 2002; 16:1537–1549.
160. Stumpf WE, Sar M, Aumuller G. The heart: a target organ for estradiol. Science 1977; 196:319–321.
161. Saunders PTK, Maguire SM, Gaughan J, et al. Expression of oestrogen receptor beta (ERβ) in multiple rat tissues visualised by immunohistochemistry. J Endocrinol 1997; 154:R13–R16.
162. Couse JF, Lindzey J, Grandien K, et al. Tissue distribution and quantitative analysis of estrogen receptor-α (ERα) and estrogen receptor-β (ERβ) messenger ribonucleic acid in the wild-type and ERα-knockout mouse. Endocrinology 1997; 138:4613–4621.
163. Grohe C, Kahlert S, Lobbert K, et al. Cardiac myocytes and fibroblasts contain functional estrogen receptors. FEBS Lett 1997; 416:107–112.
164. Lou H, Martin MB, Stoica A, et al. Upregulation of estrogen receptor-α expression in rabbit cardiac allograft. Circ Res 1998; 83:947–951.
165. Grohe C, Kahlert S, Lobbert K, et al. Expression of oestrogen receptor alpha and beta in rat heart: role of local oestrogen synthesis. J Endocrinol 1998; 156:R1–R7.
166. Pearce P, Funder JW. High affinity aldosterone binding sites (type I receptors) in rat heart. Clin Exp Pharmacol Physiol 1987; 14:859–866.
167. Myles K; Funder JW. Type I (mineralocorticoid) receptors in the guinea pig. Am J Physiol 1994; 267:E268–E272.
168. Silvestre J-S, Robert V, Heymes C, et al. Myocardial production of aldosterone and corticosterone in the rat. J Biol Chem 1998; 273:4883–4891.
169. Myles K, Funder JW. Progesterone binding to mineralocorticoid receptors: in vitro and in vivo. Am J Physiol 1996; 270:E601–E607.

170. Bidmon HJ, Gutkowska J, Murakami R, et al. Vitamin D receptors in heart: effects on atrial natriuretic factor. Experientia 1991; 47:958–962.
171. Behrendt H, Boffin H. Myocardial cell lesions caused by an anabolic hormone. Cell Tiss Res 1977; 181:423–426.
172. Melchert RB, Herron TJ, Welder AA. The effect of anabolic-androgenic steroids on primary myocardial cell cultures. Med Sci Sports Exerc 1992; 24:206–212.
173. Welder AA, Robertson JW, Fugate RD, et al. Anabolic-androgenic steroid-induced toxicitity in primary neonatal rat myocardial cell cultures. Toxicol Appl Pharmacol 1995; 133:328–342.
174. Abu-Shakra S, Alhalabi MS, Nachtman FC, et al. Anabolic steroids induce injury and apoptosis of differentiated skeletal muscle. J Neurosci Res 1997; 47:186–197.
175. Zaugg M, Jamali NZ, Lucchinetti E, et al. Anabolic-androgenic steroids induce apoptotic cell death in adult rat ventricular myocytes. J Cell Physiol 2001; 187:90–95.
176. Wang M, Tsai BM, Kher A, Role of endogenous testosterone in myocardial proinflammatory and proapoptotic signaling after acute ischemia-reperfusion Am J Physiol Heart Circ Physiol 2005; 288:H221–H226.
177. de Simone G, Devereux RB, Daniels SR, et al. Gender differences in left ventricular growth. Hypertension 1995; 26:979–983.
178. Liao Y, Cooper RS, Mensah GA, et al. Left ventricular hypertrophy has a greater impact on survival in women than in men. Circulation 1995; 92:805–810.
179. Urhausen A, Holpes R, Kindermann W. One- and two-dimensional echocardiography in bodybuilders using anabolic steroids. Eur J Appl Physiol 1989; 58:633–640.
180. De Piccoli B, Giada F, Benettin A, et al. Anabolic steroid use in body builders: an echocardiographic study of left ventricular morphology and function. Int J Sports Med 1989; 12:408–412.
181. Sachtleben TR, Berg KE, Elias BA, et al. The effects of anabolic steroids on myocardial structure and cardiovascular fitness. Med Sci Sports Exerc 1993; 25:1240–1245.
182. Thompson PD, Sadaniantz A, Cullinane EM, et al. Left ventricular function is not impaired in weight-lifters who use anabolic steroids. J Am Coll Cardiol 1992; 19:278–282.
183. Bai S, Campbell SE, Moore JA, et al. Influence of age, growth, and sex on cardiac myocyte size and number in rats. Anatom Rec 1990; 226:207–212.
184. Capasso JM, Remily RM, Smith RH, et al. Sex differences in myocardial contractility in the rat. Basic Res Cardiol 1983; 78:156–171.
185. Koenig H, Goldstone A Lu CY. Testosterone-mediated sexual dimorphism of the rodent heart. Ventricular lysosomes, mitochondria, and cell growth are modulated by androgens. Circ Res 1982; 50:782–787.
186. Rosenkranz-Weiss P, Tomek RJ, Mathew J, et al. Gender-specific differences in expression of mRNAs for functional and structural proteins in rat ventricular myocardium. J Mol Cell Cardiol 1994; 26:261–270.
187. Schaible TF, Malhotra A, Ciambrone G, et al. The effects of gonadectomy on left ventricular function and cardiac contractile proteins in male and female rats. Circ Res 1984; 54:38–49.
188. Wang S-N, Wyeth RP, Kennedy RH. Effects of gender on the sensitivity of rat cardiac muscle to extracellular calcium Eur J Pharmacol 1998; 361:73–77.
189. Morris GS, Melton SA, Hegsted M, et al. Ovariectomy fails to modify the cardiac myosin isoenzyme profile of adult rate. Horm Metabolic Res 1998; 30:84–87.

190. Golden KL, Marsh JD, Jiang Y. Testosterone regulates mRNA levels of calcium regulatory proteins in cardiac myocytes. Horm Metabolic Res 2004; 36:197–202.
191. Behrendt H. Effect of anabolic steroids on rat heart muscle cells. Cell Tiss Res 1977; 180:303–315.
192. Moore LG, McMurtry IF, Reeves JT. Effects of sex hormones on cardiovascular and hematologic responses to chronic hypoxia in rats. Proc Soc Exp Biol Med 1978; 158:658–662.
193. Scheuer J, Malhotra A, Schaible TF, et al. Effects of gonadectomy and hormonal replacement on rat hearts. Circ Res 1987; 61:12–19.
194. Malhotra A, Buttrick P Scheuer J. Effects of sex hormones on development of physiological and pathological cardiac hypertrophy in male and female rats. Am J Physiol 1990; 259:H866–H871.
195. Freshour JR, Chase SE, Vikstrom KL. Gender differences in cardiac ACE expression are normalized in androgen-deprived male mice. Am J Physiol Heart Circ Physiol 2002; 283:H1997–H2003.
196. Ikeda Y, Aihara K, Sato T, et al. Androgen receptor gene knockout male mice exhibit impaired cardiac growth anc exacerbation of angiotensin II-induced cardiac fibrosis; J Biol Chem 2005; 280:29661–29666.
197. Calovini T, Haase H, Morano I. Steroid-hormone regulation of myosin subunit expression in smooth and cardiac muscle. J Cell Biochem 1995; 59:69–78.
198. Tivesten A, Bollano E, Nystrom HC, et al. Cardiac concentric remodeling induced by non-aromatizable (dihydro-) testosterone is antagonized by oestradiol in ovariectomized rats. J Endocrinol 2006; 189:485–491.
199. Kinson GA, Layberry RA, Hebert B. Influences of anabolic androgens on cardiac growth and metabolism in the rat; Can J Physiol Pharmacol 1990; 69:1698–1704.
200. Ramo P. Anabolic steroids alter the haemodynamic responses of the canine left ventricle. Acta Physiol Scand 1987; 130:209–217.
201. Davie PS, Thorarensen H. Heart growth in rainbow trout in response to exogenous testosterone and 17-α methyltestosterone; Compar Biochem Physiol 1997; 117A:227–230.
202. Er F, Michels G, Gassanaov N, et al. Testosterone induces cytoprotection by activating ATP-sensitive K^+ channels in the cardiac mitochondrial inner membrane. Circulation 2004; 110:3100–3107.
203. Crisostomo PR, Wang M, Wairiuko GM, et al. Brief exposure to exogenous testosterone increases death signaling and adversely affects myocardial function after ischemia. Am J Physiol 2006; 290:R1188–R1174.
204. Cavasin MA, Tao Z-Y, Yu AL, et al. Testosterone enhances early cardiac remodeling after myocardial infarction, causing rupture and degrading cardiac function. Am J Physiol Heart Circ Physiol 2006; 290:H2043–H2050.
205. Nahrendorf M, Frantz S, Hu K, et al. Effect of testosterone on post-myocardial infarction remodeling and function. Cardiovasc Res 2003; 57:370–378.
206. Chainy GBN, Kanungo MS. Effects of estradiol and testosterone on the activity of pyruvate kinase of the cardiac and skeletal muscles of rats as a function of age and sex. Biochim Biophysic Acta 1978; 540:65–72.
207. Weicker H, Hagele H, Repp B, et al. Influence of training and anabolic steroids on the LDH isozyme pattern of skeletal and heart muscle fibers of guinea pigs. Int J Sports Med 1982; 3:90–96.

208. Velasco L, SÄnchez M, RubÕn JM, et al. Intracellular cAMP increases during the positive inotropism induced by androgens in isolated left atrium of rat. Eur J Pharmacol 2002; 438:45–52.

209. Drici MD, Burklow TR, Haridasse V, et al. Sex hormones prolong the QT interval and downregulate potassium channel expression in the rabbit heart. Circulation 1996; 94:1471–1474.

210. Bidoggia H, Maciel JP, Capalozza N, et al. Sex differences on the electrocardiographic pattern of cardiac repolarization: Possible role of testosterone Am Heart J, 2000; 140:678–683.

211. Brouillette J, Trépanier-Boulay, Fiset C. Effect of androgen deficiency on mouse ventricular repolarization. J Physiol 2003; 546.2:403–413.

212. Brouillette J, Rivard K, Lizotte E, et al. Sex and strain differences in adult mouse cardiac repolarization: importance of androgens. Cardiovasc Res 2005; 65:148–157.

213. Takala TES, Ramo P, Kiviluoma K, et al. Effects of training and anabolic steroids on collagen synthesis in dog heart. Eur J Appl Physiol 1991; 62:1–6.

214. Gualea MR, D'Antona G, Ceriani T, et al. Effects of testosterone on the electrical activity of rat ventricular myocardium Med Sci Res 1995; 23:705–707.

215. Sites C, Tischler MD, Rosen CJ, et al. Effect of short-term medroxyprogesterone acetate on left ventricular mass: role of insulin-like growth factor-1. Metabolism 1999; 48:1328–1331.

216. Schmieder RE, Rockstroh, JK, Aepfelbacher F, et al. Gender-specific cardiovascular adaptation due to circadian blood pressure variations in essential hypertension. Am J Hypertension 1995; 8:1160–1166.

217. Vriz O, Lu H, Visentin P, et al. Gender differences in the relationship between left ventricular size and ambulatory blood pressure in borderline hypertension. Eur Heart J 1997; 18:664–670.

218. Zabalgoitia M, Rahman NU, Haley WE, et al. Gender dimorphism in cardiac adaptation to hypertension is unveiled by prior treatment and efficacy. Am J Cardiol 1996; 78:838–840.

219. Pearson AC, Gudipati CV, Labovitz A. Systolic and diastolic flow abnormalities in elderly patients with hypertensive hypertrophic cardiomyopathy. J Am Coll Cardiol 1988; 12:989–995.

220. Celentano A, Palmieri V, Arezzi E, et al. Gender differences in left ventricular chamber and midwall systolic function in normotensive and hypertensive adults. J Hypertension 2003; 21:1415–1423.

221. Gerdts E, Zabalgoitia M, Bjornstad H, et al. Gender differences in systolic left ventricular function in hypertensive patients with electrocardiographic left ventricular hypertrophy (the LIFE study). Am J Cardiol 2001; 87:980–983.

222. Tamura T, Said S, Gerdes AM. Gender-related differences in myocyte remodeling in progression to heart failure. Hypertension 1999; 33:676–680.

223. de Simone G, Devereux RB, Roman MJ, et al. Assessment of left ventricular function by the midwall fractional shortening/end-systolic stress relation in human hypertension J Am Coll Cardiol 1994; 23:1444–1451.

224. Krumholz HM, Larson M, Levy D. Sex differences in cardiac adaptation to isolated systolic hypertension Am J Cardiol 1993; 72:310–313.

225. Aurigemma GP, Gaasch WH. Gender differences in older patients with pressure-overload hypertrophy of the left ventricle. Cardiology 1995; 86:310–317.

226. Mirsky I, Pfeffer JM, Pfeffer MA, et al. The contractile state as the major determinant in the evolution of left ventricular dysfunction in the spontaneously hypertensive rat. Circ Res 1983; 53:767–778.

227. Shiota N, Rysa J, Kovanen PT, et al. A role for cardiac mast cells in the pathogenesis of hypertensive heart disease. J Hypertension 2003; 21:1935–1944.

228. Toth MJ, Persinger R, Bell SP, et al. Sex differences in the development of cardiac hypertrophy and failure in the Dahl salt-sensitive rat. FASEB J 2003; A1273.

229. Weinberg EO, Thienelt CD, Katz SE, et al. Gender differences in molecular remodeling in pressure overload hypertrophy. J Am Coll Cardiol 1999; 34:264–273.

230. Douglas PS, Katz SE, Weinberg EO, et al. Hypertrophic remodeling: gender differences in the early response to left ventricular pressure overload. J Am Coll Cardiol 1998; 32:118–1125.

231. Dominiczak AF, Devlin AM, Brosnan MJ, et al. Left ventricular hypertrophy and arterial blood pressure in experimental models of hypertension. Adv Exp Med Biol 1997; 432:23–33.

232. Grassi de Gende AO. Relationship between systolic arterial pressure and heart mass in the rat. Jap Heart J 1993; 34:795–801.

233. Wallen WJ, Cserti C, Belanger MP, et al. Gender-differences in myocardial adaptation to afterload in normotensive and hypertensive rats. Hypertension 2002; 36:774–779.

234. Pelzer T, Jazbutyte V, Hu K, et al. The estrogen receptor-β agonist 16α-LE2 inhibits cardiac hypertrophy and improves hemodynamic function in estrogen-deficient spontaneously hypertensive rats. Cardiovasc 2005; Res; 67:604–612.

235. Booth EA, Obeid NR, Lucchesi BR. Activation of estrogen receptor-α protects the in vivo rabbit heart from ischemia-reperfusion injury. Am J Physiol Heart Circ Physiol 2005; 289:H2039–H2047.

236. Zhai P, Eurell TE, Cotthaus R, et al. Effect of estrogen on global myocardial ischemia-reperfusion injury in female rats. Am J Physiol Heart Circ Physiol 2000; 279:H2766–H2775.

237. Zhai P, Eurell TE, Cooke PS, et al. Myocardial ischemia-reperfusion injury in estrogen receptor-α knockout and wild-type mice. Am J Physiol Heart Circ Physiol 2000; 278:H1640–H1647.

238. Cavasin MA, Sankey SS, Yu A-L, et al. Estrogen and testosterone have opposing effects on chronic cardiac remodeling and function in mice with myocardial infarction. Am J Physiol Heart Circ Physiol 2003; 284:H1569–H1569.

239. Dean SA, Tan J, White R, et al. Regulation of components of the brain and cardiac rennin-angiotensin systems by 17β-estradiol after myocardial infarction in female rats. Am J Physiol Reg Integr Compar Physiol 2006; 29:R155–R162.

240. Pelzer, T., Arias Loza, P., Hu, K., Bayer, B., Dienesch, C., Calvillo, L., Couse, J.F., Korach, K., Neyses, L.and Ertl, G., Increased mortality and aggravation of heart failure in estrogen receptor-β knockout mice after myocardial infarction, Circulation, 111, 1492–1498, 2005.

241. Smith PJW, Ornatsky O, Stewart D, et al. Effects of estrogen replacement on infract size, cardiac remodeling, and the endothelin system after myocardial infraction in ovariectomized rats. Circulation 2000; 102:2983–2989.

242. Van Eickels M, Patten R, Aronovitz M, et al. 17-Beta-Estradiol increases cardiac remodeling and mortality in mice with myocardial infarction. J Am Coll Cardiol 2003; 41:2084–2092.

243. Pelzer T, Schumann M, Neumann M, et al. 17β-Estradiol Prevents Programmed Cell Death in Cardiac Myocytes, Biochem. Biophys Res Commun 2000; 268:192–200.

244. Babkiker FA, De Windt LJ, van Eickels M, et al. 17β-Estradiol antagonizes cardiomyocyte hypertrophy by autocrine/paracrine stimulation of a guanylyl cyclase a receptor-cyclic guanosine monophosphate-dependent protein kinase pathway. Circulation 2004; 109:269–276.

245. Chen Z-J, Yu L, Chang C-H. Stimulation of membrane-bound guanylate cyclase activity by 17-β estradiol. Biochem Biophys Res Comm 1998; 252:639–642.

246. Nuedling S, Kahlert S, Loebbert K, et al. 17 β-Estradiol stimulates expression of endothelial and inducible NO synthase in rat myocardium in-vitro and in-vivo. Cardiovasc Res 1999; 43:666–674.

247. Dash R, Schmidt AG, Pathak A, et al. Differential regulation of p38 mitogen-activated protein kinase mediates gender-dependent catecholamine-induced hypertrophy. Cardiovasc Res 2003; 57:704–714.

248. Xu Y, Arenas IA, Armstrong SJ, et al. Estrogen improves cardiac recovery after ischemia/reperfusion by decreasing tumor necrosis factor-α. Cardiovasc Res 2006; 69:836–844.

249. de Jager T, Pelzer T, Müller-Botz Imam A, et al. Mechanisms of estrogen receptor action in the myocardium. J Biological Chem 2001; 276:27873–27880.

250. Nuedling S, Van Eickels M, Alléra A, et al. 17 β-Estradiol regulates the expression of endothelin receptor type B in the heart. Br J Pharmacol 2003; 140:195–201.

251. Persky AM, Green PS, Stubley L, et al. Protective effect of estrogens against oxidative damage to heart and skeletal muscle in vivo and in vitro. Proc Soc Exp Biol Med 2000; 223:59–66.

252. Urata Y, Ihara Y, Murata H, et al. 17β-Estradiol protects against oxidative stress-induced cell death through the glutathione/ glutaredoxin-dependent redox regulation of akt in myocardiac h9c2 cells. J Biol Chem 2006; 281:13092–13102.

253. Hamilton KL, Gupta S, Knowlton AA. Estrogen and regulation of heat shock protein expression in female cardiomyocytes: cross-talk with NFκB signaling. J Mol Cell Cardiol 2004; 36:577–584.

254. Yu H, Shimizu T, Choudhry M, et al. Mechanisms of cardioprotection following trauma-hemorrhagic shock by a selective estrogen receptor-β agonist: up-regulation of cardiac heat shock factor-1 and heat shock proteins. J Mol Cell Cardiol 2006; 40:185–194.

255. Shinohara T, Takahashi N, Ooie T, et al. Estrogen inhibits hyperthermia-induced expression of heat-shock protein 72 and cardioprotection against ischemia/reperfusion injury in female rat heart. J Mol Cell Cardiol 2004; 37:1053–1061.

256. Anderson SE, Kirkland DM, Beyschau A, et al. Acute effects of 17β-estradiol on myocardial pH, Na^+, and Ca^{2+} and ischemia-reperfusion injury. Am J Physiol Cell Physiol 2004; 288:C57–C64.

257. Ranki HJ, Budas GR, Crawford RM., et al. 17β-Estradiol regulates expression of K_{ATP} channels in Heart-Derived H9c2 cells. J Am Coll Cardiol 2002; 40:367–374.

258. Lee T-M, Chou T-F, Tsai C-H. Differential role of K_{ATP} channels activated by conjugated estrogens in the regulation of myocardial and coronary protective effects. Circulation 2003; 107:49–54.

259. Dubey RK, Gillespie DG, Jackson EK, et al. 17β-estradiol, its metabolites, and progesterone inhibit cardiac fibroblast growth. Hypertension 1998; 31:522–528.

260. Grohe C, Kahlert S, Lobbert K, et al. Modulation of hypertensive heart disease by estrogen. Steroids 1996; 61:201–204.
261. Ishii K, Kano T, Ando J. Sex differences in [^{3}H]nitrendipine binding and effects of sex steroid hormones in rat cardiac and cerebral membranes. Jap J Pharmacol 1988; 46:117–125.
262. Pham TV, Robinson RB, Danilo P, et al. Effects of gonadal steroids on gender-related differences in transmural dispersion of L-type calcium current. Cardiovasc Res 2002; 53:752–762.
263. Berger F, Borchard U, Hafner D, et al. Effects of 17β-estradiol on action potentials and ionic currents in male rat ventricular myocytes. Arch Pharmacol 1977 356:788–796.
264. Liu B, Hu D, Wang J, et al. Effects of 17β-estradiol on early afterdepolarizations and L-type Ca^{2+} currents induced by endothelin-1 in guinea pig papillary muscles and ventricular myocytes. Meth Find Exp Clin Pharmacol 1997; 19:19–25.
265. Meyer R, Linz KW, Surges R, et al. Rapid modulation of L-type calcium current by acutely applied oestrogens in isolated cardiac myocytes from human, guinea-pig and rat. Exp Physiol 1998; 83:305–321.
266. Buitrago C, Massheimer V, De Boland AR. Acute modulation of Ca^{2+} influx on rat heart by 17β-estradiol. Cell Signal 2000; 12:47–52.
267. Dzurba A, Ziegelhoffer A, Vrbjar N, et al. Estradiol modulates the sodium pump in the heart sarcolemma. Mol Cell Biochem 1997; 176:113–118.
268. Ren J, Hintz KK, Roughead ZKF, et al. Impact of estrogen replacement on ventricular myocyte contractile function and protein kinase B/Akt activation. Am J Physiol Heart Circ Physiol 2003; 284:H1800–H1807.
269. Hara M, Danilo P, Rosen MR. Effects of gonadal steroids on ventricular repolarization and on the response to E4031. J Pharmacol Exp Therap 1998; 285:1068–1072.
270. Tanabe S, Hata T, Hiraoka M. Effects of estrogen on action potential and membrane currents in guinea pig ventricular myocytes. Am J Physiol Heart Circ Physiol 1999; 277:H826–H833.
271. Abi-Gerges N, Small B, Lawrence CL, et al. Gender differences in the slow delayed (I_{Ks}) but not in inward (I_{K1}) rectifier K+ currents of canine Purkinje fibre cardiac action potential: key roles for I_{Ks}, β-adrenoceptor stimulation, pacing rate and gender. Br J Pharmacol 2006; 147:653–660.
272. Xiao L, Zhang L, Han W, et al. Sex-based transmural differences in cardiac repolarization and ionic-current properties in canine left ventricles. Am J Physiol Heart Circ Physiol 2006; 291:H570–H580.
273. Kayes-Wandover KM, White P. Steroidogenic enzyme gene expression in the human heart. J Clin Endocrinol Metab 2000; 85:2519–2525.
274. Nakamura S, Yoshimura M, Nakayama M, et al. Possible association of heart failure status with synthetic balance between aldosterone and dehydroepiandrosterone in human heart. Circulation 2004; 13:1787–1793.
275. Tsybouleva N, Zhang L, Chen S, et al. Aldosterone, through novel signaling proteins, is a fundamental molecular bridge between the genetic defect and the cardiac phenotype of hypertrophic cardiomyopathy. Circulation 2004; 10:1284–1291.
276. Robert V, Silvestre JS, Charlemagne D, et al. Biological determinants of aldosterone-induced cardiac fibrosis in rats. Hypertension 1995; 26:971–978.
277. Young M, Fullerton M, Dilley R, et al. Mineralocorticoids, hypertension, and cardiac fibrosis. J Clin Invest 1994; 93:2578–2583.

278. Brilla CG, Pick R, Tan LB, et al. Remodeling of the rat right and left ventricles in experimental hypertension. Circ Res 1990; 67:1355–1364.
279. Robert V, Van Thiem N, Cheav SL, et al. Increased cardiac types I and III collagen mRNAs in aldosterone-salt hypertension. Hypertension 1994; 24:30–36.
280. Brilla CG, Zhou G, Matsubara L, et al. Collagen metabolism in cultured adult rat cardiac fibroblasts: response to angiotensin II and aldosterone. J Mol Cell Cardiol 1994; 26:809–820.
281. Sato A, Funder JW. High glucose stimulates aldosterone-induced hypertrophy via Type I mineralocorticoid receptors in neonatal rat cardiomyocytes. Endocrinology 1996; 137:4145–4153.
282. Korichneva I, Puceat M, Millanvoye-Van Brussel E, et al. Aldosterone modulates both the Na/H antiport and Cl/HCO3 exchanger in cultured neonatal rat cardiac cells. J Mol Cell Cardiol 1995; 27:2521–2528.
283. Ikeda U, Hyman R, Smith TW, et al. Aldosterone-mediated regulation of Na^+, K^+-ATPase gene expression in adult and neonatal rat cardiocytes. J Biol Chem 1991; 266:12058–12066.
284. Chai W, Garrelds IM, de Vries R, et al. Nongenomic effects of aldosterone in the human heart: interaction with angiotensin II. Hypertension 2005; 46:701–706.
285. La Mear NS, MacGilvray SS, Myers TF. Dexamethasone-induced myocardial hypertrophy in neonatal rats. Biol Neonate 1997; 72:175–180.
286. Muangmingsuk S, Ingram P, Gupta MP, et al. Dexamethasone induced cardiac hypertrophy in newborn rats is accompanied by changes n myosin heavy chain phenotype and gene transcription. Mol Cell Biochem 2000; 209:165–174.
287. Lindpaintner K, Jin MW, Niedermaier N, et al. Cardiac angiotensinogen and its local activation in the isolated perfused beating heart. Circ Res 1990; 67:564–573.
288. Della Bruna R, Ries S, Himmelstoss C, et al. Expression of cardiac angiotensin II AT1 receptor genes in rat hearts is regulated by steroids but not by angiotensin II. J Hyperten 1995; 13:763–769.
289. Czerwinski SM, Kurowski TT, McKee EE, et al. Myosin heavy chain turnover during cardiac mass changes by glucocorticoids. J Appl Physiol 1991; 70:300–306.
290. de Vries WB, vander Leij FR, Bakker JM, et al. Alterations in adult rat heart after neonatal dexamethasone therapy. Pediatr Res 2002; 52:900–906.
291. Tseng YT, Rockhold RW, Hoskins B, et al. Cardiovascular toxicities of nandrolone and cocaine in spontaneously hypertensive rats. Fund Appl Toxicol 1994; 22: 113–121.
292. Fleck SJ, Henke C, Wilson W. Cardiac MRI of elite junior olympic weight lifters. Int J Sports Med 1989; 10:329–333.
293. Fleck SJ, Pattany PM, Stone MH, et al. Magnetic resonance imaging determination of left ventricular mass: junior olympic weightlifters. Med Sci Sports Exerc 1993; 25–522–527.
294. Hobisch A, Eder IE, Putz T, et al. Interleukin-6 regulates prostate-specific protein expression in prostate carcinoma cells by activation of the androgen receptor. Cancer Res 1998; 58:4640–4645.
295. Bunone G, Briand PA, Miksicek RJ, et al. Activation of the unliganded estrogen receptor by EGF involves the MAP kinase pathway and direct phosphorylation. EMBO J 1996; 15:2174–2183.

12

Cardiotoxicity of Industrial Chemicals and Environmental Pollution

Nachman Brautbar[a]

Keck School of Medicine, University of Southern California, Los Angeles, California, U.S.A.

John A. Williams, II, and Michael P. Wu

Nachman Brautbar, M.D., Inc., Los Angeles, California, U.S.A.

INTRODUCTION

In the last 10 to 15 years, the scientific community has recognized that both environmental and industrial pollution play a role in cardiovascular diseases. In this chapter, we have addressed topics of public health importance and scientific interest in the genesis and contribution of cardiotoxicity. We have approached each chemical, or group of chemicals of interest, from an experimental animal point of view through the human cardiotoxicity point of view. Much has yet to be learned; however, the impact of air pollution and some industrial chemicals on cardiotoxicity is substantial. Like in any aspect of medical toxicology, we have tried to differentiate between indirect and direct cardiac toxicity; this however, is not possible in many of the chemicals studied.

---

[a] Dr. Brautbar testifies from time to time as an expert witness in toxic cases.

ENVIRONMENTAL AIR POLLUTION

Particulate Matter

Particulate air pollution comprises a heterogeneous mixture of suspended liquid and solid particles and originates from a variety of sources. The source of emission may be natural or artificial and include traffic and motor vehicle emissions, industrial combustion, smelting, agriculture, soil, soot, pollens, molds, endotoxins, forest fire, construction, volcanic emissions, commercial and residential fires, insect, plant and animal debris, and mining. Primary particles are emitted directly from a source into the atmosphere, whereas secondary particles occur from chemical reactions in the atmosphere. Numerous terms are used to describe particulate matter (PM). Animal researchers commonly use the term "residual oil fly ash" (ROFA), a fugitive-derived component of ambient PM. ROFA is an industrial combustion byproduct of residual fuel oil and contains large amounts of metals and acids. Other terms for PM are derived from the analytic or sampling technique. For example, total suspended PM is measured using high-volume air samplers and refer to air particles less than 100 μm, collectively. "Black smoke" is a term that refers typically to particulates smaller than 4.5 mm in diameter and is measured by the British smoke-shade method. Recent evidence suggests that particle size may have a determining factor in physiological response. And, because of the complexity of PM, these suspended particles have been classified principally by size. Particle diameter is a convenient method of classifying PM, because this property may indicate the likely source and composition of the particle and may determine the physiological interaction with the cardiopulmonary system. Particulate air pollutants are often categorized into three groups based on the aerodynamic diameter. Natural sources of air pollution tend to emit coarse fraction (PM_{10}), which comprise larger particles with median aerodynamic diameters between 2.5 and 10 μm. PM_{10} can readily enter the upper and lower respiratory tract. Most fine ($PM_{2.5}$) and ultrafine ($PM_{0.1}$) particles are generated as byproducts of combustion. $PM_{2.5}$ comprise particles with median aerodynamic diameters less than 2.5 μm. These smaller particles penetrate more deeply into the small airways and alveoli. $PM_{0.1}$ comprises particles with median diameters less than 0.1 μm. There exists evidence to suggest that some ultrafine particles may translocate from the respiratory tract into the systemic circulation (1,2). Studies to date have not been able to attribute specific components of air pollution to health effects (3). It is believed that fine particles ($PM_{2.5}$) play a key role, because these particles remain suspended in the air for long periods, may travel great distances, have half-life ranging from days to weeks, and are able to penetrate more deeply into the airway. Fine particles also contain toxic chemicals as sulfates, nitrates, ammonium, acids, and metals. Table 1 describes coarse particles and fine particles in detail. There is a strong body of evidence to support exposure to increased levels of airborne PM with cardiovascular morbidity and mortality. The following section reviews the

Table 1 Comparison of Airborne Fine with Coarse Particles

	Fine particles	Coarse particles
Median aerodynamic diameter	<2.5 μm	2.5–10 μm
Formed from	Gases	Large solids/droplets
Formed by	Chemical reaction or vaporization; nucleation, condensation on nuclei, and coagulation; evaporation of fog and cloud droplets in which gases have dissolved and reacted	Mechanical disruption (crushing, grinding, abrasion of surfaces, etc.); evaporation of sprays; suspension of dusts
Composed of	Sulfate, nitrate, ammonium, and hydrogen ions; elemental compounds (e.g., polyaromatic hydrocarbons); metals (e.g., lead, cadmium, vanadium, nickel, copper, zinc, manganese, iron); particle-bound water	Resuspended dust (soil dust, street dust); coal and oil fly ash; oxides of crustal elements (silicon, titanium, and iron); calcium carbonate, salt; pollen, mold, fungal spores; plant/animal fragments; tire-wear debris
Solubility	Largely soluble, hygroscopic, and deliquescent.	Largely insoluble and nonhygroscopic
Sources	Combustion of coal, oil, gasoline, diesel fuel, and wood; atmospheric transformation products of nitrogen oxides, sulfur dioxide, and organic compounds, including biogenic organic species (e.g., terpenes); high-temperature processes, smelters, steel mills, etc.	Resuspension of industrial dust and soil tracked onto roads and streets; suspension from disturbed soil (e.g., farming, mining, unpaved roads); biological sources; construction and demolition; coal and oil combustion; and ocean spray
Atmospheric half-life	Days to weeks.	Minutes to hours.
Travel distance	100s to 1000s of km.	<1 to 10s of km.

Source: From Ref. 3.

cardiotoxic effects of particulate air pollution in experimental animal and human studies.

Experimental studies on ambient PM have described a variety of cardiac responses marked by changes in autonomic function and heart rhythm. Current understanding of the role of airborne particles in the causation of adverse cardiac events remains incomplete. Most research have centered on two pathophysiological pathways by which particulate pollutants may induce cardiac response: (*i*) alteration of cardiac autonomic control, and (*ii*) direct myocardial action. The following section will describe some examples of experimental studies focused on cardiac responses to PM and understanding the biological mechanisms of cardiac toxicity.

Evidence of exposure to PM on cardiac autonomic function in animal studies has been inconsistent. Animals exposed to ambient particulates have demonstrated increases and decreases in heart rate. Tachycardiac responses have been reported in several inhalation studies using cardiopulmonary-compromised rat models (4–6). The reported increase in heart rate tended to be small compared with healthy controls. Bradycardiac responses have also been described in animals exposed to PM (7–11). There is some evidence to suggest that brachycardiac responses yield more pronounced health consequences. Campen et al. observed that normal and compromised rats exposed to ROFA exhibited cardiac arrhythmias and increased mortality in addition to bradycardia (9). While heart rate measures lack agreement, the general findings support a response of the cardiac autonomic system to PM exposure. Heart rate variability is also a useful parameter to describe the effects of PM inhalation on cardiac neural regulation. It has been shown in healthy rats that instillation of aqueous solution of $PM_{2.5}$ decreases heart rat variability (12). In this study, heart rate variability was determined by measuring the standard deviation of the intervals between normal beats (SDNN). A reduction in SDNN was observed within one hour after instillation and at doses less than 100 µg $PM_{2.5}$. Corey et al. examined this association in apolipoprotein E knockout mouse (13). Susceptible mice displayed decrease in heart rate variability parameters in association with exposure to 50 µg $PM_{2.5}$. Wellenius et al. demonstrated comparable response in rats with prior acute myocardial infarction (14). In the myocardial infarction group, rats inhaled ROFA at concentrations of 3 mg/m^3 for one hour and displayed a significant reduction in heart rate variability. Animal studies have also yielded a variety of arrhythmic responses to PM exposure noted by electrocardiograph (ECG) changes. Wold et al. showed that mice developed ventricular premature beats upon infusion of diesel engine exhaust derived-ultrafine particles (15). Wellenius et al. explored the possibility that rodents with preexisting heart conditions are at elevated risk of cardiac arrhythmia upon exposure to PM (14). Results showed that exposure to ROFA particles increased arrhythmia frequency in rats with recent heart attacks. Watkinson et al. observed similar results after exposing rats with preexisting cardiopulmonary disease to PM (16). Researchers found that normal rats and rats with pulmonary vascular inflammation and hypertension exhibited dose-related increase in frequency and severity of arrhythmias upon exposure to ROFA. Cardiac responses were more potentiated in susceptible rats and culminated in 50% mortality rate. Hypertensive rats exposed to ROFA particulates have also been shown to develop cardiomyopathy and other cardiovascular complications (17). Electrocardiographs of these exposed rats revealed depressed ST segment area, an important characteristic in the diagnosis of ventricular ischemia or hypoxia. Wichers et al. observed lengthened RR intervals, skipped beats, and bundle branch blocks in similar hypertensive rats exposed to oil combustion derived-PM (18). The presence of bundle branch block indicates conduction problems in the ventricles. In canines with coronary artery occlusion, exposure to concentrated ambient particles may exacerbate myocardial ischemia (19). Susceptible dogs demonstrated significantly elevated ST segment. Overall, these studies suggest that exposure to ambient particles may activate the autonomic system and induce cardiac arrhythmia and myocardial ischemia in healthy and susceptible animals.

Experimental studies suggest that another plausible mechanism of cardiac response to airborne particulates is via myocardial injury and disruption of cardiac cellular function. Cardiac lesions, decreased numbers of granulated mast cells, multifocal myocardial degeneration, chronic inflammation and fibrosis have been observed in rats exposed long-term to emission-related PM (20). Pathological findings of dogs residing in heavily polluted cities have also demonstrated distinct myocardial alterations, including apoptotic myocytes, endothelial and immune effector cells, degranulated mast cells, and deposition of PM in arteriolar blood vessels (21). Some studies have suggested that ambient particles affect cardiac myocytes function by disrupting ion channels involved in arrhythmogenesis (5,11,22). These studies demonstrated changes in T-waves in response to PM exposure that are suggestive of ion channel disturbance. Graff et al. examined the expression of ion channel protein in rat ventricular myocytes exposed to transition metals commonly found in PM (22). Investigators found that exposure to PM metals resulted in altered gene expression of myocyte ion channels and cytokines. These membrane proteins are important in electrical signal propagation and inflammatory response, and further demonstrate a direct cardiotoxic effect of air pollution particulates. Disruption of these cell processes may trigger cardiac arrhythmia and heart failure. There is evidence to suggest that smaller ultrafine particles are able to enter the systemic circulation and act directly on the heart (1,2). Cozzi et al. evaluated the effect of ultrafine particles (<0.1 μM) on the outcome of ischemia-reperfusion injury in mice (23). PM-exposed mice exhibited a doubling of the myocardial infarct size compared with controls. Researchers hypothesized that the change in infarct size may be attributed to increased oxidative stress observed in the myocardium of the mice after ischemia reperfusion. Kang et al. explored the relationship between $PM_{2.5}$ exposure and arrhythmogenic peptide receptors, endothelin-A, in the myocardium of infarcted rats (24). Investigators found that cardiomyocytes of infarcted rats had more endothelin-A than controls after exposure. This upregulation of the endothelin system likely explains the exacerbated cardiac response observed in PM-exposed infarcted rats. In summary, airborne particulates induce a variety of electrophysiological, morphological, and cellular changes to the heart. Observations of PM-exposed animals have confirmed alterations in cardiac autonomic regulation, as evident by presences of ECG abnormalities, bradycardia, tachycardia, and cardiac arrhythmias. Experimental studies have also demonstrated several mechanistic pathways of PM-related cardiotoxicity, such as disruption of cardiac myocyte ion channels, upregulation of arrhythmogenic processes, and increased myocardial oxidative stress.

   Many cardiac responses have been reported following exposure to elevated concentrations of ambient particulates. Several epidemiological studies on air pollution have described increases in heart rate in association with PM exposure (25–30). These effects were commonly observed following 24-hour exposure to increased levels of PM_{10} or $PM_{2.5}$. Decreases in heart rate have also been reported in response to PM exposure, however the effects have generally been small (31,32). These observed changes in heart rate have clinical significance, because heart rate is an indicator of altered autonomic response and an increase in heart rate is an independent risk factor for cardiovascular morbidity and mortality (33). Epidemiological studies have also analyzed ECG readings and heart rate variability to determine the association between PM exposure and cardiac autonomic regulation. Electrocardiographs of elderly and individuals with coronary heart disease have shown significant association between ST-segment depression during exercise and levels of ambient PM (34,35). These ECG findings provide a physiological link between ambient PM levels and increased susceptibility to myocardial ischemia. Repolarization abnormalities have also been reported after exposure to $PM_{2.5}$ in patients with ischemic heart disease (36). Electrocardiograph measures of repolarization have indicated significant increases in QT duration, decrease in T-wave complexity, and increase in T-wave amplitude 24 hours after exposure. These abnormalities signify autonomic response to PM exposure and may be useful in identifying patients at increased risk for cardiac arrhythmia and sudden death. In general, short-term exposure to elevated levels of PM is associated with reductions in most measures of heart rate variability (26,29–31,37–42). The clinical implication of a decrease in heart rate variability is that the imbalance between the parasympathetic and sympathetic nervous systems may lead to myocardial vulnerability and sudden death. And, the use of clinical parameters such as heart rate, heart rate variability, and ECG readings provide further evidence to the biological link between ambient particles and cardiac autonomic response.

   Environmental studies on air pollution have shown a positive relationship between ambient particulate concentration and various cardiovascular disease end points. This relationship does not appear to be confounded by education and income (43). Short-term exposure studies have demonstrated significant associations between elevated PM levels and increased risk of cardiac arrhythmia (44,45), onset of myocardial infarction (46–49), cardiovascular hospital admissions (50–58), and cardiovascular mortality (59–61). Long-term exposure to PM has been shown to account for a reduction in life expectancy of one to two years (62–64). Epidemiological data suggests that some early deaths are attributed to the association between long-term PM exposure and increased cardiovascular morbidity and mortality (65–70). However, epidemiological studies have not been able to identify a threshold concentration below which PM has no effect on health (71). A threshold level may be useful in establishing a standard concentration set to assure the safety of the population. If a threshold exists, it is likely below existing ambient levels. In any large population, there is likely a wide range of susceptibility in that some individuals will continue to be at risk even at the lowest concentration. While establishing an air quality standard may not be practical, public policy should aim to reduce air pollution levels and minimize cardiovascular risk to all individuals. Time-series analyses of airborne particulates suggest that pollution control may account for a reduction in rate of cardiovascular deaths. In an extended follow-up study of the Harvard Six Cities cohort, Laden et al. determined that the observed decrease in mean $PM_{2.5}$ over eight years accounted for a reduction in deaths due to cardiovascular diseases (72). Clancy et al. reported a 10.3% reduction in cardiovascular mortality 72 months following the ban of coal sales in Dublin ($p < 0.0001$) (73). Epidemiological studies on short-term and long-term exposure to ambient PM have been reviewed extensively (74). In the report, the United Kingdom Department of Health Committee on the Medical Effects of Air Pollution concluded that a clear association exists between both short-term and long-term exposure to air pollutants and effects on the cardiovascular system. Additionally, the committee states that these associations are likely causally linked. Thus despite some inconsistencies and gaps in knowledge regarding mechanism, there exists substantial evidence to support the causal association between PM and cardiotoxicity. These experimental and human data demonstrate several mechanisms by which cardiotoxicity of PM increases morbidity and mortality.

Carbon Monoxide

Carbon monoxide (CO) is an odorless, colorless, toxic gas produced from the incomplete combustion of organic substances. This diatomic gas is a byproduct of environmental and industrial processes, and is the most abundant air pollutant in the atmosphere. Ambient concentrations of CO range from 0.06 to 0.14 mg/m^3 (0.05–0.12 parts per million, ppm) worldwide (75). The main sources of CO come from internal combustion engines, motor vehicle exhaust emissions, appliances fueled by coal, gas, oil or wood, power plants, petroleum refineries, waste disposal incinerators, urban and wildfires, and tobacco smoke. CO is also produced endogenously from the breakdown of heme by the enzyme heme oxygenase. The daily production of CO in the human body is substantial, but under normal conditions CO concentration in the tissues remain rather low. Inhalation of CO is likely the only significant route of exposure. CO entering the body via dermal absorption and ingestion are likely negligible. The toxic effects of CO are primarily attributed to its preferential binding to heme components of red blood cells. The combination of CO and hemoglobin reduces the carrying capacity of oxygen by red blood cells to peripheral tissues, which is observed as a leftward shift of the oxygen-hemoglobin dissociation curve. Tissues as the heart and brain display the greatest demand for oxygen. Indeed, cardiac consequences of CO poisoning have been observed in experimental models and humans, including reports of ECG changes, arrhythmias, ischemia, histological and cellular changes, alterations in coronary blood flow and pressure, cardiac hypertrophy, myocardial infarction, heart failure, and sudden death. Tachycardia and bradycardia are common clinical findings of acute CO exposure (76). Low levels of CO exposure have also shown to exacerbate existing heart conditions (77–80). Most common diagnostic tools used to evaluate cardiopathology of individuals suspected of CO poisoning include angiocardiography, single positron emission computed tomography (SPECT), coronary angiography, and myocardial biopsy.

The mechanism for CO cardiotoxicity continues to be explored. Myocardial hypoxia is a major pathway of cardiotoxicity, however research also indicates that CO has a direct impact on the heart (81–83). CO-induced changes in the heart were first described by Klebs in 1865 (84). In lethal CO cases, he observed punctiform and diffuse hemorrhages in the endocardium, pericardium, and tips of the papillary muscles. In addition, myocardial lesions, necrosis, cardiomegaly, and other histological changes have also been observed in experimental animals and humans exposed to CO (85–89). Experimental research suggests that CO can act directly on the coronary vessels. Coronary vessels of animals exposed to CO exhibit decreased vascular resistance and increased coronary blood flow (90,91). CO-induced cardiotoxicity also occurs by disruption of cellular processes via a variety of mechanisms. It has been well established that CO has a strong affinity to hemoproteins. CO binds to cardiac myoglobin with greater affinity compared with hemoglobin. In myoglobin, CO competes with oxygen and depresses myocardial contractility (92,93). Myoglobin is also responsible for facilitating oxygen transport in cells. Disruption of this process decreases the availability of oxygen for cell respiration in the mitochondria. Indeed, isolated cardiac myocytes show decreased myoglobin-mediated oxygen uptake with incremental CO exposure (94). Cardiotoxicity also appears to be mediated by oxidative stress. Patel et al. reported that exposure to CO induces excess production of oxidants, such as hydrogen peroxide, superoxide, or derivatives of superoxide (95). The notion is supported by the findings of isolated rat hearts exposed to 0.01% and 0.05% CO buffers. CO-exposed rat hearts exhibit a dose-dependent reduction of glutathione and a decrease in perfusate flow that is suggestive of protection from oxidative stress (96). These rat hearts also display subsequent tissue damage and decrease in heart rate similar to rat hearts perfused with hydrogen peroxide (97–99). In addition, in vivo and in vitro animal studies have demonstrated that exposure to low levels of CO is associated with vascular injury induced by nitrogen oxide–derived oxidants (100,101).

Experimental animal studies of acute CO exposure have yielded a variety of ECG changes. First reports of ECG abnormalities were observed in dogs exposed to high levels of CO (102). Dogs were placed in enclosed chambers with CO levels in the order of 4500 to 7000 ppm. Prior to respiratory failure, dogs with 70% to 85% COHb levels showed ST segment depression, premature ventricular beats, T-wave inversion, loss of P wave, and progressive heart block. ST segment depression and premature beats have also been described in rabbits and monkeys with acute exposure to CO (89,103). Mikiskova et al. studied ECG changes in rats exposed to 1000 ppm CO for 120 minutes (104). At peak COHb levels of 30% to 45%, rats exhibited marked hypoxic changes of ST segment depression, QRS widening, T-wave flattening, and premature heartbeats. In the animal model, other ECG patterns have been observed following acute CO exposure, including atrioventricular block, R-wave depression, Q- and S-wave deepening, flattened and diphasic T waves, R-T segment elevation, ST segment elevation, multiple extrasystoles, and preventricular contractions (105–107). The experimental studies demonstrate direct CO effects on the myocyte, as well as indirect effects via reduced oxygen delivery. Both mechanisms play a substantial role in CO-induced cardiotoxicity.

In humans, CO exposure may induce immediate, delayed, prolonged, or reversible ECG changes. Various ECG patterns have been reported in cases involving acute poisoning, such as atrial fibrillation, atrioventricular block, extrasystoles, and P-wave changes (108–111). In 1928, Colvin observed QRS widening, T-wave flattening and T-wave inversion in a man with severe CO intoxication (112). Peak COHb measured 40%. ECG pattern returned to normal weeks later. Jaffe reported similar T-wave flattening and inversion in a group poisoned by CO (113). Reversible ECG abnormalities are not uncommon, even after severe CO poisoning. McMeekin et al. reported on a man with severe biventricular dysfunction due to CO exposure and attained full cardiac recovery after two weeks (114). Repolarization changes manifested as QT interval prolongation and ST segment depression have also been recorded upon acute exposure to CO (85,115,116). In some cases, ECG changes may persist for months or manifest long after initial exposure (117). A delayed ECG response supports the notion that CO intoxication may be associated with structural damage to the heart. Indeed, fatal cases of CO intoxication have shown papillary muscle lesions and abnormal left ventricular wall motion (118). In a prospective study of individuals with CO poisoning, Kalay et al. found mild to severe impairment of the left ventricular structure and function (119). Investigators observed that myocardial injury and dysfunction correlated with COHb level and duration of CO exposure. Myocardial injury from moderate to severe CO poisoning is common. In a review of 230 patients treated for CO poisoning, 41% of patients presented with sinus tachycardia, 30% with diagnostic ischemia, and 41% had nonspecific ST changes (120). Of the 53 patients with echocardiograms, 57% had left ventricular dysfunction, 34% had right ventricular dysfunction, and 30% had regional wall motion abnormality. Cardiac biomarkers of myocardial injury (CK-MB mass $\geq$ 5.0 ng/mL or cardiac troponin I $\geq$ 0.7 ng/mL) were available for 80% of the patients. Of these patients, 44% had measurable myocardial injury. Long-term follow-up of the 230 patients showed that myocardial injury was a significant predictor of morality (adjusted hazard ratio (HR) = 2.1, 95% confidence interval (CI) = 1.2–3.7) (121).

Recent epidemiological studies suggest that CO levels in ambient air may be associated with elevated risk of hospital admissions for angina, congestive heart failure, ischemic heart disease and other cardiovascular conditions (122–125).

The estimated annual attributable risk for hospitalizations because of congestive heart failure nationwide is in the tens of thousands (126). Individuals with preexisting cardiopulmonary conditions, those who already have elevated COHb levels (such as smokers) and the elderly are particularly vulnerable to CO toxicity. Riojas-Rodriguez et al. examined the relationship of ambient CO exposure and heart rate variability by monitoring personal CO levels in patients with known ischemic heart disease (77). Investigators found an inverse relationship between heart rate variability and personal CO levels. The results suggest that exposure to CO may alter cardiac autonomic regulation in susceptible individuals. Additionally, Allred et al. examined the short-term effects of CO exposure on individuals with coronary artery disease in a clinical setting (78). ECG responses were measured for subjects exposed to ambient room air or air containing one of two concentrations of CO (117 ppm or 253 ppm). Individuals exposed to room air, air with 117 ppm CO, and 253 ppm CO had mean COHb levels of 0.6%, 2.0%, and 3.9%, respectively. During exercise, the exposed groups demonstrated dose-dependent decreases in the length of time to threshold ischemic ST-segment change (ST end point) after CO exposure. Exposed subjects also demonstrated significantly less time to onset of angina during graded exercise ($p = 0.02$). On the basis of these data, Allred et al. conclude that exposure to low levels of CO during exercise exacerbate myocardial ischemia in individuals with coronary artery disease. These experimental human studies further demonstrate the cardiotoxic effects of CO.

Certain occupational groups are prone to CO intoxication. Among them are professional drivers, traffic and police officers, firefighters, garage mechanics, tunnel workers, welders, longshoremen, dockworkers, forklift operators, diesel engine operators, individuals working in confined or enclosed space, individuals working at high altitude, and individuals exposed to environmental tobacco smoke. Stern et al. found an elevated risk of heart disease mortality among tunnel workers exposed to historically high occupational CO levels (standardized mortality ratio, SMR = 1.35, 90% CI = 1.09–1.68) (127). In a study among foundry workers, the risk of mortality from ischemic heart disease was significantly elevated in individuals with regular CO exposure (rate ratio = 2.15, 95% CI = 1.00–4.63) (128). Bye et al. reported a positive association between employment that entailed peak CO exposure and mortality from ischemic heart disease and sudden cardiac death ($p = 0.01$) for work in those areas within 3 years from time of death) (129). In assessing occupational risk, it is important to also consider underlying smoking status. Wickramatillake et al. compared COHb levels of smokers with nonsmokers working indoors near combustion processes (130). Indoor CO levels ranged from 3 to 12 ppm throughout the day. For smokers and nonsmokers, exposed workers had a significantly higher COHb level compared with nonexposed workers. Mean COHb levels were between 2.8% and 4.0% for exposed smokers compared with 1.6% to 1.9% COHb levels for nonexposed smokers. For nonsmokers, mean COHb levels were between 1.2% and 1.4% for exposed workers compared with 0.7% COHb for nonexposed workers. These researchers suggest that for workers whose COHb levels are already elevated because of smoking, an incremental rise in COHb level from occupational CO exposure may be sufficient to induce myocardial ischemia in compromised individuals. Taken together, these studies demonstrate the adverse cardiotoxic effects of CO on human health. CO exposure is a particular concern for susceptible individuals and in the occupational setting for individuals exposed to high levels of CO. In summary, CO intoxication induces a variety of electrophysiological and morphological changes to the heart. T-wave changes are the most common ECG responses observed in animals and humans exposed to CO. While ECG is a useful measure of determining CO poisoning, it is not without limitations. ECG abnormalities are difficult to interpret, since changes are not always immediate, often nonspecific, and may not correlate with COHb levels or severity of intoxication. Despite the observation that ECG changes do not always correlate with COHb levels, these studies do support a direct effect of CO on cardiomyocytes. CO exposure has been shown to induce abnormalities in heart rate variability, increase hospitalization of cardiovascular conditions, and increase mortality of ischemic heart disease. The evidence establishes CO exposure as an independent risk factor for cardiovascular toxicity.

Diesel Exhaust Emissions

Vehicle exhaust emissions are emitted as byproducts of internal combustion of fossil fuel in gasoline and diesel-powered engines. In densely populated areas, internal combustion vehicle engines are the single greatest source of harmful air pollutants. Specific emission components depend on the fuel composition, additives, and vehicles' operating characteristics. The majority of pollutants found in exhaust emissions comprise carbon dioxide, CO, nitrogen oxides, sulfur dioxides, hydrocarbons, volatile organic compounds (including benzene, toluene, xylenes, 1,3-butadiene, acetaldehyde, and formaldehyde), and particulate matter. Engine exhaust particles are typically less than 0.1 μm in diameter with most of the particles in the range of less than 50 nm (131). Exposure typically occurs through inhalation or ingestion of suspended exhaust particles and gases in the air. Considerable research has linked inhaled gasoline engine exhaust and diesel engine exhaust with cancers and respiratory illnesses (132). While both gasoline and diesel exhaust emissions cause and contribute to morbidity and mortality, diesel exhaust remains the primary focus because diesel engines emit 20 to 100 times more particles than gasoline engines for the same load (133,134). The following section will focus on inhaled, whole diesel exhaust emissions and the toxic effects on the heart.

Diesel exhaust is a complex mixture of combustion gases and fine particle products. The gas phase fraction consists primarily of oxygen, carbon dioxide, CO, nitrogen oxides, sulfur oxides, water vapor, volatile hydrocarbons, and low–molecular weight polycyclic aromatic hydrocarbons. The solid phase fraction, also known as soot, consists primarily (92%) of carbon particles measuring less than 1.0 µm in diameter and coated with organic and inorganic substances (135). Organic component of diesel particulates accounts for 80% of the mass and comprises aliphatic hydrocarbons, hydrocarbon derivatives, polycyclic aromatic hydrocarbons, and heterocyclic compounds. The remaining 20% of diesel particulates consists of inorganic chemicals, predominately of sulfates (sulfuric acid), traces of metallic compounds and some inorganic additives and components of diesel fuel. Diesel exhaust emissions stem from three major sources: mobile sources (on-road vehicles and equipment, off-road vehicles and equipment and marine vessels), stationary area sources (oil and gas refineries, stationary engines, repair yards, shipyards, etc.), and stationary point sources (chemical manufacturing, electric utilities, etc.) (136). Personal exposure to diesel exhaust occurs mostly via inhalation and depends on duration and intensity. The highest exposures occur in the workplace. In the United States, approximately 1.35 million workers are exposed to the diesel exhaust emissions (137). Workers potentially exposed to diesel exhaust include professional drivers, truck drivers, forklift operators, railroad workers, maintenance garage workers, workers in mines and tunnels, firefighters, parking attendants, and workers on bridges, farms and loading docks. Some studies have attempted to quantify exposure levels. For instance, the highest occupational exposures to diesel PM (DPM) are with miners using diesel-operated machines. Several investigators report DPM range from 10 µg/m^3 to 1280 µg/m^3 for coal and noncoal miners (138,139). Background or environmental DPM levels are generally much lower. The U.S. Environmental Protection Agency (EPA) estimates annual DPM estimates in rural areas to be 0.3 µg/m^3 and in urban areas to be 0.7 µg/m^3 (140). In highway tunnels, particulate levels have been described to peak at 3200 µg/m^3 (141).

Although strong evidence supports a causal link between air pollution and cardiovascular diseases, few studies have examined whole diesel particulate emissions as a cardiotoxic source. Early experimental studies have not provided a clear link between diesel exhaust inhalation with cardiac workload or abnormal histopathology. Guinea pigs and rats exposed to environmentally relevant dosages of respirable diesel engine exhaust for up to two years showed no significant changes in heart mass or morphology (142,143). It is of interest that exposed animals demonstrated a consistent trend towards pulmonary arterial wall thickness for all size categories of artery, but no statistical change for heart weight and ventricular wall thickness (143). Electron microscopic studies were not available to determine whether myocytes are directly affected. Wiester et al. found no differences in heart weight ratios in animals inhaling one part exhaust diluted by 12 parts clean air for 20 hours a day up to eight weeks compared with clean air controls (144). The study should be examined in the frame of exposure-effects in infant guinea pigs. It is also important to note that electrocardiographic studies displayed P-, R-, and T-wave abnormalities. Furthermore, significant sinus bradycardia was demonstrated in the exposed animals. As with the aforementioned studies, investigators did not have ultrastructural data to rule in or rule out myocytes damage. Recent experimental studies examined histograms of RR intervals in rats exposed to five different diesel exhaust concentrations (145). The histograms were determined utilizing telemetry. On the basis of these methods and applying the understanding that RR interval changes within circadian rhythm represent autonomic system effects, the authors concluded that diesel emissions seem to influence RR variability. Apart from inhalation exposure, researchers have employed a variety of methods to investigate the effects of diesel particles on the cardiac tissue. As with the previous experimental studies, ultrastructural studies were not performed and further affecting determination of whether these changes are secondary to hypoxia or represent direct cardiac toxicity. To bypass the pulmonary effects of diesel particles, Nemmar et al. studied the systemic cardiovascular effects of rats injected intravascularly with diesel exhaust particles (146). The rationale for this methodology is based on the observation that intravascular injection of diesel particles, i.e., bypassing the pulmonary system (as compared with inhalation), have been shown to cause peripheral vascular thrombosis and platelet activation (147–149). At doses of 0.02, 0.1, and 0.5 mg/kg, a significant reduction in blood pressure and heart rate was demonstrated after 24 hours compared with saline-treated rats. The reduction in blood pressure and heart rate were explained by the production of oxygen species in the heart, as supported by previous experimental studies (150,151). The authors concluded that the presence of diesel exhaust particles in the circulation leads to both cardiovascular and prothrombotic changes. Toda et al. investigated the cardiac effects of rats injected with 12 or 120 mg/kg diesel exhaust particles and did not report indication of myocardial arrhythmia (152). Only at the higher concentration did investigators observe a decrease in blood pressure. The authors suggest that heart rate changes described in guinea pigs and not in rats are due to species differences. Additionally, the concentrations of diesel emission particles in the study were not comparable to environmental levels. While this is theoretically true, it does not follow the no-observable-adverse-effect level (NOAEL) referenced by the EPA. For minimal risk level (MRL) or NOAEL, the EPA utilizes an uncertainty factor of 10 to 100 to account for inter- and intraspecies variation (153). In the isolated heart muscle, Sakakibara et al. showed that a large dose of diesel exhaust particulate could induce negative inotropic actions on cardiac tissue, followed by cardiac arrest (154). In this model (isolated atrium of guinea pigs), the authors demonstrated direct negative inotropic actions, which were not inhibited by atropine, calcium channel blockers, diphenhydramine, indomethacin, superoxide dismutase, or catalase. Since the pharmacologic agents inhibit the negative inotropic effects via cyclic adenosine monophosphate (cAMP), the authors examined cardiac cAMP and found no significant differences between the diesel treated animals and controls. There precise mechanism by which diesel exhaust particles affect cardiac heart rate is not clear. Nevertheless, these studies demonstrate a direct cardiotoxic effect of diesel exhaust particles, independent of its effects on the lung.

Diesel exhaust emission is a great concern for healthy persons and susceptible individuals with preexisting cardiovascular conditions. Anselme et al. demonstrated that exposure to diluted diesel engine emission may cause immediate and persistent cardiac abnormalities in healthy and chronic ischemic heart failure (CHF) rats (155). The methodology utilized in the study evaluated heart rate variability, which is a well-recognized marker of autonomic function. Exposure to diesel exhaust concentrations similar to that found in urban environments caused immediate autonomic dysfunction in both healthy and CHF rats. Autonomic dysfunction was evidenced by the decrease in root mean square successive difference (RMSSD) of sinusal beats for both sham and CHF rats ($p < 0.05$). In addition, CHF rats showed an immediate 200% to 500% increase in ventricular premature beats with proarrhythmic effects lasting up to five hours after exposure. Persistent cardiac abnormalities were not observed in healthy rats. Since changes in heart rate variability occurred immediately, the authors suggest a pathway that is secondary to autonomic effects and possibly mediated by acute lung inflammation. The study provided a methodological breakthrough for examining effects of diesel exhaust exposure at low levels in unconstrained rats. Previous animal studies had evaluated proarrhythmic effects of air pollution using sedated or anesthetized animals, which made it difficult to extrapolate findings to clinical and epidemiological settings (14,147,156). Myocardial ischemia was ruled out as a possible mechanism of heart rate variability. The rapid initiation of proarrhythmic effect supports a direct action on the myocardium. Persistent ventricular extrasystoles observed after exposure termination suggests that diesel exhaust particles may trigger systemic inflammation and oxidative stress. In other compromised rats, Campen et al. reported an increased heart rate in spontaneously hypertensive rats exposed to diesel exhaust for 7 days (157). These animals also exhibited PQ interval elongation with increased exposure concentration compared with the control group. Delayed arrhythmic effects have also been noted in rats with acute myocardial ischemia/reperfusion. Research has shown rats that undergo intratracheal instillation of diesel exhaust 24 to 48 hours prior to the ischemia/reperfusion experiment die of serious arrhythmias, while rats instilled just before the brief ischemia do not show any signs of arrhythmia (158). The mechanism underlying diesel exhaust exposure and arrhythmias remain unclear, however this study suggests that oxidative stress plays an important role in the observed cardiotoxicity. Twenty-four hours after intratracheal instillation, neutrophil counts were found to be elevated. Neutrophils are known to produce reactive oxygen species (ROS) in the myocardium, and oxidative stress is thought to have major role in reperfusion arrhythmia (159–161). Okayama et al. demonstrated that ROS are also produced locally in cardiac myocytes exposed to diesel exhaust particles (162). Superoxide (O_2^-) was generated by diesel exhaust particle extracts and cardiac myocytes. These ROS induced myocardial cytotoxicity in a dose- and time-dependent manner, and the damage was attenuated by treatment with antioxidant enzymes. The results are in agreement with studies on pulmonary arteries in humans (163).

These studies demonstrate direct cardiac myocyte toxicity by diesel emission particles.

It remains unclear what components of diesel exhaust are most critical in determining cardiac toxicity. Because of the small size and mass, few analytic techniques are available to assess the composition of the diesel emission particles. Several studies have confirmed that particle mass is mostly composed of branched alkanes and alkyl-substituted cycloalkanes from unburned fuel and lubricating oils (131,164). Hirano et al. investigated the oxidative stress potency of the organic fractions of diesel exhaust particles (165). In rat hearts, these investigators showed that the organic extract of diesel exhaust has an oxidative potency to cause functional changes to microvessel endothelial cells. Minami et al. reported arrhythmias followed by death due to complete atrioventricular block in guinea pigs injected intravenously with dimethyl sulfoxide extract of diesel exhaust particles (166). Campen et al. demonstrated that nonparticulate components of whole diesel exhaust elicit ECG changes consistent with myocardial ischemia in mice (167). These animals showed significant bradycardia and T-wave depression, regardless of the presence of particulates. Overall, the experimental animal data demonstrate several plausible biological mechanisms by which diesel exhaust particles cause cardiac toxicity, including indirect actions, via pulmonary hypoxia, pulmonary reflex mediated heart rate variability and inflammatory response of the lung; and direct actions, via oxidative stress on cardiac myocytes, direct calcium overload, and reduced cAMP concentration.

Diesel exhaust emission is a great concern for human health because diesel exhaust particles remain suspended in the air for long periods and particles are generally small enough to penetrate deeply into the lung. In a double-blind, randomized, crossover study of 30 healthy men, Mills et al. found that inhalation of 300 $\mu g/m^3$ diesel exhaust impairs the regulation of vascular tone and endogenous fibrinolysis (168). These clinical findings further link diesel-exhaust exposure to certain cardiovascular conditions. Occupational and epidemiological studies also suggest that diesel exhaust exposure increases the risk of cardiovascular morbidity and mortality. Diesel exhaust is a major contributor of ultrafine particles and nanoparticles in urban areas (169,170). There is mounting evidence to support the role of small particles in the development and/or aggravation of cardiovascular conditions (171). Le Terte et al. analyzed the short-term effects of particulate air pollution on cardiovascular diseases in several European cities (52). Significant positive associations were found for 10 $\mu g/m^3$ increase in PM_{10} and black smoke on hospital admissions for cardiac causes. Black smoke is a dominant component of diesel exhaust. Regression analysis of black smoke controlling for other traffic-related pollutants had minimal effect. Likewise, the regression analysis of PM_{10} disappeared when controlling for nitrogen dioxide; nitrogen dioxide is a secondary pollutant of diesel-powered engines. These results suggest that cardiac admissions were primarily attributed to diesel exhaust. Edling et al. investigated possible adverse health effects of diesel exposure in individuals employed by a bus company. The cohort was divided into three groups: clerks, presumably with no occupational exposure to diesel exhaust; bus drivers, exposed to diesel exhaust at moderate levels; and bus garage workers, exposed to high levels of diesel exhaust. The duration of occupational exposure was at least 10 years. After controlling for smoking habits and following a latency period of at least 15 years, investigators found a significantly elevated risk of cardiovascular disease morbidity for bus garage workers (risk ratio = 4.2, $p < 0.05$) (172). A retrospective cohort study of heavy equipment operators revealed that workers commonly exposed to diesel fumes had a proportional mortality ratio of 1.32 (95% CI = 1.13–1.55) for ischemic heart disease (173). These workers maintained and operated heavy earthmoving equipment powered by diesel engines, such as cranes, bulldozers, graders, and backhoes. A recent cohort study also confirmed the association between occupational exposures to diesel exhaust fumes and elevated risk of heart disease (174). The study compared occupational and medical histories of 176,309 Swedish male construction workers exposed to diesel exhaust with 71,778 unexposed male construction workers. Researchers found that exposed workers had a higher risk of developing ischemic heart disease compared with unexposed workers (RR = 1.18, 95% CI = 1.13–1.24). Occupational studies indeed support adverse cardiovascular outcomes associated with heavy diesel exhaust exposure. However, it is difficult to attribute diesel exhaust exposure alone as a risk factor for cardiovascular disease in the occupational setting. In summary, experimental and human studies suggest that diesel exhaust exposure is probably an independent risk factor for the development and aggravation of cardiovascular conditions.

Nitrogen Oxides-Nitrogen Dioxide

Nitrogen oxides represent a mixture of gases with chemical composition of nitrogen and oxygen. The mixture consists of nitric oxide, nitrogen dioxide, nitrogen trioxide, nitrogen tetroxide, and nitrogen pentoxide. Most oxides of nitrogen are generated naturally from the chemical reaction between atmospheric nitrogen and oxygen in the presence of high temperature and pressure, as, for instance, lightening. Nitrogen oxides are also released into the atmosphere from the oxidation of nitrogen biomass. Anthropogenic contribution of nitrogen oxides comes from the combustion of fossil fuels. Nitrogen oxides are released into the air from motor vehicle exhaust and the burning of coal, natural gas, and oil, and therefore constitute an important air pollution contaminant. In the occupational setting, nitrogen oxides are emitted in electric arc welding, electroplating, engraving, and dynamite blasting. Nitrogen oxides are also found in tobacco smoke. Two most prominent oxides of nitrogen found in the air are nitric oxide and nitrogen dioxide. Nitric oxide is a very reactive, colorless gas at room temperature. Nitric oxide is a ubiquitous intracellular messenger and potent vasodilator. Its endogenous role in maintaining vascular tone and regulating cardiovascular autonomic control is well studied (175–179). Nitric oxide is unstable in air. At high concentrations, nitric oxide is oxidized by atmospheric oxidants to form nitrogen dioxide. In the presence of ozone, nitric oxide is readily converted to nitrogen dioxide. Nitrogen dioxide is a strong oxidant and is five times more oxidant than nitric oxide (180). It is a colorless-to-brown liquid at room temperature, and a reddish-brown gas above 70°F. In the environment, nitrogen dioxide exists as a gas and is at equilibrium with its dimer, nitrogen tetroxide. Nitrogen dioxide is a major urban air pollutant. The annual mean concentration of nitrogen dioxide in urban environments is typically in the range of 20 to 90 $\mu g/m^3$ (0.01–0.05 ppm), and may exceed 940 $\mu g/m^3$ (0.5 ppm) near busy roads (181). The primary route of uptake for nitrogen oxides is inhalation. Toxicity due to inhaled nitrogen oxides is mainly attributed to higher oxides formed before inhalation (182). Because of the relative abundance and stability in the air, the following section will focus on the cardiotoxic effects of nitrogen dioxide, as representative of inhalation exposure to larger class of nitrogen oxides.

Few experimental studies have examined the cardiac response in animals to inhaled nitrogen dioxide. Cardiopulmonary effects of acute nitrogen dioxide exposure have been studied in sheep (183). Conscious sheep did not demonstrate significant change in cardiac output after four-hour exposure to 15 ppm nitrogen dioxide. In rats, acute exposure to nitrogen dioxide has yielded distinct changes in cardiac function. Rats exposed to 40 ppm nitrogen dioxide for 3 hours have demonstrated ECG abnormalities with severe arrhythmias (184). Researchers have reported quicker ECG responses at even lower nitrogen dioxide concentration (185). Rats exhibited bradycardia and severe arrhythmias after 30 minutes exposure to 20 ppm nitrogen dioxide. Exposed rats also demonstrated atrioventricular blocks, premature beats, and changes in pulse interval. After three hours of exposure, rats were injected with parasympathetic nervous system inhibitor atropine sulfate. Following the injection, bradycardia and arrhythmias immediately subsided and pulse interval returned to baseline pattern. On the basis of the findings, the investigators suggest that acute cardiac response to nitrogen dioxide may be attributed to direct stimulation of the cardiac parasympathetic nervous system. It therefore appears plausible that nitrogen dioxide may induce cardiac changes directly independent of upper airway effect. Tsubone et al. studied the cardiac response in tracheostomized rats exposed to nitrogen dioxide (186). Tracheostomized rats exposed to 20 ppm nitrogen dioxide for 150 minutes demonstrated bradyarrhythmia and decreased heart rate. The cardiac response was similar to changes observed in exposed, intact rats. Tracheostomized rats also were treated with atropine sulfate at three different intervals, before and at 60-minute intervals during exposure to nitrogen dioxide. Electrocardiograph measures indicated that atropine injection prevented heart rate changes and ECG abnormalities. The results confirmed earlier findings that the parasympathetic nervous system plays an important role in cardiac response to inhaled nitrogen dioxide. These experiments demonstrate a direct cardiotoxic action of nitrogen dioxide independent of its pulmonary effects. Nitrogen dioxide-induced cardiotoxicity is further supported by the observation that atropine administration ameliorated these cardiac responses.

The Agency for Toxic Substances and Disease Registry suggests that absorption of nitrogen dioxide can lead to weak rapid pulse, dilated heart, chest congestion, and circulatory collapse (187). However, clinical studies on nitrogen dioxide have not yielded profound cardiac effects. Folinsbee et al. measured cardiopulmonary function in young male subjects exposed to 0.62 ppm nitrogen dioxide. There were no significant changes in mean blood pressure or cardiac output (188). Linn et al. monitored cardiovascular parameters of healthy and asthmatic volunteers following exposure to 4 ppm nitrogen dioxide (189). Both groups showed a small but significant decrease in systolic blood pressure ($p < 0.01$). This finding may be attributed to the conversion of inhaled nitrogen dioxide to nitric oxide, a known vasodilator, once the body absorbs nitrogen dioxide. Ecological studies on air pollution have provided support of cardiac autonomic response to nitrogen dioxide. Ruidavets et al. reported an increase in same-day resting heart rate that coincided with nitrogen dioxide concentration (p for trend $= 0.003$) (190). Chan et al. examined the association between nitrogen dioxide and heart rate variability in patients with coronary heart disease (191). In susceptible population, an increase in 10 ppb of nitrogen dioxide at moving averages was associated with 1.5% to 2.4% decrease in SDNN and 2.2% to 2.5% decrease in low frequency. No association was found for heart rate variability and other air pollutants: PM_{10}, carbon dioxide, ozone, and sulfur dioxide. Recent epidemiological studies on air pollution have attributed an increase risk of cardiovascular morbidity and mortality to elevated concentration of nitrogen dioxide (60,192–198). Time-series analyses of air pollution provide evidence of significantly elevated risk of acute myocardial infarction and cardiac arrhythmia for nitrogen dioxide. For an increase in nitrogen dioxide concentration from the 10th to 90th percentile, Poloniecki et al. report the RR of 1.0274 (95% CI $= 1.0084$–1.0479) for acute myocardial infarction and 1.0274 (95% CI $= 1.0006$–1.0984) for cardiac arrhythmia (199). Scientific findings from animal and human studies appear to support adverse cardiac response to inhaled nitrogen dioxide. The mechanism of cardiotoxicity is explained in part by the stimulation of the cardiac autonomic system. In light of the findings, nitrogen dioxide may not be a suitable proxy for other oxides of nitrogen, and, as such, we recommend additional research to explore the cardiotoxic effects due to inhalation exposure of other nitrogen oxides.

Ozone (Oxygen)

Ozone is a toxic, irritating gas composed of three atoms of oxygen. Ozone is a very reactive gas and a strong oxidizing agent. Most ozone is found in the upper atmosphere, where it provides a barrier against solar radiation. In the lower atmosphere, ozone is a secondary pollutant formed as a byproduct of fossil fuel combustion. The majority of troposheric ozone is formed by the interaction of sunlight with nitrogen dioxide and volatile organic compounds commonly found in vehicle exhaust, fossil fuel power plant emissions, and other combustion processes. The gas is a major component of smog and can cause severe health problems. Background ozone concentrations are typically in the range of 40 to 70 $\mu g/m^3$ (0.02–0.035 ppm), however peak exposure can exceed 350 $\mu g/m^3$ (0.18 ppm) for one hour (200). Estimates of background concentration vary by season, time of day, altitude, temperature, and proximity to anthropogenic activity. Ozone is also found in the workplace. In occupational setting, ozone is emitted from electric arc welding, electroplating, mercury vapor lamps, X-ray generators, photoengraving, photocopying machines, electrostatic air cleaners, high-voltage electrical equipment and indoor ultraviolet sources (201). The primary route of uptake occurs via inhalation. Ozone toxicity is in part attributed to its potent oxidative properties.

Ozone is a strong oxidizing agent, and, as such, can trigger a spectrum of biological effects. Experimental evidence suggests that ozone can cause damage to extrapulmonary tissues, including the heart. Rats exposed to 0.07 ppm ozone for five days exhibited signs of lipid peroxidation in the heart (202). Oxidative stress was evidenced by elevated levels of thiobarbituric acid reactive substance and increased antioxidant activity of hydroperoxide scavenging enzymes catalase and glutathione peroxidase. Histopathological examination of the heart revealed evidence of extracellular and intracellular edema. Similar acute cardiotoxic effects were observed in mice exposed to 800 ppb ozone for six hours (203). Investigators found elevated protein carbonyl content, a marker of protein oxidation, in the hearts of ozone-exposed mice. It is plausible that protein carbonyl compounds originate from lipid peroxidation of the lung lipids following inhalation of ozone. These animals also demonstrated a 16% decrease in cardiac protein synthesis that was attributed to a decrease in ribosomal activity. Heart tissue edema was evident by elevated cardiac wet/dry weight ratio following ozone exposure. Acute exposure to high levels of ozone has been observed to alter the rate of cellular respiration in heart mitochondria. In isolated rat heart mitochondria, Zychlinski et al. observed a significant decrease in adenosine triphosphate (ATP) synthesis efficiency (204). Heart mitochondria demonstrated significant decreases in adenosine diphosphate (ADP): oxygen and respiratory control ratios following exposure to 3 ppm ozone for eight hours. Consequently, animal studies have reported significant changes in functional parameters of the heart. One consistent finding of experimental studies is a significant decrease in heart rate following acute or short-term exposure to ozone. Watkinson et al. reported significant decrease in heart rate of rats exposed to ozone concentrations at 0.37 ppm for two hours (205). Arito et al. analyzed heart response of rats at lower concentrations (206,207). At 0.1 ppm ozone, rats exhibited significant decrease in heart rate, increase prevalence of bradyarrhythmia, and increase episodes of bradycardia. On the basis of an extrapolation of the results, the authors proposed that the NOAEL for human inhalation exposure is 0.05 ppm ozone for eight hours (207). In a follow-up study, Arito et al. administered atropine, competitive antagonist of the acetylcholine receptors, during the exposure period (208). Investigators found that atropine blocked the ozone-induced decrease in heart rate. These results suggest that ozone-induced bradycardia is attributed to stimulation of the cardiac parasympathetic nervous system. Uchiyama et al. demonstrated significant decrease in heart rate and mean arterial blood pressure following exposure to 1 ppm ozone for three hours (209). Exposed rats also showed significant prolonged PR interval ($p < 0.05$) and QRS complex ($p < 0.05$) compared with rats exposed to filtered air. All 11-week old rats displayed premature atrial contraction following ozone exposure, and four of the exposed rats showed incomplete Wenckebach's atrioventricular block. While findings from animal studies on acute ozone exposure have been mostly consistent, some studies suggest that the cardiovascular system is able to adapt to long-term exposure. Iwasaki et al. followed cardiovascular response of rats exposed to 0.1 to 0.5 ppm ozone for four consecutive days (210). Heart rate was significantly lower following the first two exposure days, however recovered to baseline on the third and fourth days of ozone exposure. Watkinson et al. also found no discernible changes in rat heart rate following the third day of exposure to 0.5 ppm ozone (211). Uchiyama et al. reported decrease in heart rate, increased PR interval, premature atrial contractions and incomplete atrioventricular block in rats exposed to 0.5 1 ppm for up to six hours (212). Another group of rats were exposed to 0.2 ppm ozone for four weeks. After the third exposure day, heart rate and PR intervals returned to preexposure values. While the mechanism of ozone cardiotoxicity is not clear, direct cardiotoxic effects are demonstrated in experimental animals.

Evidence of ozone-induced cardiotoxicity in humans is limited. The effects of ozone inhalation during exercise have been studied in volunteers with coronary heart disease (213). Volunteers were exposed to three sessions of filtered air or ozone concentrations of 0.20 or 0.30 ppm while walking on a treadmill. The results indicated that ozone-exposed subjects showed no significant signs of cardiovascular stress. Gong et al. examined cardiovascular effects of ozone exposure in hypertensive individuals (214). These individuals were exposed to 0.3 ppm ozone for three hours with intermittent exercise. Functional parameters of exposed individuals indicated increase myocardial work, as measured by significant increase heart rate (8 bpm) and rate-pressure product (1353 bpm/mm Hg) compared with those exposed to filtered air. Several studies have attempted to quantify the relationship between ambient ozone levels and heart rate variability. Gold et al. reported that exposure to ozone was associated with decreased heart rate variability (31). Heart rate variability outcome was assessed by measuring the reduction in square root of the mean square successive differences (r-MSSD) between adjacent normal RR intervals for interquartile changes in ozone. Researchers found a 5.4-millisecond reduction in r-MSSD for interquartile changes in ozone. The results suggest that exposure to ozone at elevated concentrations disrupt short-term autonomic function. Park et al. confirmed the association that exposure to ozone decreases heart rate variability (41). Their study found that 13-ppb increase in four-hour ozone decreased low-frequency power by 11.5%. The authors also reported that association between ozone levels and heart rate variability appear stronger in individuals with existing ischemic heart disease or hypertension. Changes in ventricular function have been reported in association with elevated ambient ozone levels. In a case-crossover study, interquartile range increases in 24-hour moving average for ozone was associated with 21% increased risk of ventricular arrhythmia (odds ratio, OR = 1.22, 95% CI = 1.01–1.49 in the 24 hours before arrhythmia) (215). In the same community, researchers found a statistically significant positive association between acute increases in ozone concentration and paroxysmal atrial fibrillation episodes that result in rapid ventricular rates (216). The twofold increase in risk of paroxysmal atrial fibrillation episodes was observed with each 22-ppb elevation in ozone concentration in the hour before the arrhythmia. Increase in interquartile range of ambient ozone is associated with higher risk of various cardiovascular morbidity and mortality. In South Korea, patients with congestive heart failure had higher daily mortality due to elevated ozone concentrations (60). However, this observation was only significant in men (OR = 1.159, 95% CI = 1.007–1.333), for interquartile range increase of 20.5 ppb ozone. Lee et al. reported significantly higher risk for ischemic heart disease hospital admissions in relation with incremental interquartile range of 21.7 ppb ozone (193). The association was stronger for individuals 64 years and older (RR = 1.10, 95% CI = 1.05–1.15). In a French population, a case-crossover study reported significant increased risk of acute myocardial infarction with increase of 5 $\mu g/m^3$ of ozone air pollution for current-day and one-day lag measurements ($p < 0.01$) (217). A recent meta-analysis was conducted analyzing the relationship between ozone air pollution and cardiovascular disease morbidity and mortality (74). On the basis of present epidemiological studies, the United Kingdom Department of Health Committee on the Medical Effects of Air Pollution concluded that the evidence does not strongly support (nor unequivocally refute) the relationship between ozone air pollution and cardiovascular morbidity and mortality. In summary, experimental animal and human studies have demonstrated some evidence of ozone-induced cardiotoxicity. The mechanisms of cardiotoxicity are not completely understood. Ozone-exposed animals have demonstrated myocardial injury at high doses. Ozone is a powerful oxidizing agent, and, as such, can induce a variety of physiological responses. There is sufficient evidence to support acute exposure and disruption of cardiac autonomic regulation. Consequently, both animal and human studies have demonstrated heart rate changes, ECG abnormalities, and cardiac arrhythmias in response to ozone exposure. It remains unclear whether these changes are sufficient to cause or aggravate existing cardiovascular conditions, however, some studies suggest that elderly and individuals with preexisting cardiovascular disease are more susceptible.

Sulfur Dioxide

Sulfur dioxide is a colorless, water-soluble gas at atmospheric conditions. The gas can be cooled and compressed to form liquid sulfur dioxide for industrial application. The chemical is most notable for its distinct pungent odor and is a major pollutant in the air. Environmental levels of sulfur dioxide are generally very low in the absence of human activity and range in the order of 1 ppb (218). However, the main concern is pollution stemming from artificial contributions, since sulfur dioxide is used in a variety of industrial processes. Sulfur dioxide is used in chemical industries as intermediates for the production of sulfur-containing compounds. Agricultural and food processing industries use sulfur dioxide as a bleaching agent, fumigant, and preservative for some fruits and vegetables. Municipal and water treatment facilities use it to remove residual chlorine from treated water. In the paper pulp manufacturing, sulfur dioxide is used as a stabilizing agent for mechanical pulp. Sulfite pulp workers have been exposed to sulfur dioxide levels as high as 210 ppm (219). In general, sulfur dioxide levels in the air are higher in communities near where these industrial processes occur (220). Industrial and manufacturing plants that burn coal and oil are main sources of sulfur dioxide pollution. Major stationary sources include electric power plants, petroleum refineries, cement manufacturers, metal processors, paper pulp manufacturers, and copper smelters. Mobile sources include trains, large ships, and some diesel-powered equipment.

The primary route of sulfur dioxide exposure is inhalation. Sulfur dioxide enters the body via the respiratory tract, where it is readily hydrated and dissociates to form sulfur ion derivatives, sulfite and bisulfite (221). These ions are absorbed by the blood and transported to the heart and other organs. Inhalation studies in mice confirm a dose-dependent increase of sulfite in the heart upon exposure to sulfur dioxide (222). Experimental animals studies have shown that sulfur dioxide is a systemic toxic agent that can induce cardiac abnormalities via several postulated mechanisms. Fedde et al. observed cardiopulmonary response in chickens exposed to varying concentrations of sulfur dioxide (223). Exposed chickens showed significantly elevated heart rate at 5000 ppm compared with the nonexposed group ($p < 0.01$). Heart rate remained elevated 30 minutes after exposure ($p < 0.01$). These observations were not pronounced at lower concentrations. Inhalation of sulfur dioxide has also shown to decrease blood pressure in a dose-dependent manner. Meng et al. investigated blood pressure of rats exposed to acute and subchronic dosages of sulfur dioxide and sulfur dioxide derivatives (224). Rat blood pressure was significantly lower than baseline and when compared with controls with acute inhalation exposure of 40 ppm sulfur dioxide. Similar results were found with rats inhaling 40 ppm sulfur dioxide for a week. Interestingly, at lower dosage rat blood pressure exhibited adaptive behavior from days 4 to 7. To investigate the effects of sulfur dioxide derivatives bisulfite and sulfite, researchers gave rats intraperitoneal injections of varying concentrations. Derivative-exposed rats also exhibited a dose-dependent decrease in blood pressure. These results support the notion that the cardiovascular system is highly adaptive and that sulfur dioxide derivatives may play an important role in inducing cardiovascular response. Sulfur dioxide and its derivatives have been suggested to induce free radical formation in the heart.

Oxidative stress is thought to damage the structure and alter the function of cardiac cell membranes. Additionally, lipid peroxidation has been suggested to play a role in the development of reperfusion-induced arrhythmias (225). Haider was one of the first investigators to show evidence of lipid peroxidation in the heart induced by sulfur dioxide (226). Guinea pigs exposed daily to 10 ppm sulfur dioxide for 30 days have demonstrated significantly accelerated lipid peroxidation compared with controls ($p < 0.05$). Haider also analyzed lipid profiles of the exposed guinea pigs and found that the ratio of cholesterol to phospholipids in the heart, an index of atherosclerosis, was significantly elevated in the exposed group ($p < 0.05$). Lipid peroxidation and changes in antioxidant status are also evident in the hearts of mice exposed to sulfur dioxide (227,228). Meng et al. exposed mice to sulfur dioxide at 22, 56, and 112 mg/m^3 (227). These mice showed significantly enhanced lipid peroxidation in the heart, as determined by increased concentration of thiobarbituric acid-reactive substances. Exposed groups also demonstrated decreased activities of antioxidants Cu, Zn-superoxide dismutase and glutathione. Meng et al. postulates that sulfur dioxide and its derivatives enhance the formation of sulfur- or oxygen-centered free radicals either by autooxidation of sulfur dioxide derivatives or by an enzyme-catalyzed reaction (224). These free radicals may in turn cause oxidative damage to cardiac cell membranes and ion channels. Nie et al. describe three studies investigating the effects on ion channels in isolated rat ventricular myocytes exposed to sulfur dioxide derivatives (bisulfite and sulfite) (229–231). Ventricular myocytes demonstrate changes in potassium, sodium, and voltage-gated calcium channels upon exposure to bisulfite. Researchers propose that the alteration of cardiac potassium channels may compromise the myocardial resting and action potentials, heart rate, and signaling pathways that regulate cardiac function. Cardiac sodium channels play an important role in the initiation and propagation of myocardial action potential. Disruption of this process may increase cardiac contractility or induce cardiomyopathy. Voltage-gated calcium channels are critical in determining ion homeostasis in cardiac myocytes. Calcium overload may lead to myocardial damage similar to ischemia and hypoxia. These changes present additional mechanisms for sulfur dioxide and its derivatives to induce cardiac myocytes injury. In summary, the experimental animals studies demonstrate that inhalation of sulfur dioxide may induce cardiac responses via multiple pathways. Sulfur dioxide may trigger an autonomic response that alters blood pressure and heart rate. Sulfur dioxide is metabolized to derivatives bisulfite and sulfite, which accelerate oxidative stress, damage cardiac myocyte cell structure and disrupt cell function. These mechanisms suggest direct evidence of sulfur dioxide-induced cardiotoxicity.

Studies of sulfur dioxide inhalation in humans have yielded a variety of cardiac responses. In the clinical setting, healthy volunteers inhaling sulfur dioxide concentrations in the range of 1 to 8 ppm exhibited higher pulse rate (232). Routledge et al. investigated the effect of short-term exposure to sulfur dioxide on heart rate variability and autonomic response (233). Subjects exposed to 200 ppb sulfur dioxide demonstrated a significant reduction in cardiac vagal control ($p < 0.05$). There were no observed changes in circulating markers of systemic inflammation and coagulation, suggesting that cardiac response was triggered by the autonomic nervous system. Epidemiological studies on air pollution have also reported significant cardiac response to sulfur dioxide. Peters et al. reported elevated heart rate during days of high sulfur dioxide pollution (27). The analysis indicated an increase of 70 $\mu g/m^3$ of sulfur dioxide was associated with an increase in heart rate of 1.75 bpm (95% CI = 0.93–2.57). From the same cohort, systolic blood pressure was also shown to rise with sulfur dioxide levels in the air, 0.74 mm Hg (95% CI = 0.08–1.40) per 80 $\mu g/m^3$ sulfur dioxide (234). The elevations in heart rate and blood pressure support the notion that sulfur dioxide pollution plays a role in determining autonomic control of the heart. While these responses were generally mild, slight variations in heart function and blood pressure may trigger arrhythmias and myocardial infarction in susceptible subpopulation. Several studies report a significant increased risk of developing cardiac arrhythmias in elderly and individuals with cardiovascular comorbidities (235–237). Many epidemiological studies also demonstrate that elevated sulfur dioxide levels in the air increases the risk of hospitalization and death due to cardiovascular disease as ischemic heart disease, congestive heart failure, and myocardial infarction (60,238–245). Interestingly, Hedley et al. reported a 2.0% decline in cardiovascular disease mortality ($p = 0.0214$) for five years following the introduction of low sulfur fuel in Hong Kong (246). The change in sulfur content of fuel led to a 53% reduction in sulfur dioxide pollution in the first year. The study provides evidence that environmental regulation of sulfur dioxide pollution has a direct impact on immediate and long-term cardiovascular health. Occupational studies have been conducted on populations exposed to high airborne concentration of sulfur dioxide. Englander et al. evaluated the cardiovascular disease mortality of a group of sulfuric acid plant workers (247). The median concentration of sulfur dioxide was 3.6 mg/m^3. The risk of mortality due to cardiovascular disease was significantly elevated following a five-year latency period (SMR = 1.51, $p = 0.05$). Jappinen studied the mortality of a cohort of pulp mill workers (248). During normal conditions, sulfite mill workers may be exposed to sulfur dioxide concentrations ranging from 0.1 to 50 ppm. The study reported a nonsignificant excess of cardiovascular deaths in men occupationally exposed to sulfur dioxide. Hammar et al. observed a significant increase in incidence of myocardial infarction among paper mills workers (OR = 1.6, 95% CI = 1.0–2.7) and pulp mill workers (OR = 1.3, 95% CI = 1.0–1.7) (249). The association remained significant after adjusting for age and socioeconomic status. The occupational findings are consistent with results of mortality studies on air pollution. In summary, animal and human studies have confirmed an association between inhalation of sulfur dioxide and increased risk of morbidity and mortality due to cardiovascular disease. These studies have demonstrated specific cardiac response to sulfur dioxide exposure, including changes in blood pressure, heart rate, and heart rate variability. It is likely that sulfur dioxide inhalation induces autonomic response and that sulfur dioxide derivatives cause oxidative damage to cardiac cell structure.

INDUSTRIAL CHEMICALS

Metals

Aluminum

Aluminum is the most abundant metal in the earth's crust. In the occupational setting, exposure to aluminum occurs primarily through inhalation during the refining process of the metal as well as secondary exposure to dust and particles. Dermal contact is a less significant route of exposure, although contact with other toxic exposures in an aluminum-based industrial setting can cause skin irritation and neoplastic processes. Consequently, the majority of studies regarding occupational exposure to aluminum have focused on inhalation of respirable aluminum particles. Aluminum is usually found as a mixture with other toxic chemicals, such as polycyclic aromatic hydrocarbons in coal tar pitch, and workers are rarely exposed to pure aluminum-containing dust. Industries with the largest number of workers potentially exposed to aluminum include: plumbing, heating, masonry, electrical work, medical and surgical hospitals, and warehouses.

The general population is exposed to aluminum via ambient air, ingestion of food, certain medications, and drinking water. However, unlike workers in an industrial setting, ambient air accounts for a minority of aluminum exposure. Atmospheric aluminum concentrations range from between 0.005 and 0.18 ng/m^3 (250,251). The corresponding intake of aluminum per day from inhalation, 3.6 ng, is negligible compared with that from dietary sources, 7 to 9 mg/day (252). Foods containing aluminum additives are expected to contribute the majority of dietary exposure, e.g., preservatives, coloring agents, anticaking agents, processed cheeses, and grain products. In addition, cooking in aluminum containers often increases the aluminum content of foods. Water is often treated with aluminum salts during processing to be converted into drinking water. However, aluminum concentrations in drinking water are largely insignificant, rarely exceeding 0.1 mg/L (253).

Aluminum has been shown to be a significant cardiotoxic agent in experimental animals. Zatta et al. investigated the cardiac pathology of exposure to the compound aluminum acetylacetonate in rabbits (30 µg/kg) (254). All rabbits died of congestive heart failure within 9 to 10 days following exposure. Histopathological examination of the hearts revealed biventricular lesions comprising interstitial hyperplasia, myocyte necrosis, and myocarditis, including significant swelling of the right ventricle. Interstitial spaces around myocardial fibers were hyperplastic and edematous, especially in the left ventricle. Aluminum was shown to accumulate in the myocardium in amounts 3 to 4 times that of control group exposed to free aqueous acetylacetone. Authors suggested that the observed findings provide a possible explanation for the occurrence of myocardial infarction. This study demonstrated aluminum-induced cardiotoxicity in the forms of direct myocardial injury and myocarditis. Lipid peroxidation is thought to be a mechanism of toxic injury to tissue. Bertholf et al. examined myocardial lipid peroxidation in rabbits exposed to high aluminum levels (255). The data demonstrated significant accumulation of aluminum in the heart (14.2 ± 4.03 ng/g), as well as enhanced formation of the relevant lipid peroxidation product, malondialdehyde-thiobarbiturate (MDA-TBA; 109 ± 71.6 nmol). Aluminum was shown to catalyze lipid peroxidation in rabbit cardiac tissue, thus providing a biologically plausible mechanism for cardiotoxicity. Cardiotoxic effects exhibited in rabbits by exposure to aluminum acetylacetonate were further evaluated in a later study (256). Administration of the aluminum compound (40 μg/day of total aluminum) for two weeks was shown to significantly elevate creatinine phosphokinase (CK) and lactic dehydrogenase activities. These findings were highly suggestive of cardiac damage. Histopathological studies revealed myocardial infarcts via observed contraction bands and necrotic areas, typical findings seen in human cases of myocardial infarction. Chemical and physical species of aluminum are important determinants of the cardiotoxic effects of the metal (257). The investigators utilized both aluminum lactate and aluminum acetylacetonate to compare the extent of variation in cardiac effects evoked by the two mixtures. Liposome-based administration of aluminum lactate allowed for a focused assessment of its cardiotoxic effects. Data indicated aluminum lactate to be over 300 times more cardiotoxic than the aqueous form. However, there was no appreciable difference in toxicity between aqueous and liposome-based aluminum acetylacetonate despite the synergism expected from the lipophilic character of the species. Histopathology results revealed irreversible myocardial formation of scar tissue in the infarcted areas. Prominent contraction bands and multifocal myocarditis characterized these findings. A concomitant increase in cardiac aluminum concentrations was also observed. This study demonstrated the importance of aluminum speciation in the consideration and assessment of the cardiotoxic potential of the metal. Gomes et al. described the effects of aluminum chloride on the electrical and mechanical activities of the heart in Langendorff-perfused rat hearts (258). Isovolumic systolic pressure (ISP) decreased progressively (34.3 ± 3.0 – 11.8 ± 1.5 mmHg) with increasing concentrations of aluminum chloride (1–100 μM). Atrial and ventricular rates experienced a similar pattern of reduction with increasing concentrations of aluminum chloride. After concentrations of 10 μM, aluminum chloride significantly increased the PR interval. In addition, coronary blood flow was markedly reduced by 20% and 60% at 1 and 100 μM of aluminum chloride, respectively. This dose-dependent response seen in coronary flow mirrored that of ISP reduction. The investigators suggested the decline in coronary flow to be a result of reduced ATP production. Aluminum is known to depress $Na^+ K^+$-ATPase activity. The inhibitory effect of aluminum on ATP hydrolysis was thought to be a consequence of an increased intracellular Na^+ concentration, thereby causing an exodus of calcium from intracellular stores. The resulting calcium levels would be insufficient for proper myocardial contraction activation and adversely affect ISP. The results of this study demonstrate that aluminum exerts powerful electromechanical effects on the myocardium via depression of physiological ATP hydrolysis and production. These experimental studies demonstrate aluminum to be a significant cardiotoxicant that can directly injure the myocardium and interfere with normal cardiac electromechanical activities.

The literature to date, though inconclusive, suggests roles for aluminum in the development of heart disease. Although large-scale epidemiological studies are not available, cardiac effects of aluminum exposure have been seen in hemodialysis patients. Aluminum levels are known to be high in tissues of dialysis patients. Roth et al. reported a case of a 61-year-old aluminum-intoxicated male patient on chronic hemodialysis with congestive cardiomyopathy (259). The cardiomyopathy was characterized by increased left ventricular end-diastolic volume and pressure, as well as decreased ejection fraction. Following his death, an autopsy revealed a myocardial aluminum concentration of 5.4 µg/g. In addition, the hypertrophied heart had left ventricular wall thickening without dilatation. It was suggested that the deposition of aluminum precipitates in the form of salts to myocardial lysosomes might have caused the congestive cardiomyopathy. The specific mechanism and adverse effects for this deposition on the cardiomyocytes were undetermined. However, this study demonstrated that aluminum intoxication in some dialysis patients could result in significant cardiomyopathy. Another study was conducted to investigate the role of aluminum on the myocardium in hemodialysis patients (260). The results revealed that there was a correlation between two parameters of aluminum load [deferoxamine test (DFO) and stainable cortical bone aluminum (SCBA)] and increased left ventricular mass (LVM). Patients with SCBA had significantly increased LVM. The correlations were independent of the duration of dialysis therapy. Of the four factors significantly related to LVM (body surface area, systolic arterial pressure, immunoreactive parathyroid hormone, and increment in serum aluminum after DFO), aluminum accumulation (ΔAl DFO) was thought to be the most important. The investigators suggested that an association exists between aluminum load and cardiotoxicity, principally left ventricular hypertrophy, in hemodialysis patients. Although primarily limited to hemodialysis patients, the data from these studies suggest a relationship between aluminum accumulation in the myocardium and the development of cardiac abnormalities. The experimental animal data and the case reports from human studies suggest that under certain conditions (*i*) aluminum accumulates in the heart; (*ii*) this accumulation affects myocyte metabolic activities; and (*iii*) under certain conditions (such as chronic hemodialysis), aluminum may contribute to cardiomyopathy.

Antimony

The majority of the exposure to antimony in the United States is from impure metallic antimony or recycled antimony scrap. A thorough assessment of industrial antimony toxicity is difficult because it is usually found with lead and arsenic (261). Moreover, separation of exposures from a toxicological standpoint is often difficult or impossible. Antimony oxide fumes is a major route of exposure. Antimony trioxide is a chemical component of fire retardants (262). This can been seen as a potential, albeit low level, source of occupational exposure to firefighters. Workers in the glass industry use antimony trioxide during the refining process. Blood and urine levels of exposed workers have been reported to be elevated.

The general population is exposed to antimony via food and water, with an average daily intake of 100 µg/day (262). Individuals residing near industrial sources of antimony are exposed to higher levels of antimony. Environmental exposures typically occur through inhalation of contaminated air or ingestion of contaminated soil or vegetation. Antimonial compounds have important uses in medications for acute promyelocytic leukemia, leishmaniasis, protozoal infections, helminthic infections, schistosomiasis, and filariasis (264).

The heart is one of the target organs for antimony compounds. Animal studies report adverse cardiovascular events to antimony exposure at the lowest levels tested. On the other hand, inhalational exposure to antimony in rats (3.07 mg/m^3), dogs (5.55 mg/m^3), and rabbits (5.6 mg/m^3) resulted in definite myocardial injury and ECG changes (265). Autopsies performed on 2 of 10 rats revealed myocardial dilatation and flabbiness. All exposed rabbits demonstrated similar findings. Histopathological examination revealed swelling of the myocardial fibers and marked cytoplasmic granules. In effect, the degenerative changes of the myocardium seen in the rats and rabbits were consistent over the six-week exposure period at concentrations of 3.07 to 5.6 mg/m^3. However, the findings in the dogs over the course of 10 weeks were not as definite. The maximum allowable concentration (MAC) of antimony was 0.5 mg/m^3. Trivalent compounds such as sodium antimony dimercaptosuccinate and potassium antimony tartrate (PAT) have been observed to cause bradycardia and decreased contractile force in anesthetized dogs following injection of only high concentrations of the compounds (64 mg/kg) (266). However, blood pressures progressively decreased with increasing doses of 1, 2, 4, 8, and 16 mg/kg, respectively. The cause of the hypotension was unclear but was surmised to be the result of venous pooling. Guinea pigs treated with intramuscular injections of trivalent (10 mg/kg) and pentavalent (16 mg/kg) antimony experienced ECG changes such as T-wave flattening and/or inversion, depression of ST segment, elongation of RR and QT intervals, and marked bradycardia (267). These observations, especially the ECG changes, occurred as a direct result of the conversion of pentavalent antimony [Sb^{5+}] to trivalent antimony [Sb^{3+}]. Ventricular myocytes exposed to Sb^{3+} had depressed plateaus and prolonged durations compared with myocytes from a control group injected with saline. This was determined to result from a reduction in the calcium current. The authors observed no changes in the QRS duration, as neither the conduction or depolarization processes were affected, however, repolarization was adversely impacted. Oxidative stress was thought to play a significant role in Sb^{3+} cardiotoxicity. In a related study, investigators utilized a neonatal rat in vitro cardiac myocyte model to research the effects of PAT on calcium during excitation/ contraction (268). Twenty-four-hour exposure to PAT concentrations between 2 and 8 μm significantly reduced spontaneous beating rates of antimony-burdened myocytes in a concentration-dependent fashion, the reduction becoming consistent at concentrations of 6 μm. The mechanism thought to be responsible for the reduction in cardiac output was a decrease of systolic calcium levels. Diastolic calcium was unaffected. Moreover, 24-hour exposure to point concentrations of 5 or 10 μm also significantly reduced spontaneous beating. PAT was found to effectively reduce calcium concentrations in the myocytes. It was suggested that several mechanisms might be responsible for this finding including: lipid peroxidation, a reduced sarcoplasmic reticulum calcium store, and a reduced release of calcium from a normal calcium store. In a later study on isolated guinea pig ventricular myocytes, therapeutic levels of both PAT and Sb^{5+} prolonged the action potential duration (269). Delays in cardiac repolarization are known triggers of QT prolongation and torsade de pointes. As with other experiments, cardiac calcium currents proved to be more vulnerable to the Sb^{3+}compound PAT. Therefore, this study supported the hypothesis that the conversion of Sb^{5+} to Sb^{3+} is the primary mechanism by which therapeutic antimony drugs produce cardiotoxic consequences.

Similar to experimental animals, humans have been shown to experience electrocardiographic changes in response to inhalational antimony trisulfide exposure (265). Among workers in an abrasives manufacturing plant, 37 of the 75 workers examined experienced T-wave changes deemed significant by the consultant cardiologist. Additionally, investigators reported 14 of 113 men exposed to airborne levels between 0.58 and 5.5 mg/m^3 of this compound experienced blood pressure increases to 150/90 mmHg. This effect is in contrast to that seen in experimental animals, where a decrease in blood pressure has been observed. In addition to electrocardiographic effects, it has been demonstrated that antimony compounds can damage the heart. A case of Stokes-Adams attack was described following intravenous administration of 190 mg of sodium antimonylgluconate (Triostam) on four successive days (270). Direct myocardial injury and ECG abnormalities (flattened T-waves and prominent U-waves) suggestive of an inferior myocardial infarct were observed. Suggested mechanisms for antimony cardiotoxicity in this case were: direct myocardial toxicity, suppression of intracellular enzymatic activities, vagus or sympathetic nervous system disturbances, and alterations in myocardial electrolyte balances. Antimony has been shown to accumulate in the heart. Pandey et al. observed reversible ST-T changes with prolongation of corrected QT (QTc) intervals in patients undergoing prolonged treatment for kala-azar with sodium stibogluconate, a pentavalent antimonial compound (271). The ECG changes were presumed to be the result of a gradual accumulation of antimony in the myocardium, because of slow elimination time of a portion of the antimonial, which lead to myocarditis. Patients with idiopathic dilated cardiomyopathy (DCM) were observed to have elevated antimony concentrations in myocardial tissue of 19,260 ng/g versus 1.5 ng/g in control subjects (272). Among these patients, the mean antimony concentration of those with valvular heart disease was 6 ng/g and 6.5 ng/g in patients with ischemic heart disease. In this study on the pathogenic role of myocardial trace elements (TE), the increased antimony concentration was suggested to affect mitochondrial activity and myocardial metabolism thus decreasing sarcomere contraction. Antimony and other heavy metals are known to induce the formation of oxygen free radicals that may inhibit the cardiac sodium pump (272). A concomitant increase in ventricular arrhythmias was correlated with increases in TE concentrations, particularly for antimony. The mechanism for TE accumulation in idiopathic DCM patients is unknown. The investigators speculated that a cardiac viral infection might affect the influx or outflow of specific TE with resultant cardiotoxic outcomes. Six patients being treated with sodium antimony gluconate for kala-azar developed congestive heart failure and/or a sequence of ventricular ectopics, ventricular tachycardia, torsade de pointes, and ventricular fibrillation with three deaths (273). The investigators discovered that the cardiotoxicity observed was due to a particularly toxic formulation of the drug, which contained an osmolarity 300 mOsm/L higher than normal. However, they surmised that antimony cardiotoxicity might affect a similar sequence of adverse events.

Antimony compounds are recognized cardiac toxicants. Evidence for cardiotoxicity has come from experimental studies and human studies investigating therapeutic treatments of parasitic diseases and occupational exposures. In this regard, the conversion of pentavalent antimonial compounds to trivalent compounds is responsible for both shared clinical efficacy as well as cardiotoxicity. In addition to electrocardiographic changes, several mechanisms of antimony cardiotoxicity have been examined, i.e., direct myocardial toxicity, oxidative stress leading to lipid peroxidation, and disruption of Ca^{2+} homeostasis. These experimental and human studies demonstrate that antimony has a direct cardiotoxic effect.

Arsenic

Arsenic has significant uses in several industries. The production of glass, paper, semiconductors, wood preservatives, and certain pesticides utilize arsenic to varying degrees. Nonferrous metal smelting is a major contributor to arsenic contamination of air, water, and soil (274). Occupational exposure occurs mainly through inhalational and dermal contact. The National Institute for Occupational Safety and Health (NIOSH) National Occupational Exposure Survey reported 55,000 workers were potentially exposed to arsenic between 1981 and 1983 (275). As arsenic is no longer produced in the United States and increasing numbers of arsenical pesticides are being banned, occupational exposures have significantly decreased.

Arsenic is a naturally occurring element in soil and minerals. It is able to contaminate air, water, and land from wind-blown dust. Environmental exposures are seen secondary to drinking well water contaminated from arsenic containing products disposed in a manner with potential seepage into the groundwater. Arsenic air levels increase as the population lives closer to industrial sources. Air concentrations can range from less than 1 to 2000 ng/m^3 (276). Water concentrations have been generally described as less than 10 µg/L in lakes and rivers, although individual samples may range much higher (277–280). Nevertheless, contamination of drinking water secondary to groundwater contamination from arsenic and pesticide wastes can increase these levels. Arsenic is ubiquitous in nature and exposure occurs by food, drinking water, and inhalation. However, food, particularly seafood, is the largest source of exposure to less toxic organic arsenic forms. Groundwater is a greater potential source of arsenic exposure than surface water. Roughly 80% of U.S. drinking water supplies contain less than 2 ppb of arsenic, while 2% of supplies contain 20 ppb (281). Food generally contains between 20 and 140 ppb of arsenic, with levels of the toxic inorganic arsenic being much lower.

Trivalent arsenic, or As^{3+}, is more toxic than pentavalent arsenic, or As^{5+}. Guinea pig ventricular myocytes that underwent several hours' exposure to arsenic trioxide (As$_2$O$_3$) experienced increased cardiac calcium currents and reduced trafficking of the hERG (human Ether-a-go-go-Related Gene) cardiac potassium channel (282). Furthermore, the suppression of this channel at clinical concentrations of 0.1 to 1.5 µm As$_2$O$_3$ reduced I_{Kr} (rapidly activating delayed rectifier K current), thus prolonging the action potential durations of the myocytes. This caused QT prolongation and torsade de pointes. In another study utilizing arsenic trioxide in guinea pig papillary heart muscle, QT prolongation was progressive and both dose and reverse frequency-dependent (283). A low stimulation frequency of 0.1 Hz caused the greatest percent prolongation in action potential duration compared with higher frequencies. These effects were seen for both parenteral and intravenous administrations of arsenic trioxide. Moreover, it has been observed that parenteral administration of arsenic trioxide to rabbits induced similar effects as those seen in the guinea pigs of the Chiang study, in addition to ventricular tachycardia and accumulation of arsenicals in cardiac tissue (284). The QT interval of the rabbits was prolonged by acute As$_2$O$_3$ exposure at extremely high concentrations (300 µm from 362 ± 19 to 414 ± 23 milliseconds, $p = 0.02$), as well as chronic exposure of daily administration of As$_2$O$_3$ for 30 days. In a study designed to compare the two primary forms of arsenic, three groups of male rats were exposed to 50 µg/mL of As^{3+} or As^{5+} and two groups of female rabbits were exposed to 50 µg/mL of As^{3+} (285). All groups exposed to As^{3+} experienced decreased stroke volume and cardiac output with increased vascular resistance. Pentavalent arsenic–exposed rats exhibited no cardiovascular changes. The study by Ficker was comparable to that described in patients receiving As$_2$O$_3$ for refractory acute promyelocytic leukemia (APL), QT prolongation, torsade de pointes, and sudden cardiac death (282). The study by Chiang further demonstrates a direct effect of As_2O_3 on cardiac repolarization and potential prolongation of the QT interval (283). Wu suggests the effects at extremely high doses in a chronic toxicity study demonstrate QT prolongation and cardiac arrhythmias secondary to accumulation of arsenic in the myocardium (284). Overall, these experimental studies demonstrate that (*i*) arsenic affects cardiac repolarization; (*ii*) the cardiotoxicity of arsenic is mediated via direct effects on ion transport; (*iii*) chronic accumulation of arsenic in cardiac tissue is another probable mechanism of toxicity; and (*iv*) these effects may be preventable and to some extent, reversible.

Wang et al. examined drinking water from wells contaminated with arsenic (286). They found a close link between long-term exposure to ingested arsenic in contaminated drinking water and carotid atherosclerosis. Significant dose-response relationships with coronary atherosclerosis indices marked positive relationships between duration, concentration, and cumulative arsenic exposure with the prevalence of the carotid atherosclerosis indices (CAIs). Multivariate ORs adjusted for age, sex, hypertension, diabetes, dyslipidemia, cigarette smoking, and alcohol consumption were significant for individuals with the highest cumulative arsenic exposure ($\geq$20 mg/L years): 3.1 (95% CI = 1.3–7.4) and 2.9 (95% CI = 1.2–6.9), for CAI-1 and CAI-2, respectively. The importance of this study is that since the carotid artery atherosclerosis index is a marker for generalized atherosclerosis and since atherosclerosis increases the risk of coronary artery disease, long-term ingestion of arsenic in drinking water can accelerate underlying atherosclerosis. The researchers suggested that the EPA should further assess the current maximum contaminant level (MCL) for arsenic of 10 mg/L, in the interests of public health. Zierold et al. examined adults exposed to arsenic-contaminated well water, at levels over 10 mg/L (287). The individuals were found to have a higher prevalence of cardiovascular diseases as compared with those with levels less than 2 mg/L. The adjusted ORs for heart attack, high blood pressure and circulatory problems were 2.08 (95% CI = 1.10–4.31), 1.68 (95% CI = 1.13–2.49, and 2.64 (95% CI = 1,17–5.95), respectively. There were significant dose-response relationships between cumulative arsenic exposure and carotid atherosclerosis prevalence. Arsenic is believed to act as a modifying factor in atherogenesis and related cardiovascular diseases via increased oxidative stress, inflammatory activity of vasculature, and altered nitric oxide homeostasis (288). In vitro studies with cultured cells suggested that arsenic affects several cellular functions, including DNA synthesis and increased oxidative stress (289–291). The experimental and human data demonstrate mechanistically and epidemiologically that arsenic mediates atherosclerosis. Arsenic-related atherosclerosis is a systemic disease that may also involve the coronary arteries. Indeed, researchers have demonstrated a dose-response relationship between long-term arsenic exposure from drinking artesian well water and ischemic heart disease (292). Glass blowers were observed to have increased risks of ischemic heart disease due to arsenic exposure (293). Male workers exposed to lead arsenate pesticide spray showed an almost twofold increased risk of dying of coronary artery disease (294). Arsenic-induced cardiomyopathy was initially recognized among beer drinkers in 1900 (295). Sugarcane shipped to a single brewery supplier contained arsenic-contaminated sulfuric acid. The affected beer contained arsenic concentrations between 2 and 4 ppm. Among the resultant cases and fatalities, congestive heart failure was a noted outcome. In accordance with animal studies demonstrating the ability of arsenic to affect cardiac repolarization, arsenic has also been shown to alter myocardial depolarization in humans. Specifically, prolonged QT intervals and nonspecific ECG ST segment changes are frequently seen. However, these changes in cardiac rhythm seen in humans occur at much higher exposure levels and are typically less severe. Typical dosages for As_2O_3 are 0.15 mg As/kg/day. On the basis of the experimental and human studies, it is reasonable to conclude that exposure to arsenic, primarily via ingestion of contaminated drinking water, increases the risk of atherosclerotic disease. In addition, arsenic may be contributory to cardiac depolarization abnormalities.

Cadmium

Industrial use of cadmium (Cd) began 60 years ago. Cadmium is a by-product of lead and zinc mining and smelting operations. It has many applications in the pigment, battery, plastics, alloy production, and metal-plating industries. These industries offer particularly high risk for cadmium inhalation because of high atmospheric concentrations and large numbers of workers. The highest numbers of workers are exposed to cadmium sulfide and cadmium oxide. Exposure to cadmium compounds in industry occurs through inhalation of fumes and dust, primarily in the form of cadmium oxide. Unfortunately, the majority of airborne cadmium is respirable. Typical airborne cadmium concentrations found in the workplace are 0.05 $\mu g/m^3$ or less in the contaminated areas, while the uncontaminated areas are less than 0.1 $\mu g/m^3$.[1] Moreover, the lungs absorb roughly 15% to 30% of inhaled cadmium (297).

Cadmium is also readily found in the environment. The major species found in air is cadmium oxide in the form of particulate matter, tire wear, and burned fuel. Incinerator processes may also release cadmium chloride. Fallout from the air and cadmium-containing irrigation water serve to maintain cadmium's presence in soil. Phosphate fertilizers may contain up to 20 mg/kg of cadmium (298). An important source of cadmium toxicity is commercial sludge used in agriculture. This sludge may contain up to 1500 mg of Cadmium/kg (299). Cigarette smoke is another major source of respirable cadmium. One cigarette may contain 1 to 2 μg cadmium of which 0.1 to 0.2 μg is inhaled (297). Additionally, smoking is known to double the body burden of cadmium. For nonsmokers, food is the greatest source of cadmium exposure. Pipes in water distribution systems may become contaminated by cadmium, thereby allowing an avenue to drinking water. However, owing to very low levels, drinking water is not considered an important source of cadmium exposure.

Cadmium is a known cardiotoxic agent. Isolated Langendorff rat heart preparations exposed to cadmium sulfate (3×10^{-2} mM) experienced prolonged PR intervals and complete atrioventricular block (300). Additionally, heart rates were significantly reduced by cadmium concentrations greater than 3×10^{-4} mM. In another study, the investigators demonstrated that moderate accumulation of cadmium in heart tissue could result in cardiotoxicity (301). The investigators further demonstrated an increased heart cadmium concentration, and that this accumulation mediates the observed electrophysiological changes. Moreover, this can occur even in the absence of clinical signs of cadmium poisoning. Female rats orally exposed to a low-dose cadmium diet experienced biphasic blood pressure changes (302). Low doses of cadmium, 10 μg/day, caused a 20% increase in blood pressure, while intakes 10 to 100 times higher caused reductions in blood pressure to normal readings or below. There was a dose-dependent association between cadmium dose and blood pressure effect. The cadmium levels responsible for the toxic effects and lesions in cardiovascular tissues were similar to exposure levels in the general population. Purkinje fibers from calf hearts have been dissected to assess cadmium-induced effects on cardiac fast Na^+ channels (303). Cadmium ions caused a voltage-independent blockade of the Na^+ channels. The investigators observed that two cadmium ions were required to block one channel, a finding confirmed in other studies. Additionally, the cadmium ions affected channel-blocking action on the outer side of the Na^+ channel membrane in the His bundle region. Histopathological lesions were seen to develop in the hearts of male rats exposed to 50 ppm dietary cadmium for seven weeks (304). The lesions were consistent with varying degrees of myocardial congestion and muscle fiber splitting. The mean cadmium heart concentrations of 0.55 to 1.22 μg Cd^{g-1} were influenced by dietary copper levels and were unrelated to the observed cardiac lesions. It was determined that the heart was a target organ for cadmium toxicity via a mechanism operating independently of increased cadmium-induced tissue peroxidation. Additionally, cadmium also affects coronary blood flow in the perfused rat heart (305). Cadmium consistently reduced coronary flow at low perfusate concentrations. Particularly, significant reductions were seen at levels as low as 0.5 μM of $CdCl_2$. Cadmium concentrations between 1 and 10 μM $CdCl_2$ caused 58 to 63% reductions in coronary blood flow. Cadmium began affecting myocardial contractile activity at 1 μM of $CdCl_2$ and became a significant depressant at cadmium concentrations of 5 μM and greater. It was proposed that decreases in coronary blood flow mirrored decreases in myocardial oxygen consumption through a mechanism by which cadmium inhibited mitochondrial respiration. Male rhesus monkeys exposed to low doses of cadmium (0 and 3 ppm) experienced increases in systolic blood pressure for the duration of the experiment. The monkeys exposed to high doses of cadmium (30 and 100 ppm) experienced an inhibition of age-related hypertension later in life (306).

From experimental animal studies, it was suggested that cadmium binds to sulfhydryl (SH) groups at the membrane level and thereby suppresses the excitability of the atrioventricular cardiac system (307–310). One of the mechanisms suggested is reduction of ATPase activity at the cardiac conduction system (311,312). The mechanism of cadmium cardiotoxicity is the result of reducing blood flow to the coronary arteries at lower levels and interference with mitochondrial function at higher levels (305). The observation of direct effect on cardiac mitochondrial function, which in turn affects coronary blood flow, is a result of disturbances in vasoactive substances that are mechanistically complementary. A recent study summarizes cardiac effects of cadmium toxicity (313). At very high levels, cadmium directly affects the endothelium, secondary to necrotic cell mechanisms. The acute cellular toxicity of cadmium has been studied and results suggest an inactivation of SH groups, disruption of Ca^{2+}, and other concentration-dependent mechanisms and mitochondrial functions. The effects of cadmium on cell apoptosis; cell adhesion molecules, metal ion transporters, and protein kinase signaling pathways have been described (313). Electron microscopic studies have demonstrated cellular degeneration at the atrioventricular location. These findings are of importance mechanistically since they demonstrate, in vivo, ultrastructural changes to the heart at low levels of 5 ppm.

It has been shown that chronic low doses can cause cadmium to accumulate in the heart (314). This accumulation is associated with reduced cellular energy production (compatible with mitochondrial effects of cadmium), and initially with prolongation of the PR interval despite a rapid, mean heart rate. Furthermore, it has been suggested that cadmium may be an unrecognized cause of DCM. In a recent study, cadmium was shown to act on the endothelium of the heart causing decreased vascularization (313). It is no surprise that cadmium has been suggested as another metal capable of causing DCM. This observation is based on human studies demonstrating elevated urinary cadmium in patients with heart failure (315). The investigators discovered significantly high mortality risks for heart failure in both men and women with high levels of urinary cadmium. Another study found significantly elevated blood cadmium levels in DCM patients (316). Cadmium is a known component of cigarette smoke. However, when compared with smokers, nonsmokers, and ex-smokers, nonsmoking DCM patients exhibit significantly higher levels of cadmium in their blood. Taken together, the experimental animal and human studies further support cadmium's role in the development of DCM through antagonistic action on the vascular endothelium of the heart. Other important effects of cadmium on the heart are direct cardiac toxicity and arrhythmias.

Cobalt

The largest use of cobalt is in the production of superalloys used in gas turbine aircraft engines (317). Cobalt compounds are also used in pigments for glass, paints, and ceramics. Occupational exposure to cobalt occurs primarily in the hard metal, coal mining, metal mining, smelting, and refining industries. Inhalation is an important route of exposure. Concentrations of cobalt in hard metal industries can range from 1 to 300 μg/m³, whereas normal atmospheric concentrations are between 0.4 and 2.0 ng/m³ (318). Workers at nuclear facilities, irradiation facilities, and nuclear waste storage sites may be exposed to radioactive cobalt. Cobalt-induced contact dermatitis is seen in industry and is exhibited by erythematous papules occurring on the hands of workers in the hard metal industry (319). Ingestion of contaminated food and water are also means by which the general population is exposed to cobalt. Drinking water supplies may contain between less than 2.0 μg/L and 107 μg/L of cobalt (320). Foods such as bakery goods and cereals, vegetables, mean and poultry, soups, and fruit can contribute as much as 5.0 to 40.0 μg/day. Small amounts of cobalt can also be found in rocks, plants, soil, and animals.

Cobalt cardiomyopathy in experimental animals has been shown to possess similar features to the disease as it occurs in humans. Mohiuddin et al. described the cardiac effects of cobalt sulfate in guinea pigs (321). Guinea pigs were gavaged with 20 mg cobalt/kg/day for five weeks. Investigators reported changes consistent with cardiomyopathy. The cardiomyopathy was characterized by abnormal ECGs (bradycardia, decreased QRS voltage, repolarization abnormalities), pericardial effusions, pancardiopathic heart lesions (myocardial, pericardial, and endocardial), and disfigured mitochondria. Electron microscopy also demonstrated dilated sarcoplasmic reticulum and portions of rough endoplasmic reticulum. This study confirmed the results of previous studies that cobalt can lead to a distinctive cardiomyopathy consisting of specific morphologic and electrocardiographic changes (322,323). The mechanism is probably a combination of sarcoplasmic reticulum damage and mitochondrial damage. Alcohol is known to induce cardiomyopathy as an outcome of chronic alcoholism. The potential cardiotoxic interaction between alcohol and cobalt was investigated in rats (324). Rats administered drinking water containing 50 mg/kg cobalt chloride exhibited multifocal myocytolysis. The simultaneous administration of 10% alcohol increased the damage caused by the cobalt chloride. Myofibrillar damage was also seen to occur. Cobalt chloride and alcohol additively decreased arterial blood pressure, cardiac output, and nutritive blood flow of the heart. The results of this study showed alcohol to potentiate the cardiac damaging effects of cobalt exposure. Histopathology showed swollen mitochondria and dilated sarcoplasmic reticulum compatible with hypoxic effects of alcohol, while damage to the contractile elements was connected with hypoxia-mediated cobalt cytotoxicity. In addition, support for a potentiation effect was seen in the myocardial damaging effects of the simultaneous exposure to the two substances at levels considered nontoxic for either. Clyne et al. analyzed the effects of 24 weeks of chronic cobalt exposure on myocardial antioxidant enzyme activities and mitochondrial ATP production in rats (325). The manganese-superoxide dismutase activity (Mn-SOD) activity was markedly reduced in the myocardium. Enzymatic respiratory chain activities were also reduced. The observed declining rate of myocardial ATP production per gram of myocardium was thought to be a secondary effect to decreased Mn-SOD activity.

The results of this study demonstrate that cobalt can induce a significant decrease in Mn-SOD activity that subsequently causes a decrease in myocardial mitochondrial ATP production. The data from experimental studies demonstrates a directly cardiotoxic effect of cobalt, which in turn causes disruption of normal cardiac enzymatic activities. The confirmatory studies demonstrating ATP effects suggest that cobalt cardiotoxicity is preliminarily via mitochondrial damage.

Barborik et al. introduced the first case of occupational cobalt cardiomyopathy (326). A 41-year-old hard metal worker was exposed to dust containing cobalt. Upon admission for general malaise and other symptoms, an ECG revealed widened QRS and PR intervals suggestive of right ventricular hypertrophy. Further deterioration led to death and an autopsy revealed a grossly enlarged heart with dilation of both atria and ventricles. The left ventricular wall also showed marked thickening. Histopathological results revealed myofibrillar changes, a thickened endocardium, and parietal thrombi. A left ventricular myocardium sample contained 0.37 μg cobalt per gram of tissue, an amount thought to represent a significant accumulation. The authors suggested that cobalt interferes with cardiac metabolism thereby causing myocardial insufficiency and dilatation and parietal thrombosis. Because of the massive accumulation of cobalt in the myocardium and clinical absence of causal factors for the observed cardiac lesions, the authors suggested the data revealed an important case of cobalt-induced cardiomegaly with cardiomyopathy. Cardiomyopathy has been shown to develop in patients undergoing maintenance hemodialysis who are exposed to cobalt (327). A 17-year-old who was administered 25 mg cobalt chloride twice daily exhibited cardiomegaly, pericardial effusion, and left ventricular insufficiency. A pericardial window demonstrated a pale myocardium with poor contractions. Upon death, necropsy revealed marked cardiac dilatation. A myocardial sample contained 8.9 ppm cobalt, whereas 0.2 ppm is seen as a normal value for patients exposed to cobalt in maintenance hemodialysis. It was suggested that the metabolic impact of hemodialysis concomitant with nutritional deficiencies might render the myocardium more sensitive to cobalt. The authors determined on the basis of the clinical data that cobalt was the primary cause for the patient's cardiomyopathy. Another paper describes cardiac disease in a 48-year-old hard metal worker exposed to excessive amounts of cobalt (328). The patient developed cardiac failure and expired. An autopsy revealed extensive myocardial fibrosis, thickened endocardium, and chronic ventricular dilatation. A myocardial cobalt sample contained 7 μg/g. This finding, in light of the absence of coronary artery disease, led the investigators to conclude that the patient's cardiomyopathy was due to industrial cobalt poisoning. Jarvis et al. described two cases of inflammatory cardiomyopathy in men employed in mineral assay industry (329). Case 1 was a 27-year-old male admitted with congestive heart failure. An EKG revealed nonspecific ST-T changes and left atrial enlargement. Echocardiography demonstrated increased right and left sided pressures, global hypokinesis, enlargement of both atria and ventricles, and an ejection fraction of 26.5%. A heart biopsy showed hypertrophic myocardial cells and myofibrillar changes. There was insufficient tissue for a cardiac cobalt sample. However, a pubic hair sample contained 1.5 µg cobalt/g hair. Case 2 was admitted in cardiac failure and underwent transplantation a week later. The explant heart was flabby and enlarged with a hemorrhagic surface. Both ventricles revealed dilated cardiomyopathy and signs of myocyte hypertrophy and necrosis. The cardiac cobalt level was 1.09 µg/g. On the basis of the exclusion of infectious etiology, clinical pathology, and cardiac cobalt levels, the researchers concluded that cobalt exposure was responsible for these cardiomyopathies. A review article suggested that perhaps the most well known cases of cobalt-induced cardiac effects occurred among beer drinkers in the 1960s (330). The cobalt was used as a foam-stabilizing agent. Heavy beer drinkers (10 L/day) consumed an average of 0.04 to 0.14 mg cobalt/kg/day for a number of years and were documented to develop a peculiar dilated cardiomyopathy and other symptoms of general illness. This cardiomyopathy was characterized by sinus tachycardia, left and right ventricular failure, cardiogenic shock, diminished myocardial compliance, pericardial effusion, and cardiomegaly. The presentations were similar to alcoholic cardiomyopathy but the onset was strikingly more abrupt (331–334). The literature from experimental and human studies has documented cobalt to be a cardiotoxic agent, with the most common clinical presentation of cardiomyopathy. The accumulation of cobalt in the myocardium has been demonstrated from electrocardiographic, echocardiographic, and histopathological studies, to have detrimental effects on cardiac functioning. Suggested mechanisms responsible for cobalt cardiotoxicity are hypoxia, inhibition of cellular respiration via decreased mitochondrial ATP production, and decreased calcium concentrations that adversely affect cardiac contraction.

Lead

Exposure to lead may occur in several industries: smelting and refining, battery manufacturing, steel welding, construction, rubber and plastics, automotive repair shops, printing, and others. Other significant exposures occur in occupational exposures to soldering, ceramic glazing, caulking, radiation shields, circuit boards, military equipment (jet turbines and military tracking systems), IV pumps, fetal monitors, and some surgical equipment (335). According to NIOSH, 580,000 workers were exposed to some form of lead in 1980. Occupational exposure to lead is primarily inhalational, although ingestion of lead-containing dusts and fumes is another important route. NIOSH has set a standard for airborne lead levels at 0.05 mg/m^3 (336). Activities such as the mining and smelting of ore, manufacture of lead-containing products, fossil fuel combustion, and waste incineration are the primary means by which lead is dispersed throughout the environment.

Lead is a nonbiodegradable chemical and persists throughout environment. As such, many sources of former lead use continue to contribute to the lead concentrations in the environment. Lead has been identified in over 1280 of the 1,662 EPA National Priorities List (NPL) hazardous waste sites (337). Additionally, lead is the most frequently found metal at NPL sites. Lead-containing paint has been banned since 1978. Even so, deteriorating housing complexes and buildings remain a significant source of lead exposure. As power sanding is a common practice before repainting, lead releases occur when paint dust is disturbed.

Children and pregnant women face the highest risk of lead exposure. Exposure in food, ambient air, drinking water, soil, and dust are frequent vehicles of exposure for the general population. While adults absorb between 3% and 10% of ingested lead, children are known to absorb an average of 40 to 50% (337). Therefore, children are especially susceptible to toxic levels of lead found in paint or in other lead-polluted environments. Deteriorating lead found in paint further contributes to lead levels in house dust and soil, which are more common means for lead exposure in children than paint chips. Consumption of a single chip of lead-based paint may contain lead concentrations of 1 to 5 mg/cm^2 (338). Children in particular can be afflicted with pica (the compulsive eating of nonfood items). Therefore, these concentrations can provide a major source of short-term exposure to lead in children. Moreover, one study revealed that in a series of 454 children, 88% had a history of paint pica (339).

The majority of the U.S. population receives 20% of daily lead exposure from drinking water (335). Lead-containing plumbing components used in schools continue to be a source of lead exposure. Moreover, the EPA revealed in 2004 that a majority of 23,000 homes with leaded pipes had lead levels exceeding the EPA's current 15 ppb action level (340). The study highlighted problems inherent in urban water systems nationwide. Lead-contaminated drinking water is of most concern in either very old or very new buildings. Plumbing installed before 1930 is likely to contain lead pipes, while the "lead-free" declaration of newer homes refers to solders and pipe fittings that may not contain more than 0.2% lead and 8% lead, respectively (337).

Rats provided drinking water containing 1% lead acetate experienced degenerative changes in the myocardium consisting of myofibrillar fragmentation and separation by edema fluid (341). It was unclear whether these changes directly affected myocardial function. Moreover, at the ultrastructure level, the changes resembled those seen from exposure to other toxic agents such as cobalt and alcohol. This study is important since it demonstrates myocardial ultrastructural changes of the heart after short-term lead ingestion. The changes precede findings of congestive heart failure and electrolyte abnormalities. This study is in line with the observations of interstitial myocardial fibrosis associated with conduction abnormalities in a patient with lead toxicity (342). Clinical reports of myocarditis in patients with lead toxicity and atrioventricular conduction defects, and angina are intertwined and supported by experimental studies. Hypertension, as a mechanism for lead-induced cardiac changes, has been suggested in a study showing ultrastructural changes at toxic levels of lead (60 μg/100 mL) that demonstrated myofibrillar degeneration (342). Since lead toxicity, chronic lead exposure, and increased body burden have been demonstrated to cause hypertension; it is reasonable to suggest blood pressure changes as a mechanism for the myofibrillar changes and cardiac toxicity. Investigators have reported blood-lead level-dependent ultrastructural changes in the myocardium of mice. Nuclear changes of the myocardium were seen in lead acetate-treated mice with blood lead levels over 20 µg/100 mL; mitochondrial and endoplasmic reticulum enlargement and dilatation were seen with blood lead levels over 40 µg/100 mL; and focal myofibrillar degeneration and disorganization were observed with blood lead levels over 60 µg/100 mL. It was suggested that the initial nuclear changes observed at the lowest levels were due to a dysfunction in cellular RNA metabolism. The tendency of lead to congregate in mitochondrial segments of cells resulted in impaired oxidative phosphorylation and energy metabolism processes. Hypertension has been demonstrated to be causal from lead toxicity and lead-induced kidney failure. Several mechanisms have been examined. A common mechanism for hypertension involves the renin-angiotensin system. This axis has been examined and demonstrates that lead-induced hypertension in experimental animals reaching blood lead levels of 40 to 70 mg/100 mL were not associated with hyperreactivity of the renin angiotensin system (343). It was also demonstrated that rats fed with low levels of lead in their diet exhibited increases in blood pressure (344). The mean systolic blood pressure increased without evidence of systemic toxicity and in the absence of renal dysfunction. A study was conducted on the mechanisms of lead-induced hypertension (345). The data indicated that short-term exposure (two weeks) to modest lead levels could induce blood pressure elevations in rats genetically predisposed to develop hypertension. This acute model of lead-induced hypertension skewed from traditional mechanisms of chronic lead exposure-induced hypertension. These mechanisms, in addition to the aforementioned renin-angiotensin axis, include lead's effects on vascular tension and contractility, Na^+-K^+-ATPase activity, and intracellular Ca^{2+} homeostasis. The association between low-level lead exposure at levels seen in the general population and high blood pressure, renin angiotensin system changes, and cardiac changes have been studied (346). These investigators concluded on the basis of the experimental animal and human studies that lead causes selective cardiac tropism capable of causing systemic hemodynamic abnormalities when adjusted for other morbidities, i.e., coronary artery disease and other toxic metals) (347–350). These studies are demonstrative of direct cardiac toxicity of lead and indirect cardiac toxicity via adrenergic, catecholamines changes, and high blood pressure. In agreement with other studies, researchers have observed that rats attained maximum blood pressure elevation after three months exposure to 0.01% lead acetate in drinking water (351). Rats with higher lead exposure (0.5% lead acetate) did not experience any changes in blood pressure. A 12 kDa protein band was discovered in the plasma of rats after three months of .01% lead acetate exposure. The investigators determined this band was associated with hypertension development in experimental animals as well as in humans with essential hypertension.

A group of 27 male workers in a battery storage factory were exposed to lead dust with concentrations ranging from 21 to 45 $\mu g/m^3$ (352). Workers in the plant with the highest lead levels (the shatter check site) experienced significantly increased systolic and diastolic blood pressures. Although the airborne lead concentrations were considered safe according to ACGIH standard, the investigators findings were consistent with others studies showing modest increases in blood pressure with low-level lead exposures. There has been some disagreement among researchers concerning the effects lead exposure has on heart frequency and absolute sinus arrhythmia (SA_a). A cohort of 109 male workers experienced decreased heart rate variability and higher SA_a after 19.1 ± 9.0 years of lead exposure (353). This effect was exacerbated in a retest four years later on a sub-cohort of 17 men who were exposed to high levels of lead on a continuous basis. While the cardiac disturbances could not be directly attributed to lead exposure, a focus of the exposure on the vagus branch of the autonomic nervous system was deemed prudent. The investigators interpreted the depressive effect of lead on the vagus branch to be responsible for the decrease in heart rate variability, independent of age or other exogenous factors. Ultimately, it was suggested that several factors such as the findings of lower heart rate and higher SA_a were considered coincidental. Bone lead levels are thought to be better indicators of long-term lead toxicity as compared with blood lead levels that help determine exposure that is more recent. It has been suggested that increased bone lead levels are associated with cardiac conduction disturbances (354). In this study, disturbances such as prolonged QT intervals and intraventricular/atrioventricular node defects were in agreement with previous epidemiological studies (355,356). Additionally, this study specifically established that bone lead, a marker of cumulative exposure, could be responsible for current adverse ECG outcomes. The pertinent mechanisms involved through which lead alters the cardiac conduction system are disturbances in calcium homeostasis leading to disorganized neural and vasomotor functions, inhibition of key hemoglobin-synthesizing enzymes, and direct myocardial injury. Indeed, these findings are supported in experimental studies with lead-intoxicated animals displaying myocardial degeneration and ultrastructural changes (357). The researchers proposed that lead prolongs myocardial contractility while inhibiting the conduction system. Another study also investigated the impairment by lead on the myocardium in a study on employees of a zinc and lead steelworks plant (358). Those workers exposed to lead had a mean blood level of 30.4 ± 1.06 mg/dL. The lead-exposed group experienced a 3% decrease in the ejection fraction of the left ventricle, a 6% increase in the left ventricular enddiastolic diameter, and an 11% increase in heart muscle mass. From the experimental data, case studies, and epidemiological studies, it is reasonable to conclude that lead has both direct and indirect cardiotoxic effects. Several mechanisms including high blood pressure, autonomic nervous system, and mitochondrial damage have been demonstrated to mediate lead cardiotoxicity.

Mercury

Occupational exposure to mercury occurs in numerous workplace environments such as: chloralkai production facilities, cinnabar mining and processing operations, commercial artists and crafts people, chemists and facilities that utilize liquid mercury. Occupations with a high potential of exposure are electrical equipment manufacturers, metal processing, construction workers, chemical processing plants, and the medical professions through exposure to mercury-containing equipment. Fossil fuels can contain up to 1 ppm of mercury and processes such as burning coal and natural gas and petroleum refining emit 5000 tons of mercury per year (297). The primary route of exposure in the workplace is through vapor inhalation. Painters in particular, are exposed in this manner during the application of exterior latex paints containing phenylmercuric acetate. Commercial artists, crafts people, and chemists are other groups that experience mercury exposure. It has been estimated that 95% of urine samples from workers exposed to mercury contain less than 20 µg/L (ppb) (359).

Environmental mercury exists in several forms that can be classified under three categories: metallic mercury, inorganic mercury, and organic mercury. Atmospheric metallic mercury is the primary means for global transport of the metal. Inorganic mercury is formed when mercury is combined with other elements such as chlorine, sulfur, or oxygen. The resulting mercury salts are mainly white powders or crystals. Although methylmercury is the most common organic compound in the environment, dimethylmercury is the only organomercurial found at hazardous waste sites. Methylmercury is known to accumulate in the food chain and build up to toxic levels in freshwater and saltwater fish, and other marine mammals. Ambient air, drinking water, and food contamination are important potential sources of environmental exposure to mercury. Dietary exposures to mercury through fish and shellfish are the most important means of nonoccupational exposure. This observation is mediated by the variability in consumption habits of fish among the population. However, the largest nonoccupational contributor to mercury exposure in terms of total body burden is dental amalgams, particularly in individuals with large numbers (>8) of fillings (360). Dental amalgams contain a mixture of 50% metallic mercury, 35% silver, 9% tin, 6% copper, and trace amounts of zinc. Once hardened, amalgams slowly release minute amounts of mercury because of the natural mastication process. The released mercury may either enter the air as vapor or become dissolved in saliva. It has been estimated that dental amalgams release between 3 to 17 µg of mercury per day (361).

Mercury has been shown to distribute to all organs and tissues. Although the toxic effects and mechanisms responsible for the influence of mercury on the heart are poorly understood, there are several relevant studies. Wojciechowski et al. examined rabbits exposed to mercury vapors in an experimental chamber for four hours/day for three months at concentrations of 2 to 3 mg/m^3 (362). This concentration was considered representative of chronic occupational exposure conditions in man. The investigators observed bradycardia, myocardial lesions, and thickening of endocardial papillary muscles. This study was one of the first to show that metallic mercury vapor can directly damage the endocardium and indirectly damage the myocardium through vascular changes, as well as act on the autonomic system causing bradycardia. Carmignani et al. examined the effects of mercury in drinking water on the cardiovascular system of rats administered 50 mg/mL of mercury [HgCl₃] for 320 days (363). Among other parameters, they have examined blood pressure, left ventricle pressure, heart rate, and electrocardiographic monitoring. They reported increased cardiac inotropism and demonstrated that chronic exposure to mercuric chloride affects specifically, the cardiovascular reactivity to catecholamines. They suggested a mechanism for this observation: mercuric chloride opposing the vasoconstrictive effect of α-adrenergic stimulation. They further demonstrated reversal of moderate systolic hypertension and increased diastolic hypertension. This was explained by a potentiation of vasodilator effects of β-adrenergic stimulation. Another study determined that several of the biochemical changes known to occur in other tissues in response to mercury, such as the kidney and brain, also occur in myocardial tissue (364). In this study, rat papillary muscle developed a positive inotropic response from mercury concentrations equivalent to those found in plasma of poisoned humans. It was suggested that mercury exerted toxic effects on the myocardium through actions on the sarcolemma, sarcoplasmic reticulum, and contractile proteins. In addition to effects on mechanical activity, a study observed that mercury also has arrhythmogenic effects, slows the heart rate, decreases arterial blood pressure, and causes atrioventricular conduction block (365). This study highlighted the cellular level toxic effects of mercury in causing arrhythmias, i.e., inhibition of inward sodium current, depression of Na^+K^+-ATPase and sarcoplasmic reticulum activity. Another important finding of this study was to reinforce that one of the main cardiovascular changes resulting from mercury exposure is reduction in arterial blood pressure. In a related study, anesthetized rats that were administered 5 mg/kg $HgCl_2$ experienced decreased left ventricular systolic pressure and increased right ventricular systolic pressure (366). The goal of this study was to elucidate the mechanisms responsible for the known mercury-mediated decrease in arterial blood pressure. The investigators suggested two possibilities to explain the phenomenon: cardiac mechanical failure and/or pulmonary hypertension caused by pulmonary vasoconstriction. The effects of $HgCL_2$ on the contractile activity of the right ventricular myocardium have been observed in rat hearts (367). It was determined that mercury's effects on the right ventricular myocardium are unique. Increasing concentrations of mercury caused a marked reduction of tetanic force. Mercury depressed the contractile function when strips of right ventricular wall were used, however, this effect was not seen in Langendorff-perfused rat hearts or in vivo. It was thought that an increase in coronary perfusion pressure resulting in positive inotropism was the primary factor in this finding. Diastolic pressure increased on a concentration-dependent basis, with the increase becoming significant between concentrations 0.1 and 3 μM $HgCl_2$.

Similar results were obtained in another study (368). However, the reduction in the tetanic tension seen in the ventricular strips was preceded by a significant increase in tetanic tension. In summary, although the mechanisms responsible for these cardiac effects are not completely understood, it is fairly well documented that mercury exerts its toxic effects in general through a process involving the combining of SH groups (369). These groups play vital roles in the normal functioning of key proteins, enzymes, ion channels, and receptors (370). Additionally, mercury reduces activity of the Na^+K^+-ATPase as well as the Ca^{2+}-ATPase activity in the sarcoplasmic reticulum, leading to an increase in Ca^{2+} release (364). Myocardial cells are able to accumulate and concentrate mercury. This may lead to a reduction in the activity of contractile proteins and myosin ATPase causing loss of tetanic tension development. These experimental studies demonstrate direct toxicity in the cardiac cell via several proposed mechanisms.

The consumption of mercury-containing fish has been associated with increased risks of acute myocardial infarction and death from coronary heart disease and cardiovascular disease (371). In this study, men grouped in the highest tertile (≥ 2.03 µg/g) of hair mercury content had an adjusted risk of an acute coronary event, RR = 1.60 (95% CI = 1.24–2.06) and of cardiovascular disease, RR = 1.68 (95% CI = 1.15–2.44). Adjusting for risk of cardiovascular death returned an RR of 2.9 (95% CI = 1.2–6.6). These increased risks were believed to be due to increased mercury-mediated lipid peroxidation via several mechanisms including: the reduction of antioxidative capacity in plasma and cells, the promotion of free radicals, mercury's high affinity to SH groups, and the formation of a mercury selenide complex. The hypothesis that mercury contributed to increased risk of myocardial infarction was supported by documented associations between the high mercury content of sampled hair and elevated titers of oxidized LDL-containing immune complexes. This study revealed the important finding that mercury, even in low levels, was still a significant risk factor for coronary heart disease. In another cohort study, 6784 male mercury miners experienced increased hypertension rates, SMR = 1.46, (95% CI = 1.08–1.93), as well as increased heart diseases other than ischemic, SMR = 1.36, (95% CI = 1.20–1.53) (372). The mortality rates for these cardiovascular conditions increased with estimated cumulative mercury exposure. Because of the strong dose-response relationship between mercury exposure and hypertension, as well as the subsequent increased mortality, it was suggested that a kidney-mediated mechanism was responsible for the hypertension rates. Interestingly, the investigators believed that misclassification of workers and exposures resulted in an underestimation of the association between mercury mining and cardiovascular outcomes. A case-control study studied men first diagnosed with myocardial infarction (373). Men with average toenail mercury levels of 0.25 µg/g demonstrated a dose-response, significant risk for myocardial infarction after adjusting for docosahexaenoic acid level in adipose tissue and coronary risk factors, OR = 2.16, (95% CI = 1.09–4.29). Exposure to mercury was thought to be a result of relatively high consumption of Mediterranean fish. In a later study, the intake of mercury from food, primarily fish, has also been demonstrated to cause systolic hypertension (374). Pulse pressure was positively correlated and increased with higher mercury content in the blood. However, blood mercury was negatively and significantly correlated with diastolic pressure. The investigators suggested that mercury consumption via fish introduced vascular lesions of the aorta and other large arteries. This formed the foundation for atherosclerotic processes and increased systolic blood pressure. These observations support the proposition that certain mercury contaminated fish consumption is contributory to cardiovascular disease. Mercury may also accumulate in the heart through self-injections of metallic mercury (375). Upon cardiac ultrasound, the investigators discovered metal dense deposits in the right ventricle and distal septum of a young man who self-injected mercury obtained from a thermometer. It was proposed that mercury within the heart could induce the formation of cardiac granulomas and abnormal ECG readings from the resulting fibrosis. This observation is in line with the experimental animal studies demonstrating mercury accumulation in heart cells. Mercury used in dental amalgams has been found to be contributory to the development of heart disease (376). In this study, subjects with dental amalgams had significantly higher blood pressures and lower heart rates than control subjects. The amalgam subjects also exhibited greater incidences of chest pains, heart murmur, and tachycardia. Upon removal of amalgams, subjects reported improvement in the cardiovascular symptoms. The symptoms experienced by the amalgam group are typical of mercury toxicity. The authors suggested that the continual release of mercury vapor from the amalgam might lead to the observed cardiac physiological changes.

Although direct causality cannot be drawn, the evidence to date from experimental animal studies and epidemiological studies lends support to the hypothesis that a range of mercury levels in the body can be cardiotoxic and increase the risk of cardiovascular disease. Several possible mechanisms have been noted to be effectors of mercury's cardiac toxicity. A threshold value for mercury exposure, after which cardiotoxicity begins, has yet to be determined. One reason for lack of more data on chronic mercury body build up (body burden) is that private practitioners, as well as practicing academicians, are not always looking into environmental, dietary, and occupational exposures. As a result, many more cases are probably underestimated and underdiagnosed.

Organic Solvents

A hydrocarbon or organic solvent is a chemical compound consisting solely of hydrogen and carbon that is capable of dissolving another substance (377). Solvents are ubiquitous in nature and nearly everyone is exposed to them. The classes of organic solvents are derived from petroleum and have boiling points ranging from 35 to 320°C.

Aromatic Solvents

Benzene

Benzene is the parent compound for the aromatic class of organic solvents, being composed of a single benzene ring. As such, it is the prototype for other solvents such as styrene, phenol, and cyclohexane. The OSHA permissible limit for benzene exposure is 1 ppm for an eight-hour time-weighted average (TWA) exposure and 5 ppm for any 15-minute period short-term exposure limit (378). Several industries use benzene, including petrochemicals, petroleum refining, coke/coal chemical manufacturing, rubber tire manufacturing, and storage/ transport of chemicals made from benzene. Other workers with potential benzene exposure are steel industry workers, printers, rubber workers, shoemakers, firefighters, gas station employees, and medical/surgical hospital employees.

The inhalation of contaminated air is the main route of exposure. Industry, motor vehicles, and gasoline service stations are the main contributors to benzene in the environment and levels in the air. Natural sources are also important contributors of environmental benzene and include: gas emissions from volcanoes and forest fires, crude oil, and cigarette smoke. Of these, tobacco smoke is the largest source. Benzene levels in air generally range from 0.02 to 34 ppb from rural environments to urban, heavily congested roads. People residing near hazardous waste sites or petrochemical manufacturing plants can be exposed to significantly higher levels. Additionally, private residences with attached garages and/or tobacco-using inhabitants have been shown to increase exposure. Oral intake of benzene through food and water is a substantially less significant route of exposure. Cigarette smoke is an important contributing source for benzene exposure. It has been calculated that mainstream tobacco smoke contains 50 μg benzene per cigarette, which is equivalent to 0.89 mg benzene/day in the average smoker (379). Bottled water, benzene-contaminated well water, and the consumption of foods prepared with contaminated tap water have been reported means of exposure. Dermal exposure to benzene can also occur through contaminated water used during showering and bathing, as well as the industrial use of solvents to remove paint from the skin or to wash the hands to remove grease.

There is a paucity of data pertaining to the cardiotoxicity of benzene exposure. Organic solvents are generally known to induce arrhythmias. Vidrio et al. examined possible cardiac sensitizing effects of near lethal doses of benzene and toluene on chloralose-anesthetized rats using a static inhalation procedure (380). While both solvents produced tachycardia, benzene decreased P-wave duration and increased the number of epinephrine-induced ectopic beats, while toluene increased QRS duration and decreased ectopic beats. Benzene was judged to have a particular myocardial-sensitizing property not shared by toluene. In a follow-up study, pentobarbital-anesthetized rats subject to more severe ventricular arrhythmias demonstrated identical outcomes following benzene and toluene exposures (381). The mechanism by which benzene causes arrhythmia is not clear. However, increasing the catecholamine receptors' sensitivity in the heart has been suggested.

Human studies regarding benzene cardiotoxicity are limited to human poisoning cases (382,383). In these studies, the mechanism of death was suspected to be the production of fatal arrhythmias or a direct, toxic effect on the myocardium. In addition to pathologic ECG changes, another study demonstrated that benzene caused an increased prevalence of arterial hypertension among petrochemical workers (384). Kotseva et al. reported increased blood pressure in workers exposed to benzene (385,386). On the basis of their epidemiological studies, Kotseva et al. concluded that at high levels of exposure to benzene, increased blood pressure, ECG changes, and arrhythmias can be observed. Clinically, benzene poisoning commonly presents with irritant signs, central nervous symptoms, and hematologic malignancies. It is possible that the cardiac effects may have not been reported often due to an emphasis on these signs. Nevertheless, experimental animal and human studies support cardiotoxic effects of benzene exposure.

Styrene

Styrene is a highly volatile hydrocarbon used in the production of several polymers, copolymers, and glass-reinforced plastics. Styrene linked together in long chains to form polystyrene is used in the production of packaging, insulation, fiberglass, pipes, automobile parts, drinking cups, and carpet backing. Occupational settings provide the highest levels of styrene exposure primarily through inhalation. Ingestion and dermal absorption are other potential routes for exposure. The reinforced plastics industry represents the single highest potential for styrene exposure. Workers in this industry may be exposed up to 3 g of styrene/day (387–389).

In a study conducted for the EPA, styrene concentrations in ambient air were found to range, at different locations and times, from 0.09 to 0.89 ppb (390). Styrene is released in the air from industries that make use of the solvent. Residual amounts of styrene can also be found in vehicle exhaust (both gasoline and diesel engines), cigarette smoke, building materials, and consumer products. Although styrene is not commonly found in water sources, industrial effluents are the principal contributors to water levels. Concentrations ranging from less than 10 to 970 μg/L have been detected in coal gasification and chemical plants (391–393). Moreover, styrene has been detected at landfills, as well as the surface and groundwater of hazardous waste sites.

The literature regarding styrene exposure and cardiovascular disease in experimental animals is sparse. Reports documenting cardiotoxic effects of the styrene have been inconclusive.

Occupational epidemiologic studies have shown an increased risk of ischemic heart disease among styrene-exposed workers, particularly in those with short employment periods (<4 years) (394,395). It is theorized that styrene may be found in low levels in ambient air and be adherent to PM. Matanoski et al. examined workers in styrene-butadiene rubber-manufacturing plants who died from ischemic heart disease (396). In this study, styrene was shown to significantly influence the development of ischemic heart disease in both short-term and long-term workers. However, active workers with two or more years of employment had the highest risk of death from ischemic heart disease: relative hazard (RH) = 2.95 (95% CI = 1.02–8.57) at a TWA styrene concentrations of 0.2 to less than 0.3 ppm and RH = 4.30 (95% CI = 1.56–11.84) at TWA greater than or equal to 0.3 ppm. Another study found increased risk of arteriosclerotic heart disease only in black styrene-butadiene polymer workers (397). These studies support the hypothesis that workers with both acute and long-term industrial styrene exposure may be susceptible to increased risks of ischemic heart disease.

Toluene

Toluene is a clear, colorless solvent that is typically added to gasoline with benzene and xylene. Workers in the plastics industry, waste water workers, gasoline station attendants, and nail and hair salons are regularly exposed to toluene. Printers, in particular, are routinely exposed to high levels of toluene. In the occupational setting, exposure to toluene occurs primarily by inhalation. Reported concentrations of 5 to 50 ppm are common in the workplace with levels reaching as high as 250 ppm in some settings (398).

The uses of toluene-containing materials allow the solvent to enter the environment. For example, paints, paint thinners, adhesives, fingernail polish, and gasoline are widely used and known to contain toluene. Leaking underground gasoline storage tanks and solvent spills are responsible for the entrance of toluene into groundwater and surface water. However, toluene is not commonly found in drinking water supplies. In 1998, the EPA reported that 99% of hazardous waste sites contained toluene-contaminated well water (399). Moreover, 77% of sites reported toluene in soil samples. Similar to occupational exposure, the general population is exposed to toluene most often by inhalation. Cigarette smoke contains small amounts of toluene on the order of 80 μg/cigarette (400).

One of the benchmarks for determining the extent of solvent cardiac toxicity is the sensitization of the myocardium to the arrhythmogenic properties of epinephrine. While it is known that solvents generally induce some form of rhythm disturbance, the nature and severity of the arrhythmia can vary. Morvai et al. studied the electrical activity in rat hearts exposed to benzene, toluene, and xylene either intraperitoneally or subcutaneously, or administered by inhalation (401). In anesthetized rats, acute toluene inhalation produced bradyarrhythmia and asystole, while subacute toluene poisoning induced repolarization disorders and arrhythmias. The ECG changes were seen to occur only after prolonged exposures and high concentrations of 6000 mg/m^3. The repolarization disorders were suggested to be the result of myocardial damage, either direct or indirect, and the arrhythmias were thought to be the result of a disturbance in the cardiac conduction system. The repolarization disturbances were thought to develop through several mechanisms depending on the length of exposure. For example, acute poisonings were thought to induce repolarization disorders by alterations in metabolic and oxidative systems or damage to mitochondrial membranes. Subacute and chronic intoxications operated through increased oxidative processes responsible for solvent detoxification. Other factors were direct solvent-induced intracellular membrane damage, animal age, body weight, and the deleterious effect of vascular lesions on the autonomic nervous system responsible for normal repolarization. Another study observed that while both benzene and toluene brought about electrocardiographic changes in rat hearts, toluene increased the QRS complex duration and PR interval, while benzene decreased the P-wave duration (380). This study showed significant differences in the ECG influences of toluene and benzene. Toluene decreased intraventricular and atrioventricular conduction, while benzene increased atrial conduction. It has been speculated that the lipophilicity of toluene and subsequent nonspecific membrane action may give the solvent an antiarrhythmic quality. This finding was replicated in a study that also compared the ventricular arrhythmic potentials of benzene and toluene in rats (381). Toluene was observed to decrease the number of ectopic ventricular beats, while benzene increased the number of beats. As was seen in Vidrio et al. study, the two solvents displayed differential electrophysiological effects. Goldstein suggested that similar membrane-stabilizing factors might affect membrane fluidity differently because of varying molecular shapes and hydrogen bond and spatial orientations (402). This could account for the disparate myocardial sensitizing properties of the two solvents. Another study proposed that toluene-induced arrhythmias in rat ventricular myocytes could be the result of low levels of toluene (μM concentrations) causing blockage of sodium channels (403). The inhibition of sodium channels was observed to be similar to that done by local anesthetics. The novel findings of a recent study using radio telemetry observed a biphasic cardiac response to toluene doses given by oral gavage (404). An initial dose-related tachycardic response was followed by a lower, stable heart rate that was significantly elevated above controls. There was an additional observed hypertensive response that appeared to track the toluene-induced tachycardia, i.e., rises and falls in blood pressure followed rises and falls in heart rate. Toluene has also been shown to cause direct myocardial injury. Ikeda et al. subjected 25 dogs to toluene vapor rebreathing (405). The ECG analyses revealed a direct effect of toluene on the septal and ventricular muscles of the heart. These ECG changes were consistent with left bundle branch block of a myocardial infarction. The fatal ventricular arrhythmia in the dogs was determined to be the result of a direct effect of toluene on the heart. These experimental studies demonstrate direct arrhythmogenic and cardiotoxic effects.

Most of the human studies come from cases of toluene abuse, intoxication, and occupational studies. Toluene intoxication has been shown to cause arrhythmias, and in some cases sudden death.[383,2] Poisonings comprise the majority of reports on toluene toxicity (407,408). The hallmark of toluene cardiotoxicity is thought to be the development of tachyarrhythmias (409,410). Research pertaining to toluene-induced cardiomyopathy is lacking. Toluene has been implicated in a number of cases of inhalation leading to myocardial infarction. Cunningham et al. described a case of anterior myocardial infarction and ventricular fibrillation in a 16-year-old boy that abused large amounts (4 to 6 L) of glue containing toluene (411). Although a chest X-ray showed no abnormalities, an ECG revealed anterior myocardial infarction. A subsequent echocardiogram showed an anteroapical aneurysm with normal ejection fraction of 69%. The investigators suggested that coronary artery spasm precipitated the infarct and were able to rule out toxic myocarditis because of ECG readings displaying changes specific to anterior myocardial infarction. A case of recurrent non-Q-wave myocardial infarction was reported in a 55-year-old toluene abuser (412). It was suggested that coronary vasospasm resulted from the increased response to catecholamines, thereby causing the myocardial infarction. It is however of interest, that this same patient with recurrent non Q-wave myocardial infarction, had normal coronary arteries, while his electrolytes demonstrated hypokalemia and non-anion acidosis. The authors concluded that acute exposure to toluene led to coronary vasospasm secondary to sensitivity to catecholamines with subsequent non Q-wave myocardial infarction. Hypokalemia and metabolic acidosis also play a role in the arrhythmogenic effect of chronic toluene exposure since intracellular concentrations of sodium and potassium are altered which further derange myocyte electroneutrality. Carder et al. reported a 22-year-old male who spent the day stripping varnish formulated with pure toluene and experienced an acute myocardial infarction (413). The patient was not provided with protective respiratory gear and used the pure toluene in a confined area, thereby increasing his toluene exposure. It is of interest that during the acute phase of toxicity, the ECG changes were those of subacute lateral myocardial infarction, and his 2-D echocardiogram demonstrated anterolateral hypokinesis and a reduced ejection fraction of 40%. His coronary angiogram displayed normal coronary arteries. The mechanism of acute myocardial infarction in this case was probably the result of the cardiac depressive effects of toluene on the heart. This in turn, caused reduced cardiac output, and reduced blood flow to the coronary arteries, leading to myocardial infarction. Acute and chronic arrhythmogenic effects of toluene causing reduced perfusion of the myocardium cannot be ruled out. As this was the patient's first exposure to the solvent, the investigators suggested that his myocardial infarction stemmed from toluene-induced coronary artery spasm. Toluene has been shown to decrease the heart rate and stroke volume, thus depriving the coronary arteries of adequate blood flow. Wiseman et al. addressed the issue of toluene toxicity and dilated cardiomyopathy (414). In this case, a 15-year-old boy was admitted to the hospital with nonspecific chest pains and a two-year history of intermittent glue sniffing. The primary solvent contained in the glue was toluene. The boy had evidence of biventricular dilatation and pansystolic murmur, as well as, normal cardiac enzymatic activity. The left ventricular ejection fraction was 17% and catheterization demonstrated signs of chronic myocarditis and interstitial fibrosis without inflammatory changes. The patient was referred for and successfully underwent cardiac transplantation. Pathological examination of the heart revealed no unique histological features of the diseased heart despite toluene's toxic insult. In a later study, Vural et al. investigated a case of dilated cardiomyopathy in a 21-year-old toluene abuser (415). ECG readings revealed extrasystoles and incomplete right bundle branch block. This study is important since it also addresses toluene toxicity and cardiomyopathy, an issue of growing concern. This patient displayed evidence of cardiomyopathy with an ejection fraction of 40%. A 2-D echo taken six months following treatment demonstrated resolution of the cardiomyopathy, as did the ECG studies. In summary, while electron microscopy studies of the myocyte are not available, the experimental studies and case studies demonstrate a stress cardiotoxic effect of toluene on the heart via several mechanisms including arrhythmia, vasospasm, and electrolyte changes.

Xylene

Xylene or dimethylbenzene is a synthetic chemical produced from petroleum. It ranks in the top 30 of chemicals produced in the United States (416). It is used extensively as a solvent in the printing, rubber, and leather industries as well as raw material in the chemical, plastics, and synthetic fiber industries. The major routes of exposure to xylene are dermal or inhalation. Other significant exposures to xylene occur in the painting industry, wood processing plant workers, automobile garage workers, and metal workers. Although xylene is primarily released from industrial sources, exposure can occur through automobile exhaust, hazardous waste disposals, and solvent spills. Outdoor air levels of xylene typically range from 1 to 30 ppb, whereas indoor air levels range from 1 to 10 ppb (417). Exposures to xylene can occur from paint, gasoline, and cigarette smoke. Xylene has been known to leach into groundwater, where the half-life of the compound is between 25 and 287 days versus the half-life in air of 8 to 14 hours (418–420). Fewer than 6% of drinking water samples in the United States have tested positive for xylene content. Levels in drinking water are typically below 2 ppb, while foods can contain between 1 to 100 ppb xylene (417). However, inhalation is the most important route of exposure. Pumping gasoline, car travel, painting, scale model building, and pesticide use provide important sources of xylene.

Although the experimental data is limited, it has been suggested that xylene can induce cardiovascular disorders. Acute, subacute, and chronic benzene, toluene, and xylene poisoning was investigated in male rats (401). Xylene injected intraperitoneally or subcutaneously or administered by inhalation had no effect on ECG readings. However, inhaled xylene induced bradyarrhythmia and asystole during the acute phase of intoxication. Subacute xylene poisoning adversely affected repolarization and evoked arrhythmia. These cardiac consequences were duration and dose-dependent. Although deemed detrimental to the cardiovascular system, xylene was shown to be a far less potent cardiotoxicant than benzene. Morvai et al. investigated the effect of inhalational xylene on coronary microvessels in rats (421). Xylene was observed to alter the myocardial contractility of the heart via alterations in the concentration of vasoactive substances. Xylene is also an adjuvant to emulsifiable-concentrate herbicides. A recent study demonstrated that xylene, as a formulated adjuvant, induced marked vasodilation in intact and denuded rat aortas (422). In addition, xylene caused significant inhibition of contraction in the isolated rat hearts. The investigators suggested that cases of hypotension and cardiac arrest seen in accidental ingestions and poisonings might be the result of the effects of formulated adjuvants. These experimental studies provide evidence that xylene is a significant arrhythmogenic agent capable of depressing the myocardium.

The cardiotoxic effects of xylene exposure in humans have not been a topic of extensive investigation. However, a report investigated cases of xylene poisoning in laboratory workers (423). All cases were women who worked in unventilated rooms and were exposed to xylene from between 1.5 and 18 years. Signs and symptoms included nondescript chest pain, ECG abnormalities, and cardiovascular disturbances in workers with longer exposure periods. There was no elaboration or explanation offered. Although the literature is sparse, xylene as an aromatic solvent has been shown to cause some cardiovascular disturbances, including ECG abnormalities.

Halogenated Solvents

The addition of halogens to a hydrocarbon compound improves its solvency. Combined with their nonflammability and low acute toxicity, halogenated solvents are widely used in several industries (424). Major uses for this solvent class include metal degreasing and the dissolving of oils and other materials. Chlorinated solvents in particular, are used in the dry-cleaning industry. Some common examples of this class of solvent include trichloroethylene, tetrachloroethylene, 1,1,1-trichloroethane, methylene chloride, and the fluorocarbons. Carbon tetrachloride and vinyl chloride have minor and no current use as solvents, respectively.

Carbon Tetrachloride

Carbon tetrachloride is a clear liquid that does not burn easily. Occupational exposure to carbon tetrachloride is most likely to occur by inhalation of vapors. Workers exposed to 0.1 ppm carbon tetrachloride will have an eight-hour day intake equivalent to 35 µg/kg/day (425). Industrial uses for carbon tetrachloride were seen in the manufacture of refrigerants and aerosol can propellants. The solvent was widely used as a degreaser in the dry cleaning industry and as a cleaning fluid in industry. The manufacture and use of carbon tetrachloride has drastically declined since being identified as a threat to the ozone layer.

Carbon tetrachloride evaporates easily and moves from either the ground or water to reside in the air. It is typically found in drinking water supplies at levels of less than or equal to 0.5 ppb (426). Carbon tetrachloride has been detected in water and soil samples at 26% of Superfund waste sites at concentrations of less than 50 to greater than 1000 ppb (425). Although banned from consumer products in 1970, the long life of carbon tetrachloride in the atmosphere is responsible for a background level of 0.1 µg/kg/day (427,428). People that live near industries that produce or use carbon tetrachloride can have significantly increased intakes from air and water ranging from 12 to 511 µg/day and 0.2 to 60 µg/day, respectively (429). Tap water used for bathing and other purposes can also be important sources of exposure via dermal and inhalation routes. Carbon tetrachloride was used in fire extinguishers and in fumigants used to kill grain insects; however, most of these uses were discontinued in the 1960s. Additionally, carbon tetrachloride's use as a pesticide was discontinued in 1986.

Evidence from experimental studies suggests that carbon tetrachloride can be injurious to the heart. Ali et al. investigated cardiac effects of carbon tetrachloride via lipid peroxidation in rats (430). ECG readings revealed significant sinus bradycardia. Histological examination of the myocardium revealed myofibril swelling. There was a significant increase in myocardial lipid peroxidation and serum transaminases, specifically serum glutamate-oxaloacetate transaminase (SGOT) that were indicative of cardiac damage. This study demonstrated that carbon tetrachloride administration was able to induce significant lipid peroxidation in the myocardium. Lipid peroxidation is known to damage subcellular organelles and biomembranes. This has important implications for the endoplasmic reticulum in cardiomyocytes, as well as the sarcoplasmic reticulum where the calcium for excitation-contraction resides. A later study demonstrated that carbon tetrachloride could damage the myocardium. Dziadecki administered 0.6 mL/100g carbon tetrachloride to rats (431). Electron microscopic studies revealed damage to myocardial mitochondria and endoplasmic reticulum, as well as to myofibrils. In a previously described study, Tse et al. researched the issue of lipid peroxidation via free radicals (432). This study concluded that carbon tetrachloride was a particularly powerful inducer of lipid peroxidation, more so than the other chlorinated solvents under investigation. A synergistic relationship between iron and carbon tetrachloride was considered to be key to the propagation of lipid peroxidation and subsequent chronic cardiotoxic effect of the solvent. A study was conducted to investigate the depressant effects of carbon tetrachloride in cardiomyocytes (433). Carbon tetrachloride (2.5 mM) was shown to have a negative chronotropic effect on the myocytes, reducing beat frequency via prolongation of the relaxation phase of beating. However, the solvent did not affect the duration of contraction, regardless of the addition of extracellular calcium. An important observation was the complete recovery to spontaneous beating of the cardiomyocytes upon withdrawal from the carbon tetrachloride medium. The authors suggested the extent and speed of this recovery were dependent on the solvent's vapor pressure, a measure of a solvent's potency. Low vapor pressures correspond to lower doses required to adversely affect the heart. It can be inferred from this study that carbon tetrachloride is a strong cardiac sensitizer because of the observed myocardial depressant action of 2.5 mM exposure seen in cultured cardiomyocytes. Cardiovascular disturbances involving pathological changes are largely the result of altered endothelial cell function. Increased endothelemia, an important marker for endothelial cell injury, is frequently implicated in ischemic and valvular heart diseases. Carbon tetrachloride–mediated oxidative stress can cause massive endothelial cell damage via the production of free radicals. Babal et al. evaluated carbon tetrachloride-induced damage to endothelial cells in rats (434). Rats administered 0.5 mL/kg carbon tetrachloride for eight weeks demonstrated a nearly threefold increase in endothelial cell concentration. There was no evidence of significant change in the increased endothelemia during a subsequent three-week spontaneous recovery period. Vascular histopathology revealed cytoplasmic vacuolization with areas of subendothelial edema and cell detachment. Similar endothelial changes are known to occur following prolonged ischemia and ischemia after reperfusion (435). In summary, this study demonstrates that carbon tetrachloride can inflict irreversible damage to vascular endothelium through increased endothelemia that was not observed to recede, following a three-week recovery period. These experimental studies suggest a direct cardiotoxic effect of carbon tetrachloride. Considered as a chlorinated compound, the cardiotoxicity observed is consistent with cardiotoxicity observed in several other chlorinated compounds discussed in this chapter.

Carbon tetrachloride's widespread use, as a pesticide, was abandoned in 1986 and most of its industrial uses were abandoned in the 1970s. The available studies conducted in humans exposed to carbon tetrachloride have not provided findings of significant cardiac injury. Sporadic case histories comprise the bulk of cardiotoxic outcomes of carbon tetrachloride exposure. Kennaugh described a 30-year-old man who ingested 120 mL of carbon tetrachloride (436). Upon admission, the patient developed atrial fibrillation from which he eventually recovered. Another series of case histories of carbon tetrachloride poisoning was examined retrospectively (437). In this report, 9 of 12 patients exhibited adverse changes indicative of myocardial damage from carbon tetrachloride exposure. These reports support the data from experimental animal studies that carbon tetrachloride is an arrhythmogenic solvent that can cause direct injury to the myocardium. At current environmental levels, cardiotoxic effects are not anticipated, although large-scale studies are not available.

Fluorocarbons

Fluorocarbons, or chlorinated fluorocarbons (CFCs), are chemically stable compounds derived from aliphatic hydrocarbons such as methane, ethane, and ethylene. In addition to fluorine, chlorine is often the component of fluorocarbons that replace the hydrogen atoms of the organic compound. Fluorocarbons are commonly used as aerosol propellants, refrigerants, and industrial solvent degreasers. They are also widely used as foam blowing agents, solvents, and chemical intermediates in polymers and resins manufacturing. In California, the primary emitters of CFCs are manufacturers of miscellaneous plastic products, ophthalmic goods, and electronic components and services.

CFCs persist in the air for long periods of time, thereby making inhalation an important route of exposure for the general population. The ingestion of contaminated water and dermal contact with these compounds comprise alternative ways for exposure. Chlorinated fluorocarbons are typically photolyzed to release chlorine atoms in the stratosphere. The compounds can persist in the troposphere for 50 to 150 years (438).

Chlorinated fluorocarbons have a demonstrated toxic effect on the heart. A large portion of research into the cardiotoxic effects of these agents has been conducted on experimental animals. Taylor et al. studied the cardiac effects of inhaled dichlorodifluoromethane (Freon 12) and dichlorotetrafluoroethane (Freon 114) on monkeys (439). All 14 monkeys were observed to develop ventricular premature beats within a mean of 39 ± 4.2 seconds. Moreover, in 11 monkeys, ventricular extrasystoles became more frequent following cessation of propellant inhalation. Three monkeys exhibited bigeminy without ventricular tachycardia and four others did indeed develop ventricular tachycardia. The authors suggested the gases operated by sensitizing the myocardium to endogenous catecholamines in a synergistic fashion, an effect seen following administration of other hydrocarbons. However, in this experiment, epinephrine was not injected into the monkeys, and it was thought that the gases might have sensitized the myocardium via absorption into the bloodstream. Alternatively, it was deemed biologically plausible that the fluoroalkane gases had a direct, toxic effect on the heart that was independent of myocardial sensitization. Adding to arrhythmogenic effects, another study described a direct depressive action on myocardial contractility from Freon 12 exposure on rat left ventricular papillary muscles (440). Freon 12 reversibly decreased the isometric force production and velocity of isotonic shortening in all muscles tested. These dose-related effects were noted to occur at a minimum concentration of 1.06 mg/100 mL Freon 12 at which a 20% depression in isometric force development was observed. The presence or absence of hypoxic conditions of the surrounding Freon 12 medium had no effect on the development of observed effects. Since hypoxemia may often be expected in CFC intoxication, the investigators noted that hypoxia would potentiate the negative inotropic action of Freon 12. These results further demonstrated that the aerosol propellant gas Freon 12 is a potent myocardial depressant. The proarrhythmic effect of an aerosol propellant was observed in cats following inhalation of high concentrations of the gas (441). Each cat exhibited epinephrine-evoked ventricular tachyarrhythmias following inhalation of 37% dichlorodifluoromethane. This effect was seen to persist for as long as

10 minutes following cessation of exposure. It was suggested that the post-inhalation period is a critical time for the development of cardiotoxic sequelae, the development of which are independent of removal from exposure to the noxious compound. A later study tested the minimal effective cardiotoxic concentrations of aerosol propellants in anesthetized dogs (442). Inhalation of the propellants caused depression of myocardial contractility, aortic hypotension, and decreased cardiac output. Freon 11, Freon 114, and Freon 12 began to elicit these effects at 1%, 2.5%, and 10%, respectively. The researchers suggested that the most consistent effects seen at these minimal concentrations were a fall in systemic arterial pressure coupled with an even greater reduction in myocardial contractile force. Kilen et al. provided data that further supported the synergistic relationship between the administration of Freon 12 and hypoxia in depressing the myocardial contractility of rat papillary muscle (443). Freon 12 combined with hypoxia more profoundly and selectively depressed contraction force and peak shortening velocity than hypoxia or Freon 12 alone. It was, however, unclear by what mechanism hypoxia potentiates the effects of Freon 12. The investigators suggested that Freon 12 might interfere with the calcium influx accompanying excitation-contraction during the depolarization process. Kawakami et al. corroborated these results in a later study using Freon 113 in isolated perfused rat hearts (444). Atrioventricular conduction delay and heart rate decrease were enhanced by 75% in the coadministration of Freon 113 and hypoxia. It was suggested that Freon 113 exhibited direct toxicity to cardiomyocytes via antagonistic actions on passive and active membranous ionic movements. The experimental data demonstrate that fluorocarbons are known proarrhythmic agents that can depress the myocardium and potentially exert directly toxic effects on the heart.

Most of the data about fluorocarbon cardiotoxicity in humans comes from case reports of intoxication, occupational solvent exposure, and recreational drug use. Brady et al. documented a case involving a 15-year-old boy who intentionally inhaled Freon 12 from an automobile air conditioner recharge unit (445). After collapsing, the boy was admitted to the hospital and a cardiac monitor revealed coarse ventricular fibrillation. A later ECG showed a sinus tachycardia with left bundle branch configuration followed by an anterior myocardial injury pattern. The authors suggested that the most clinically significant cardiotoxic response to Freon exposure is the development of potentially life threatening arrhythmias. The arrhythmias can range from benign atrial tachycardias to ventricular tachycardias and sudden death. Kaufman et al. described two cases of atrial fibrillation, and one sudden death, in workers exposed to trifluorotrichloroethane (Freon 113) (446). The atrial fibrillation cases resolved to normal sinus rhythm and no further cardiac abnormalities. The medical examiner determined that the fatality was caused by cardiac arrhythmia induced by Freon 113, without evidence of preexisting heart disease. The estimated Freon 113 exposure concentrations for the fatality were between 5000 and 20,000 ppm. The investigators noted that the inherently lower toxicity of fluorocarbons allow higher levels of exposure, which thereby increases the risk for cardiac arrhythmias. Lessard et al. have suggested that fluorocarbons, by virtue of enhanced liposolubility, decrease the ionic permeability of cellular membranes and set the stage for cardiac conduction block, altered refractory periods, and disturbances of pacemaker activity (447,448). Arrhythmias may then develop in a situation of increased catecholamine outflow. A later study focused on the inhalation of decomposed chlorodifluoromethane (Freon 22) and the development of myocardial infarction (449). A 65-year-old man employed as a refrigerator repairman for 30 years was chronically exposed to freon. Exposure to Freon 22 in particular for eight hours a day caused respiratory symptoms that worsened to the point of needing hospital care. Electrocardiogram revealed signs suggestive of a myocardial infarction. A subsequent echocardiogram showed decreased ventricular function and a defect in the ventricular septum. His cardiac symptoms worsened and he expired. Autopsy revealed biventricular thickening, pericardial effusion, and fibrinous deposits on the epicardium. The right coronary vessel contained an adherent thrombus and the left chamber area exhibited myofibrillar changes as well as myocytolysis. The researchers suggested that the histological results favored the depositions of subacute inflammatory fibrin deposits that proceeded to myocardial infarction. Fibrinogen is a well-known marker of inflammation and, in this case, was felt to be the pathogenic mechanism responsible for the fatal myocardial infarction. Freon 152a, or 1,1-difluoroethane, was the cause of an accidental death following repeated exposure to the propellant (450). A 42-year-old man was found dead in his car with several canisters of CRC Duster, a consumer product containing Freon 152a. An autopsy revealed arteriosclerotic coronary disease, fibrosis, and an acute infarction of the left ventricle. On the basis of these findings, the cause of death was determined to be fatal cardiac arrhythmia due to Freon 152a intoxication with contributory atherosclerotic disease. Taken together, the experimental and human exposure studies indicate that fluorocarbons can cause the development of potentially fatal arrhythmias via sensitization of the myocardium. Different fluorocarbons exhibit varying degrees of cardiotoxicity, however, most organic solvents share a proarrhythmic potential if exposure is sufficiently high.

Methylene Chloride

Methylene chloride is a colorless, volatile liquid with a sweet odor that evaporates easily. There are a number of industries that make use of methylene chloride as a common industrial solvent. However, the production and processing operations of the solvent offer the most important exposures. Other significant exposures can occur during occupational activities such as spray painting, spray gluing, metal painting, paint stripping, and aerosol packing. NIOSH estimated that over one million workers were exposed to methylene chloride in the early 1980s (275). Decreased production and use as well as threshold-limit values have resulted in fewer workers being exposed since the mid-1980s. Methylene chloride concentrations as low as 1 ppm have been detected in workplace areas, while breathing-zone concentrations of workers exposed to the solvent have returned 1400 ppm (451). This clearly exceeds the current OSHA permissible exposure limit (PEL) of 25 ppm (452).

Methylene chloride is an artificial chemical that is produced from methane gas or wood alcohol. Inhalation of fumes is the most common route of exposure, which may also occur via the slower route of skin absorption. The fastest route of exposure is through the drinking of contaminated water and subsequent absorption via the stomach. Since methylene chloride releases CO in the body, the toxicological effects of methylene chloride are attributed to CO cardiotoxicity and direct effects of CO. The reader is referred to the section on CO cardiotoxicity in this chapter.

Reinhardt et al. examined the arrhythmogenic effect of vapor mixtures of halogenated hydrocarbons in anesthetized dogs (453). Measurements of gas concentration and cardiac rhythm were conducted. The baseline was administration of a single compound, followed by epinephrine challenge. The dogs developed arrhythmias ranging from isolated abnormal beats to multiple ventricular beats preceding ventricular fibrillation. In anesthetized dogs, it was found that exposure depressed myocardial contractility, which in turn decreased cardiac output and lowered systemic arterial blood pressure. The authors concluded that the mechanism of cardiac sensitization is probably the result of disturbances in conduction and electrical impulse through the heart. The sensitization required epinephrine for the cardiac arrhythmia to develop. However, the authors could not rule out the contribution of hypoxemia toward cardiac sensitization. This observation is indicative that methylene chloride may contribute direct cardiotoxicity in synergism with the CO effects and reduced oxygen delivery to the myocyte. Aviado examined the cardiopulmonary effects of chlorinated solvents in anesthetized dogs (454). The primary action was depression of myocardial contractility and reduced blood pressure. To further examine the effects of methylene chloride, the investigators administered inosine (a cardiotropic drug) and measured the effects on cardiac function produced by methylene chloride. Among the parameters measured were mean arterial blood pressure, heart rate, left ventricular functions, coronary blood flow, and coronary artery resistance. Administration of methylene chloride caused decreased myocardial contractility, but no change in coronary artery flow, demonstrating direct effects of methylene chloride on the heart. Since the level of coronary blood flow is dictated primarily by myocyte metabolic requirements, which in turn affect cardiac contractility, the slight observed change in the coronary artery tone represents physiological vascular adjustment of the myocardium. Therefore, this indicates that methylene chloride cardiotoxicity is primarily mediated via direct cardiac muscle effects that, together with the proarrhythmic effects, may cause fatal changes. The negative inotropic effect of methylene chloride was reversed by inosine, further demonstrating a direct cardiotoxic effect of methylene chloride. Muller et al. examined exposure to methylene chloride in rats via gavage (455). Cardiac functions were monitored, as were methylene chloride and epinephrine. Myocardial changes included alterations in adrenergic cardiac response and augmentation of the negative inotropic effects of catecholamines. It was suggested that the increased catecholamines' effect on the heart was a direct result of methylene chloride. In this model, the authors did not find cardiac arrhythmias, contrary to previous studies (456,457). The lack of arrhythmias in the experiments was attributed to the use of urethane as a narcotic. Nevertheless, these studies further demonstrate direct cardiotoxicity of methylene chloride, independent of CO. The direct arrhythmogenic effect of methylene chloride was studied in Wistar rats that were anesthetized (458). Atrioventricular blockage and heart metabolites were measured in parallel to levels of methylene chloride in blood. The blood levels of methylene chloride were comparable to those found in human intoxication cases. The incidence of atrioventricular block during reperfusion was markedly increased by methylene chloride administration. In addition to its negative inotropic effects, methylene chloride demonstrated an arrhythmogenic effect. These studies in isolated perfused hearts demonstrate direct cardiotoxic effects, mostly independent of CO. In a study of Sprague-Dawley rats exposed to methylene chloride it was found that the amount of calcium found in the cardiac myocytes was decreased after the exposure (459). This decrease in sarcoplasmic reticulum calcium stores depresses the cardiac myocyte thus making them more prone to the negative inotropic and arrhythmogenic properties of methylene chloride. This study was probably as near to accurately examining the cardiac myocyte as available at the time. The authors examined single neonatal myocytes electric activity and calcium transients at various concentrations of methylene chloride. These effects were reversible. Studying methylene chloride effects in isolated myocytes allows the examination of direct cardiotoxicity and further supports prior studies that negative inotropic and arrhythmogenic effects are a recognized effect of the solvent. Follow up studies by Hoffman et al. also support the observation that methylene chloride cardiotoxicity is mediated via its effects on calcium fluxes (460,461).

After inhalation, over 70% of methylene chloride enters the bloodstream and quickly spreads to the liver, kidney, brains, lungs, and fatty tissues. About 50% of methylene chloride leaves the bloodstream in 40 minutes. Unchanged methylene chloride and its breakdown products are primarily removed by breathed air, while small amounts are excreted through urine and stool. The body metabolizes between one-quarter to one-third of methylene chloride to CO and carbon dioxide. Other important metabolic intermediates are formaldehyde and formic acid, which are thought to be involved in the carcinogenicity of methylene chloride. The carboxyhemoglobin produced from the breakdown of methylene chloride has a longer half-life in the body than that after direct CO inhalation (462). Methylene chloride is a lipophilic solvent. As such, fat and other tissues may continue to release accumulation of methylene chloride for several hours following cessation of exposure. According to Baselt, the elevated carboxyhemoglobin that is metabolized from methylene chloride exposure has a half-life of 13 hours, or 2.5 times that of carboxyhemoglobin resulting from CO inhaled directly (463). The CO displaces oxygen available to the heart tissue, reducing oxygen delivery to cardiac myocytes, and increases the risk of heart damage. In normal individuals, there is less than 1% of carboxyhemoglobin in the bloodstream. Smokers of 1 pack/day can have levels of 4% to 5%, while heavy smokers have been known to have carboxyhemoglobin levels of 8% to 12%. When exposed to methylene chloride at the permissible workplace level of 500 ppm and above, the carboxyhemoglobin level can reach 15% or more in smokers. These levels are below the hazardous mark, but persons with coronary artery disease can experience additional stress to an already-compromised cardiovascular system. The cardiotoxicity of methylene chloride has been studied via its release of CO in the body. The cardiotoxicity of CO is discussed in the subheading "Carbon Monoxide" in this chapter, and therefore will not be discussed here. The reader is referred to that section.

Methylene chloride is suggested to increase cardiovascular stress in persons suffering from coronary heart disease. Stewart et al. reported a case of a 66-year-old man who suffered three heart attacks following exposure to liquid gel paint and varnish remover containing 80% methylene chloride (464). The patient was initially admitted complaining of severe, crushing chest pain that radiated to his left shoulder and arm. Although no correlation was made with exposure to the varnish remover, a diagnosis of acute anterior myocardial infarction was made. Two weeks following discharge, the patient reapplied the varnish remover and suffered a second myocardial infarction. This episode was complicated by cardiogenic shock, dysrhythmia, and heart failure. Six months following recovery, the patient again returned to his paint stripping efforts. However, after experiencing chest pains the patient collapsed and died. Although the patient had no prior history of heart disease, the authors suggested that undiagnosed, presently occurring heart disease may have rendered the patient unable to withstand the cardiovascular toxic effects of methylene chloride exposure. It is reasonable to conclude that following exposure to methylene chloride, the patient's carboxyhemoglobin levels were elevated to saturations greater than 5%, a level known to adversely affect patients with cardiovascular disease. Additionally, the physical exertion experienced during the paint stripping may have been contributory to the third and fatal myocardial infarction. This study showed methylene chloride to be a precipitator of myocardial infarctions. Methylene chloride exposure has also been shown to cause myocardial damage. Bonventre et al. have described a methylene chloride exposure case involving the death of a 13-year boy (465). The boy was using paint remover containing methylene chloride as the primary agent. The autopsy revealed dilation of the heart and multiple petechiae of the epicardial surface. The myocardium was observed to have a peculiar tiger-stripped appearance. Ultrastructural changes of the heart consisted of centers of loss of cross striations and deep cytoplasmic staining in areas of greatest congestion. This study demonstrated the potential of methylene chloride to cause direct myocardial injury. These studies provide support that methylene chloride is a biologically plausible cardiotoxin. In addition to sensitizing the heart to epinephrine, methylene chloride may also induce myocardial infarctions, as seen in a case report. Persons with coronary heart disease appear to be particularly susceptible to methylene chloride exposure.

These studies, both in experimental animals and humans, demonstrate direct cardiotoxic effects of methylene chloride, both inotropic and arrhythmogenic, which are mediated via inhibition of calcium dynamics at the myocyte level. Future studies should focus on the detection of cardiovascular disease risk from methylene chloride exposures in those with preexisting heart disease.

Tetrachloroethylene (Perchloroethylene)

Tetrachloroethylene is a synthetic chemical most widely known for its use in the dry-cleaning industry. Other names for tetrachloroethylene include perchloroethylene (PCE), pert, tetrachloroethane, perclene, and perchlor. Dry cleaners employees such as machine operators have experienced TWA exposures to tetrachloroethylene ranging from 4.0 to 149 ppm; pressers, seamstresses, and front counter workers can be exposed to mean levels between 3.0 and 3.3 ppm (466). The examination of venous blood samples in dry cleaning workers has shown increasing concentrations of tetrachloroethylene as the workweek progresses. It has been determined that humans have a limited capacity for metabolizing tetrachloroethylene, the ceiling being 100 ppm (467). After this point, metabolite excretion of trichloroacetic acid leveled off. Tetrachloroethylene also finds use as a metal degreaser, a function that employees can be expected to have a high exposure. Other significant exposures may occur during wood processing, working at a textile plant, during pesticide use, and working in a paint store.

Tetrachloroethylene becomes introduced to the environment through its use and subsequent evaporation. Secondary exposures occur through contaminated water and soil during disposal of sewage sludge and factory waste or underground storage tanks. Background levels of tetrachloroethylene exposure, in air, water, and food, are far less significant than occupational sources. Tetrachloroethylene can be detected in air at 1 ppm and 0.3 ppm in water (468). The average amount of tetrachloroethylene the general population might breathe is between 0.08 and 0.2 mg/day (469). The amount that might be ingested from water range between 0.0001 and 0.002 mg/day (468). Consumer products such as water repellants, silicone lubricants, fabric finishers, spot removers, adhesives, and wood cleaners may contain the solvent.

Halogenated solvents have demonstrated a tendency to sensitize the myocardium to epinephrine-induced arrhythmias (453). An investigation was undertaken on the effects of tetrachloroethylene on cardiac rhythm and performance. Rabbits, cats, and dogs were intravenously injected with tetrachloroethylene under anesthesia (470). In the anesthetized state, the animals developed ventricular arrhythmias and increased myocardial susceptibility to epinephrine-induced ventricular premature contractions, bigeminal rhythms, and tachycardia. The mean thresholds doses of arrhythmia-producing epinephrine and tetrachloroethylene for rabbits, cats, and dogs were 10, 24, and 13 mg/kg, respectively. However, tetrachloroethylene administered alone produced arrhythmias in 30% of animals. Relatively low IV doses between 20 and 40 mg/kg were sufficient to produce myocardial depression. This was revealed in dogs exposed at this dosage that experienced significant depressions of $dP/dt_{(max)}$, a known indicator of myocardial contractility. The evidence from this study demonstrated tetrachloroethylene is arrhythmogenic and capable of depressing the myocardium. Although solvents generally produce arrhythmias, they are not all created equal in terms of potency. A study was conducted to determine if a particular inhibitor of drug metabolism, 2,4-dichloro-6-phenylphenoxyethyldiethylamine-HBr, could potentiate the cardiac effects of tetrachloroethylene (471). Male rabbits were exposed to 5200 ppm tetrachloroethylene to enhance the opportunity for arrhythmogenic effects without inducing untoward central nervous system (CNS) depressant outcomes. It was determined that tetrachloroethylene had relatively low ability to sensitize the myocardium. In the animals in which arrhythmias occurred, the arrhythmias appeared within 15 to 30 minutes of the exposure and disappeared because of a perceived adaptation in the rabbits. This study demonstrated tetrachloroethylene to be weakly arrhythmogenic, even at maximal exposure levels. Hypoxia has known influences on cardiac impulse conduction, reducing ATP production and inducing atrioventricular block. Investigators examined the interactions between tetrachloroethylene, ethanol, and hypoxia using ECG readings to evaluate the heart conduction system of perfused rat hearts (472). The simultaneous coadministration of ethanol and hypoxia with 0.1 mM tetrachloroethylene caused significant PQ prolongation. Because of the use of ethanol, the effect of endogenous catecholamines was negated. Therefore, cardiac sensitization was not the mechanism responsible for the PQ prolongation. This study supported the hypothesis that tetrachloroethylene has direct, local, and synergistic effects with ethanol and hypoxia on the heart conduction system. It has been suggested that halogen solvents induce myocardial depression and arrhythmia through toxic effects on calcium dynamics across the sarcolemmal and sarcoplasmic reticulum membranes. A study investigated eight commonly used chlorinated solvents, including tetrachloroethylene, to assess their effects on calcium fluxes during excitation-contraction coupling in electrically stimulated rat cardiomyocytes (459). The effects the solvents had on calcium during KCl-induced depolarization were also studied to assess the function of the sarcolemmal membrane in solvent-induced effects on calcium dynamics. Tetrachloroethylene was shown to reversibly depress calcium transients in cardiac myocytes, as well as inhibit the sarcolemmal calcium influx after KCl depolarization. The subsequent depression of calcium release from the sarcoplasmic reticulum decreased the calcium available for excitation-contraction coupling. The results of this study provide further evidence to support the hypothesis that decreased calcium stores used for excitation-contraction coupling adversely affect myocardial contraction capability. The resulting changes in calcium dynamics provide a reasonable explanation for negative inotropism and tetrachloroethylene arrhythmogenicity. These studies provide evidence for arrhythmogenic and cardiac depressant effects of tetrachloroethylene, further demonstrating direct cardiac toxicity.

Investigations concerning tetrachloroethylene cardiotoxicity are few and largely consist of case reports and occupational studies. One of the earlier reports investigated a 24-year-old dry-cleaner worker who presented with a six-month history of "skipping heart beats" (473). He was exposed to tetrachloroethylene for seven months and developed multiple ventricular beats (VPBs). As the VPBs appeared one month after employment, tetrachloroethylene exposure was suggested to be the focus of attention. However, the researchers were cautious not to causally link the solvent to the cardiac symptoms and suggested avoidance of the agent to those with heart conditions. Hara et al. examined the cardiovascular status of dry-cleaning workers who were directly exposed to Perc (474). The workers experienced significantly increased heart wall thickness to radius ratios, fractional shortening of the internal dimensions of the left ventricle, and depression of mean velocity of circumferential fiber shortening. The demonstrated depression in myocardial shortening capacity, although not sufficient to infer causality, was suggestive of cardiotoxicity.

The evidence to date has shown tetrachloroethylene to be an arrhythmogenic, myocardial depressant in both experimental animals and humans. Although uncertain as with other solvents, the mechanism by which tetrachloroethylene is cardiotoxic is believed to operate by sympathetic stimulation of the myocardium to endogenous catecholamines. The resulting cardiac sensitization can potentially lead to ventricular arrhythmias and death as seen in the literature. Moreover, it can be conceived that activities such as rigorous exercise and alcoholic drink consumption may potentiate the cardiac effects of tetrachloroethylene. Further experimental and epidemiological studies are needed to further appreciate the role of tetrachloroethylene in the development of cardiotoxic consequences. Nevertheless, the data are sufficient to suggest a direct tetrachloroethylene cardiotoxicity.

Trichloroethylene

The majority of uses seen for trichloroethylene are in degreasing operations. According to a study conducted by NIOSH from 1981 to 1983, over 400,000 workers employed in the United States were exposed to trichloroethylene (475). Mean TWA concentrations range from less than 50 to 100 ppm in the breathing zones of workers (476). The major routes of exposure to trichloroethylene for the general population are inhalation and the ingestion of drinking water. Urban area concentrations of the compound in ambient air tend to be higher than those of rural areas. A study compared trichloroethylene levels in the blood of workers from both cities representative of both regions and found levels of 0.180 ng/L in rural workers versus 0.763 ng/L observed in occupational workers (477). Indoor air typically contains higher concentrations than outdoor air, including that sampled in areas near chemical plants. Wallace measured median indoor air values ranging from 0.2 to 4.8 ppb, while outdoor concentrations were hardly measurable (390). Consumer products such as wood stains, varnishes, finishes, lubricants, adhesives, typewriter correction fluids, paint removers, and cleaners can provide exposure to trichloroethylene. The EPA has discontinued the use of trichloroethylene as an anesthetic, fumigant, and solvent for decaffeinating coffee. The chlorination process of wastewater has been shown to produce small amounts of trichloroethylene (478). Groundwater used for drinking water generally contains higher levels of trichloroethylene than surface water used for drinking purposes.

Investigations in experimental animals have revealed that halogenated solvents, including trichloroethylene, are capable of sensitizing the heart to epinephrine resulting in cardiac arrhythmias. These arrhythmias are typically ventricular and may result in sudden death. Reinhardt et al. suggested that cardiac sensitization is the cause of death in aerosol-sniffing fatalities in dogs (479). Dogs administered a control dose of epinephrine injections did not develop arrhythmias. The challenge dose of epinephrine was injected five minutes after breathing the test compound. Trichloroethylene was found to be a cardiac sensitizer at the 0.5% concentration level. Higher concentrations at the 1% level evoked ventricular fibrillations following epinephrine challenge. Autopsies performed on dogs that developed fatal arrhythmias revealed no pathological or anatomical changes compatible with other causes of arrhythmia. Therefore, trichloroethylene was suggested to be directly arrhythmogenic. Ethanol has been found to potentiate the arrhythmogenic properties of trichloroethylene. White et al. examined the effect of ethanol on epinephrine-induced cardiac arrhythmias in rabbits exposed to high levels (6000 ppm) of trichloroethylene (480). After one-hour of exposure to trichloroethylene, rabbits treated with ethanol (1 g/kg, IV or orally 30 minutes prior to exposure) developed arrhythmias sooner and at lower doses than control rabbits, as did rabbits treated with ethanol intravenously. However, more arrhythmias occurred in rabbits treated intravenously. The arrhythmias consisted of premature ventricular contractions. It was demonstrated that concomitant administration of trichloroethylene and alcohol resulted in an inhibition of the metabolism of both compounds. This observation was seen at ethanol blood concentrations as low as 65 mg%, which is a level that persons working with trichloroethylene could conceivably encounter. This study demonstrated a unique interaction between trichloroethylene and ethanol and further demonstrated the arrhythmogenic effect of trichloroethylene. Similar to ethanol, there is evidence that caffeine is also an important potentiator of epinephrine-induced arrhythmias in rabbits exposed to trichloroethylene (481). Caffeine (10 mg/kg, IV 30 min prior to exposure) induced premature ventricular contractions in rabbits exposed to high doses of trichloroethylene (6000 ppm).

More arrhythmias developed in the caffeine-treated rabbits than in those treated with trichloroethylene alone, while also appearing sooner and at lower doses of epinephrine. Caffeine is a known cardiac stimulant that, like trichloroethylene, is able to potentiate the endogenous release of catecholamines. Westfall et al. demonstrated that caffeine might also stimulate norepinephrine release from adrenergic nerve endings in mammalian hearts, thus providing an additive effect in the development of arrhythmias during trichloroethylene exposure (482). Carlson et al. showed benzo(a)pyrene to be an inducer of arrhythmias in tri-chloroethylene-exposed rabbits (483). Rabbits administered benzo(a)pyrene (40 mg/kg, IV) 72 and 48 hours prior to exposure to 8100 ppm trichloroethylene developed more arrhythmias and at lower doses of epinephrine than control rabbits. Pretreatment of the rabbits with benzo(a)pyrene increased the arrhythmias observed during trichloroethylene administration despite decreasing blood levels of trichloroethylene. Although the mechanism for this effect was unclear, the investigator suggested that benzo(a)pyrene may itself be a weak arrhythmogenic agent or a facilitator of trichloroethylene-mediated sensitization of the myocardium to epinephrine. Coronary artery ligation has been utilized for investigating the cardiotoxic effects of trichloroethylene (484). In this study, urethane-anesthetized rats were monitored for arrhythmias, heart rate changes, and mortality after administration of 16.7 mmol/kg trichloroethylene. The rats were observed to have a high occurrence of complete and incomplete atrioventricular block episodes over a significant time period, resulting in bradycardia. An atrioventricular block was defined as 75% of the "other forms of arrhythmia" category. This study further confirms the cardiotoxic effects of trichloroethylene and demonstrated that the solvent caused a reduced survival rate in urethane-anesthetized rats. Free radicals via lipid peroxidation have been postulated to be important mechanistic mediators of chlorinated solvents' cardiotoxicity. Tse et al. researched this issue with trichloroethylene being one of several agents of concern (432). The formation of thiobarbiturate acid reactive products was used as index of lipid peroxidation. Incubation of cultured arterial endothelial cells with low levels of iron (3.1–25 μM Fe^{3+} chelated by ADP) and trichloroethylene was shown to stimulate lipid peroxidation. This synergistic interaction was also seen in aortic smooth muscle cells. Furthermore, aortic smooth muscle cells incubated with two different valences of iron (6.2 μM Fe^{2+} chelated by ADP or 6.2 μM Fe^{3+} chelated by ADP) induced lipid peroxidation in a similar fashion. Although cytochrome P-450 is found in endothelial cells, it was suggested that concentrations of the cytochrome in the myocardium might be too low to significantly metabolize trichloroethylene. The addition of iron, however, synergistically enhanced the lipid peroxidation effect of incubated mixtures containing cultured vascular cells and trichloroethylene. This nonspecific reaction proceeded regardless of differences in the metabolic capabilities between endothelial cells and aortic smooth muscle cells. The evidence from this study led the researchers to suggest some plausible mechanisms for chlorinated solvent-induced lipid peroxidation: membrane partitioning of the solvent thereby affecting membrane fluidity or alternatively, interaction of the solvent with lipid radicals or peroxides that form secondary radicals to propagate the lipid peroxidative chain. It was indicated that the chlorine substitution of a particular solvent was important in determining its lipid peroxidation-inducing potential. This study suggested that lipid peroxidation in the presence of iron and trichloroethylene may cause myocardial necrosis and further demonstrated the chronic cardiotoxic potential of trichloroethylene. Hoffmann et al. demonstrated that trichloroethylene might depress the myocardium and induce arrhythmias through effects on calcium dynamics across the sarcolemmal and sarcoplasmic reticulum membranes (459). This study researched eight chlorinated solvents, including trichloroethylene, to assess toxic effects on calcium fluxes during excitation-contraction coupling in electrically stimulated rat cardiomyocytes. Trichloroethylene was observed to reversibly depress calcium transients in cardiac myocytes, as well as inhibit the sarcolemmal calcium influx after KCl depolarization. The depression of calcium release from the sarcoplasmic reticulum reduced the calcium available for excitation-contraction coupling. The results of this study provide further support to the hypothesis that decreased calcium stores used for excitation-contraction coupling may adversely affect myocardial contraction. The subsequent changes in calcium dynamics provide a plausible explanation for negative inotropic effects and trichloroethylene arrhythmogenicity. These studies in experimental animals have demonstrated trichloroethylene to be a potent cardiac sensitizing solvent. There is evidence that key metabolic interactions with potentiators such as caffeine and ethanol may increase its arrhythmogenic potential.

Dimitrova et al. studied the phases of the heart's systole in workers exposed to trichloroethylene who excreted trichloroacetic acid (TCA), the solvent's metabolite (485). Chronic exposure to trichloroethylene has been shown to lead to ventricular fibrillation and sudden death in exposed workers (486). In the Dimitrova study, significant electrocardiographic changes were observed in workers exposed to trichloroethylene. Workers also experienced shortened cardiac cycles, while the tension phase and isometric period were prolonged. This showed decreased myocardial activity and an inhibition of increased intraventricular tension. In addition to depressed myocardial function, the investigators measured diminished systole. Mean TCA levels in urine in trichloroethylene-exposed workers were significantly increased (40.71 mg/L compared with 1.58 mg/L in controls). TCA levels in workers fell to below normal after the 30th exposure-free day and a concomitant normalization of electrocardiographic indicators. These changes were suggested to reflect functional effects on the cardiovascular system and were indicative of an interaction between the altered phase structure of the ventricular systole and elevated levels of TCA. This study offered support for the effectiveness of the polycardiographic method to determine the presence and extent of hemodynamic changes in trichloroethylene-exposed workers. A patient with a several years' habit of solvent abuse was admitted with a one-day history of breathlessness, wheeze, and cough productive of bloody sputum (487). The shoe cleaning solvent used in this intoxication contained 67% trichloroethylene. The patient experienced a continuously deteriorating hospital course of over three weeks' duration complicated by drastically elevated cardiac enzymes and increasing heart failure, leading to death. Autopsy results revealed an enlarged and thickened left ventricle. The myocardium was hypertrophied with attenuation of fibers and widening of the interstitium. The general appearance of the heart led to the diagnosis of congestive dilated cardiomyopathy. Trichloroethylene was deemed the major contributor to the patient's cardiomyopathy in accordance with the long-standing solvent abuse. Hantson et al. investigated two cases of acute trichloroethylene intoxication that were complicated by cardiac conduction disturbances (488). A 23-year-old man voluntarily ingested 50 mL of trichloroethylene, amyl acetate (SASSI). An initially normal ECG later revealed atrioventricular block four hours later. Arrhythmias persisted for 10 hours but returned to normal a week following exposure. A 30-year-old man who was addicted to SASSI was admitted following the sniffing of three bottles of the substance the previous day. An ECG administered three hours following admission demonstrated irregular sinus rhythm and subsequent sinoatrial block (type I). This observation was followed by an ectopic atrial rate three days later. These cases demonstrate the basis for the severity of trichloroethylene cardiac intoxications. Although uncommon compared with descriptions of ventricular arrhythmias, cardiac conduction disturbances can occur in trichloroethylene exposures and appear to be acute reversible phenomena.

The literature supports the assertion that trichloroethylene is a significant cardiotoxicant in both acute and chronic exposures. Experimental animal studies, as well as human exposure studies, have demonstrated the ability of the solvent to induce arrhythmias in fashion similar to other halogenated hydrocarbons. Cardiac arrest and sudden death have been reported following accidental or suicidal ingestions or acute exposure to high concentrations of trichloroethylene vapors. Chronic exposure to trichloroethylene may lead to irreversible myocardial damage suggestive of congestive cardiomyopathy.

1,1,1-Trichloroethane

1,1,1-Trichloroethane is a synthetic chemical that had many industrial uses. It was used as a solvent, oil remover, and degreaser. The United Sates ceased use of 1,1,1-trichloroethane after January 1, 2002, and until 2005, small amounts were still produced for essential purposes, i.e., as the primary precursor for hydrofluorocarbons, in medical devices, and aviation safety (489). The majority of 1,1,1-trichloroethane exposures occurred in sewing machine operators, registered nurses, maids, janitors and cleaners in hospitals, electricians, technicians, assemblers, installers, machinists, and repairers in electrical and electronic industry. Inhalation is the primary route of exposure. Because of the phasing out of 1,1,1-trichloroethane, exposures are expected to decrease. Environmental exposures to 1,1,1-trichloroethane are typically too small to cause adverse health effects. In the United States, city air was found to contain 0.1 to 1.0 ppb, while rural air normally contains less than 0.1 ppb (489). These measures translate to average human daily nonoccupational intakes of 10.8 to 108 µg/day. When 1,1,1-trichloroethane was frequently used in home and office environments, air concentrations were significantly higher (0.3–4.4 ppb) than levels found outside (490). Glues, household cleaners, and sprays were typical consumer products that contained 1,1,1-trichloroethane. Liquid Paper or typewriter correction has been implicated in numerous intoxication cases in people who deliberately inhaled vapors of the solvent. Drinking water from underground wells has contained 1,1,1-trichloroethane levels ranging from 0.0035 to 5.4 ppm, with one private well once measured to contain 12 ppm (489).

Experimental investigations have revealed that halogenated solvents are capable of inducing ventricular fibrillation via the sensitization of the myocardium to circulating epinephrine following inhalation of the solvent (453). Reinhardt et al. further studied this phenomenon of cardiac sensitization in dogs inhaling commonly used solvents, including 1,1,1-trichloroethane (479). The researchers demonstrated 1,1,1-trichloroethane to be a strong cardiac sensitizer at concentrations of 0.5% as well as capable of inducing ventricular fibrillation at the 1.0% level. 1,1,1-trichloroethane was discovered to possess a sensitizing potential nearly equal to the other compounds tested—trichloroethylene and trichlorotrifluoroethane. This study supported the evidence that moderate concentrations of halogenated solvents are capable of inducing ventricular arrhythmias via cardiac sensitization. Herd et al. reported a more direct effect on the cardiovascular system from 1,1,1-trichloroethane exposures (491). Exposure of 1,1,1-trichloroethane in anesthetized dogs caused a dose-dependent, biphasic decline in blood pressure, the second phase in particular, marked with a decline in cardiac output and decreases in both stroke volume and heart rate. In addition to the vascular effects, depression in myocardial contractility was also observed. Extracellular calcium levels, known to affect contractility, were examined to assess correlations with 1,1,1-trichloroethane-mediated decline in myocardial function. The injection of endogenous calcium caused a significant increase in myocardial contractility thereby negating the influence of 1,1,1-trichloroethane on the myocardium, specifically, the rate of force generation defined by V_{max} and dT/dt. Therefore, it was suggested that the myocardial depression might reflect an inability of the cardiac mitochondria to supply sufficient amounts of ATP. Elevated extracellular calcium could then augment the contractile efficiency of the existing, subnormal levels of ATP. A previously described study investigated the ability of 1,1,1-trichloroethane, among other chlorinated solvents, to promote lipid peroxidation (432). While 1,1,1-trichloroethane alone did not increase the formation of thiobarbiturate reactive products (the index for assessing lipid peroxidation), when combined with a mixture endothelial and aortic smooth muscle cells with low levels of iron chelated by ADP, lipid peroxidation was increased up to 200% of control levels. Hoffmann et al. described the mechanism by which 1,1,1-trichloroethane depressed the myocardium by examining the influence of the solvent on calcium dynamics during KCl-induced depolarizations (492). Video motion analysis demonstrated that 1,1,1-trichloroethane was able to reversibly depress calcium transients in rat ventricular cardiac myocytes, as well as inhibit the sarcolemmal calcium influx after KCl depolarization. The inhibition of calcium release from the sarcoplasmic reticulum decreased the calcium available for excitation-contraction coupling. The results of this investigation showed that decreased calcium stores used for excitation-contraction coupling adversely affect myocardial contractility, thus providing a plausible explanation for negative inotropism and 1,1,1-trichloroethane arrhythmogenicity. Moreover, a nearly identical study later conducted by Hoffmann et al. confirmed the results of their previous study (459). This study, however, investigated the cardiotoxic mechanism of seven other solvents besides 1,1,1-trichloroethane. The alteration calcium dynamics was seen as a common mechanism of halogenated solvent cardiotoxicity. These experimental studies demonstrate that 1,1,1-trichloroethane is a potent cardiac sensitizer, which can induce ventricular arrhythmias and depress myocardial contractility. In addition to lipid peroxidation, an alteration in intracellular calcium dynamics is an important mechanism behind 1,1,1-trichloroethane cardiotoxicity.

Occupational and intentional use case reports represent the vast majority of sources of information concerning 1,1,1-trichloroethane cardiotoxicity. The use of 1,1,1-trichloroethane as a degreaser, as well as a component of typewriter correction fluid, has led to a number of intoxications and deaths. Concentrations of the solvent can quickly reach anesthetic and toxic levels within confined spaces. Travers reported a case involving an 18-year-old navy sailor who collapsed following inhalation of vapors from a 1,1,1-trichloroethane-soaked rag (493). An ECG revealed widening of the QRS complex and ventricular fibrillation. Despite intubation with supportive and treatment measures, hypotension and bradycardia developed that were resistant to norepinephrine and isoproterenol. Cardiac arrest and death occurred 24 hours after his collapse. Autopsy showed evidence of ventricular dilatation and subendocardial hemorrhage. Microscopic examination of the myocardium demonstrated evidence of widespread, massive infarction that was suggested to be a result of prolonged hypoxia and hypotension followed by vigorous treatment efforts. It was thought that the norepinephrine infusions might have been contributory to the development of ventricular arrhythmias. Since halogenated solvents are known to sensitize the myocardium to catecholamines, including norepinephrine, the authors suggested the use of propranolol as an option for future treatment protocol. The cardiotoxic effects of low levels of 1,1,1-trichloroethane have been shown to persist for weeks following cessation of exposure (494). In this report, a 45-year-old truck repairman was admitted because of cardiac arrhythmias. His job entailed nearly continuous, low-level exposure to 1,1,1-trichloroethane used to clean parts. Urine drug screen revealed 20 µg/100 mL of 1,1,1-trichloroethane. A 24-hour Holter monitor revealed ventricular ectopic beats, tachycardia, and unifocal premature ventricular contractions. The patient was discharged on a regimen of quinidine gluconate and then re-evaluated two weeks later. He was found to be asymptomatic and antiarrhythmics were discontinued. Seventy-two hours following withdrawal from antiarrhythmic medications, repeat Holter monitor showed the return of normal sinus rhythm. Although the patient reported the installation of an exhaust ventilation system at his work area and the use of rubber gloves, a follow-up Holter monitor six weeks later revealed three benign premature ventricular contractions. It was suggested that ongoing low-level exposure to 1,1,1-trichloroethane was a factor in the appearance of the extra-systoles. This study demonstrated the persistence of significant arrhythmias despite low urine levels of the solvent and a complete cessation two weeks from exposure. Typewriter correction fluid is known to contain 1,1,1-trichloroethane and has been implicated in sudden cardiac death following inhalation of vapors. Ranson et al. examined a 13-year-old boy who died suddenly following exercise (495). The boy was a known abuser of typewriter correction fluid for the previous four or five months. The autopsy determined the cause of death to be ventricular arrhythmia following 1,1,1-trichloroethane inhalation. The engagement in vigorous exercise was thought to additively precipitate the onset of the arrhythmias because exercise is known to increase circulating levels of the catecholamine adrenalin. McLeod et al. described two cases of chronic cardiac toxicity of 1,1,1-trichloroethane involving acute intoxication and long-term occupational exposure (496). The deterioration in cardiac performance in these cases was observed following the administration of halothane anesthesia for conditions unrelated to the solvent exposure. Histological examination of ventricular biopsy samples revealed a severely hypertrophied myocardium and evidence of preexisting myocarditis. These cases demonstrated the development of two forms of chronic myocardial damage following short- and long-term exposure to 1,1,1-trichloroethane. In addition, a toxic cross-reaction with another known myocardial sensitizer, halothane, was suggested to be contributory to the varying severity of cardiac damage. Another case described the first known case of 1,1,1-trichloroethane causing direct myocardial injury (497). A 15-year-old boy collapsed while inhaling Liquid Paper and became unresponsive. Ventricular fibrillation was noted and serial electrocardiograms performed the next morning revealed an acute antero-septal myocardial injury. A resting echocardiogram showed an area of hypokinesis, and an echocardiogram revealed septal wall motion abnormalities involving the distal interventricular septum. This finding corroborated the results of the earlier electrocardiogram showing antero-apical subendocardial infarction. Because of the absence of myocardial ischemia, the authors suggested temporary coronary artery spasm was the mechanism responsible for the myocardial injury. However, another study did ascribe the development of asymptomatic myocardial infarction to myocardial ischemia (498). A 37-year-old female was admitted with an abnormal initial ECG that suggested myocardial injury. She had been cleaning stainless steel with a product containing 30% 1,1,1-trichloroethane and collapsed. A repeat ECG 10 hours later revealed atrioventricular block, T-waves inversion, and Q waves in III and aVF, followed by bigeminy at 20 hours post exposure. The investigators believed the solvent exposure caused coronary spasm leading to myocardial necrosis in coronary vessels with preexisting atherosclerosis. The ischemia that led to the infarction may have been harmless in a person without coronary disease was suggested to present a particular challenge to the patient because of her compromised coronary vessels. The data from experimental studies and human case reports suggests that both acute and chronic exposures to 1,1,1-trichloroethane can cause myocardial damage in various forms ranging from ventricular arrhythmias to myocardial infarction. Human reports also indicate a possible toxic interaction with commonly used anesthetics that can lead to adverse cardiac events. Although large scale epidemiological studies are not available, the experimental data and human case reports suggest that exposure to 1,1,1-trichloroethane may be substantially cardiotoxic in patients with underlying cardiac disease (coronary artery disease, ventricular hypertrophy, preexisting cardiac arrhythmias).

Carbon Disulfide

Carbon disulfide is a toxic, colorless, volatile, flammable liquid with a sweet, aromatic odor. Impure carbon disulfide used in industrial processes is a yellowish liquid with a strong, disagreeable odor. The largest use of carbon disulfide is as raw material in the production of viscose rayon fibers. Carbon disulfide is also used to make cellophane, carbon tetrachloride, and some pesticides, and is a common solvent for rubber, sulfur, oils, resins, and waxes. The primary source of carbon disulfide in the environment is from manufacturing and processing facilities, such as viscose rayon plants, oil refineries, and coal blast furnaces. Environmental concentrations of carbon disulfide have been estimated in the range from 0.1 to 6 mg/m^3 near viscose plants (499,500). Carbon disulfide is also found in groundwater and soil near these facilities. Occupational exposure to carbon disulfide is a great concern. Individuals who work with carbon disulfide may be exposed to concentrations ranging from 9 mg/m^3 to peaks above 6200 mg/m^3 (501). The primary route of exposure to carbon disulfide is via inhalation, however individuals may be exposed to carbon disulfide from ingestion of contaminated drinking water and food and via dermal absorption in the workplace. The following organizations have set occupational standards for carbon disulfide exposure: the ACGIH threshold limit value is TWA 31 mg/m^3; the NIOSH recommended exposure limit is TWA 3 mg/m^3; and the OSHA PEL value is TWA 62 mg/m^3 (502,503).

Carbon disulfide has been known to be a vasotropic toxin and may induce atherosclerosis (504–508). A number of experimental studies have also shown that carbon disulfide causes direct cardiac changes in exposed animals. Rats inhaling 700 mg/m^3 of carbon disulfide for six hours daily for 14 weeks have demonstrated increased arterial blood pressure and cardiac index, decreased cardiac output and increased relative heart mass (509). Decelerated intracardiac impulse conduction, modified cardiac arrhythmia and reduced survival rate have been shown in rats exposed short-term to carbon disulfide (510). Hoffman et al. found that single administration of carbon disulfide in rats prolonged PR and QTc intervals and reduced heart rate in a dose-dependent manner (511). Grodeckaja et al. demonstrated dose-dependent ECG response in rats after chronic carbon disulfide exposure, such as decreased heart rate and lowered T wave (512). Some reports indicate that carbon disulfide may induce cardiac response by altering catecholamine metabolism. Chandra et al. examined the cardiotoxic effects of carbon disulfide in relation to treatment with phenobarbitone and noradrenaline (513). Investigators found large areas of left ventricular necrosis. The histological changes were similar to phenobarbitone-treated rats given two doses of noradrenaline without exposure to carbon disulfide. To study the effect of endogenous catecholamine, another group of rats were placed in stressful cold environment. Following carbon disulfide exposure, these rats also demonstrated extensive myocardial necrosis similar to rats treated with exogenous noradrenaline. Functional changes to the heart have been observed following exposure to carbon disulfide and exogenous injection of catecholamines. Hoffmann et al. reported delayed atrioventricular impulse conduction and increased number of extrasystoles in animals exposed to carbon disulfide (514). The injection of catecholamines caused dose-dependent increases in number of extrasystoles and transient T-wave elevation, indicating more pronounced myocardial ischemia that is possibly mediated by the catecholamine inactivation and inhibitory actions of carbon disulfide on energy production. Klapperstuck et al. studied the cardiac effects of epinephrine and norepinephrine in rats subacutely exposed to carbon disulfide (515). Compared with the control group, exposed rats demonstrated enhanced catecholamine-induced myocardial necrosis, diminished left ventricular inotropic response, elevated transient T-wave, and enhanced myocardial ischemia. The results support the notion that carbon disulfide disturbs the transport and utilization of energy by the heart. Indeed, Chandra et al. displayed patchy areas of loss of cytochrome oxidase, phosphorylase, and succinic dehydrogenase activity in the myocardium of carbon disulfide-exposed rats (513). Tan et al. evaluated the functional effects of carbon disulfide on cultured cardiac myocytes (516,517). The investigators observed an increase in beating arrest rate and a decrease in succinic dehydrogenase activity with increasing exposure levels. Succinic dehydrogenase is an enzyme involved in the citric acid cycle and is an indicator of the ability to produce ATP. It is suggested that the reduction in energy supply to cardiac myocytes may decrease heart contractility. These experimental studies confirm that exposure to carbon disulfide has a direct and dose-dependent cardiotoxic effect. Although, the exact mechanism by which carbon disulfide induced cardiotoxicity cannot be determined on the basis of the present data, some evidence suggests that carbon disulfide may alter catecholamine metabolism and energy supply to the heart, and affect the cardiac catecholamine receptor sensitivity.

Industrial workers who are exposed to chronic low levels of carbon disulfide have a significant increased prevalence of ECG abnormalities (518–521). Ventricular arrhythmias have been reported among workers with over 20 years of exposure and repolarization disturbances have been evident in workers with 10 to 20 years exposure history (522). A case-control study of 121 individuals exposed to carbon disulfide demonstrated in exposed workers dysrhythmia, disturbances in conduction, and presence of focal changes of cardiac muscle (523). These cardiac responses were not present in the control group. A study of male workers exposed to carbon disulfide at rayon manufacturing plants found a dose-dependent relationship between cumulative carbon disulfide exposure and ECG abnormalities (524). Exposure history of 31 to 57 ppm-year of carbon disulfide was associated with an OR of 7.2 (95% CI = 1.5–36.7). Franco et al. measured ECG changes in viscose rayon workers exposed to carbon disulfide concentrations below the threshold limit value of 60 mg/m^3 at the time (525). Exposed workers demonstrated shortened left ventricular ejection time and prolonged isovolumetric contraction time, indicative of impaired left ventricular contractility that is comparable to mild coronary dysfunction. Bortkiewicz et al. examined male workers at a chemical fiber plant who were continuously exposed to carbon disulfide at levels of 0 to over 18 mg/m^3 (526). Carbon disulfide-exposed workers displayed significant dysfunction of the autonomic nervous system, as evident by increased resting heart rate, decreased total power spectrum and its particular frequency ranges (HF, LF, and VLF), and absence of correlation between heart rate variability parameters and workers' ages. Persistent ECG abnormalities have been reported after exposure has been ceased. Guidotti et al. followed 13 chemical workers with average exposure history of 3.2 years, 18 hours a week at levels ranging from 20 to 50 ppm, and intermittent peak exposure between 100 and 200 ppm (527). Five of the thirteen workers had persistent ECG abnormalities during the six months of follow-up. Exposed workers exhibited delayed right ventricular conduction, left axis deviation, and changes in ST-T waves. A study of former viscose rayon factory workers was conducted seven years after the factory was closed (528). Multivariate linear analysis showed that previous exposure history was related to decreased heart rate variability and reduced LF power, which are risk factors for increased cardiovascular mortality. Indeed, several epidemiological studies have demonstrated the association between occupational carbon disulfide exposure and significant increased cardiovascular morbidity and mortality (529–536). Nurminen et al. conducted a cohort study of Finnish men exposed to carbon disulfide in a viscose rayon plant for at least five years (537). For the first five years of follow-up, workers showed a 4.7-fold increase in cardiovascular mortality. An intervention program was implemented at the rayon plant after five years. The plant reduced carbon disulfide exposure to the set hygienic standard of 10 ppm and removed all workers with coronary risk factors from exposure to carbon disulfide. For the eight years after the intervention, the relative risk of mortality for ischemic and other heart diseases reduced to 1.0.

The ECG abnormalities observed at chronic low levels provide evidence of direct cardiotoxic action of carbon disulfide. Experimental studies show that carbon disulfide alters catecholamine metabolism and energy supply to the heart. Epidemiological studies of exposed workers demonstrate persistent changes in heart function and increased risk of cardiovascular morbidity and mortality. Carbon disulfide exposure is a risk factor for cardiovascular disease and prudent intervention, such as worker education, engineering controls, protective devices, and monitoring of exposure levels are important components in improving health outcome of exposed workers.

Pesticides

Pesticides comprise any substance or mixture of substances used for preventing, destroying, repelling, or mitigating pests. Exposure to pesticides can be either occupational or environmental. Accidental and suicidal poisonings can also occur in occupational and environmental exposure settings. Occupational exposures to pesticides occur chiefly among workers in the agriculture industry, including migrant farmworkers. Industrial workers, pest control exterminators, greenhouse workers/florists, office workers, health care workers, veterinary employees, and others also can be significantly exposed to pesticides (538). Exposure to pesticides in industry occurs via inhalation, absorption into skin, and ingestion in the form of chemical vapors, solid particulates, or water-based aerosols. For most workers however, the primary route of exposure is through the skin.

General population and environmental exposures to pesticides demand particular attention because of the lack of uniformity among those affected, i.e., people of all ages, health status, and socioeconomic status (539). For example, with regard to sensitive populations, fetuses and children are the most susceptible to the health effects of pesticides. Rapidly developing bodily systems combined with increased respiratory rates and hand-oral contacts increase the risks of otherwise low-level, but significant exposure. Other potentially sensitive groups of considerable interest are women, minorities, those from low socioeconomic groups, and the immunocompromised. Important situations involving environmental exposure to pesticides include residential exposure, agricultural take-home exposure, close farm proximity, aerial spraying, public places, contaminated organ donor, and chemical warfare.

Organophosphates and Carbamates

Organophosphates cause an irreversible inhibition of acetylcholinesterase and are generally neurotoxic. This inhibition results in elevated levels of the substrate acetylcholine, hence the neurotoxicity caused by the formation of a phosphorylated-acetylcholinesterase intermediate. Carbamates operate on a mechanistically similar basis, affecting the formation of a carbamylated-acetylcholinesterase intermediate. However, the carbamate intermediate is hydrolyzed to an active enzyme more rapidly, resulting in less severe, self-limiting effects (540). In addition to CNS white matter and the pancreas, plasma acetylcholinesterase is also found in the heart.

Organophosphates are known to be cardiotoxic in three phases: (*i*) sinus tachycardia resulting from increased sympathetic tone; (*ii*) pronounced parasympathetic tone expressed as S-T segment changes, atrioventricular conduction disturbances, and arrhythmias; and (*iii*) QT interval prolongation leading to sudden cardiac death (541). A study was undertaken to research the long-term complications of organophosphorus compounds sarin and soman in rats (542). Both sarin and soman significantly prolonged the QT intervals of the rats. Additionally, there were signs of direct myocardial injury in the form of myopathic foci, hyaline fibers, and fibrotic tissue. These cardiac lesions were especially severe in the sarin-exposed rats. Thus, sarin and soman induced similar effects characteristic of organophosphates with the additional consequence of causing myocardial degeneration. The cardiotoxicity of methidathion (MD) has been investigated (543). The researchers hypothesized that the rat heart may be particularly sensitive to the lipid peroxidative damage caused by an enhanced production of ROS. In this study, subchronic administration of MD-induced oxidative stress as revealed by enhanced malondialdehyde (MDA) production in the rat heart, an important and previously unknown finding. The cardiomyocytes experienced loss of striation and underwent myocytolysis. However, combination treatment with the important antioxidants vitamins E and C reduced heart damage caused by MD. Therefore, protection was conferred on the heart muscle cells against myocardial injury. Cardiac arrhythmias have also developed in rats exposed to methylphosphonothiolate (544). However, the rats developed arrhythmias as early as 50 minutes after exposure. This is in sharp contrast to other studies documenting abnormalities beginning two to three hours or two to three days after the challenge. This study confirmed that at least some organophosphates are indeed capable of inducing arrhythmias. Several routes have been suggested including (*i*) a marked overflow of catecholamines causing arrhythmias; (*ii*) direct, myocardial neurogenic effects; (*iii*) lipid peroxidative damage via ROS; (*iv*) Na^+K^+-ATPase inhibition; (*v*) calcium overload; and (*vi*) direct myocardial injury from oxidative processes. The toxic effects on the heart may differ between organophosphates, dosage, exposure route, and species affected (545).

Carbamate compounds have a mechanism of action similar to organophosphates. However, the inhibition of cholinesterase is reversible, unlike the effects of organophosphates. The cardiotoxicity of methomyl, a common carbamate insecticide was examined in rabbits administered methomyl by oral intubation at dosages of 4 mg/kg and 5 mg/kg on days 1 and 2, respectively (546). The rabbits experienced reversible, dose-dependent T-wave inversions. One of the four rabbits was observed to have significant ST segment depressions in leads I, II, aVL, and aVF. The study was remarkable because anticholinesterase compounds are not known to cause T-wave changes. The investigators deemed the dose-dependent T-wave changes as evidence of a direct cardiotoxic effect of methomyl exposure.

The majority of human cardiotoxic outcomes from organophosphate exposures have been a result of intentional or accidental ingestion. As in experimental animals, organophosphates act biochemically to inhibit acetylcholinesterase in the nervous system. Surely, acetylcholinesterase is a major player in the cardiovascular system. Organophosphates affect myocardial peripheral nerves as well as central nervous system centers controlling heart rhythm. As such, it is known that the toxic consequences of excess acetylcholine can lead to cardiac slowing, arrhythmias, and sudden cardiac death (545). However, precious few studies have stressed the ability of organophosphates to be directly arrhythmogenic apart from acid-base disturbances or electrolyte imbalances. Researchers conducted a study on a series of organophosphates poisonings with a special focus on 56 cases of arrhythmias (547). This study brought to attention the importance of long-term monitoring of organophosphate poisoning cases for arrhythmias and ECG changes in the absence of observable toxic clinical symptoms. Of particular concern is the development of prolonged QT interval with torsade de pointes, a pleomorphic ventricular arrhythmia that commonly triggers sudden cardiac death (548). This syndrome can have both early and late manifestations, appearing between 3 and 15 days after intoxication. Although the precise mechanism is unknown, torsades de pointes is thought to result from the interspersion of normal myocardium with focal areas, which produces myriad areas of reentry and nonhomogeneous repolarization (549). Lung function may be adversely affected, leading to insufficiency and subsequent cardiac outcomes. Typical effects have been seen in recent studies involving adult patients who were subject to severe organophosphate intoxication (550,551). The cardiac complications included noncardiogenic pulmonary edema, ECG abnormalities, prolonged QTc intervals, ST-T changes, conduction defects, tachycardia, and bradycardia. In addition to electrophysiological considerations, organophosphates can also cause direct myocardial injury. In particular, methyl parathion has caused gross and microscopic histopathological changes in the heart such as micronecrosis and pericapillary hemorrhage (552,553). Both parasympathetic and sympathetic phases of organophosphate toxicity can lead to myocardial damage. In another study, rats were found to have focal necrosis of the myocardium and endocardium following exposure to intrathion (554). There is also support for neurogenic effects of organophosphate toxicity in the development of cardiac lesions (555). The cardiac lesions were surmised to be either secondary to brain lesions or to have developed following prolonged sympathetic overstimulation. Topacoglu et al. investigated a case of atrial fibrillation in a 26-year-old male employed in a carbamate production factory (556). The patient was exposed to methomyl dust for five minutes and presented to the hospital with an irregular heart rhythm. Electrocardiogram confirmed atrial fibrillation with normal ventricular response. The authors suggested atrial fibrillation to be an unusual consequence of insecticide intoxication.

The literature has shown that organophosphate-induced cardiotoxicity is an area that merits further research. While there has been support for several relevant hypotheses, cardiac-specific mechanisms of organophosphate toxicity are still being elucidated. Arguably, one of the most important consequences of organophosphate intoxication is the late occurrence of cardiac complications and potential sudden death. The frequency of dysrhythmias is positively correlated with the severity of the toxic insult. Such electrophysiological changes can range from ST-T changes to the malignant arrhythmia torsade de pointes. Nevertheless, ultrastructural heart changes and morphologic damage have been known to occur during the acute stage of toxicity. Important considerations in assessing cardiotoxic effects include the organophosphate in question, dosage, and route of exposure.

Organochlorines

Organochlorines such as lindane, endosulfan, methoxychlor, and dicofol are frequently used in the United States. This type of pesticide has been known to produce hypertension and tachycardia with associated arrhythmias. A study was conducted to explore the myocardial damage caused by endosulfan and lindane (557). Rabbits were exposed to either endosulfan or lindane in identical amounts (2.5 or 5.0 mg) dissolved in propylene glycol. Both groups experienced significant increases in blood pressure, PR, QT, QRS, and RR intervals. Moreover, rabbits exposed to 5.0 mg lindane or endosulfan for 12 months suffered severe myocardial damage in the form of muscle fiber degeneration with vacuolization and leukocytic infiltration. Another study focused specifically on the morphological and electrical consequences of rat hearts chronically exposed to low doses of lindane between 0.5 to 2 ppb (558). Rat hearts in the highest exposure group (2 ppb) displayed hypertrophied, thinning left ventricular walls, atrophied papillary muscles, and unorganized, hemorrhagic interspaces. The action potential duration of the 1 ppb group demonstrated shortened plateaus while the 2 ppb group exhibited shortened plateaus and slow depolarizing phases. In addition to the inducements of direct myocardial injury and electrical activity disturbances, lindane also has the capacity to induce oxidative stress on the heart (559). Rats given lindane orally (1.5 and 7 mg/kg/day for 21 days) experienced increased lipid peroxidation of the heart, as well as myocardial edema. Specific ultrastructural changes were evident in the loss of myofibril integrity, Z-band disruption, and mitochondrial damage. These studies offer support that endosulfan and lindane can cause significant myocardial damage in the form of cardiac lesions and coronary insufficiency.

Organochlorines compounds were widely used between the 1940s and 1970s. However, most of them have been banned because of recognized environmental effects (560). One of the most widely studied organochlorines, DDT, is considered of moderate human toxicity. The mechanism of action of a currently used organochlorine, lindane is to induce rapid convulsions by blocking the chloride channel in GABA receptor complexes. Lindane is in the process of being phased out in favor of less toxic pyrethroids but is still in use in shampoos designed to treat head lice. Human cardiotoxicity studies relating to organo-chlorine exposures are limited and near completely focused on suicidal and unintentional ingestions. Myocardial insufficiency developed in one of two cases of acute intentional endosulfan intoxication (561). Pulmonary insufficiency and cardiac failure were also seen to develop. Earlier studies reported cardiovascular collapse and cardiac failure (562,563). These findings are in support of previous investigations of endosulfan poisoning, where it was observed that the myo-cardium was especially susceptible to malignant dysrhythmia from organo-chloric compound exposure.

Organochlorines have been shown to cause electrocardiographic effects and direct, myocardial damage. Experimental studies have revealed severe morphological alterations and necrosis of cardiac tissue in organochlorine-exposed animals. There is evidence that accumulation of organochlorines, such as lindane, in heart tissue can cause the action potential duration to be shortened. A suggested mechanism for organochlorine cardiotoxicity is the development of oxidative stress via lipid peroxidation. Suicidal ingestions and poisoning have revealed cases of myocardial insufficiency, a known prelude to cardiac failure. Therefore, these studies and others to follow are of prime clinical interest.

Pyrethroids

Pyrethroids are synthetic neurotoxins used as insecticides. They are known to be substantially more effective than other classes of insecticides such as organo-phosphates, carbamates, and organochlorines. These synthetic compounds are derivatives of natural pyrethroids of *Chrysanthemum cinaeriaefolium* and share similar abilities to inhibit the enzyme $Na^+ K^+$-ATPase and affect Na^+ channels of excitable tissues. Pyrethroids are known for their low mammalian toxicity compared with organophosphorus compounds. Pyrethroids are divided into two major classes, type II and type I (560). Type II compounds possess an α-cyano substituent which invokes the C-S response (choreoathetosis, salivation, and seizures). Type I compounds do not have this CN group and cause the T syn-drome (tremors, aggressive sparring, and enhanced startle response). Research however, has not adequately addressed the interactions between pyrethroids and potential cardiac consequences of exposure. It has been suggested that pyreth-roids may produce cardiotoxicity via I_{Na}-mediated (sodium current) prolongation of cardiac myocytes (564). This study evaluated the cardiotoxic actions of the type I pyrethroid tefluthrin and the type II pyrethroids fenpropathrin and α-cypermethrin. Both classes of pyrethroids demonstrated an ability to prolong the action potential duration and stimulate early afterdepolarizations (EADs). This is important because EADs significantly disperse the action potential dura-tion, a potential precursor to arrhythmia development. It was suggested that the observed arrhythmias were a result of a direct effect of the pyrethroids on the myocardium. A later study on isolated rat ventricular myocytes and perfused, whole rat hearts confirmed that pyrethroid exposure caused significant, consistent prolongations of action potentials and after-depolarizations (565). Moreover, the pyrethroids showed proarrhythmic activity that had direct effects on the myocardium. The researchers determined that the pyrethroid under study, tefluthrin, which is a type I compound, and other compounds that affect Na^+ channel inactivation might directly depolarize cardiac cells and indirectly support Ca^{2+} overloading. Furthermore, Ca^{2+} is a known risk factor in the development of arrhythmias. Coskun et al. examined frogs exposed to cypermethrin, a type II compound (566). Following 30 and 60 minutes of exposure, the frogs experienced striking reductions in the contractions forces of the atrial and ventricular muscles and amplitudes of the P waves and QRS complexes. Histopathologically, the hearts revealed hyperchromatic nuclei changes, breaches of cell membrane integrity, and destruction of smooth endoplasmic reticulum and other endothelial organelles. Therefore, cypermethrin was shown to damage the heart muscle, decrease atrial and ventricular contraction forces, and cause significant reductions in heart rate causing prolongation of the cardiac cycle. Suggested mechanisms responsible for study findings include hypoxia, parasympathetic stimulation, destruction of mitochondria, and damage to myocardial cells. Taken together, these observations demonstrate the potential for pyrethroids to cause significant disruption of the normal cardiac rhythm. In addition to disturbances in the electrical activity, pyrethroids may cause substantial decreases in the contractile ability of the heart, as well as direct myocardial injury.

Pyrethroids are less toxic to mammals, including humans, than other pesticides. However, systemic toxicity can still occur. The clinical course of pyrethroid intoxication remains unclear. It has been speculated that the mechanism of toxicity is similar in experimental animals and humans, that being, the disruption of nerve membrane sodium channels. Previous reports of human toxicity admit co-exposure with solvents, surfactants, and organophosphates. For example, permethrin, a type I pyrethroid, contains 20% permethrin, 70% xylene, and 10% surfactants. Therefore, there may be a share of responsibility for clinical health effects. Cardiac toxicology reports from pyrethroid exposure is scattered and have been observed in occupational exposures, suicide attempts, and accidental ingestions (567). A recent study reported cardiac symptoms such as arrhythmias (sinus tachycardia) and shock in 3 of 48 patients poisoned with insecticides containing permethrin formulations (568). However, the majority of clinical signs of permethrin toxicity in this study were gastrointestinal. Another study compiled acute pyrethroid poisoning reports from the Chinese medical literature during 1983–1988 (569). The investigators found 8 of 71 patients with ECG changes including ST-T changes; sinus tachycardia in 10 patients; and ventricular premature beat and sinus bradycardia in two patients (570–573). These studies, although informative, provide an inadequate foundation for a reliable clinical description of cardiotoxicity attributable to permethrin and other pyrethroids.

The pyrethroids class of insecticides is known to be generally less toxic than other compounds, i.e., organophosphates, and considerably more effective.

Both classes of pyrethroids, types I and II, have been shown to cause neuronal-based, systemic symptoms resulting from prolonged action potential durations and to invoke similar cardiotoxic effects. However, research on cardiac toxicity and mechanisms has not been adequately addressed. It is thought that modifications of the cardiac Na^+ channel, together with alterations in intracellular Ca^{2+} levels, may be responsible for pyrethroid-induced arrhythmias. Additionally, the ability to directly depolarize cardiac cells has shown pyrethroids to be positively inotropic. Experimental studies on frogs and other amphibians have shown that pyrethroids can affect the heart muscle directly, causing widespread ultrastructural, myocardial damage resembling cardiomyopathy. These animals are considered bioindicators whose health reflects the health of an ecosystem in general (566).

Until recently, the cardiac toxicology of pesticides has received less attention compared with other well-known systemic complications. The mechanism by which pesticides induce cardiac toxicity is unclear. However, calcium overload to the heart and sodium pump inhibition are suspected. It has been shown in experimental and human studies that the early stages of intoxication can result in morphologic lesions with a neurogenic foundation and sinus bradycardia. On the other hand, cardiotoxic symptoms often manifest during the later stages of insult, when other signs of clinical intoxication have disappeared. The development of arrhythmias is the third stage of cardiac toxicity and the most important consequence of pesticide cardiac pathophysiology, involving complex electrophysiological and histopathological interactions. This stage can appear from two days to two weeks after the initial insult. QT-prolongation followed by pleomorphic tachycardia often lead to sudden cardiac death. There is a direct relationship between the severity of intoxication and the development of fatal arrhythmias and other cardiac consequences. Therefore, it is imperative that further experiments and studies on both animal and humans be conducted to clarify the role of pesticide intoxication on the cardiac system.

Dioxins

Chlorinated dibenzo-*p*-dioxins (dioxins) comprise a family of 75 different compounds divided into eight groups (574). On the basis of the number of chlorine atoms, group 1 contains one chlorine atom (mono), while groups 2 to 8 contain the respective numbers of chlorine atoms (di, tri, tetra, penta, hexa, hepta, and octa). Industrial exposures to dioxins occur mainly through inhalation and dermal contact. Workers with significant exposures to dioxins include firefighters, incinerator operators, metal reclamation operators, and pesticide handlers. Exposure to the compounds can place workers at risk for the development of chloracne and other illnesses. However, occupational exposures to most dioxin compounds have been significantly reduced in recent years.

Dioxins are present at low levels in the environment in measurements known as nanograms and picograms (one billionth of a gram, and one trillionth of a gram, respectively). Background levels of dioxins are inhaled in ambient air and consumed in food or milk. The majority of exposure comes from foods such as meat, dairy products, fish, fruits, and vegetables. Infants may be exposed through mother's milk and formula. Skin contact with dioxins can occur from the handling of chlorinated pesticides and herbicides, contaminated soils, or PCP-treated woods. The presence of dioxins in all samples of adipose tissue and blood (serum lipids) in persons without known previous exposure establishes the compounds' ubiquity. Levels of 2,3,7,8-tetrachlorodibenzo-*p*-dioxin (TCDD) in serum from the general population can range from 3 to 7 ppt (parts per trillion) (574).

There have been a number of studies designed to investigate the cardiotoxicity of 2,3,7,8-TCDD. Monkeys fed a diet containing low levels of TCDD (500 ppt) displayed signs of direct myocardial injury (575). Petechial hemorrhages were observed in the atria, ventricles, and papillary muscles. These hemorrhage sites contained collections of intact partially disrupted red blood cells that altered the structural pattern of the myocardium. The authors indicated that TCDD is capable of inducing detrimental tissue-level changes in the heart of monkeys following nine months of exposure. Brewster et al. examined guinea pig atrial muscles isolated from animals singly injected with 1 μg TCDD/kg (576). Atrial muscle from animals treated with TCDD for 20 days exhibited significantly a decreased basal force of contraction, despite the positive inotropic effect of isoproterenol. It was suggested that the decreased sensitivity of the heart to isoproterenol was due to alterations in the β-adrenergic system as a result of influences of TCDD on cAMP concentrations. Canga et al. assessed possible TCDD cardiotoxicity in guinea pig right ventricular papillary muscle (577). Cardiac β-adrenergic responsiveness was found to be decreased in guinea pigs exposed to TCDD. In addition, isoproterenol (0.03–0.3 μM) experienced a 65% decrease in its positive inotropic effect on cardiac contractility. Intracellular calcium concentrations were increased in papillary muscle; however, TCDD did not block low calcium-channel activity. The researchers suggested these specific findings to be indicative of a TCDD-mediated pattern of cardiac dysfunction and that mammalian species may be targets for TCDD cardiotoxicity. A later investigation studying TCDD cardiotoxicity in chick embryo hearts produced confirmatory results (578). The cardiotoxicity and histopathology of 3,3′,4,4′-tetrachloroazoxybenzene (TCAOB) was described in gavaged rats and mice (579). TCAOB is a dioxin-like compound that has been studied on a limited basis in previous studies. Rats exhibited changes consistent with an exacerbation of cardiomyopathy. A normally occurring, spontaneous lesion was observed to contain a grater number of degenerative foci, with more widespread distribution and involvement of the right atrium and ventricles. In addition, further injury was manifest as myocardial hemorrhage, acute inflammation, and endocardial proliferation. The mice under investigation experienced no cardiac effects. The cardiomyopathy in rats was thought to be secondary to changes in pulmonary vasculature causing pulmonary hypertension and increased load on the right side of the heart. The authors speculated that cardiotoxic effects on the heart, via a cardiopulmonary pathway, were mediated by toxic metabolites of TCAOB. Rats in a TCDD study displayed spontaneous cardiomyopathy (580). The incidence of cardiomyopathy was significantly increased and dose-related, however, the severity of observed lesions was based on the amount of myocardium affected. The incidence was seen to increase and the severity was minimal or slightly greater than seen in controls. Xie et al. studied the cardiac effects of TCDD on action potentials and afterdepolarizations in rat ventricular myocytes (581). TCDD concentrations of 1 to 100 nM significantly prolonged action potential duration at 90% repolarization (APD_{90}) on a concentration-dependent basis. Exposure to TCDD (10 nM) caused delayed afterdepolarizations (DADs) in a majority of cells. The administration of isoproterenol markedly potentiated the amplitude and frequency of DADs. Co-exposure to TCDD and isoproterenol also induced EADs. DADs and EADs following prolongation of action potential duration are known to be pro-arrhythmic, with EADs being particularly dangerous. This observation coupled with an increased calcium flux suggests TCDD exposure to be arrhythmogenic and potentially dangerous for patients suffering from cardiomyopathies and calcium overload. The data from experimental studies suggests that dioxins such as TCDD exhibit significant cardiotoxic effects. Of particular importance are negative inotropic and cardiac calcium level impacts that may predispose experimental animals to arrhythmias and sudden death.

Human studies focusing on TCDD cardiotoxicity are limited. Kim et al. conducted an investigation among Korean Vietnam veterans exposed to Agent Orange (582). Agent Orange was a phenoxyherbicide used in the Vietnam War that contained between 1 and 50 ppm TCDD. Among other medical problems, the veterans exposed to higher levels of Agent Orange exhibited a significantly increased frequency of ischemic heart disease ($p < 0.01$) and valvular heart disease ($p < 0.01$). The researchers suggested that these observations be studied further in future investigations. A similar study examined U.S. Army Chemical Corps Veterans who were exposed to Agent Orange during Vietnam (583). Veterans who sprayed the herbicide were found to have significantly increased rates of heart disease (OR = 1.52; CI = 1.18–1.94). Although limited and primarily concerned with carcinogenesis, the literature on the cardiotoxic impacts of dioxins exposure suggests the compounds promote the development of hypertension and various forms of heart disease.

Organic Nitrates

Nitrates and nitrites are compounds with wide industrial and consumer uses. Workers in construction who handle dynamite and those in the explosives and munitions industries can be exposed to considerable levels of nitrates. The composition of dynamite is approximately 60% organic nitrates, 25% blasting oil, and 10% dinitrotoluene (584). Exposure levels are highest during the mixing of explosives and cartridge filling. Plasma concentrations of nitroglycerin in gunpowder production workers have been measured at 98.1 nM compared with 5.7 nM from sublingual administration of 1.0 mg nitroglycerin (585).

Food and water can contain high concentrations of nitrates. However, the United States Department of Agriculture approved the use of inorganic nitrates and nitrites in foods as food-coloring agents and food preservatives despite concerns about potential carcinogenicity (586). Of the two compounds, nitrites are more potent oxidizing agents and in inorganic form, are found in contaminated well water supplies. Inorganic nitrates are contained in plants such as cauliflower, spinach, collard greens, and broccoli. Antidiarrheal agents, diuretics, and topical burn treatments are but a few medical uses of inorganic nitrates. Examples of organic nitrates are ethylene nitrate, dinitrotoluene, and trinitrotoluene used in the manufacture of explosives and munitions.

There is limited data on the cardiotoxic effects of organic nitrates in experimental studies. In rats, exposed animals experienced more frequent ventricular ectopic beats and increased mortality following repeated injections with ethylene glycol dintrate (587). Investigators attributed the findings to heightened sensitivity of rat heart to epinephrine after exposure to nitrate esters. Fish and other aquatic animals can accumulate high concentrations of nitrites in ambient water via the gill epithelium. Jensen conducted research on rainbow trout to explore cardiovascular effects of nitrite exposure (588). Trout were observed to have a rapid, persistent increase in heart rate that could not be ascribed to decreased levels of blood oxygen, reduced pacemaker cell depolarization, or stress responses such as catecholamine release. There were also important decreases in heart rate variability in fish particularly sensitive to nitrites. This finding was seen to be a consequence of altered autonomic control of the heart indicative of physiological dysfunction. Cows that consumed hay containing 2500 ppm of nitrate-nitrogen and 11 ppm of nitrite-nitrogen exhibited tachycardia and cardiac hyperemia (589). These studies suggest that nitrates and nitrites are vasoactive, arrhythmogenic agents that can potentially disrupt physiological cardiac processes.

Occupational exposure to organic nitrates and explosives has been association with acute episodes of angina, myocardial infarction, and sudden death (590–596). Klock et al. describes a case of a 38-year-old explosives foreman that was admitted for recurrent, crushing chest pain (597). He reported exposure to dynamite and nitroglycerin of more than 10 years duration. Further tests revealed the presence of a nitroglycerin dependence syndrome. The angina-like pain was determined to be nonocclusive heart disease and coronary spasm associated with chronic exposure, followed by sudden withdrawal, to nitrates. The frequency and severity of ischemic pain improved over time following cessation of exposure to nitrates and administration of sublingual nitroglycerin as needed. Another series of cardiotoxic manifestations of industrial nitroglycerin withdrawal was observed in an explosives factory worker (598). Complaints of angina led to the diagnoses of dilated cardiomyopathy, transmural anteroseptal and anterolateral myocardial infarction, and total occlusion of the left anterior descending branch of the left coronary artery. The investigators suggested that coronary vasospasm led to formation of a thrombus, thereby causing the myocardial infarction and subsequent aggravation of the cardiomyopathy. Levine et al. discovered a surprising excess (SMR = 143; CI = 107–187) of ischemic heart disease in workers exposed to dinitrotoluene in ammunition plants (599). The duration and intensity of dinitrotoluene exposure was consistent with observed mortality from ischemic heart disease. An earlier study by Benditt suggested a significant biological plausibility of atherosclerotic plaque formation due to nitrate-mediated injury to the coronary arteries (600). Later studies on workers exposed to ammonia nitrate revealed myocardiodystrophy and electrocardiographic T-wave changes (601,602). Those observations were associated with respiratory changes, such as bronchitis, and whether cardiac response is secondary to the pulmonary effects has not been clarified. In summary, experimental animal and human studies suggest nitrate and nitrite exposure to be cardiotoxic. In addition to vasodilative and arrhythmogenic effects, organic nitrates have been observed to induce a peculiar withdrawal syndrome upon sudden cessation of exposure. Reports suggestive of cardiomyopathy and myocardial infarction lend further support to the cardiotoxicity of organic nitrate exposure.

Ammonia

Ammonia is a naturally occurring chemical found in water, soil, and air. It is a major source of nitrogen for plants and animals and is naturally produced from the breakdown of dead animals and plants. Ammonia is used in the production of many common chemicals. It is used to make explosives, pharmaceuticals, pesticides, textiles, leather, flare-retardants, plastics, pulp and paper, rubber, petroleum products, cyanide, glass cleaners, toilet bowl cleaners, metal polishers, floor strippers, wax removers, and smelling salts. Eighty percent of all manufactured ammonia is used in fertilizer. Industrial exposure to ammonia may occur from leakage of pressurized liquid ammonia during transportation or from industrial accidents. Firefighters are at risk of exposure to ammonia as it is released when nylon, silk, wood, and melamine are burned in fires. Ammonia is a colorless gas with a very sharp smell. Odor threshold for ammonia is at 30 ppm (603). Eye and nasal irritation may occur at 50 ppm. Severe pulmonary symptoms may arise at level of 1000 ppm and sudden death may occur 1500 ppm. In 2002, the United States Poison Control Center reported nearly 6000 cases of toxic ammonia exposure (604). Of these cases, 93% were caused by unintentional exposure, 70% occurred in adults and 20% occurred in children younger than six years old. The general population is constantly being exposed to low levels of ammonia from the air, soil, and water. Ammonia is present in air at concentrations in the range of 1 to 5 ppb and levels fluctuate by season and time of day (605). Ammonia is also found in rainwater. The concentration of ammonia in rivers and bays are generally less than 6 ppm. In soil, ammonia is typically present at levels ranging from 1 to 5 ppm and may be found as high as 1000 ppm at hazardous waste sites.

Studies in animals indicate that exposure to ammonia may induce cardiotoxic effects. Myocardial fibrosis has been observed in rats, guinea pigs, dogs, and rabbits continuously exposed up to 470 mg/m^3 of ammonia for 90 days (606). Kapeghian et al. reported on acute inhalation toxicity of ammonia in mice (607). Mice inhaling ammonia concentrations exceeding 4000 ppm for 14 days displayed pericardial fat atrophy. Electrocardiographic changes have been demonstrated in female Saanen goats poisoned with ammonium compounds (608). Ammonia-infused goats revealed cardiovascular changes, including sinus arrhythmia, atrioventricular dissociation, ventricular premature beats, transitory rise in blood pressure with decrease in PaO$_2$ and ventricular fibrillation. In rabbits, acute inhalation of ammonia has shown to cause bradycardia at 2500 ppm and hypertension and arrhythmias leading to cardiovascular collapse at 5000 ppm (609). The mechanism of ammonia cardiotoxicity remains unclear, however recent study on antioxidant enzymes of the rat heart suggests that ammonia intoxication may induce oxidative stress (610). Venediktova et al. observed an increase in superoxide dismutase, catalase and glutathione peroxidase activity in the rat heart upon acute ammonia inhalation. These data indicate an adaptive response of the heart to oxidative stress under hyperammonemic conditions.

Several case reports have cited ammonia-induced cardiotoxicity due to accidental intoxication. Myocardial lesions have been detected in patients with acute ammonia poisoning (611). A 20-year-old male was described as experiencing elevated blood pressure and pulse after being found unconscious in a room filled with ammonia vapor (612). At the six-month follow-up, the patient showed no ill effects of ammonia intoxication. Individuals exposed to massive amounts of ammonia gas have also reportedly displayed elevated pulse, shock, and cardiac failure (613). Tachycardia was present in 4 of 14 fisherman exposed to high concentration of ammonia gas from a refrigeration system leak (614). Cardiopulmonary arrest and tachycardia was reported in a six-month-old infant heavily exposed to ammonia fumes (615). The patient required intubation and was discharged from the hospital after 22 days. A 47-year-old patient developed unexplained bradycardia after being exposed to ammonia for over 45 minutes (616). In 2001, a chemical plant in France storing ammonium nitrate exploded and released an unknown amount of ammonia and nitrogenous compounds into the atmosphere (617). Inhabitants within a 3-km radius of the explosion showed significantly higher incidence of acute coronary syndromes for up to 10 days following the explosion.

Ammonia is a corrosive, toxic irritant. Its main effects are generally restricted to the sites of direct contact. However, experimental studies and case reports suggest that ammonia can induce cardiac consequences, such as arrhythmias (bradycardia and tachycardia), changes in pulse rate and blood pressure and cardiac arrest. Investigators have not established a direct mechanism of ammonia-induced cardiotoxicity, however some data indicate that the heart experiences increased oxidative stress. It remains unclear if the cardiovascular changes are attributed to direct cardiotoxic effects or secondary to injury to the cardiopulmonary system, however clinicians should be aware of possible cardiovascular consequences of acute ammonia poisoning.

Hydrogen Cyanide

Cyanides are compounds that can be potent and rapid-acting poisons. Hydrogen cyanide (HCN) gas is a typical example of this class of compounds. Inhalation and skin absorption are the expected routes of occupational exposures. Industrial exposure to cyanide can occur in workers involved in electroplating, metallurgy, cyanotype printing, pesticide application, firefighting, steel manufacturing, and gas works operations. Surveys of plating facilities measured concentrations of cyanide ranging from 0.0009 to 4.0 ppm (618). Medical and emergency personnel may be exposed to elevated levels of cyanide through resuscitation attempts or removal of gastric contents of deceased victims. The NIOSH has set a recommended exposure limit to cyanide of 4.7 ppm (619). Exposures to the general population can occur from inhalation of cyanide in ambient air and ingestion of food and drinks containing cyanide. Hydrogen cyanide is the primary representative of the cyanide compounds found in air, with concentrations ranging from 160 to 166 ppt in nonurban areas (620,621). The nonurban, nonsmoking U.S. population is generally exposed 3.8 to µg/day of hydrogen cyanide (622). The daily consumption of cyanide in drinking water of the average adult is equivalent to 0.002 to 0.22 mg, and the maximum contaminant level set by the EPA is 0.2 mg/L (623). The daily cyanide intake from food has not been estimated. However, the EPA has established tolerances for potential exposure in various foods ranging from 5 to 250 ppm (624).

Cyanide has demonstrated varying cardiotoxic effects in experimental animals. Suzuki observed direct myocardial injury leading to adverse effects on myocardial contractility in rats administered 10 mg/kg of potassium cyanide (625). Electron microscope studies of exposed rats revealed myofibrillar distortion, mitochondrial destruction, swollen sarcoplasmic reticulum vesicles, and capillary endothelial cell swelling. Electrocardiogram recorded sinus irregularity, disappearance of P waves, elevation of S-T segments, and eventual terminal tachycardia and fibrillation. The results demonstrate that cyanide exposure has detrimental effects consisting of ultrastructural changes and ECG abnormalities on the rat heart. The authors suggest that some ultrastructural changes were indirectly mediated by histotoxic anoxia because of the inactivation of cytochrome oxidase. In awake dogs, intra-aortic injections of sodium cyanide (0.3 mg/kg NaCN) evoked significant elevations in cardiac output, heart rate, and arterial blood pressure, and anoxic hypoxia (626). Vascular resistance remained unchanged. Previous reports of anesthetized dogs exhibited contrasting results, such as marked reductions in blood pressure and vascular resistance (627–629). It is also possible that the route of administration had a different effect from a cardiac point of view. Research suggests that cardiotoxic circulatory response to cyanide is mechanistically rooted within the central nervous system and not sinoaortic reflexogenic zones. Purser et al. conducted a study on monkeys to assess the HCN incapacitating effects of fire atmospheres (630). Hydrogen cyanide gas exposures caused bradycardia with arrhythmias and T-wave abnormalities. Vick et al. examined ECG changes following intravenous administration of sodium cyanide (2.5 mg/kg) in beagle dogs (631). Exposed animals showed severe bradycardia, arterial hypotension, and hypoxic ECG changes. Death occurred within 5 to 7 minutes following injection. It was suggested that cyanide induces coronary arteriolar vasoconstriction leading to decreases in cardiac output. Degeneration of the myocardium in dogs fed a diet of cassava containing the cyanogenic glucoside linamarin has been described in the literature (632). Linamarin releases HCN following hydrolysis in the intestinal tract of animals and man. Histopathological examination revealed significant hemorrhage between swollen myofibrils. In sum, experimental animal studies reveal cyanide to be a detrimental cardiotoxicant. The data demonstrate the ability of cyanide to induce arrhythmias, atrioventricular block, ventricular fibrillation, and eventual asystole as a result of direct cardiotoxicity.

The heart, as an ATP-dependent organ, is one of the primary target organs of cyanide toxicity. Mechanistically, cyanide exerts particularly toxic effects on cardiac cytochrome oxidase (633). The literature relevant to cyanide-induced cardiotoxicity is sporadic and limited primarily to case reports. Lasch et al. discusses two children involved in cyanide poisoning following the ingestion of apricot kernels (634). Apricot kernels contain varying amounts of amygdalin (8.9 to 217 mg/100 gm) that hydrolyzes to HCN. Children experienced tachycardia and severe hypotension. A case report summarized findings of a 23-year-old man who accidentally ingested a mouthful of cyanide-containing metal cleaning solution (635). ECG reported that the patient experienced sinus tachycardia, and he subsequently recovered from a sequence of severe cardiovascular collapse. Johnson et al. reported on a 30-year-old patient with depression and suicidal ideation who ingested 3 gm of granular sodium cyanide (636). On admission, the patient exhibited atrial fibrillation and ST segment depression in inferior and lateral leads. Peddy et al. also reported cardiovascular collapse in a 17-year-old victim of cyanide poisoning (637). Results taken from experimental studies and case reports demonstrate that cyanide has profound cardiotoxic consequences, ranging from ultrastructural changes to ventricular arrhythmias and death. The mechanism is primarily via inhibition of the cellular respiratory chain and disruption of ATP production.

REFERENCES

1. Nemmar A, et al. Passage of intratracheally instilled ultrafine particles from the lung into the systemic circulation in hamster. Am J Respir Crit Care Med 2001; 164: 1665.
2. Nemmar A, et al. Passage of inhaled particles into the blood circulation in humans. Circulation 2002; 105:411.

3. Wilson WE, Suh HH. Fine particles and coarse particles: concentration relationships relevant to epidemiologic studies. J Air Waste Manag Assoc 1997; 47:1238.
4. Gordon T, et al. Pulmonary and cardiovascular effects of acute exposure to concentrated ambient particulate matter in rats. Toxicol Lett 1998; 96–97:285.
5. Gordon T, et al. Effects of concentrated ambient particles in rats and hamsters: an exploratory study. Res Rep Health Eff Inst 2000; 93:5.
6. Wichers LB, et al. Effects of acute exposure to concentrated ambient particulates on cardiopulmonary, thermoregulatory, and biochemical parameters in healthy and monocrotaline-treated Sprague-Dawley rats. Am J Respir Crit Care Med 2003; 167:A107.
7. Campen MJ, et al. Cardiovascular and thermoregulatory effects of inhaled PM-associated transition metals: a potential interaction between nickel and vanadium sulfate. Toxicol Sci 2001; 64:243.
8. Campen MJ, et al. Cardiac and thermoregulatory effects of instilled particulate matter-associated transition metals in healthy and cardiopulmonary-compromised rats. J Toxicol Environ Health A 2002; 65:1615.
9. Campen MJ, Costa DL, Watkinson WP. Cardiac and thermoregulatory toxicity of residual oil fly ash. Inhal Toxicol 2000; 12(supplement 2):7.
10. Cheng TJ, et al. Effects of concentrated ambient particles on heart rate and blood pressure in pulmonary hypertensive rats. Environ Health Perspect 2003; 111:147.
11. Godleski JJ, et al. Mechanisms of morbidity and mortality from exposure to ambient air particles. Res Rep Health Eff Inst 2000; 91:5.
12. Rodriguez Ferreira Rivero DH, et al. PM (2.5) induces acute electrocardiographic alterations in healthy rats. Environ Res 2005; 99:262.
13. Corey LM, Baker C, Luchtel DL. Heart-rate variability in the apolipoprotein E knockout transgenic mouse following exposure to Seattle particulate matter. J Toxicol Environ Health A 2006; 69:953.
14. Wellenius GA, et al. Electrocardiographic changes during exposure to residual oil fly ash (ROFA) particles in a rat model of myocardial infarction. Toxicol Sci 2002; 66:327.
15. Wold LE, et al. In vivo and in vitro models to test the hypothesis of particle-induced effects on cardiac function and arrhythmias. Cardiovasc Toxicol 2006; 6:69.
16. Watkinson WP, Campen MJ, Costa DL. Cardiac arrhythmia induction after exposure to residual oil fly ash particles in a rodent model of pulmonary hypertension. Toxicol Sci 1998; 41:209.
17. Kodavanti UP, et al. The spontaneously hypertensive rat as a model of human cardiovascular disease: evidence of exacerbated cardiopulmonary injury and oxidative stress from inhaled emission particulate matter. Toxicol Appl Pharmacol 2000; 164:250.
18. Wichers LB, et al. Effects of instilled combustion-derived particles in spontaneously hypertensive rats. Part I: Cardiovascular responses. Inhal Toxicol 2004; 16: 391.
19. Wellenius GA, et al. Inhalation of concentrated ambient air particles exacerbates myocardial ischemia in conscious dogs. Environ Health Perspect 2003; 111:402.
20. Kodavanti UP, et al. Inhaled environmental combustion particles cause myocardial injury in the Wistar Kyoto rat. Toxicol Sci 2003; 71:237.
21. Calderon-Garciduenas L, et al. Canines as sentinel species for assessing chronic exposures to air pollutants: part 2. Cardiac pathology. Toxicol Sci 2001; 61:356.

22. Graff DW, et al. Metal particulate matter components affect gene expression and beat frequency of neonatal rat ventricular myocytes. Environ Health Perspect 2004; 112:792.
23. Cozzi E, et al. Ultrafine particulate matter exposure augments ischemia-reperfusion injury in mice. Am J Physiol Heart Circ Physiol 2006; 291:H894.
24. Kang YJ, et al. Elevation of serum endothelins and cardiotoxicity induced by particulate matter (PM2.5) in rats with acute myocardial infarction. Cardiovasc Toxicol 2002; 2:253.
25. Dockery DW, et al. Daily changes in oxygen saturation and pulse rate associated with particulate air pollution and barometric pressure. Res Rep Health Eff Inst 1999; 83:1.
26. Pope CA 3rd, et al. Heart rate variability associated with particulate air pollution. Am Heart J 1999; 138:890.
27. Peters A, et al. Increases in heart rate during an air pollution episode. Am J Epidemiol 1999; 150:1094.
28. Pope CA 3rd, et al. Oxygen saturation, pulse rate, and particulate air pollution: A daily time-series panel study. Am J Respir Crit Care Med 1999; 159:365.
29. Magari SR, et al. The association between personal measurements of environmental exposure to particulates and heart rate variability. Epidemiology 2002; 13:305.
30. Liao D, et al. Association of higher levels of ambient criteria pollutants with impaired cardiac autonomic control: a population-based study. Am J Epidemiol 2004; 159:768.
31. Gold DR, et al. Ambient pollution and heart rate variability. Circulation 2000; 101:1267.
32. Ibald-Mulli A, et al. Effects of particulate air pollution on blood pressure and heart rate in subjects with cardiovascular disease: a multicenter approach. Environ Health Perspect 2004; 112:369.
33. Task Force of the European Society of Cardiology and the North American Society of Pacing and Electrophysiology, Heart rate variability: standards of measurement, physiological interpretation and clinical use. Circulation 1996; 93:1043.
34. Pekkanen J, et al. Particulate air pollution and risk of ST-segment depression during repeated submaximal exercise tests among subjects with coronary heart disease: the Exposure and Risk Assessment for Fine and Ultrafine Particles in Ambient Air (ULTRA) study. Circulation 2002; 106:933.
35. Gold DR, et al. Air pollution and ST-segment depression in elderly subjects. Environ Health Perspect 2005; 113:883.
36. Henneberger A, et al. Repolarization changes induced by air pollution in ischemic heart disease patients. Environ Health Perspect 2005; 113:440.
37. Adar SD, et al. Focused exposures to airborne traffic particles and heart rate variability in the elderly. Epidemiology 2007; 18:95.
38. Chuang KJ, et al., Effects of particle size fractions on reducing heart rate variability in cardiac and hypertensive patients. Environ Health Perspect 2005; 113:1693.
39. Lipsett MJ, et al. Coarse particles and heart rate variability among older adults with coronary artery disease in the Coachella Valley, California. Environ Health Perspect 2006; 114:1215.
40. Magari SR, et al. Association of heart rate variability with occupational and environmental exposure to particulate air pollution. Circulation 2001; 104:986.

41. Park SK, et al. Effects of air pollution on heart rate variability: the VA normative aging study. Environ Health Perspect 2005; 113:304.
42. Vallejo M, et al. Ambient fine particles modify heart rate variability in young healthy adults. J Expo Sci Environ Epidemiol 2006; 16:125.
43. Cakmak S, Dales RE, Judek S. Do gender, education, and income modify the effect of air pollution gases on cardiac disease? J Occup Environ Med 2006; 48:89.
44. Peters A, et al. Air pollution and incidence of cardiac arrhythmia. Epidemiology 2000; 11:11.
45. Dockery DW, et al. Association of air pollution with increased incidence of ventricular tachyarrhythmias recorded by implanted cardioverter defibrillators. Environ Health Perspect 2005; 113:670.
46. Peters A, et al. Increased particulate air pollution and the triggering of myocardial infarction. Circulation 2001; 103:2810.
47. von Klot S, et al. Ambient air pollution is associated with increased risk of hospital cardiac readmissions of myocardial infarction survivors in five European cities. Circulation 2005; 112:3073.
48. Pope CA 3rd, et al. Ischemic heart disease events triggered by short-term exposure to fine particulate air pollution. Circulation 2006; 114:2443.
49. Zanobetti A, Schwartz J. Air pollution and emergency admissions in Boston, MA. J Epidemiol Community Health 2006; 60:890.
50. Ballester F, et al. Air pollution and cardiovascular admissions association in Spain: results within the EMECAS project. J Epidemiol Community Health 2006; 60:328.
51. Dominici F, et al. Fine particulate air pollution and hospital admission for cardiovascular and respiratory diseases. JAMA 2006; 295:1127.
52. Le Tertre A, et al. Short-term effects of particulate air pollution on cardiovascular diseases in eight European cities. J Epidemiol Community Health 2002; 56:773.
53. Metzger KB, et al. Ambient air pollution and cardiovascular emergency department visits. Epidemiology 2004; 15:46.
54. Samet JM, et al. The National Morbidity, Mortality, and Air Pollution Study. Part II: Morbidity and mortality from air pollution in the United States. Res Rep Health Eff Inst 2000; 94:5.
55. Schwartz J, Morris R. Air pollution and hospital admissions for cardiovascular disease in Detroit, Michigan. Am J Epidemiol 1995; 142:23.
56. Schwartz J. Air pollution and hospital admissions for cardiovascular disease in Tucson. Epidemiology 1997; 8:371.
57. Schwartz J. Air pollution and hospital admissions for heart disease in eight U.S. counties. Epidemiology 1999; 10:17.
58. Zanobetti A, Schwartz J, Dockery DW. Airborne particles are a risk factor for hospital admissions for heart and lung disease. Environ Health Perspect 2000; 108:1071.
59. Analitis A, et al. Short-term effects of ambient particles on cardiovascular and respiratory mortality. Epidemiology 2006; 17:230.
60. Kwon HJ, et al. Effects of ambient air pollution on daily mortality in a cohort of patients with congestive heart failure. Epidemiology 2001; 12:413.
61. Omori T, et al. Effects of particulate matter on daily mortality in 13 Japanese cities. J Epidemiol 2003; 13:314.
62. Brunekreef B. Air pollution and life expectancy: is there a relation? Occup Environ Med 1997; 54:781.

63. Nevalainen J, Pekkanen J. The effect of particulate air pollution on life expectancy. Sci Total Environ 1998; 217:137.
64. Rabl A. Interpretation of air pollution mortality: number of deaths or years of life lost? J Air Waste Manag Assoc 2003; 53:41.
65. Dockery DW, et al. An association between air pollution and mortality in six U.S. cities. N Engl J Med 1993; 329:1753.
66. Miller KA, et al. Long-term exposure to air pollution and incidence of cardiovascular events in women. N Engl J Med 2007; 356:447.
67. Pope CA 3rd, et al. Particulate air pollution as a predictor of mortality in a prospective study of U.S. adults. Am J Respir Crit Care Med 1995; 151:669.
68. Pope CA 3rd, et al. Cardiovascular mortality and long-term exposure to particulate air pollution: epidemiological evidence of general pathophysiological pathways of disease. Circulation 2004; 109:71.
69. Pope CA 3rd, et al. Lung cancer, cardiopulmonary mortality, and long-term exposure to fine particulate air pollution. JAMA 2002; 287:1132.
70. Samet JM, et al. Fine particulate air pollution and mortality in 20 U.S. cities, 1987 to 1994. N Engl J Med 2000; 343:1742.
71. World Health Organization Working Group. Health aspects of air pollution with particulate matter, ozone and nitrogen dioxide. World Health Organization, Copenhagen, Denmark, 2003.
72. Laden F, et al. Reduction in fine particulate air pollution and mortality: Extended follow-up of the Harvard Six Cities study. Am J Respir Crit Care Med 2006; 173:667.
73. Clancy L, et al. Effect of air-pollution control on death rates in Dublin, Ireland: an intervention study. Lancet 2002; 360:1210.
74. Ayres JG. Cardiovascular disease and air pollution. Presented as a report by the Committee on the Medical Effects of Air Pollutants, United Kingdom, Department of Health, February 2006.
75. World Health Organization Regional Office for Europe. Carbon monoxide. In: WHO Air Quality Guidelines. 2nd ed. Copenhagen, Denmark: WHO, 2000: chap. 5.5.
76. Thompson N, Henry JA. Carbon monoxide poisoning: poisons unit experience over five years. Hum Toxicol 1983; 2:335.
77. Riojas-Rodriguez H, et al. Personal PM2.5 and CO exposures and heart rate variability in subjects with known ischemic heart disease in Mexico City. J Expo Sci Environ Epidemiol 2006; 16:131.
78. Allred EN, et al. Short-term effects of carbon monoxide exposure on the exercise performance of subjects with coronary artery disease. N Engl J Med 1989; 321:1426.
79. Allred EN, et al. Effects of carbon monoxide on myocardial ischemia. Environ Health Perspect 1991; 91:89.
80. Kleinman MT, et al. Effects of short-term exposure to carbon monoxide in subjects with coronary artery disease. Arch Environ Health 1989; 44:361.
81. Wittenberg BA, Wittenberg JB. Effects of carbon monoxide on isolated heart muscle cells. Res Rep Health Eff Inst 1993; 62:1.
82. McFaul SJ, McGrath JJ. Studies on the mechanism of carbon monoxide-induced vasodilation in the isolated perfused rat heart. Toxicol Appl Pharmacol 1987; 87:464.
83. McGrath JJ, Martin LG. Effects of carbon monoxide on isolated heart muscle. Proc Soc Exp Biol Med 1978; 157:681.

84. Klebs E. Uber die Wirkung des Kohlenoxyds auf den thierische Organismus. Virchows Arch Pathol Anat Physiol 1865; 32:450.
85. Anderson RF, Allensworth DC, DeGroot WJ. Myocardial toxicity from carbon monoxide poisoning. Ann Intern Med 1967; 67:1172.
86. Fineschi V, et al. Myocardial findings in fatal carbon monoxide poisoning: a human and experimental morphometric study. Int J Legal Med 2000; 113:276.
87. Kjeldsen K, Thomsen HK, Astrup P. Effects of carbon monoxide on myocardium. Ultrastructural changes in rabbits after moderate, chronic exposure. Circ Res 1974; 34:339.
88. Penney DG, Barthel BG, Skoney JA. Cardiac compliance and dimensions in carbon monoxide-induced cardiomegaly. Cardiovasc Res 1984; 18:270.
89. Takahashi K. Cardiac disturbances due to CO poisoning in experimental animals. I. Electrocardiographic changes due to CO poisoning and those under the influences of fluid infusion. Tohoku J Exp Med 1961; 74:211.
90. Einzig S, Nicoloff DM, Lucas RV Jr. Myocardial perfusion abnormalities in carbon monoxide poisoned dogs. Can J Physiol Pharmacol 1980; 58:396.
91. Kleinert HD, Scales JL, Weiss HR. Effects of carbon monoxide or low oxygen gas mixture inhalation on regional oxygenation, blood flow, and small vessel blood content of the rabbit heart. Pflugers Arch 1980; 383:105.
92. Erickson HH, Buckhold DK. Coronary blood flow and myocardial function during exposure to 100 ppm carbon monoxide. Physiologist 1972; 15:128.
93. James WE, Tucker CE, Grover RF. Cardiac function in goats exposed to carbon monoxide. J Appl Physiol 1979; 47:429.
94. Wittenberg BA, Wittenberg JB, Myoglobin-mediated oxygen delivery to mitochondria of isolated cardiac myocytes. Proc Natl Acad Sci U S A 1987; 84:7503.
95. Patel AP, et al. Carbon monoxide exposure in rat heart: evidence for two modes of toxicity. Biochem Biophys Res Commun 2004; 321:241.
96. Patel AP, et al. Carbon monoxide exposure in rat heart: glutathione depletion is prevented by antioxidants. Biochem Biophys Res Commun 2003; 302:392.
97. Dulchavsky SA, et al. Effects of deferoxamine on H2O2-induced oxidative stress in isolated rat heart. Basic Res Cardiol 1996; 91:418.
98. Onodera T, et al. Effect of exogenous hydrogen peroxide on myocardial function and structure in isolated rat heart. Can J Cardiol 1992; 8:989.
99. Harrison GJ, Jordan LR, Willis RJ. Deleterious effects of hydrogen peroxide on the function and ultrastructure of cardiac muscle and the coronary vasculature of perfused rat hearts. Can J Cardiol 1994; 10:843.
100. Maines MD. The heme oxygenase system: a regulator of second messenger gases. Annu Rev Pharmacol Toxicol 1997; 37:517.
101. Thom SR, et al. Role of nitric oxide-derived oxidants in vascular injury from carbon monoxide in the rat. Am J Physiol 1999; 276:H984.
102. Haggard HW. Studies in carbon monoxide asphyxia: I. The behavior of the heart. Am J Physiol 1921; 56:390.
103. Wieland H. Experimental research on the problem of carbon monoxide and oxygen deficiency. Zentralblatt Arbeitsmedizin Arbeitsschutz Erogon 1956; 6:77.
104. Mikiskova H, Frantik E. Animal model of cardiotoxicity: carbon monoxide induced ECG hypoxia masked in light narcosis. Act Nerv Super (Praha) 1987; 29:274.
105. Ehrich WE, Bellet S, Lewey FH. Cardiac changes from CO poisoning. Am J Med Sci 1944; 208:511.

106. Preziosi TJ, et al. An experimental investigation in animals of the functional and morphologic effects of single and repeated exposures to high and low concentrations of carbon monoxide. Ann N Y Acad Sci 1970; 174:369.
107. Swann HG, Brucher M. The cardiorespiratory and biochemical events during rapid anoxic death; carbon monoxide poisoning. Tex Rep Biol Med 1949; 7:569.
108. Beck HG, Suter GM. Role of carbon monoxide in causation of myocardial disease. JAMA 1938; 11:1982.
109. Stearns WH, Drinker CK, Shaughnessy TJ. The electrocardiographic changes found in 22 cases of carbon monoxide (illuminating gas) poisoning. Am Heart J 1938; 15: 434.
110. Middleton GD, Ashby DW, Clark F. Delayed and longlasting electrocardiographic changes in carbon-monoxide poisoning. Lancet 1961; 1:12.
111. Davies DM, Smith DJ. Electrocardiographic changes in healthy men during continuous low-level carbon monoxide exposure. Environ Res 1980; 21:197.
112. Colvin LT. Electrocardiographic changes in a case of severe carbon monoxide poisoning. Am Heart J 1928; 3:484.
113. Jaffe N. Cardiac injury and carbon monoxide poisoning. S Afr Med J 1965; 39:611.
114. McMeekin JD, Finegan BA. Reversible myocardial dysfunction following carbon monoxide poisoning. Can J Cardiol 1987; 3:118.
115. Carnevali R, et al. Electrocardiographic changes in acute carbon monoxide poisoning. Minerva Med 1987; 78:175.
116. Cosby RS, Bergeron M. Electrocardiographic changes in carbon monoxide poisoning. Am J Cardiol 1963; 11:93.
117. Shafer N, Smilay MG, MacMillam FP. Primary myocardial disease in man resulting from acute carbon monoxide poisoning. Am J Med 1965; 38:316.
118. Corya BC, Black MJ, McHenry PL. Echocardiographic findings after acute carbon monoxide poisoning. Br Heart J 1976; 38:712.
119. Kalay N, Ozdogru I, Cetinkaya Y, et al. Cardiovascular effects of carbon monoxide poisoning. Am J Cardiol 2007; 99:322.
120. Satran D, et al. Cardiovascular manifestations of moderate to severe carbon monoxide poisoning. J Am Coll Cardiol 2005; 45:1513.
121. Henry CR, et al. Myocardial injury and long-term mortality following moderate to severe carbon monoxide poisoning. JAMA 2006; 295:398.
122. Hosseinpoor AR, et al. Air pollution and hospitalization due to angina pectoris in Tehran, Iran: a time-series study. Environ Res 2005; 99:126.
123. Burnett RT, et al. Association between ambient carbon monoxide levels and hospitalizations for congestive heart failure in the elderly in 10 Canadian cities. Epidemiology 1997; 8:162.
124. Yang W, Jennison BL, Omaye ST. Cardiovascular disease hospitalization and ambient levels of carbon monoxide. J Toxicol Environ Health A 1998; 55:185.
125. Hexter AC. Ambient carbon monoxide and hospitalizations for heart failure: earlier findings. Am J Public Health 1996; 86:1031.
126. Morris RD, Naumova EN, Munasinghe RL. Ambient air pollution and hospitalization for congestive heart failure among elderly people in seven large US cities. Am J Public Health 1995; 85:1361.
127. Stern FB, et al. Heart disease mortality among bridge and tunnel officers exposed to carbon monoxide. Am J Epidemiol 1988; 128:1276.

128. Koskela RS, et al. Factors predictive of ischemic heart disease mortality in foundry workers exposed to carbon monoxide. Am J Epidemiol 2000; 152:628.

129. Bye T, et al. Health survey of former workers in a Norwegian coke plant: Part 2. Cancer incidence and cause specific mortality. Occup Environ Med 1998; 55:622.

130. Wickramatillake HD, Gun RT, Ryan P. Carbon monoxide exposures in Australian workplaces could precipitate myocardial ischaemia in smoking workers with coronary artery disease. Aust N Z J Public Health 1998; 22(3 suppl.):389.

131. Kittelson DB. Engines and nanoparticles: a review. J Aerosol Sci 1998; 29:575.

132. Mauderly JL. Toxicological and epidemiological evidence for health risks from inhaled engine emissions. Environ Health Perspect 1994; 102(suppl. 4):165.

133. World Health Organization, Diesel Fuel and Exhaust Emissions, Geneva, Switzerland, 1996.

134. Mauderly JL. Diesel exhaust. In: Lippmann M, ed. Environmental Toxicants. Human Exposures and Their Health Effects. New York, NY: Van Nostrand Reinhold Company, 1992:119.

135. California Air Resources Board. Emission Inventory 1995. Technical Support Division, Sacramento, CA, 1997.

136. National Toxicology Program. Diesel exhaust particulates. Rep Carcinog 2002; 10:94.

137. Centers for Disease Control, Publication of NIOSH Current Intelligence Bulletin on carcinogenic effects of diesel exhaust. MMWR Morb Mortal Wkly Rep 1989; 38:76.

138. Rogers A. Whelan B. Exposures in Australian mines. In: HEI Communication No.7—Diesel Workshop: Building a Research Strategy to Improve Risk Assessment (Stone Mountain, GA). Cambridge, MA: Health Effects Institute, 1999.

139. Saverin R, et al. Diesel exhaust and lung cancer mortality in potash mining. Am J Ind Med 1999; 36:415.

140. United States Environmental Protection Agency. Health Assessment Document for Diesel Engine Exhaust. Washington, DC: EPA, 2002.

141. Waller RE, Commins BT, Lawther PJ. Air pollution in road tunnels. Br J Ind Med 1961; 18:250.

142. Penney DG, et al. A study of heart and blood of rodents inhaling diesel engine exhaust particulates. Environ Res 1981; 26:453.

143. Vallyathan V, et al. Effect of diesel emissions and coal dust inhalation on heart and pulmonary arteries of rats. J Toxicol Environ Health 1986; 19:33.

144. Wiester MJ, Iltis R, Moore W. Altered function and histology in guinea pigs after inhalation of diesel exhaust. Environ Res 1980; 22:285.

145. Kyoso M, et al. Influence of exposure to diesel emissions in rats and distribution profile for R-R interval. Conf Proc IEEE Eng Med Biol Soc 2005; 5:5544.

146. Nemmar A, et al. Cardiovascular and lung inflammatory effects induced by systemically administered diesel exhaust particles in rats. Am J Physiol Lung Cell Mol Physiol 2006; 292(3):L664. [Epub ahead of print].

147. Nemmar A, et al. Diesel exhaust particles in lung acutely enhance experimental peripheral thrombosis. Circulation 2003; 107:1202.

148. Nemmar A, et al. Pharmacological stabilization of mast cells abrogates late thrombotic events induced by diesel exhaust particles in hamsters. Circulation 2004; 110:1670.

149. Nemmar A, et al. Pulmonary inflammation and thrombogenicity caused by diesel particles in hamsters: role of histamine. Am J Respir Crit Care Med 2003; 168:1366.

150. Gurgueira SA, et al. Rapid increases in the steady-state concentration of reactive oxygen species in the lungs and heart after particulate air pollution inhalation. Environ Health Perspect 2002; 110:749.

151. Rhoden CR, et al. PM-induced cardiac oxidative stress and dysfunction are mediated by autonomic stimulation. Biochim Biophys Acta 2005; 1725:305.

152. Toda N, et al. Effects of diesel exhaust particles on blood pressure in rats. J Toxicol Environ Health A 2001; 63:429.

153. United States Environmental Protection Agency. Diesel engine exhaust (CASRN N.A.). Integrated Risk Information System. Washington, DC: EPA, 2003.

154. Sakakibara M, et al. Biological effects of diesel exhaust particles (DEP) on isolated cardiac muscle of guinea pigs. Res Commun Mol Pathol Pharmacol 1994; 86:99.

155. Anselme F, et al. Inhalation of diluted diesel engine emission impacts heart rate variability and arrhythmia occurrence in a rat model of chronic ischemic heart failure. Arch Toxicol 2006. [Epub ahead of print].

156. Wellenius GA, et al. Cardiac effects of carbon monoxide and ambient particles in a rat model of myocardial infarction. Toxicol Sci 2004; 80:367.

157. Campen MJ, et al. Cardiovascular effects of inhaled diesel exhaust in spontaneously hypertensive rats. Cardiovasc Toxicol 2003; 3:353.

158. Yokota S, et al. Delayed exacerbation of acute myocardial ischemia/reperfusion-induced arrhythmia by tracheal instillation of diesel exhaust particles. Inhal Toxicol 2004; 16:319.

159. Fantone JC, Ward PA. Role of oxygen-derived free radicals and metabolites in leukocyte-dependent inflammatory reactions. Am J Pathol 1982; 107:395.

160. Dhein S, et al. The contribution of neutrophils to reperfusion arrhythmias and a possible role for antiadhesive pharmacological substances. Cardiovasc Res 1995; 30:881.

161. Shen YC, Chen CF, Sung YJ. Tetrandrine ameliorates ischaemia-reperfusion injury of rat myocardium through inhibition of neutrophil priming and activation. Br J Pharmacol 1999; 128:1593.

162. Okayama Y, et al. Role of reactive oxygen species on diesel exhaust particle-induced cytotoxicity in rat cardiac myocytes. J Toxicol Environ Health A 2006; 69:1699.

163. Bai Y, Suzuki AK, Sagai M. The cytotoxic effects of diesel exhaust particles on human pulmonary artery endothelial cells in vitro: role of active oxygen species. Free Radic Biol Med 2001; 30:555.

164. Tobias HJ, et al. Chemical analysis of diesel engine nanoparticles using a nano-DMA/thermal desorption particle beam mass spectrometer. Environ Sci Technol 2001; 35:2233.

165. Hirano S, et al. Oxidative-stress potency of organic extracts of diesel exhaust and urban fine particles in rat heart microvessel endothelial cells. Toxicology 2003; 187:161.

166. Minami M, et al. Electrocardiographic changes induced by diesel exhaust particles (DEP) in guinea pigs. Res Commun Mol Pathol Pharmacol 1999; 105:67.

167. Campen MJ, et al. Nonparticulate components of diesel exhaust promote constriction in coronary arteries from ApoE-/- mice. Toxicol Sci 2005; 88:95.

168. Mills NL, et al. Diesel exhaust inhalation causes vascular dysfunction and impaired endogenous fibrinolysis. Circulation 2005; 112:3930.

169. Kim S, Shen S, Sioutas C. Size distribution and diurnal and seasonal trends of ultrafine particles in source and receptor sites of the Los Angeles basin. J Air Waste Manag Assoc 2002; 52:297.

170. Shi JP, et al. Sources and concentration of nanoparticles (<10 nm diameter) in the urban atmosphere. Atmos Environ 2001; 35:1193.

171. Delfino RJ, Sioutas C, Malik S. Potential role of ultrafine particles in associations between airborne particle mass and cardiovascular health. Environ Health Perspect 2005; 113:934.

172. Edling C, Axelson O. Risk factors of coronary heart disease among personnel in a bus company. Int Arch Occup Environ Health 1984; 54:181.

173. Finkelstein MM, et al. Ischemic heart disease mortality among heavy equipment operators. Am J Ind Med 2004; 46:16.

174. Toren K, et al. Occupational exposure to particulate air pollution and mortality due to ischemic heart disease and cerebrovascular disease. Occup Environ Med 2007; [Epub ahead of print].

175. Cannon RO 3rd. Role of nitric oxide in cardiovascular disease: focus on the endothelium. Clin Chem 1998; 44:1809.

176. Chowdhary S, Townend JN. Role of nitric oxide in the regulation of cardiovascular autonomic control. Clin Sci (Lond) 1999; 97:5.

177. Balbatun A, Louka FR, Malinski T. Dynamics of nitric oxide release in the cardiovascular system. Acta Biochim Pol 2003; 50:61.

178. Jugdutt BI. Nitric oxide and cardiovascular protection. Heart Fail Rev 2003; 8:29.

179. Cengel A, Sahinarslan A. Nitric oxide and cardiovascular system. Anadolu Kardiyol Derg 2006; 6:364.

180. Troncy E, Francoeur M, Blaise G. Inhaled nitric oxide: clinical applications, indications, and toxicology. Can J Anaesth 1997; 44:973.

181. World Health Organization Regional Office for Europe. Nitrogen dioxide. In: WHO Air Quality Guidelines. 2nd ed. Copenhagen, Denmark: WHO, 2000: chap 7.1.

182. Hayward CS, Kelly RP, Macdonald PS. Inhaled nitric oxide in cardiology practice. Cardiovasc Res 1999; 43:628.

183. Abraham WM, et al. Cardiopulmonary effects of short-term nitrogen dioxide exposure in conscious sheep. Environ Res 1980; 22:61.

184. Tsubone H, et al. Alteration of cardiac function in rats acutely exposed to nitrogen dioxide. Nippon Eiseigaku Zasshi 1981; 36:550.

185. Tsubone H, et al. Electrocardiographic abnormalities in rats by acute exposure to nitrogen dioxide. Toxicol Lett 1982; 12:125.

186. Tsubone H, et al. Changes of cardiac and respiratory rhythm in non- and tracheostomized rats exposed to nitrogen dioxide. Environ Res 1984; 35:197.

187. Agency for Toxic Substances and Disease Registry. Medical Management Guidelines for Nitrogen Oxides. Atlanta, GA: ATSDR, 2007.

188. Folinsbee LJ, et al. Effect of 0.62 ppm NO2 on cardiopulmonary function in young male nonsmokers. Environ Res 1978; 15:199.

189. Linn WS, et al. Effects of exposure to 4 ppm nitrogen dioxide in healthy and asthmatic volunteers. Arch Environ Health 1985; 40:234.

190. Ruidavets JB, et al. Increased resting heart rate with pollutants in a population based study. J Epidemiol Community Health 2005; 59:685.

191. Chan CC, et al. Association between nitrogen dioxide and heart rate variability in a susceptible population. Eur J Cardiovasc Prev Rehabil 2005; 12:580.

192. Wong TW, et al. Associations between daily mortalities from respiratory and cardiovascular diseases and air pollution in Hong Kong, China. Occup Environ Med 2002; 59:30.

193. Lee JT, et al. Air pollution and hospital admissions for ischemic heart diseases among individuals 64+ years of age residing in Seoul, Korea. Arch Environ Health 2003; 58:617.

194. Grazuleviciene R, et al. Exposure to urban nitrogen dioxide pollution and the risk of myocardial infarction. Scand J Work Environ Health 2004; 30:293.

195. Nafstad P, et al. Urban air pollution and mortality in a cohort of Norwegian men. Environ Health Perspect 2004; 112:610.

196. Maheswaran R, et al. Outdoor air pollution, mortality, and hospital admissions from coronary heart disease in Sheffield, UK: a small-area level ecological study. Eur Heart J 2005; 26:2543.

197. Rosenlund M, et al. Long-term exposure to urban air pollution and myocardial infarction. Epidemiology 2006; 17:383.

198. Naess O, et al. Relation between concentration of air pollution and cause-specific mortality: four-year exposures to nitrogen dioxide and particulate matter pollutants in 470 neighborhoods in Oslo, Norway. Am J Epidemiol 2007; 165:435.

199. Poloniecki JD, et al. Daily time series for cardiovascular hospital admissions and previous day's air pollution in London, UK. Occup Environ Med 1997; 54:535.

200. World Health Organization Regional Office for Europe. Ozone and other photochemical oxidants. In: WHO Air Quality Guidelines. 2nd ed., Copenhagen, Denmark: WHO, 2000.

201. Canadian Centre for Occupational Health and Safety. Basic information on ozone. OSH Answers. February 19, 1999. Available at: http://www.ccohs.ca/oshanswers/chemicals/chem_profiles/ozone/basic_ozo.html.

202. Rahman I, Massaro GD, Massaro D. Exposure of rats to ozone: evidence of damage to heart and brain. Free Radic Biol Med 1992; 12:323.

203. Kelly FJ, Birch S. Ozone exposure inhibits cardiac protein synthesis in the mouse. Free Radic Biol Med 1993; 14:443.

204. Zychlinskim L, et al. Age-related difference in bioenergetics of lung and heart mitochondrial from rats exposed to ozone. J Biochem Toxicol 1989; 4:251.

205. Watkinson WP, et al. Acute effects of ozone on heart rate and body temperature in the unanesthetized, unrestrained rat maintained at different ambient temperatures. Inhal Toxicol 1993; 5:129.

206. Arito H, et al. Ozone-induced bradycardia and arrhythmia and their relation to sleep-wakefulness in rats. Toxicol Lett 1990; 52:169.

207. Arito H, et al. Age-related changes in ventilatory and heart rate responses to acute ozone exposure in the conscious rat. Ind Health 1997; 35:78.

208. Arito H, Uchiyama I, Yokoyama E. Acute effects of ozone on EEG activity, sleep-wakefulness and heart rate in rats. Ind Health 1992; 30:23.

209. Uchiyama I, Simomura Y, Yokoyama E. Effects of acute exposure to ozone on heart rate and blood pressure of the conscious rat. Environ Res 1986; 41:529.

210. Iwasaki T, et al. Adaptation of extrapulmonary responses to ozone exposure in conscious rats. Ind Health 1998; 36:57.

211. Watkinson WP, Wiester MJ, Highfill JW. Ozone toxicity in the rat. I. Effect of changes in ambient temperature on extrapulmonary physiological parameters. J Appl Physiol 1995; 78:1108.

212. Uchiyama I, Yokoyama E. Effects of short- and long-term exposure to ozone on heart rate and blood pressure of emphysematous rats. Environ Res 1989; 48:76.

213. Superko HR, Adams WC, Daly PW. Effects of ozone inhalation during exercise in selected patients with heart disease. Am J Med 1984; 77:463.
214. Gong H Jr., et al. Cardiovascular effects of ozone exposure in human volunteers. Am J Respir Crit Care Med 1998; 158:538.
215. Rich DQ, et al. Association of short-term ambient air pollution concentrations and ventricular arrhythmias. Am J Epidemiol 2005; 161:1123.
216. Rich DQ, et al. Increased risk of paroxysmal atrial fibrillation episodes associated with acute increases in ambient air pollution. Environ Health Perspect 2006; 114:120.
217. Ruidavets JB, et al. Ozone air pollution is associated with acute myocardial infarction. Circulation 2005; 111:563.
218. Brook RD, et al. Air pollution and cardiovascular disease: a statement for healthcare professionals from the Expert Panel on Population and Prevention Science of the American Heart Association. Circulation 2004; 109:2655.
219. International Agency for Research on Cancer. Sulfur dioxide and some sulfites, bisulfites and metabisulfites (Group 3). IARC Summaries and Evaluations 1992; 54:131.
220. Yao X, et al. Use of stationary and mobile measurements to study power plant emissions. J Air Waste Manag Assoc 2006; 56:144.
221. Shapiro R. Genetic effects of bisulfite (sulfur dioxide). Mutat Res 1977; 39:149.
222. Meng Z, Li R, Zhang X. Levels of sulfite in three organs from mice exposed to sulfur dioxide. Inhal Toxicol 2005; 17:309.
223. Fedde MR, Kuhlmann WD. Cardiopulmonary responses to inhaled sulfur dioxide in the chicken. Poult Sci 1979; 58:1584.
224. Meng Z, et al. Blood pressure of rats lowered by sulfur dioxide and its derivatives. Inhal Toxicol 2003; 15:951.
225. Hearse DJ, Tosaki A. Free radicals and reperfusion-induced arrhythmias: protection by spin trap agent PBN in the rat heart. Circ Res 1987; 60:375.
226. Haider SS. Effects of exhaust pollutant sulfur dioxide on lipid metabolism of guinea pig organs. Ind Health 1985; 23:81.
227. Meng Z, et al. Oxidative damage of sulfur dioxide inhalation on lungs and hearts of mice. Environ Res 2003; 93:285.
228. Meng Z. Oxidative damage of sulfur dioxide on various organs of mice: sulfur dioxide is a systemic oxidative damage agent. Inhal Toxicol 2003; 15:181.
229. Nie A, Meng Z. Sulfur dioxide derivative modulation of potassium channels in rat ventricular myocytes. Arch Biochem Biophys 2005; 442:187.
230. Nie A, Meng Z. Study of the interaction of sulfur dioxide derivative with cardiac sodium channel. Biochim Biophys Acta 2005; 1718:67.
231. Nie A, Meng Z. Modulation of L-type calcium current in rat cardiac myocytes by sulfur dioxide derivatives. Food Chem Toxicol 2006; 44:355.
232. Amdur MO, Melvin WW Jr., Drinker P. Effects of inhalation of sulphur dioxide by man. Lancet 1953; 265:758.
233. Routledge HC, et al. Effect of inhaled sulphur dioxide and carbon particles on heart rate variability and markers of inflammation and coagulation in human subjects. Heart 2006; 92:220.
234. Ibald-Mulli A, et al. Effects of air pollution on blood pressure: a population-based approach. Am J Public Health 2001; 91:571.
235. Dockery DW, et al. Particulate air pollution and nonfatal cardiac events. Part I. Air pollution, personal activities, and onset of myocardial infarction in a case-crossover study. Particulate air pollution and nonfatal cardiac events. Part II. Association of

air pollution with confirmed arrhythmias recorded by implanted defibrillators. Rep Health Eff Inst 2005; 124:83.

236. Sarnat SE, et al. Ambient particulate air pollution and cardiac arrhythmia in a panel of older adults in Steubenville, Ohio. Occup Environ Med 2006; 63:700.

237. Vedal S, et al. Air pollution and cardiac arrhythmias in patients with implantable cardioverter defibrillators. Inhal Toxicol 2004; 16:353.

238. Ballester F, et al. The EMECAM project: a multicentre study on air pollution and mortality in Spain: combined results for particulates and for sulfur dioxide. Occup Environ Med 2002; 59:300.

239. Ciccone G, Faggiano F, Falasca P. SO2 air pollution and hospital admissions in Ravenna: a case-control study. Epidemiol Prev 1995; 19:99.

240. Fung KY, et al. Air pollution and daily hospital admissions for cardiovascular diseases in Windsor, Ontario. Can J Public Health 2005; 96:29.

241. Krewski D, et al. Overview of the reanalysis of the Harvard Six Cities Study and American Cancer Society Study of Particulate Air Pollution and Mortality. J Toxicol Environ Health A 2003; 66:1507.

242. Sharovsky R, Cesar LA, Ramires JA. Temperature, air pollution, and mortality from myocardial infarction in Sao Paulo, Brazil. Braz J Med Biol Res 2004; 37:1651.

243. Sunyer J, et al. The association of daily sulfur dioxide air pollution levels with hospital admissions for cardiovascular diseases in Europe (The Aphea-II study). Eur Heart J 2003; 24:752.

244. Venners S, et al. Particulate matter, sulfur dioxide, and daily mortality in Chongqing, China. Environ Health Perspect 2003; 111:562.

245. Wong TW, et al. Air pollution and hospital admissions for respiratory and cardiovascular diseases in Hong Kong. Occup Environ Med 1999; 56:679.

246. Hedley AJ, et al. Cardiorespiratory and all-cause mortality after restrictions on sulphur content of fuel in Hong Kong: an intervention study. Lancet 2002; 360:1646.

247. Englander V, et al. Mortality and cancer morbidity in workers exposed to sulphur dioxide in a sulphuric acid plant. Int Arch Occup Environ Health 1988; 61:157.

248. Jappinen P, Tola S. Cardiovascular mortality among pulp mill workers. Br J Ind Med 1990; 47:259.

249. Hammar N, et al. Differences in the incidence of myocardial infarction among occupational groups. Scand J Work Environ Health 1992; 18:178.

250. Hoffman GL, Duce RA, Zoller WH. Vanadium copper, and aluminum in the lower atmosphere between California and Hawaii. Environ Sci Technol 1969; 3:1207.

251. Sorenson JR, et al. Aluminum in the environment and human health. Environ Health Perspect 1974; 8:3.

252. Agency for Toxic Substances and Disease Registry. Toxicological Profile for Aluminum. Atlanta, GA: ATSDR, September 2006.

253. Miller RG, et al. The occurrence of aluminum in drinking water. J Am Water Works Assoc 1984; 76:84.

254. Zatta P, et al. A neutral lipophilic compound of aluminum(III) as a cause of myocardial infarct in the rabbit. Toxicol Lett 1987; 39:185.

255. Bertholf RF, et al. Measurement of lipid peroxidation products in rabbit brain and organs (response to aluminum exposure). Ann Clin Lab Sci 1987; 17:418.

256. Corain B, et al. Cardiotoxicity of the lipophilic compound aluminum acetylacetonate in rabbits. Biomed Environ Sci 1988; 1:283.

257. Bombi GG, et al. Experimental aluminum pathology in rabbits: effects of hydrophilic and lipophilic compounds. Environ Health Perspect 1990; 89:217.
258. Gomes MG, et al. Effects of aluminum on the mechanical and electrical activity of the Langendorff-perfused rat heart. Braz J Med Biol Res 1994; 27:95.
259. Roth A, et al. Multiorgan aluminium deposits in a chronic haemodialysis patient. Electron microscope and microprobe studies. Virchows Arch A Pathol Anat Histopathol 1984; 405:131.
260. London GM, et al. Association between aluminum accumulation and cardiac hypertrophy in hemodialyzed patients. Am J Kidney Dis 1989; 13:75.
261. McCallum RI. Occupational exposure to antimony compounds. J Environ Monit 2005; 7:1245.
262. Cavallo D, et al. Genotoxic risk and oxidative DNA damage in workers exposed to antimony trioxide. Environ Mol Mutagen 2002; 40:184.
263. Wiersema JM, et al. Human exposure to potentially toxic elements through ambient air in Texas. Proc Air Pollut Contr Assoc 1984; 1:84.
264. Winship KA. Toxicity of antimony and its compounds. Adverse Drug React Acute Poisoning Rev 1987; 2:67.
265. Brieger H, et al. Industrial antimony poisoning. Ind Med Surg 1954; 23:521.
266. Cotten MD, Logan ME. Effects of antimony on the cardiovascular system and intestinal smooth muscle. J Pharmacol Exp Ther 1966; 151:7.
267. Alvarez M, et al. Antimony-induced cardiomyopathy in guinea-pig and protection by L-carnitine. Br J Pharmacol 2005; 144:17.
268. Toraason M, et al. Altered Ca2+ mobilization during excitation-contraction in cultured cardiac myocytes exposed to antimony. Toxicol Appl Pharmacol 1997; 146:104.
269. Kuryshev YA, et al. Antimony-based antileishmanial compounds prolong the cardiac action potential by an increase in cardiac calcium currents. Mol Pharmacol 2006; 69:1216.
270. Dancaster CP, Duckworth WC, Matthews REP. Stokes-Adams attacks following sodium antimonylgluconate (Triostam). S Afr Med J 1966; 7:99.
271. Pandey AK, Kumar M, Thakur CP. ECG changes in prolonged treatment of kala-azar with antimony compounds. J Assoc Physicians India 1988; 36:398.
272. Frustaci A, et al. Marked elevation of myocardial trace elements in idiopathic dilated cardiomyopathy compared with secondary cardiac dysfunction. J Am Coll Cardiol 1999; 33:1578.
273. Sundar S, et al. A cluster of cases of severe cardiotoxicity among kala-azar patients treated with a high-osmolarity lot of sodium antimony gluconate. Am J Trop Med Hyg 1998; 59:139.
274. Jarup L. Hazards of heavy metal contamination. Br Med Bull 2003; 68:167.
275. National Institute for Occupational Safety and Health. National Occupational Exposure Survey, Cincinnati, OH: NIOSH, 1990.
276. Schroeder WH, et al. Toxic trace elements associated with airborne particulate matter: a review. JAPCA 1987; 37:1267.
277. National Academy of Sciences. Arsenic. Drinking water and health, Washington, DC: NAS, 1977.
278. Page GW. Comparison of groundwater and surface water for patterns and levels of contamination by toxic substances. Environ Sci Technol 1981; 15:1475.

279. Smith RA, Alexander RB, Wolman MG. Water-quality trends in the nation's rivers. Science 1987; 235:1607.
280. Welch AH, Lico MS, Hughes JL. Arsenic in groundwater of the western United States. Ground Water 1988; 26:333.
281. Agency for Toxic Substances and Disease Registry, Toxicological Profile for Arsenic. Atlanta, GA: ATSDR, September 2005.
282. Ficker E, et al. Mechanisms of arsenic-induced prolongation of cardiac repolarization. Mol Pharmacol 2004; 66:33.
283. Chiang CE, et al. Prolongation of cardiac repolarization by arsenic trioxide. Blood 2002; 100:2249.
284. Wu MH, et al. Direct cardiac effects of As$_2$O$_3$ in rabbits: evidence of reversible chronic toxicity and tissue accumulation of arsenicals after parenteral administration. Toxicol Appl Pharmacol 2003; 189:214.
285. Carmignani M, Boscolo P, Castellino N. Metabolic fate and cardiovascular effects of arsenic in rats and rabbits chronically exposed to trivalent and pentavalent arsenic. Arch Toxicol Suppl 1985; 8:452.
286. Wang CH, et al. Biological gradient between long-term arsenic exposure and carotid atherosclerosis. Circulation 2002; 105:1804.
287. Zierold KM, Knobeloch L, Anderson H. Prevalence of chronic diseases in adults exposed to arsenic-contaminated drinking water. Am J Public Health 2004; 94:1936.
288. Simeonova PP, Luster MI. Arsenic and atherosclerosis. Toxicol Appl Pharmacol 2004; 198:444.
289. Barchowsky A, et al. Arsenic induces oxidant stress and NF-kappa B activation in cultured aortic endothelial cells. Free Radic Biol Med 1996; 21:783.
290. Barchowsky A, et al. Stimulation of reactive oxygen, but not reactive nitrogen species, in vascular endothelial cells exposed to low levels of arsenite. Free Radic Biol Med 1999; 27:1405.
291. Hirano S, et al. Difference in uptake and toxicity of trivalent and pentavalent inorganic arsenic in rat heart microvessel endothelial cells. Arch Toxicol 2003; 77:305.
292. Tseng CH, et al. Long-term arsenic exposure and ischemic heart disease in arseniasis-hyperendemic villages in Taiwan. Toxicol Lett 2003; 137:15.
293. Wingren G, Axelson O. Mortality in the Swedish glassworks industry. Scand J Work Environ Health 1987; 13:412.
294. Tollestrup K. Mortality in a cohort of orchard workers exposed to lead arsenate pesticide spray. Arch Environ Health 1995; 50:221.
295. Reynolds ES. An account of the epidemic outbreak of arsenical poisoning occurring in beer drinkers in the North of England and the Midland counties in 1900. Lancet 1901; i:166.
296. Agency for Toxic Substances and Disease Registry, Toxicological Profile for Cadmium. Atlanta, GA: ATSDR, 1999.
297. Goyer RA. Toxic effects of metals. In: Klaasen CD, Amdur MO, Doull J, eds., Casarett and Doull's Toxicology: The Basic Science of Poisons. 5th ed. McGraw-Hill, 1996: chap. 23.
298. Singh BR. Trace element availability to plants in agricultural soils, with special emphasis on fertilizer imputs. Environ Rev 1994; 2:133.

299. United States Environmental Protection Agency, Cadmium contamination of the environment: an assessment of nationwide risk. United States Environmental Protection Agency, Office of Water Regulations and Standards, EPA-440/4-85-023, Washington, DC, 1985.
300. Kopp SJ, Hawley PL. Factors influencing cadmium toxicity in A-V conduction system of isolated perfused rat heart. Toxicol Appl Pharmacol 1976; 37:531.
301. Kopp SJ, Hawley PL. Cadmium feeding: apparent depression of atrioventricular-his-Purkinje conduction system. Acta Pharmacol Toxicol (Copenh) 1978; 42:110.
302. Kopp SJ, et al. Cardiovascular actions of cadmium at environmental exposure levels. Science 1982; 217:837.
303. DiFrancesco D, Ferroni A, Zaza A. Cadmium-induced blockade of the cardiac fast Na channels in calf Purkinje fibres. Proc R Soc Lond B Biol Sci 1985; 223:475.
304. Jamall IS, et al. A comparison of the effects of dietary cadmium on heart and kidney antioxidant enzymes: evidence for the greater vulnerability of the heart to cadmium toxicity. J Appl Toxicol 1989; 9:339.
305. Kisling GM, et al. Cadmium-induced attenuation of coronary blood flow in the perfused rat heart. Toxicol Appl Pharmacol 1993; 118:58.
306. Akahori F, et al. A nine-year chronic toxicity study of cadmium in monkeys. II. Effects of dietary cadmium on circulatory function, plasma cholesterol and triglyceride. Vet Hum Toxicol 1994; 36:290.
307. Toda N. Inhibition by cadmium ions of the electrical activity of sinoatrial nodal pacemaker fibers and their response to norepinephrine. J Pharmacol Exp Ther 1973; 184:357.
308. Toda N. Influence of cadmium ions on contractile response of isolated aortas to stimulatory agents. Am J Physiol 1973; 225:350.
309. Rifkin RJ. In vitro inhibition of Na+-K+ and Mg2+ ATPases by mono, di and trivalent cations. Proc Soc Exp Biol Med 1965; 120:802.
310. Rothstein A. Cell membrane as site of action of heavy metals. Fed Proc 1959; 18:1026.
311. Smith HM. Effects of sulfhydryl blockade on axonal function. J Cell Physiol 1958; 51:161.
312. Kleinfeld M, Stein E, Aguillardo D. Divalent cations on action potentials of dog heart. Am J Physiol 1966; 211:1438.
313. Prozialeck WC, Edwards JR, Woods JM. The vascular endothelium as a target of cadmium toxicity. Life Sci 2006; 79:1493.
314. Kopp SJ, et al. Electrocardiographical, biochemical and morphological effects of chronic low level cadmium feeding on the rat heart. Proc Soc Exp Biol Med 1978; 159:339.
315. Nakagawa H, et al. Urinary cadmium and mortality among inhabitants of a cadmium-polluted area in Japan. Environ Res 2006; 100:323.
316. Smetana RH, Glogar DH. Role of cadmium and magnesium in pathogenesis of idiopathic dilated cardiomyopathy. Am J Cardiol 1986; 58:364.
317. Agency for Toxic Substances and Disease Registry, Toxicological profile for cobalt, Atlanta, GA, April 2004.
318. Koponen M, Gustafsson T, Kalliomaki P-L. Cobalt in hard metal manufacturing dusts. Am Ind Hyg Assoc J 1982; 43:645.
319. Barceloux DG. Cobalt. J Toxicol Clin Toxicol 1999; 37:201.

320. Smith IC, Carson BL. Trace Metals in the Environment. Ann Arbor, MI: Ann Arbor Science Publishers, 1981.
321. Mohiuddin SM, et al. Experimental cobalt cardiomyopathy. Am Heart J 1970; 80:532.
322. Grice HC, et al. Myocardial toxicity of cobalt in the rat. Ann N Y Acad Sci 1969; 156:189.
323. Hall JL, Smith EB. Cobalt heart disease. An electron microscopic and histochemical study in the rabbit. Arch Pathol (Chic) 1968; 86:403.
324. Morvai V, et al. The effects of simultaneous alcohol and cobalt chloride administration on the cardiovascular system of rats. Acta Physiol Hung 1993; 81:253.
325. Clyne N, et al. Chronic cobalt exposure affects antioxidants and ATP production in rat myocardium. Scand J Clin Lab Invest 2001; 61:609.
326. Barborik M, Dusek J. Cardiomyopathy accompanying industrial cobalt exposure. Br Heart J 1972; 34:113.
327. Manifold IH, Platts MM, Kennedy A. Cobalt cardiomyopathy in a patient on maintenance haemodialysis. Br Med J 1978; 2:1609.
328. Kennedy A, Dornan JD, King R. Fatal myocardial disease associated with industrial exposure to cobalt. Lancet 1981; 1:412.
329. Jarvis JQ, et al. Cobalt cardiomyopathy. A report of two cases from mineral assay laboratories and a review of the literature. J Occup Med 1992; 34:620.
330. Seghizzi P, et al. Cobalt myocardiopathy. A critical review of literature. Sci Total Environ 1994; 150:105.
331. McDermott PH, et al. Myocardosis and cardiac failure in men. JAMA 1966; 198:163.
332. Bonenfant JL, Miller G, Roy PE. Quebec beer-drinkers' cardiomyopathy: pathological studies. Can Med Assoc 1967; 97:910.
333. Kesteloot H, et al. An enquiry into the role of cobalt in the heart disease of chronic beer drinkers. Circulation 1968; 37:854.
334. Morin Y, Tetu A, Mercier G. Cobalt cardiomyopathy: clinical aspects. Br Heart J 1971; 33:175.
335. Patrick L. Lead toxicity, a review of the literature. Part I: Exposure, evaluation, and treatment. Altern Med Rev 2006; 11:2.
336. National Institute for Occupational Safety and Health. NIOSH Pocket Guide to Chemical Hazards. Atlanta, GA: NIOSH, 2005.
337. Agency for Toxic Substances and Disease Registry. ATSDR's Hazardous Substance Release and Health Effects (HazDat) Database. Atlanta, GA: ATSDR April 13, 2005.
338. Farfel MR, Chisolm JJ Jr. An evaluation of experimental practices for abatement of residential lead-based paint: report on a pilot project. Environ Res 1991; 55:199.
339. McDonald JA, Potter NU. Lead's legacy? Early and late mortality of 454 lead-poisoned children. Arch Environ Health 1996; 51:116.
340. Centers for Disease Control and Prevention (CDC), Blood lead levels in residents of homes with elevated lead in tap water–District of Columbia, 2004. MMWR Morb Mortal Wkly Rep 2004; 53:268.
341. Asokan SK. Experimental lead cardiomyopathy: myocardial structural changes in rats given small amounts of lead. J Lab Clin Med 1974; 84:20.
342. Khan MY, Buse M, Louria DB. Lead cardiomyopathy in mice: a correlative ultrastructural and blood level study. Arch Pathol Lab 1977; 101:89.

343. Victery W, et al. Lead, hypertension, and the renin-angiotensin system in rats. J Lab Clin Med 1982; 99:354.
344. Perry HM, Erlanger MW, Perry EF. Increase in the blood pressure of rats chronically fed low levels of lead. Environ Health Perspect 1988; 78:107.
345. Nakhoul F, et al. Rapid hypertensinogenic effect of lead: studies in the spontaneously hypertensive rat. Toxicol Ind Health 1992; 8:89.
346. Carmignani M, et al. Kininergic system and arterial hypertension following chronic exposure to inorganic lead. Immunopharmacology 1999; 44:105.
347. Boscolo P, et al. Cardiovascular function and urinary kallikrein excretion in rats chronically exposed to mercury, arsenic, lead, cadmium or cadmium and lead. Acta Med Rom 1980; 18:211.
348. Boscolo P, et al. Urinary vanillylmandelic acid and kallikrein and cardiovascular parameters in rats chronically exposed to different toxic metals. Acta Med Rom 1985; 23:208.
349. Porcelli G, et al. Urinary kininase and kallikrein activities and cardiovascular function in rats chronically exposed to cadmium, lead or cadmium and lead. Agents Actions 1982; 9:413.
350. Staessen J, et al. Blood lead concentration, renal function, and blood pressure in London civil servants. Br J Ind Med 1990; 47:442.
351. Khalil-Manesh F, et al. Lead-induced hypertension: possible role of endothelial factors. Am J Hypertens 1993; 6:723.
352. Fenga C, et al. Relationship of blood lead levels to blood pressure in exhaust battery storage workers. Ind Health 2006; 44:304.
353. Bockelmann I, et al. Assessing the suitability of cross-sectional and longitudinal cardiac rhythm tests with regard to identifying effects of occupational chronic lead exposure. J Occup Environ Med 2002; 44:59.
354. Cheng Y, et al. Electrocardiographic conduction disturbances in association with low-level lead exposure (the Normative Aging Study). Am J Cardiol 1998; 82:594.
355. Read J, Williams J. Lead myocarditis: report of a case. Am Heart J 1952; 44:797.
356. Myerson R, Eisenhauer J. Atrioventricular conduction defects in lead poisoning. Am J Cardiol 1963; 11:409.
357. Kopp SJ, et al. Simultaneous recording of His bundle electrogram, electrocardiogram, and systolic tension from intact modified Langendorff rat heart preparations. II. Dose-response relationship of cadmium. Toxicol Appl Pharmacol 1978; 46:475.
358. Kasperczyk S, et al. Function of heart muscle in people chronically exposed to lead. Ann Agric Environ Med 2005; 12:207.
359. United States Environmental Protection Agency. Mercury health effects updates: health issue assessment. Final report, Office of Health and Environmental Assessment, Document no. EPA 600/8-84-019F, Washington, DC, 1984.
360. Agency for Toxic Substances and Disease Registry, Toxicological profile for mercury, Atlanta, GA, March 1999.
361. World Health Organization, Inorganic mercury, International Programme on Chemical Safety, Geneva, Switzerland, 1991; 118:168.
362. Wojciechowski J, Kowalski W. Cardiac and aortic lesions in chronic experimental poisoning with mercury vapors. Pol Med Sci Hist Bull 1974; 15:255.
363. Carmignani M, Finelli VN, Boscolo P. Mechanisms in cardiovascular regulation following chronic exposure of male rats to inorganic mercury. Toxicol Appl Pharmacol 1983; 69:442.

364. Oliveira EM, et al. Mercury effects on the contractile activity of isolated heart muscle. Toxicol Appl Pharmacol 1994; 128:86.
365. Massaroni L, et al. Haemodynamic and electrophysiological acute toxic effects of mercury in anaesthetized rats and in langendorff perfused rat hearts. Pharmacol Res 1995; 32:27.
366. Rossoni LV, et al. Effects of mercury on the arterial blood pressure of anesthetized rats. Braz J Med Biol Res 1999; 32:989.
367. Cunha FN, et al. Effects of mercury on the contractile activity of the right ventricular myocardium. Arch Environ Contam Toxicol 2001; 41:374.
368. de Assis GP, et al. Effects of small concentrations of mercury on the contractile activity of the rat ventricular myocardium. Comp Biochem Physiol C 2003; 134:475.
369. Halbach S. Mercury compounds: lipophilicity and toxic effects on isolated myocardial tissue. Arch Toxicol 1990; 64:315.
370. Clarkson TW. The pharmacology of mercury compounds. Toxicol Appl Pharmacol 1972; 12:375.
371. Virtanen JK, et al. Mercury, fish oils, and risk of acute coronary events and cardiovascular disease, coronary heart disease, and all-cause mortality in men in eastern Finland. Arterioscler Thromb Vasc Biol 2005; 25:228.
372. Boffetta P, et al. Mortality from cardiovascular diseases and exposure to inorganic mercury. Occup Environ Med 2001; 58:461.
373. Guallar E, et al. Mercury, fish oils, and the risk of myocardial infarction. N Engl J Med 2002; 347:1747.
374. Pedersen EB, et al. Relationship between mercury in blood and 24-h ambulatory blood pressure in Greenlanders and Danes. Am J Hypertens 2005; 18:612.
375. Davey P, Benson M. A young man with a heavy heart. Heart 1999; 82:e11.
376. Siblerud RL The relationship between mercury from dental amalgam and the cardiovascular system. Sci Total Environ 1990; 99:23.
377. McKee RH, Medeiros AM, Daughtrey WC. A proposed methodology for setting occupational exposure limits for hydrocarbon solvents. J Occup Environ Hyg 2005; 2:524.
378. United States Department of Labor, Occupational Safety and Health Administration, Benzene, Code of Federal Regulations, 29CFR1910.1028, 2003.
379. National Industrial Chemicals Notification and Assessment Scheme, Benzene: priority existing chemical assessment report no. 21, Commonwealth of Australia, September 2001.
380. Vidrio H, Magos GA, Lorenzana-Jimenez M. Electrocardiographic effects of toluene in the anesthetized rat. Arch Int Pharmacodyn Ther 1986; 279:121.
381. Magos GA, Lorenzana-Jimenez M, Vidrio H. Toluene and benzene inhalation influences on ventricular arrhythmias in the rat. Neurotoxicol Teratol 1990; 12:119.
382. Avis SP, Hutton CJ. Acute benzene poisoning: a report of three fatalities. J Forensic Sci 1993; 38:599.
383. Winek CL, Collom WD. Benzene and toluene fatalities. J Occup Med 1971; 13:259.
384. Kotseva K, Popov T. Study of the cardiovascular effects of occupational exposure to organic solvents. Int Arch Occup Environ Health 1998; 71:S87.
385. Kotseva K. Prevalence de l'hypertension arterielle chez les travailleurs d' unites de production de benzene. Arch Mal Prof 1993; 54:43.

386. Kotseva K. Prevalence of arterial hypertension and coronary artery disease in xylene production workers. Presented at: the 21 Medichem Congress, Melbourne, Australia, October 18–24, 1994.

387. Engstrom J, Astrand I, Wigaeus E. Exposure to styrene in a polymerization plant. Uptake in the organism and concentration in subcutaneous adipose tissue. Scand. J. Work Environ. Health 1978; 4:324.

388. National Institute for Occupational Safety and Health. Criteria for a recommended standard: occupational exposure to styrene. United States Department of Health and Human Services, Public Health Service, Centers for Disease Control, DHHS (NIOSH) Publication No. 83-119, NTIS No. PB84-148295, Cincinnati, OH, 1983.

389. Rappaport SM, Fraser DA. Air sampling and analysis in a rubber vulcanization area. Am Ind Hyg Assoc J 1977; 38:205.

390. Wallace LA. Personal exposures, indoor and outdoor air concentrations, and exhaled breath concentrations of selected volatile organic compounds measured for 600 residents of New Jersey, North Dakota, North Carolina, and California. Environ Toxicol Chem 1986; 12:215.

391. Pellizzari ED, et al. Identification of organic components in aqueous effluents from energy-related processes. In: Van Hall CE, ed. Measurement of Organic Pollutants in Water and Wastewater, ASTM Special Technical Publication No. 686. Philadelphia, PA: American Society for Testing and Materials, 1979:256.

392. Perry DL, et al. Identification of organic compounds in industrial effluent discharges. Battelle Columbus Laboratories, EPA-600/4-79-016, NTIS No. PB-294794, Columbus, OH, 1979.

393. King L, Sherbin G. Point sources of toxic organics to the upper St. Clair River. Water Poll Res J Canada 1986; 21:433.

394. Bond GG, et al. Mortality among workers engaged in the development or manufacture of styrene-based products–an update. Scand J Work Environ Health 1992; 18:145.

395. Wong O, Trent LS, Whorton MD. An updated cohort mortality study of workers exposed to styrene in the reinforced plastics and composites industry. Occup Environ Med 1994; 51:386.

396. Matanoski GM, Tao XG. Styrene exposure and ischemic heart disease: a case-cohort study. Am J Epidemiol 2003; 158:988.

397. Matanoski GM, Santos-Burgoa C, Schwartz L. Mortality of a cohort of workers in the styrene-butadiene polymer manufacturing industry (1943–1982). Environ Health Perspect 1990; 86:107.

398. National Cancer Institute. Monograph on human exposure to chemicals in the workplace: toluene. Bethesda, MD: Division of Cancer Etiology, 1985.

399. Agency for Toxic Substances and Disease Registry. ATSDR's Hazardous Substance Release and Health Effects (HazDat) Database. Atlanta, GA: ATSDR, 2000.

400. Grob K. Gas chromatography of cigarette smoke. Part III. Separation of the overlap region of gas and particulate phase by capillary columns. J Gas Chromatogr 1965:52.

401. Morvai V, et al. ECG changes in benzene, toluene and xylene poisoned rats. Acta Med Acad Sci Hung 1976; 33:275.

402. Goldstein DB. The effects of drugs on membrane fluidity. Annu Rev Pharmacol Toxicol 1984; 24:43.

403. Cruz SL, et al. Inhibition of cardiac sodium currents by toluene exposure. Br J Pharmacol 2003; 140:653.
404. Gordon CJ, et al. Cardiovascular effects of oral toluene exposure in the rat monitored by radiotelemetry. Neurotoxicol Teratol 2007; 29:228.
405. Ikeda N, et al. The course of respiration and circulation in 'toluene-sniffing'. Forensic Sci Int 1990; 44:151.
406. Ameno E, et al. A fatal case of oral ingestion of toluene. Forensic Sci Int 1989; 41:255.
407. Meulenbelt J, de Groot G, Savelkoul TJ. Two cases of acute toluene intoxication. Br J Ind Med 1990; 47:417.
408. Einav S, et al. Bradycardia in toluene poisoning. J Toxicol Clin Toxicol 1997; 35:298.
409. Bass M. Sudden sniffing death. JAMA 1970; 212:2075.
410. Streicher HZ, et al. Syndromes of toluene sniffing in adults. Ann Intern Med 1981; 94:758.
411. Cunningham SR, et al. Myocardial infarction and primary ventricular fibrillation after glue sniffing. Br Med J (Clin Res Ed) 1987; 294:739.
412. Hussain TF, Heidenreich PA, Benowitz N. Recurrent non-Q-wave myocardial infarction associated with toluene abuse. Am Heart J 1996; 131:615.
413. Carder JR, Fuerst RS. Myocardial infarction after toluene inhalation. Pediatr Emerg Care 1997; 13:117.
414. Wiseman MN, Banim S. "Glue sniffer's" heart? Br Med J (Clin Res Ed) 1987; 294:739.
415. Vural M, Ogel K. Dilated cardiomyopathy associated with toluene abuse. Cardiology 2006; 105:158.
416. SRI International. Directory of chemical producers: United States of America. Menlo Park, CA: SRI International, 2004.
417. Agency for Toxic Substances and Disease Registry. Draft Toxicological Profile for Xylene. Atlanta, GA: ATSDR, 2005.
418. Atkinson R. Gas-phase tropospheric chemistry of organic compounds: A review. Atmos Environ 1990; 24A:1.
419. Wilson JT, Kampbell DH, Armstrong J. Natural bioreclamation of alkylbenzenes (BTEX) from a gasoline spill in methanogenic groundwater. In: Hinchee RE, ed. Hydrocarbon Bioremediation. Boca Raton, FL: Lewis Publishers, 1994:210.
420. Beller HR, Ding WH, Reinhard M. Byproducts of anaerobic alkylbenzene metabolism useful as indicators of in situ bioremediation. Environ Sci Technol 1995; 29:2864.
421. Morvai V, et al. Effects of quantitative undernourishment, ethanol and xylene on coronary microvessels of rats. Acta Morphol Hung 1987; 35:199.
422. Chan YC, et al. Cardiovascular effects of herbicides and formulated adjuvants on isolated rat aorta and heart. Toxicol In Vitro 2007; 21:595.
423. Hipolito RN. Xylene poisoning in laboratory workers: case reports and discussion. Lab Med 1980; 11:593.
424. Armstrong SR, Green LC. Chlorinated hydrocarbon solvents. Clin Occup Environ Med 2004; 4:481.
425. Agency for Toxic Substances and Disease Registry. Toxicological Profile for Carbon Tetrachloride. Atlanta, GA: ATSDR, August 2005.

426. Letkiewicz F. Occurrence of carbon tetrachloride in drinking water, food and air. Prepared by: JRB Associates, Inc. PB95183174. McLean, VA:1983.
427. Wallace LA. Comparison of risks from outdoor and indoor exposure to toxic chemicals. Environ Health Perspect 1991; 95:7.
428. Integrated Risk Information System. Carbon tetrachloride. Washington, DC: EPA, June 6, 2003.
429. Howard PH, et al. Handbook of Environmental Degradation Rates. Chelsea, MI: Lewis Publishers, Inc., 1991:34.
430. Ali SF, Tariq M. Effect of carbon tetrachloride on cardiac lipid peroxidation, serum lipids and enzymes of albino rats. Toxicol Lett 1982; 11:229.
431. Dziadecki J. Toxic effect of carbon tetrachloride on the myocardium. II. Experimental part. B. Ultrastructure of the myocardium of rats in acute carbon tetrachloride poisoning. Med Pr 1984; 35:317.
432. Tse SY, et al. Chlorinated aliphatic hydrocarbons promote lipid peroxidation in vascular cells. J Toxicol Environ Health 1990; 31:217.
433. Toraason M, et al. Depression of contractility in cultured cardiac myocytes from neonatal rat by carbon tetrachloride and 1,1,1-trichloroethane. Toxic In Vitro 1990; 4:363.
434. Babal P, et al. Red wine polyphenols prevent endothelial damage induced by CCl4 administration. Physiol Res 2006; 55:245.
435. Chetham PM, et al. Segmental regulation of pulmonary vascular permeability by store-operated Ca2+ entry. Am J Physiol 1999; 276:L41.
436. Kennaugh RC. Carbon tetrachloride overdosage. A case report. S Afr Med J 1975; 49:635.
437. Dziadecki J. Toxic effect of carbon tetrachloride on the myocardium. I. Clinical aspects. Med Pr 1984; 35:191.
438. Wilcosky TC, Simonsen NR. Solvent exposure and cardiovascular disease. Am J Ind Med 1991; 19:569.
439. Taylor GJ, Harris WS, Bogdonoff D. Ventricular arrhythmias induced in monkeys by the inhalation of aerosol propellants. J Clin Invest 1971; 50:1546.
440. Kilen SM, Harris WS. Direct depression of myocardial contractility by the aerosol propellant gas, dichlorodifluoromethane. J Pharmacol Exp Ther 1972; 183:245.
441. Thompson EB, Harris WS. Time course of epinephrine-induced arrhythmias in cats exposed to dichlorodifluoromethane. Toxicol Appl Pharmacol 1974; 29:242.
442. Simaan JA, Aviado DM. Hemodynamic effects of aerosol propellants. I. Cardiac depression in the dog. Toxicology 1975; 5:127.
443. Kilen SM, Harris WS. Effects of hypoxia and Freon 12 on mechanics of cardiac contraction. Am J Physiol 1976; 230:1701.
444. Kawakami T, Takano T, Araki R. Enhanced arrhythmogenicity of Freon 113 by hypoxia in the perfused rat heart. Toxicol Ind Health 1990; 6:493.
445. Brady WJ, et al. Freon inhalational abuse presenting with ventricular fibrillation. Am J Emerg Med 1994; 12:533.
446. Kaufman JD, Silverstein MA, Moure-Eraso R. Atrial fibrillation and sudden death related to occupational solvent exposure. Am J Ind Med 1994; 25:731.
447. Lessard Y, Begue J, Paulet G. Fluorocarbons and cardiac arrhythmia: does difluorodichloromethane (FC 12) inhibit cardiac metabolism? Acta Pharmacol Toxicol (Copenh) 1986; 58:71.

448. Lessard Y, Paulet G. A proposed mechanism for cardiac sensitisation: electrophysiological study of effects of difluorodichloromethane and adrenaline on different types of cardiac preparations isolated from sheep hearts. Cardiovasc Res 1986; 20:807.

449. Sjogren B, Gunnare S, Sandler H. Inhalation of decomposed chlorodifluoromethane (freon-22) and myocardial infarction. Scand J Work Environ Health 2002; 28:205.

450. Avella J, Wilson JC, Lehrer M. Fatal cardiac arrhythmia after repeated exposure to 1,1-difluoroethane (DFE), Am J Forensic Med Pathol; 2006; 27:58.

451. International Agency for Research on Cancer. Dichloromethane, IARC monograph on the evaluation of the carcinogenic risk of chemicals to humans. Some halogenated hydrocarbons and pesticide exposures. Lyon, France: World Health Organization, 1986:41:43.

452. Occupational Safety and Health Administration. Occupational exposure to methylene chloride. Federal Register 1997; 62:1494.

453. Reinhardt CF et al. Cardiac arrhythmias and aerosol "sniffing." Arch Environ Health 1971; 22:265.

454. Aviado DM. Effects of fluorocarbons, chlorinated solvents, and inosine on the cardiopulmonary system. Environ Health Perspect 1978; 26:207.

455. Muller S et al. Adrenergic cardiovascular actions in rats as affected by dichloromethane exposure. Biomed Biochim Acta 1991; 50:307.

456. Clark DG, Tinston DJ. Correlation of the cardiac sensitizing potential of halogenated hydrocarbons with their physicochemical properties. Br J Pharmacol 1973; 49:355.

457. Rantanen J. Occupational exposure to organic solvents. Presented at: Joint International Symposium on Environmental Consequences of Hazardous Waste Disposal, Berlin, 1983.

458. Scholz J et al. Acute effects of dichloromethane on arrhythmia development during the early phase of myocardial ischemia and reperfusion in the rat. Arch Toxicol Suppl 1991; 14:128.

459. Hoffmann P et al. Depression of calcium dynamics in cardiac myocytes: a common mechanism of halogenated hydrocarbon anesthetics and solvents. J Mol Cell Cardiol 1994; 26:579.

460. Hoffmann P et al. Cardiotoxicity of dichloromethane in rats and in cultured rat cardiac myocytes, Toxic In Vitro 1995; 9:489.

461. Hoffmann P et al. Calcium dynamics in cardiac myocytes as a target of dichloromethane cardiotoxicity. Arch Toxicol 1996; 70:158.

462. Ellenhorn MJ et al. Respiratory toxicology. In: Ellenhorn MJ et al., ed. Ellenhorn's Medical Toxicology: Diagnosis and Treatment of Human Poisoning. 2nd ed. New York, NY: Elsevier, 1997:chap. 66.

463. Baselt RC. Disposition of Toxic Drugs and Chemicals in Man. 5th ed. Foster City, CA: Chemical Toxicology Institute, 2000:255.

464. Stewart RD and Hake CL. Paint-remover hazard. JAMA 1976; 235:398.

465. Bonventre J et al. Two deaths following accidental inhalation of dichloromethane and 1,1,1-trichloroethane. J Anal Toxicol 1977; 1:158.

466. Ludwig HR et al. Worker exposure to perchloroethylene in the commercial dry cleaning industry. Am Ind Hyg Assoc J 1983; 44:600.

467. Ohtsuki T et al. Limited capacity of humans to metabolize tetrachloroethylene. Int Arch Occup Environ Health 1983; 51:381.

468. Agency for Toxic Substances and Disease Registry. Toxicological Profile for Tetrachloroethylene. Atlanta, GA: ATSDR, September 1997.
469. Kawata K, Fujieda Y. Volatile chlorinated hydrocarbons in ambient air at Niigata area. Japn J Toxicol Environ Health 1993; 39:474.
470. Kobayashi S, Hutcheon DE, Regan J. Cardiopulmonary toxicity of tetrachloroethylene. J Toxicol Environ Health 1982; 10:23.
471. Carlson GP. Epinephrine-induced cardiac arrhythmias in rabbits exposed to tetrachloroethylene. Toxicol Lett 1983; 19:113.
472. Kawakami T, Takano T, Araki R. Synergistic interaction of tri- and tetrachloroethylene, hypoxia, and ethanol on the atrioventricular conduction of the perfused rat heart. Ind Health 1988; 26:25.
473. Abedin Z, Cook RC, Milberg RM. Cardiac toxicity of perchloroethylene (a dry cleaning agent). South Med J 1980; 73:1081.
474. Hara M et al. Cardiovascular effects of organic solvents (perchloroethylene) (perc). Presented at: the Proceedings of the 49th Annual Scientific Meeting of the Japanese Circulation Society. Jpn Circ J 1985; 49:741 (abstr).
475. National Institute for Occupational Safety and Health. National Occupational Exposure Survey (1981–1983). Cincinnati, OH: United States Department of Health and Human Services, December 7, 1990.
476. Santodonato J. Monograph on human exposure to chemicals in the workplace: trichloroethylene. NTIS PB86–134574/GAR, 1985.
477. Brugnone F et al. Blood and urine concentrations of chemical pollutants in the general population. Med Lav 1994; 85:370.
478. Bellar TA, Lichtenberg JJ, Kroner RC. The occurrence of organohalides in chlorinated drinking waters. J Am Water Works Assoc 1974; 66:703.
479. Reinhardt CF, Mullin LS, Maxfield ME. Epinephrine-induced cardiac arrhythmia potential of some common industrial solvents. J Occup Med 1973; 15:953.
480. White JF, Carlson GP. Epinephrine-induced cardiac arrhythmias in rabbits exposed to trichloroethylene: potentiation by ethanol. Toxicol Appl Pharmacol 1981; 60:466.
481. White JF, Carlson GP. Epinephrine-induced cardiac arrhythmias in rabbits exposed to trichloroethylene: potentiation by caffeine. Fundam Appl Toxicol 1982; 2:125.
482. Westfall DP, Fleming WW. The sensitivity of the guinea-pig pacemaker to norepinephrine and calcium after pretreatment with reserpine. J Pharmacol Exp Ther 1968; 164:259.
483. Carlson GP, White JF. Cardiac arrhythmogenic action of benzo(a)pyrene in the rabbit. Toxicol Lett 1983; 15:43.
484. Hoffmann P. Cardiotoxicity testing of organic solvents by coronary artery ligation in closed-chest rats. Arch Toxicol 1987; 61:79.
485. Dimitrova M, Usheva G, Pavlova S. The work environment's influence on the cardiovascular system. Polycardiographic investigations in workers exposed to trichloroethylene. Int Arch Arbeitsmed 1974; 32:145.
486. Lilis R et al. Chronic effects of trichloroethylene exposure. Med Lav 1969; 60:595.
487. Mee AS, Wright PL. Congestive (dilated) cardiomyopathy in association with solvent abuse. J R Soc Med 1980; 73:671.
488. Hantson PH et al. Trichloroethylene and cardiac toxicity: report of two consecutive cases. Acta Clin Belg 1990; 45:34.
489. Agency for Toxic Substances and Disease Registry. Toxicological Profile for 1,1,1-Trichloroethane. Atlanta, GA: ATSDR, July 2006.

490. Pellizzari ED et al. Comparison of indoor and outdoor residential levels of volatile organic chemicals in five US geographical areas. Environ Int 1986; 12:619.
491. Herd PA et al. Cardiovascular effects of 1,1,1-trichloroethane. Arch Environ Health 1974; 28:227.
492. Hoffmann P, Breitenstein M, Toraason M. Calcium transients in isolated cardiac myocytes are altered by 1,1,1-trichloroethane. J Mol Cell Cardiol 1992; 24:619.
493. Travers H. Death from 1,1,1-trichloroethane abuse: case report. Mil Med 1974; 139:889.
494. Wright MF, Strobl DJ. 1,1,1-Trichloroethane cardiac toxicity: report of a case. J Am Osteopath Assoc 1984; 84:285.
495. Ranson DL, Berry PJ. Death associated with the abuse of typewriter correction fluid. Med Sci Law 1986; 26:308.
496. McLeod AA, et al. Chronic cardiac toxicity after inhalation of 1,1,1-trichloroethane. Br Med J (Clin Res Ed) 1987; 294:727.
497. Wodka RM, Jeong EW. Myocardial injury following the intentional inhalation of typewriter correction fluid. Mil Med 1991; 156:204.
498. Bailey B, et al. Two cases of chlorinated hydrocarbon-associated myocardial ischemia. Vet Hum Toxicol 1997; 39:298.
499. Izmerov NF. Carbon disulfide. Centre of International Projects (GKNT). Scientific reviews of Soviet literature on toxicity and hazards of chemicals. No. 41, Moscow, Russia, 1983.
500. Struwe W, Sprinzl G. Transmission von H_2S und CS_2. Osterreichisches Bundesinstitut fur Gesundheitswesen, Vienna, Austria, 1984.
501. National Institute for Occupational Safety and Health. Criteria for a recommended standard occupational exposure to carbon disulfide. United States Department of Health, Education, and Welfare, Washington, DC, 1977.
502. American Conference of Governmental Industrial Hygienists. 1999 TLVs and BEIs. Threshold limit values for chemical substances and physical agents: carbon disulfide. Biological Exposure Indices, Cincinnati, OH, 1999.
503. National Institute for Occupational Safety and Health. Pocket Guide to Chemical Hazards: Carbon Disulfide. United States Department of Health and Human Services, Public Health Service, Centers for Disease Control and Prevention, NIOSH Publication No. 2005–149, Cincinnati, OH, 1997.
504. Wesolowska T. Effects of chronic inhalation intoxication with carbon disulfide on the content of various lipid metabolism indices in the serum, aorta and cardiac muscle in rabbits. II. Lipid phosphorus and phospholipid fractions in the serum, aorta and cardiac muscle. Med Pr 1979; 30:323.
505. Wegrowski, J., Effect of carbon disulfide on the metabolism of connective tissue of rats' aorta and lungs. Med Pr 1980; 31:13.
506. Wronska-Nofer T, Szendzikowski S, Obrebska-Parke M. Influence of chronic carbon disulphide intoxication on the development of experimental atherosclerosis in rats. Br J Ind Med 1980; 37:387.
507. Antov G, et al. Effect of carbon disulphide on the cardiovascular system. J Hyg Epidemiol Microbiol Immunol 1985; 29:329.
508. Lewis LG, et al. Exposure of C57BL/6 mice to carbon disulfide induces early lesions of atherosclerosis and enhances arterial fatty deposits induced by a high fat diet. Toxicol Sci 1999; 49:S124.

509. Morvai V, Szakmary E, Ungvary G. The effects of carbon disulfide and ethanol on the circulatory system of rats. J Toxicol Environ Health A 2005; 68:797.

510. Hoffmann P, et al. Short term effects of carbon disulfide on the intracardial irritation development and transmission in the rat. Arch Exp Veterinarmed 1989; 43:515.

511. Hoffmann P, Klapperstuck M. Effects of carbon disulfide on cardiovascular function after acute and subacute exposure of rats. Biomed Biochim Acta 1990; 49:121.

512. Grodeckaja NS, et al. Characteristics of the combined effect of carbon disulfide in minimal concentrations and repeated stress. Z Gesamte Hyg 1987; 33:237.

513. Chandra SV, Butler WH, Magos L. The effect of carbon disulphide on the myocardium of the rat. Exp Mol Pathol 1972; 17:249.

514. Hoffmann P, Muller S. Subacute carbon disulfide exposure modifies adrenergic cardiovascular actions in rats. Biomed Biochim Acta 1990; 49:115.

515. Klapperstuck M, Muller S, Hoffmann P. Carbon disulfide exposure attenuates adrenergic inotropic response in rats. J Hyg Epidemiol Microbiol Immunol 1991; 35:113.

516. Tan X et al. Carbon disulfide cytotoxicity on cultured cardiac myocytes of rats. Environ Toxicol 2002; 17:324.

517. Tan X, et al. Carbon disulfide cytotoxicity on cultured cardiac myocyte cell of rats. Ecotoxicol Environ Saf 2003; 55:168.

518. Kamal AA, et al. Quantitative evaluation of ECG components of workers exposed to carbon disulfide. Environ Health Perspect 1991; 90:301.

519. Kuo HW, et al. Effects of exposure to carbon disulfide (CS2) on electrocardiographic features of ischemic heart disease among viscose rayon factory workers. Int Arch Occup Environ Health 1997; 70:61.

520. Takebayashi T, et al. A six-year follow up study of the subclinical effects of carbon disulphide exposure on the cardiovascular system. Occup Environ Med 2004; 61:127.

521. Jhun HJ, et al. Electrocardiographic features of Korean carbon disulfide poisoned subjects after discontinuation of exposure. Int Arch Occup Environ Health 2007; 80:547.

522. Bortkiewicz A, Gadzicka E, Szymczak W. Cardiovascular disturbances in workers exposed to carbon disulfide. Appl Occup Environ Hyg 2001; 16:455.

523. Murawska T. ECG picture in persons exposed to carbon disulfide. Med Pr 1977; 28:275.

524. Chang SJ, et al. Electrocardiographic abnormality for workers exposed to carbon disulfide at a viscose rayon plant. J Occup Environ Med 2006; 48:394.

525. Franco G, Malamani T. Systolic time intervals as a measure of left ventricular function in viscose rayon workers exposed to carbon disulfide. Scand J Work Environ Health 1976; 2:107.

526. Bortkiewicz A, Gadzicka E, Szymczak W. Heart rate variability in workers exposed to carbon disulfide. J Auton Nerv Syst 1997; 66:62.

527. Guidotti TL, Hoffman H. Indicators of cardiovascular risk among workers exposed to high intermittent levels of carbon disulphide. Occup Med (Lond) 1999; 49:507.

528. Jhun HJ, et al. Heart-rate variability of carbon disulfide-poisoned subjects in Korea. Int Arch Occup Environ Health 2003; 76:156.

529. Tiller JR, Schilling RS, Morris JN. Occupational toxic factor in mortality from coronary heart disease, Br Med J 1968; 4:407.

530. Tolonen M Nurminen M, Hernberg S. Ten-year coronary mortality of workers exposed to carbon disulfide. Scand J Work Environ Health 1979; 5:109.

531. Balcarova O, Halik J. Ten-year epidemiological study of ischaemic heart disease (IHD) in workers exposed to carbon disulphide. Sci Total Environ 1991; 101:97.
532. Kotseva K, et al. Cardiovascular effects in viscose rayon workers exposed to carbon disulfide. Int J Occup Environ Health 2001; 7:7.
533. Peplonska B, et al. A mortality study of workers with reported chronic occupational carbon disulfide poisoning. Int J Occup Med Environ Health 1996; 9:291.
534. Pepllonska B, et al. Mortality pattern in the cohort of workers exposed to carbon disulfide. Int J Occup Med Environ Health 2001; 14:267.
535. Swaen GM, Braun C, Slangen JJ. Mortality of Dutch workers exposed to carbon disulfide. Int Arch Occup Environ Health 1994; 66:103.
536. Tan X, et al. Cardiovascular effects of carbon disulfide: meta-analysis of cohort studies. Int J Hyg Environ Health 2002; 205:473.
537. Nurminen M, Hernberg S. Effects of intervention on the cardiovascular mortality of workers exposed to carbon disulphide: a 15-year follow up. Br J Ind Med 1985; 42:32.
538. Jaga K, Dharmani C. Sources of exposure to and public health implications of organophosphate pesticides. Rev Panam Salud Publica 2003; 14:171.
539. Fleming LE, Herzstein JA. Emerging issues in pesticide health studies. Occup Med 1997; 12:387.
540. Kwong TC. Organophosphate pesticides: biochemistry and clinical toxicology. Ther Drug Monit 2002; 24:144.
541. Roth A et al. Organophosphates and the heart. Chest 1993; 103:576.
542. Abraham S, et al. QTc prolongation and cardiac lesions following acute organophosphate poisoning in rats. Proc West Pharmacol Soc 2001; 44:185.
543. Yavuz T, et al. Cardiotoxicity in rats induced by methidathion and ameliorating effect of vitamins E and C. Hum Exp Toxicol 2004; 23:323.
544. Robineau P. Cardiac abnormalities in rats treated with methylphosphonothiolate. Toxicol Appl Pharmacol 1987; 87:206.
545. Baskin SI. The cardiac toxicology of organophosphorus agents. In: Baskin SI, ed. Principles of Cardiac Toxicology. Boca Raton, FL: CRC Press, 1991:chap. 7.
546. Saiyed HN, et al. Cardiac toxicity following short-term exposure to methomyl in spraymen and rabbits. Hum Exp Toxicol 1992; 11:93.
547. Kiss Z, Fazekas T. Arrhythmias in organophosphate poisonings. Acta Cardiol 1979; 34:323.
548. Ludomirsky A, et al. Q-T prolongation and polymorphous ("torsade de pointes") ventricular arrhythmias associated with organophosphorus insecticide poisoning. Am J Cardiol 1982; 49:1654.
549. Bardy GH, et al. A mechanism of torsades de pointes in a canine model. Circulation 1983; 67:52.
550. Karki P, et al. Cardiac and electrocardiographical manifestations of acute organophosphate poisoning. Singapore Med J 2004; 45:385.
551. Saadeh AM, Farsakh NA, Al-Ali MK. Cardiac manifestations of acute carbamate and organophosphate poisoning. Heart 1997; 77:461.
552. Fazekas IG. Macroscopic and microscopic alterations in Wofatox poisoning (methyl parathion). Z Rechtsmed 1971; 68:189.
553. Limaye MR. Acute organophosphorous compound poisoning. A study of 76 necropsies J Indian Med Assoc 1966; 47:492.

554. Biernat S, Giermaziak H. Myocardial and endocardial lesions in rabbit after acute poisoning with Intration and after treatment with some detoxifying agents. Pol Med Sci Hist Bull 1975; 15:249.

555. McDonough JH et al. Atropine and/or diazepam therapy protects against soman-induced neural and cardiac pathology. Fundam Appl Toxicol 1989; 13:256.

556. Topacoglu H et al. An unusual cause of atrial fibrillation: exposure to insecticides. Am J Ind Med 2007; 50:48.

557. Anand M, et al. Hypertension and myocarditis in rabbits exposed to hexa-chlorocyclohexane and endosulfan. Vet Hum Toxicol 1990; 32:521.

558. Sauviat MP, et al. Electrical activity alterations induced by chronic absorption of lindane (gamma-hexachlorocyclohexane) trace concentrations in adult rat heart. Can J Physiol Pharmacol 2005; 83:243.

559. Ananya R et al. Oxidative stress and histopathological changes in the heart following oral lindane (gamma hexachlorohexane) administration in rats. Med Sci Monit 2005; 11:BR325.

560. Costa LG. Basic toxicology of pesticides. Occup Med 1997; 12(2):251.

561. Eyer F, et al. Acute endosulfan poisoning with cerebral edema and cardiac failure. J Toxicol Clin Toxicol 2004; 42:927.

562. Shemesh Y et al. Survival after acute endosulfan intoxication. J Toxicol Clin Toxicol 1988;26:265.

563. Tasai YJ et al. Acute massive endosulfan poisoning: a study of 14 cases. Vet Hum Toxicol 1988; 30:170.

564. Spencer CI, et al. Actions of pyrethroid insecticides on sodium currents, action potentials, and contractile rhythm in isolated mammalian ventricular myocytes and perfused hearts. J Pharmacol Exp Ther 2001; 298:1067.

565. Spencer CI, Sham JS. Mechanisms underlying the effects of the pyrethroid teflu-thrin on action potential duration in isolated rat ventricular myocytes. J Pharmacol Exp Ther 2005; 315:16.

566. Coskun B, et al. Evaluation of the toxic effects of cypermethrin inhalation on the frog heart. Ecotoxicol Environ Saf 2004; 57:220.

567. Chen SY, et al. An epidemiological study on occupational acute pyrethroid poisoning in cotton farmers. Br J Ind Med 1991; 48:77.

568. Yang PY, et al. Acute ingestion poisoning with insecticide formulations containing the pyrethroid permethrin, xylene, and surfactant: a review of 48 cases. J Toxicol Clin Toxicol 2002; 40:107.

569. He F, et al. Clinical manifestations and diagnosis of acute pyrethroid poisoning. Arch Toxicol 1989; 63:54.

570. He F. Clinical observations on acute pyrethroids poisoning. Chin Rural Med 1985; 5:31.

571. Mu R. A severe case of fenvalerate-parathion mixture poisoning. Clin Med 1987; 1:60.

572. Tan J. Six cases report of acute Decis poisoning. J Adv Study Phys 1987; 5:55.

573. Wang S, Liu L, He F. Clinical manifestations of 61 cases of acute pyrethroids poisoning. Hyg Res 1988; 3.

574. Agency for Toxic Substances and Disease Registry. Toxicological profile for chlorinated dibenzo-p-dioxins (CDDs). Atlanta, GA: ATSDR, December 1998.

575. Allen JR, et al. Morphological changes in monkeys consuming a diet containing low levels of 2,3,7,8-tetrachlorodibenzo-p-dioxin. Food Cosmet Toxicol 1977; 15:401.

576. Brewster DW, Matsumura F, Akera T. Effects of 2,3,7,8-tetrachlorodibenzo-p-dioxin on guinea pig heart muscle. Toxicol Appl Pharmacol 1987; 89:408.

577. Canga L, Levi R, Rifkind AB. Heart as a target organ in 2,3,7,8-tetrachlorodibenzo-p-dioxin toxicity: decreased beta-adrenergic responsiveness and evidence of increased intracellular calcium. Proc Natl Acad Sci U S A 1988; 85:909.

578. Canga L, et al. 2,3,7,8-Tetrachlorodibenzo-p-dioxin increases cardiac myocyte intracellular calcium and progressively impairs ventricular contractile responses to isoproterenol and to calcium in chick embryo hearts. Mol Pharmacol 1993; 44:1142.

579. van Birgelen AP, et al. Toxicity of 3,3′,4,4′-tetrachloroazoxybenzene in rats and mice. Toxicol Appl Pharmacol 1999; 56:206.

580. Jokinen MP, et al. Increase in cardiovascular pathology in female Sprague-Dawley rats following chronic treatment with 2,3,7,8-tetrachlorodibenzo-p-dioxin and 3,3′,4,4′,5-pentachlorobiphenyl. Cardiovasc Toxicol 2003; 3:299.

581. Xie A, Walker MJ, Wang D. Dioxin (2,3,7,8-tetrachlorodibenzo-p-dioxin) enhances triggered afterdepolarizations in rat ventricular myocytes. Cardiovasc Toxicol 2006; 6:99.

582. Kim J.S. et al. Impact of Agent Orange exposure among Korean Vietnam veterans. Ind Health 2003; 41:149.

583. Kang HK, et al. Health status of Army Chemical Corps Vietnam veterans who sprayed defoliant in Vietnam. Am J Ind Med 2006; 49:875.

584. Benowitz NL. Cardiotoxicity in the workplace. Occup Med 1992; 7:465.

585. Gjesdal K, et al. Exposure to glyceryl trinitrate during gun powder production: plasma glyceryl trinitrate concentration, elimination kinetics, and discomfort among production workers. Br J Ind Med 1985; 42:27.

586. Ellenhorn MJ, Barceloux DG. Medical Toxicology: Diagnosis and Treatment of Human Poisoning, New York, NY: Elsevier, 1988:844.

587. Clark DG. The supersensitivity of the rat cardiovascular system to epinephrine after repeated injections of ethylene glycol dinitrate. Toxicol Appl Pharmacol 1970; 17:433.

588. Jensen FB. Nitrite disrupts multiple physiological functions in aquatic animals. Comp Biochem Physiol A Mol Integr Physiol 2003; 135:9.

589. Ozmen O, Mor F, Ayhan U. Nitrate poisoning in cattle fed Chenopodium album hay. Vet Hum Toxicol 2003; 45:83.

590. Carmichael P, Lieben J. Sudden death in explosives workers. Arch Environ Health 1963; 7:424.

591. Forman SA, Helmkamp JC, Bone CM. Cardiac morbidity and mortality associated with occupational exposure to 1,2 propylene glycol dinitrate. J Occup Med 1987; 29:445.

592. Hogstedt C, Axelson O. Nitroglycerine-nitroglycol exposure and the mortality in cardio-cerebrovascular diseases among dynamite workers. J Occup Med 1977; 19:675.

593. Lange RL, et al. Nonatheromatous ischemic heart disease following withdrawal from chronic industrial nitroglycerin exposure. Circulation 1972; 46:666.

594. Lund RP, Haggendal J, Johnsson, G. Withdrawal symptoms in workers exposed to nitroglycerine. Br J Ind Med 1968; 25:136.

595. Morton WE. Occupational habituation to aliphatic nitrates and the withdrawal hazards of coronary disease and hypertension. J Occup Med 1977; 19:197.

596. Symanski H. Severe health the damage by occupational contact with nitroglycol. Arch Hyg Bakteriol 1952; 136:139.

597. Klock JC. Nonocclusive coronary disease after chronic exposure to nitrates: evidence for physiologic nitrate dependence. Am Heart J 1975; 89:510.
598. Przybojewski JZ. Myocardial infarction complicating dilated (congestive) cardiomyopathy in an industrial nitroglycerin worker. A case report. S Afr Med J 1986; 69:381.
599. Levine RJ, et al. Heart disease in workers exposed to dinitrotoluene. J Occup Med 1986; 28:811.
600. Benditt EP. The origin of atherosclerosis. Sci Am 1977; 236:74.
601. Tsimakuridze M, Saakadze V, Tsereteli M. The characteristic state of health of ammonia nitrate producing workers. Georgian Med News 2005; 122:80.
602. Tsimakuridze MP. Characterization of labor conditions and state of health among ammonia nitrate producing workers. Georgian Med News 2005; 124–125:87.
603. Ellenhorn MJ, Barceloux DG. Metical Toxicology: Diagnosis and Treatment of Human Poisoning. New York, NY: Elsevier, 1988:871.
604. Issley S, Lang E. Toxicity, ammonia, eMedicine World Medical Library, WebMD. January 8, 2007; Available at: http://www.emedicine.com/emerg/topic846.htm.
605. Agency for Toxic Substances and Disease Registry. Toxicological Profile for Ammonia. Atlanta, GA: ATSDR, September 2004.
606. Coon RA, et al. Animal inhalation studies on ammonia, ethylene glycol, formaldehyde, dimethylamine, and ethanol. Toxicol Appl Pharmacol 1970; 16:646.
607. Kapeghian JC, et al. Acute inhalation toxicity of ammonia in mice. Bull Environ Contam Toxicol 1982; 29:371.
608. Itabisashi T. Electrocardiographic observation on goats with urea-ammonia poisoning and a consideration on the main cause of death. Natl Inst Anim Health Q (Tokyo) 1977; 17:151.
609. Richard D, Jouany JM, Boudene C. Acute inhalation toxicity of ammonia in rabbits. C R Acad Sci Hebd Seances Acad Sci D 1978; 287:375.
610. Venediktova NI, et al. Antioxidant enzymes of the rat liver, brain, heart and erythrocytes in ammonia intoxication. Biomed Khim 2005; 51:185.
611. Zhang YX et al. Detection of myocardial lesion in patients with acute ammonia poisoning. Zhonghua Lao Dong Wei Sheng Zhi Ye Bing Za Zhi 2003; 21:247.
612. White ES. A case of near fatal ammonia gas poisoning. J Occup Med 1971; 13:549.
613. Slot GM. Electrocardiograms in 80 cases of angina of effort. Lancet 1938; 2:1356.
614. Montague TJ, Macneil AR. Mass ammonia inhalation. Chest 1980; 77:496.
615. Hatton DV, et al. Collagen breakdown and ammonia inhalation. Arch Environ Health 1979; 34:83.
616. George A, et al. Liquid ammonia injury. Burns 2000; 26:409.
617. Ruidavets JB, et al. Triggering of acute coronary syndromes after a chemical plant explosion. Heart 2006; 92:257.
618. National Institute for Occupational Safety and Health. In-Depth Survey Report of American Airlines Plating Facility. United States Department of Health and Human Services, Public Health Service, Centers for Disease Control and Prevention, NIOSH Publication No 83187799, Cincinnati, OH, 1982.
619. National Institute for Occupational Safety and Health. NIOSH recommendations for occupational safety and health. Compendium of policy documents and statements. United States Department of Health and Human Services, Public Health Services, Centers for Disease Control, National Institute for Occupational Safety and Health, Division of Standards Development and Technology Transfer, Cincinnati, OH, 1992.

620. Cicerone RJ, Zellner R. The atmospheric chemistry of hydrogen cyanide (HCN). J Geophys Res 1983; 88:10689.
621. Jaramillo M, et al. Measurements of stratospheric hydrogen cyanide and McMurdo Station, Antarctica: further evidence of winter stratospheric subsidence? J Geophys Res 1989; 94:16773.
622. Agency for Toxic Substances and Disease Registry, Toxicological profile for cyanide. Atlanta, GA: ATSDR, July 2006.
623. United States Environmental Protection Agency. Exposure and risk assessment for cyanide. United States Environmental Protection Agency, Office of Water, EPA440485008, PB85220572, Washington, DC, 1981.
624. United States Environmental Protection Agency. Code of Federal Regulations 40 CFR 185.3600, Washington, DC, 1975.
625. Suzuki T. Ultrastructural changes of heart muscle in cyanide poisoning. Tohoku J Exp Med 1968; 95:271.
626. Krasney JA. Cardiovascular responses to cyanide in awake sinoaortic denervated dogs. Am J Physiol 1971; 220:1361.
627. Deburghdaly M, Scott MJ. The cardiovascular effects of hypoxia in the dog with special reference to the contribution of the carotid body chemoreceptors. J Physiol 1964; 173:201.
628. Kahler RL, Goldblatt A, Braunwald E. The effects of acute hypoxia on the systemic venous and arterial systems and on myocardial contractile force. J Clin Invest 1962; 41:1553.
629. Korner PI. Circulatory adaptations in hypoxia. Physiol Rev 1959; 39:687.
630. Purser DA. A bioassay model for testing the incapacitating effects of exposure to combustion product atmospheres using cynomolgus monkeys. J Fire Sci 1984; 2:20.
631. Vick JA, Froehlich HL. Studies of cyanide poisoning, Arch Int Pharmacodyn Ther 1985; 273:314.
632. Kamalu BP. Pathological changes in growing dogs fed on a balanced cassava (Manihot esculenta Crantz) diet. Br J Nutr 1993; 69:921.
633. Ballantyne B. An experimental assessment of the diagnostic potential of histo-chemical and biochemical methods for cytochrome oxidase in acute cyanide poisoning. Cell Mol Biol Incl Cyto Enzymol 1977; 22:109.
634. Lasch EE, El Shawa R. Multiple cases of cyanide poisoning by apricot kernels in children from Gaza. Pediatrics 1981; 68:5.
635. Krieg A, Saxena K. Cyanide poisoning from metal cleaning solutions. Ann Emerg Med 1987; 16:582.
636. Johnson RP, Mellors JW. Arteriolization of venous blood gases: a clue to the diagnosis of cyanide poisoning. J Emerg Med 1988; 6:401.
637. Peddy SB, Rigby MR, Shaffner DH. Acute cyanide poisoning. Pediatr Crit Care Med 2006; 7:79.

13

Passive Smoking Causes Heart Disease

Stanton A. Glantz

*Division of Cardiology, Department of Medicine, Center for Tobacco Control
Research and Education, Cardiovascular Research Institute,
University of California, San Francisco, California, U.S.A.*

INTRODUCTION

While most of the discussion of the health effects of passive smoking on non-smokers has concentrated on lung cancer (1), heart disease is a much more important endpoint (2–4). Whereas passive smoking–induced lung cancer accounts for about 3000 deaths a year, passive smoking–induced heart disease accounts for up to 62,000 deaths annually (3), with about an equal number of nonfatal events (5–8). Epidemiological studies of the effects of passive smoking on both fatal and nonfatal endpoints associated with heart disease reveal about a 30% increase in risk (9), and the American Heart Association has formally concluded that passive smoking is an important risk factor for heart disease in both adults (10) and children (11).

The primary issue related to passive smoking and heart disease has been the size of this effect compared with the effect of active smoking on smokers. Active smoking, which involves a dose of the toxins in smoke, which is substantially greater than what a nonsmoker receives from secondhand smoke, only about doubles the risk of heart disease compared with a 30% increase associated with passive smoking. Thus, the effect of secondhand smoke seems large for the dose, assuming a linear dose-response relationship. This assumption does not, however, consider the fact that sidestream smoke (which is emitted from the lit end of the cigarette) is richer in a wide variety of toxins than the mainstream smoke that the smoker inhales (1–3). Indeed, per unit mass, fresh sidestream smoke is three to four times more toxic than mainstream smoke (12). Moreover, the smoke becomes another three to four times more toxic as it ages (13); so, per unit mass, the aged sidestream smoke (which comprises about 90% of second-hand smoke) is about an order of magnitude more toxic than the mainstream smoke that the smoker inhales. Most important, there are a wide variety of clinical and experimental studies that demonstrate that the effects of secondhand smoke on the cardiovascular system occur at low doses in nonsmokers, with the effects in many cases almost as large as those observed in active smokers (9,14,15) (Table 1). A significant part of the cardiovascular toxicity is mediated by effects on platelets, vascular function, and inflammation, among other factors. The dose-response relationship between tobacco smoke exposure and heart disease is not linear; it is superlinear.

EPIDEMIOLOGICAL STUDIES: LONG-TERM EFFECTS

Epidemiological data on the relationship between passive smoking and heart disease have been accumulating since the mid-1980s. Eight meta-analyses have been published (5,7–9,16–19), which, except for one funded by the tobacco industry (19), consistently yielded relative risks of heart disease from passive smoking around 1.3. Figure 1 shows that the pooled relative risk from 29 studies of the risk of ischemic heart disease in never smokers chronically exposed to secondhand smoke compared with those with minimal exposure is 1.31 (95% CI: 1.21–1.41), similar to the estimates of earlier meta-analyses (5,7,8,16–18). [This analysis excludes one cohort study because of serious misclassification bias (20,21).]

In 2004, Whincup et al. (22) published an important 20-year prospective study of passive smoking and coronary heart disease, which found that the risk associated with passive smoking was from 1.45 (1.10–2.08) and 1.57 (1.08–2.28), depending on the level of exposure. These estimates are about twice as high as earlier estimates (Fig. 1) and nearly as high as observed in light (1–9 cigarettes/day) active smokers (1.66; 1.04–2.68). The reason for the higher relative risk estimate is the fact that the authors used cotinine [a stable metabolite of nicotine (23)] as the measure of secondhand smoke exposure, rather than simply comparing heart disease rates in nonsmokers married to smokers with non-smokers married to nonsmokers. Earlier epidemiological studies that used marriage to a smoker as a surrogate for exposure did not capture the entire exposure to secondhand smoke, including from workplaces and public places (such as restaurants and bars). This exposure misclassification error biases the risk estimate of the effect of secondhand smoke toward the null. By using cotinine as the measure of exposure, Whincup et al. (22) were able to capture more of the total secondhand smoke exposure. These results suggest that passive smoking leads to between 68% and 86% of the risk of light smoking, depending on the level of secondhand smoke exposure (Table 1).

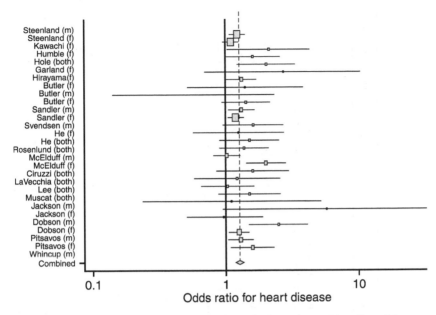

Figure 1 Relative risk estimates (with 95% confidence intervals), adjusted for age and sex, from 29 studies comparing ischemic heart disease in lifelong nonsmokers whose spouse currently smokes with those whose spouse never smoked. *Source*: From Ref. 9.

PLATELETS

Secondhand smoke activates blood platelets, which increases the likelihood of formation of a thrombus, and can damage the lining of the coronary arteries and facilitate the development of atherosclerotic lesions (14,15,24–29). Increased platelet activity is associated with increased relative risk for ischemic heart disease (30), and the increases in platelet activity observed in passive smokers would be expected to have acute effects, increasing the risk by 34% (16), about what is observed in the epidemiological studies.

In one experiment, smokers and nonsmokers were asked to smoke two cigarettes (27) (Fig. 2). The smokers' platelets, which were "stickier" than the nonsmokers' platelets at the beginning of the experiment, did not significantly change activity in response to the two cigarettes. Most likely, the effects on smokers' platelet activation had saturated because of the chronic exposure to the toxins in cigarette smoke, so the addition of the relatively small amount of toxins in two cigarettes had no additional effects. In contrast, smoking just two cigarettes (compared with what a smoker receives on an ongoing basis) significantly increased nonsmokers' platelet activity, to the point that it was not significantly different from habitual smoker.

Table 1 Comparative Effects of Passive and Active Smoking[a]

	SHS effect[b]	Exposure	Active effect[c]	SHS/active effect[d]
Risk of heart disease (95% CI)				
Figure 1 of this chapter	1.31 (1.21, 1.41)	Chronic	1.78 (1.31, 2.44)[e]	40%
20 yr (22)	1.57 (1.08, 2.28)[f]	Cotinine at study entry	1.66 (1.04, 2.68)	86%
First 4 yr (22)	3.73 (1.32, 10.98)	Cotinine at study entry	3.32 (0.87, 12.64)	122%
Platelet function				
Platelet activation (27) (SI PGI$_2$)[g]	0.55 ± 0.059	20 min	0.54 ± 0.069	96%
Platelet aggregate ratio (25,31) (change)	−0.09	20 min	−0.15	60%
Fibrinogen (128) (95% CI) (mg/dL)	5.2 (−1.2, 12)	Chronic	6.9 (−0.9, 14)	75%
Fibrinogen (44) (mg/dL) (SE)	11.2 ± 4.1	Chronic	18.1 ± 6.7	62%
Plasma thromboxane (46) (pg/mL)	3.30 ± 0.35	Acute	2.93 ± 0.07	114%
Plasma malondialdehyde (46) nmol/L/10^9 platelets	4.2 ± 0.17	Acute	3.9 ± 0.07	108%
Endothelium and arterial function				
Endothelial cell count (change) (25,31) (mean number of anuclear cell carcasses on 0.9 μL chamber)	0.9	20 min	2.0	45%
Coronary flow velocity reserve (59) (cm/s)	68.8 ± 22.7	30 min	67.1 ± 15.0	91%
Flow-mediated dilation (55)%	3.1 ± 2.7	3 yr	4.4 ± 3.1	134%
Endothelial cell count (change) (25,31) (mean number of anuclear cell carcasses on 0.9 μL chamber)	0.9	20 min	2.0	45%
Aortic stiffness (129,130) (mm Hg/mm)	58	4 min	49	110%
HDL (131) (mg/dL)	48.26 ± 3.47	Chronic	45.59 ± 4.6	73%
Increase in intimal media thickness (132) (μm/3 yr)	5.9	Chronic	14.3	41%

Inflammatory markers (128) (95% CI)				
White blood cells (×10³ per µL)	0.6 (0.3, 0.8)	Chronic	0.6 (0.5, 0.7)	100%
CRP (mg/dL)	0.08 (0.02, 0.1)	Chronic	0.1 (0.08, 0.2)	80%
Homocysteine (µmol/L)	0.4 (0.2, 0.6)	Chronic	0.5 (0.1, 0.9)	80%
Oxidized LDL (mg/dL)	3.3 (0.5, 6)	Chronic	3.9 (1.4, 7)	85%
Antioxidants				
Vitamin C µmol/L (98) Median (interquartile range)	53 (41, 79)	Chronic	40 (25, 58)	57%
Hypovitaminosis (98) (vitamin C <23 µmol/L)	12%	Chronic	24%	50%
Ratio of DHAA[h] to ascorbic acid (133)	10.3 ± 7.00	>6 mo	11.2 ± 6.9	78%
Vitamin C in children (99) mmol/L (mean ± SE)	−8.8 ± 1.5[i]	Chronic	−9.0 ± 2.3	98%
β-carotene (101) µmol/L mean (SE)	0.129 ± 0.022	Chronic	0.155 ± 0.021	174%
β-carotene (103) µmol/L	0.15	Chronic	0.17	128%
Red blood cell folate mean decrease (134) nmol/L (95% CI)[j]	−50 (−69, −31)	Chronic	−86 (−101, −71)	58%

Notes:
[a]Data presented as mean ± SD unless otherwise noted.
[b]Change in variable associated with passive smoking among nonsmokers (after minus before SHS exposure).
[c]Difference in variable between smokers and nonsmokers (smoker minus nonsmoker).
[d]Represents the difference between passive smoking effect divided by active smoking effect times 100%.
[e]Risk of death at age 65 smoking 20 cigarettes/day (16).
[f]Cotinine levels 2.8 to 14.0 ng/mL.
[g]Sensitivity index to prostacyclin.
[h]Dehydroascorbic acid.
[i]High dose SHS group .
[j]High exposure to SHS.
Abbreviation: SHS, secondhand smoke.
Source: From Ref. 9.

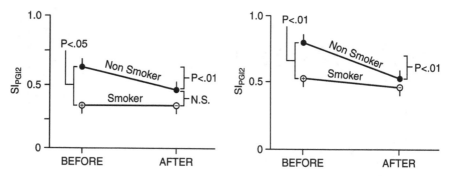

Figure 2 Effect of active (*left*) and passive (*right*) smoking on platelet aggregation in smokers and nonsmokers. The sensitivity index, SI_{PGI2}, is defined as the inverse of the concentration of prostaglandin I_2 necessary to inhibit ADP-induced platelet aggregation by 50%. Lower values of SI_{PGI2} indicate greater platelet aggregation. *Source*: From Refs. 8, 27.

More important, the same investigator (27) measured platelet activity in smokers and nonsmokers before and after they sat in a room for 20 minutes, where cigarettes had been smoked just before the experimental subjects entered (Fig. 2). Again, there was no significant change in the platelet activity among the smokers, but a significant increase in platelet stickiness among the nonsmokers, to the point that their platelet activation was not discernibly different from the smokers. These data, together with other human experiments (25,31–35), indicate that nonsmokers are much more sensitive to secondhand smoke than smokers and that very low levels of secondhand smoke exposure can have major impact on nonsmokers' platelet activity. It also appears that the process saturates at low doses: once the nonsmoker has been exposed to even a low dose of secondhand smoke, the platelets are maximally activated, similar to that of a habitual smoker. In vitro experiments on human platelets extracts of sidestream smoke show that, at equal doses, sidestream smoke is about 1.5 times more potent platelet activator than extracts of mainstream smoke (36).

Animal data support this conclusion. Studies of the effects of passive smoking on heart disease reveal that bleeding time (another measure of platelet activity) is significantly shortened (meaning more activated platelets) in both rabbits (37,38) and rats (39) exposed at even the lowest doses of secondhand smoke, with no additional effects at higher doses.

At a biochemical level, studies of cigarette smoke extract on the effects of platelet activity suggest that the toxins in the cigarette smoke increase platelet activation factor by interfering with the activity of the plasma enzyme platelet-activating factor acetylhydrolase (PAF-AH) (40). Nicotine does not appear to be the only active agent in tobacco smoke that contributes to these effects on the platelets (32,40). This biochemical result is reinforced by clinical studies, which find that smokers treated with nicotine patches show fewer changes in platelet activity than continuing smokers despite having similar nicotine levels (41).

Increased levels of cadmium and strontium, known to alter endothelial function, have also been found in young smokers and passive smokers (42).

Fibrinogen, a mediator of platelet activation and an inflammatory marker associated with a higher risk of heart disease (43), is elevated in passive smokers (16,44,45) (Table 1). In addition, thromboxane, another marker of platelet activation, is also increased in passive smokers and, with repeated one-hour daily exposures, can reach levels observed in active smokers (46) (Table 1).

Platelet activation is not, however, the only player in thrombus formation. Blood vessel integrity is vital to prevent thrombus formation. A pathological event, such as rupture of an atherosclerotic plaque, will lead to platelet adhesion to the arterial wall and platelet activation, culminating in the formation of a platelet plug (thrombus) and potentially vessel occlusion and ischemia or infarction (47,48).

ENTHOTHELIAL FUNCTION

Arteries have a one-cell thick lining known as the vascular endothelium. The endothelium plays an important role in maintaining vascular integrity, including controlling the ability of arteries to dilate and constrict (and so regulate blood flow), inhibiting intimal hyperplasia, and regulating platelet and leukocyte adhesion. In addition, damage to the vascular endothelium is characterized by endothelial dysfunction with vasoconstriction and a procoaggulant and proinflammatory milieu on the vessel wall. Platelets activated by secondhand smoke also damage the endothelium; secondhand smoke interferes with endothelium-dependent vasodilation in animals (49–52) and humans (53–55). Moreover, it is possible to block these effects by increasing the amount of l-arginine, an amino acid that is a precursor for nitric oxide (NO), the compound that mediates endothelium-dependent vasodilation (56–58). This result indicates that secondhand smoke specifically interferes with the production of NO production, which mediates endothelium-dependent vasodilation.

These effects are manifested clinically within 15 to 30 minutes (35,59–61). Using the coronary flow velocity reserve, a clinical surrogate measure of endothelial function, Otsuka et al. (59) showed that 30 minutes of breathing secondhand smoke (at levels comparable to a bar) impaired endothelium-dependent vasodilation in coronary arteries of nonsmokers almost to the same extent as seen in habitual smokers (Table 1).

In passive and active smokers (62), decreased production of endothelial NO is one of the mechanisms by which the risk of heart disease is increased. Light (<1 pack/wk) and heavy smokers (1 pack/wk) have similarly decreased levels of endothelial NO (63), indicating that cigarette smoke has an effect at low exposure, which saturates at high exposures.

Direct endothelial cell injury has also been described. Secondhand smoke exposure for 20 minutes is associated with increased levels of circulating endothelial cell carcasses (25) (Table 1). Mullick et al. (64) exposed rats to six weeks of secondhand smoke (6 hr/day, 5 days/wk) and found damage to carotid artery endothelial cells. There was disruption of the junctional complexes between adjacent cells and elevation of the basal surface of endothelial cells off the internal elastic membrane (64). These injuries in the endothelial cells in the artery wall lead to increase vascular permeability and atherosclerosis.

Endothelial function partially recovers in humans after chronic exposure to secondhand smoke ends. One year after long-term exposure to secondhand smoke had ended, endothelial-dependent dilation was significantly better in former passive smokers than in current passive smokers, although both groups were impaired compared with controls (65). Only partial endothelium recovery might be attained because of the damage that secondhand smoke produces in the endothelial repair mechanism (66,67).

ATHEROSCLEROSIS

In addition to short-term toxicity of cigarette smoke, there are long-term per-manent effects. As discussed above, endothelial dysfunction represents the key event in the development of atherosclerosis. Cigarette smoke extract impairs NO-mediated endothelial function in isolated endothelial cells from both humans and animals because of increased production of superoxide anion (68,69). Acrolein, an important constituent of secondhand smoke (2), is one of the compounds in secondhand smoke that causes these effects (69). Acrolein, as well as other gas phase oxidants in cigarette smoke, remain stable in blood, and so are capable of acting directly on the vascular endothelium. Xanthine oxidase, an enzyme that produces reactive oxygen species, leading to oxidative stress, is upregulated by very low doses of tobacco smoke condensate (70), important in the development of atherosclerosis (29,71,72).

Once there is damage to the arterial endothelium, either through mechan-ical or chemical factors, platelets interact with or adhere to the subendothelial connective tissue and initiate a sequence that leads to formation of athero-sclerotic plaque. When platelets interact with or adhere to subendocardial con-nective tissue, they are stimulated to release their granule contents. Endothelial cells normally prevent platelet adherence because of the nonthrombogenic character of their surface and their capacity to form antithrombotic substances such as prostacyclin and NO. Once the endothelial cells have been damaged, the platelets can stick to them and release mitogens such as platelet-derived growth factor, which encourages migration and proliferation of smooth muscle cells in the region of the endothelial injury.

If platelet aggregation is increased because of exposure to secondhand smoke, the chances of platelets building up at that endothelial injury site will be increased. Experiments in humans have indicated that even short-term exposure to secondhand smoke—like active smoking (73)—significantly increases the appearance of anuclear endothelial cell carcasses in the blood of people exposed to secondhand smoke (or other tobacco products) constituents (25). The appearance of these cell carcasses indicates damage to the endothelium, which is the initiating step in the atherosclerotic process. The appearance of endothelial cells after passive smoking in nonsmokers is almost as great as in primary smoking in nonsmokers.

Passive smoking both among adolescents whose parents smoke and also in adults working in places where smoking is permitted exhibit lower levels of high-density lipoprotein (HDL) than children breathing clean air (74,75). Similar results have been reported in adults who work in smoky environments (76). This effect on cholesterol and the ratio of HDL to total cholesterol also increases the risk of developing atherosclerosis. Adults breathing secondhand smoke for only 5.5 hours exhibit compromised antioxidant biochemical defenses and increased accumulation of low-density lipoprotein (LDL) cholesterol in macrophages (77). As discussed below, free radicals oxidize LDL cholesterol, making it more prone to oxidation, therefore more likely to become part of the plaque.

Many atherosclerotic plaques in humans are either monoclonal (meaning they arose from a single cell) or possess a predominantly monoclonal component, which indicates that the smooth muscle cells of each plaque have a predominant cell type. Several animal studies (78–89) demonstrated that polycyclic aromatic hydrocarbons (PAHs), in particular 7,12-dimethylbenz(a,h)anthracene (DMBA), 1-3 butadiene, and benzo(a)pyrene (BAP), accelerate the development of atherosclerosis. BAP is an important constituent of secondhand smoke. The PAHs appear to bind preferentially to both the LDL and HDL subfragments of cholesterol, which may facilitate incorporation of the carcinogenic compounds into the cells lining the coronary arteries and hence contribute to both cell injury and the hyperplasia, in the atherosclerotic process.

Humans exposed to secondhand smoke at work exhibit increased production of 8-hydroxy-2'-deoxyguanosine, an indicator of DNA damage that has been linked to increased risk of cancer and heart disease (90).

In addition to this biochemical evidence demonstrating the effects of specific components in secondhand smoke on the development of atherosclerotic lesions at a cellular and molecular level, animal experiments have demonstrated that short-term exposure to secondhand smoke significantly speeds the atherosclerotic process. Zhu et al. (37) exposed three groups of rabbits on a high cholesterol diet to 10 weeks of exposure to secondhand smoke from Marlboro cigarettes. The animals were exposed to the secondhand smoke six hours a day, five days a week for just 10 weeks. One group was exposed to smoke at levels that would be observed in a smoky bar and the others were exposed to levels about three times as high. The high-dose group was exposed to pollution levels comparable to those observed in a Mazda 626 with the windows rolled up and four cigarettes per hour being smoked (91). With just 10 weeks of exposure (a total of 300 hours), the fraction of the pulmonary artery and aorta covered with lipid deposits nearly doubled (Fig. 3). This result demonstrates that even short-term exposure can substantially accelerate the atherosclerotic process. This effect appears to be directly due to elements in the cigarette smoke itself, rather

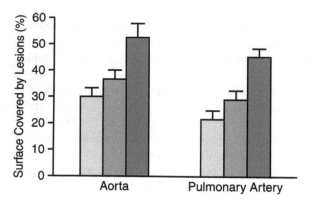

Figure 3 Passive smoking increases lipid deposits in arteries of rabbits, in a dose-dependent manner. Bars are for control (clean air), low dose, and high dose secondhand smoke exposures. *Source*: From Ref. 37

than a reaction to the secondhand smoke, which might have increased circulating catecholamines. (Increased levels of circulating catecholamines is one of the mechanisms by which cigarette smoking increases the risk of heart disease in active smokers.) Sun et al. (38) exposed rabbits in an experiment similar to that just described to secondhand smoke but gave half the rabbits the β-blocking drug metropolol. As expected, the animals receiving metropolol developed fewer lipid deposits than those who were receiving a placebo (saline), but this effect was independent of whether the rabbits were breathing secondhand smoke. Therefore, the secondhand smoke effects on the development of atherosclerotic-type lesions in the arteries were not mediated by the increased levels of catecholamines.

In addition, it is unlikely that these effects are due to the carbon monoxide in the smoke, because experiments in which chickens were exposed to high doses of pure carbon monoxide did not produce increased atheroschlerosis (82). In contrast, exposure to secondhand smoke for a relatively brief time (corresponding to about 0.4% of their life span) significantly accelerated the development of plaques (83,85). The fact that it is possible to induce atherosclerotic-like changes in two different species of experimental animals with only a few weeks' exposure to secondhand smoke similar to that experienced by people in normal day-to-day life is an important finding linking the epidemiological and biochemical evidence that passive smoking causes heart disease. The experimental studies on rabbits and cockerels, which do not suffer from the potential confounding variables in epidemiological studies, bridge this gap by showing that it is possible to induce atherosclerosis in experimental animals with secondhand smoke. Finally, there are also data in humans showing that passive smokers have significantly thicker carotid artery walls than people who never were exposed to passive or active smoking, with a dose-response relationship (92). Moreover, He et al. (93) observed that the number of stenotic (blocked or narrowed) coronary arteries observed in patients during coronary angiography was related to the amount of secondhand smoke to which they were exposed. These results are consistent with what one would expect from the animal experiments.

FREE RADICALS AND ISCHEMIC DAMAGE

Free radicals are highly reactive oxygen products (94,95), which, among others, are produced in cells as a result of the respiratory process in mitochondria that uses oxygen (96) to oxidize LDL cholesterol and directly depress NO production by the endothelium (69). Under normal conditions, endogenous antioxidants protect the vascular system from oxidative stress damage. In addition to free radicals produced in the body, free radicals from secondhand smoke can deplete these antioxidants (77,97–104) (Table 1).

Passive smoking worsens the outcome of an ischemic event in the heart through the activity of free radicals during reperfusion injury. The nicotine of just one cigarette doubled the reperfusion injury in dogs (105). This is so low a dose of nicotine that it had no effect on heart rate, blood pressure, regional myocardial shortening, or other hemodynamic measures of cardiac function commonly affected by nicotine in active and passive smokers (106). After an ischemic episode in which the left anterior descending coronary artery was litigated for 15 minutes, the regional shortening during reperfusion was reduced by 50% of the preischemic values. When the dog was exposed to the nicotine from just a single cigarette, the muscle shortened by 25% of control values. When the dog was given a free radical scavenger with the nicotine, this effect was obliterated. Thus, exposure to a very low dose of nicotine doubled the impact of the reperfusion injury.

The effects of free radicals induced by passive smoking have been explored at the cellular level (107,108). Rats exposed to secondhand smoke from two cigarettes a day for two months exhibited severely damaged mitochondrial function during reperfusion injury so that the ability of cardiac mitochondria to convert oxygen into ATP was much more compromised during reperfusion injury among rats exposed to these low doses of secondhand smoke than among control rats. Similar results were found in mice at low levels of smoke exposure (109). This is another way that the toxins in secondhand smoke interfere with myocardial energy metabolism. There is also some evidence that smokers are less sensitive to free radical damage from cigarette smoke than nonsmokers because of changes in the levels of enzymes that control free radicals (110). When hamsters were exposed to the secondhand smoke from six cigarettes a day for eight weeks, the activity of antioxidant enzymes in their lungs nearly doubled. Similar changes were found in the lungs of smokers compared with nonsmokers. This is another piece of evidence that the effects of passive cigarette smoking on smokers and nonsmokers may be different. Chronic exposure to cigarette smoke appears to increase the free radical scavenging systems in smokers, a benefit that nonsmokers would not have when breathing someone else's smoke.

In addition, passive smoking by humans sensitizes lung neutrophils (111). As with platelets, neutrophils are an important element of the body's defenses against infection and damage. Inappropriately activated neutrophils, however, release oxidants, and these elements can play a role in tissue damage in passive smokers. In a group of passive smokers exposed to just three hours of sidestream smoke, there were significant increases in the circulating leukocyte counts and stimulated neutrophil migration. (This study deals with neutrophils in the lungs, but it is reasonable to assume that the neutrophils exhibit similar effects throughout the body, since they are transported by the blood.) Like the other responses, the responses to secondhand smoke were greater in nonsmokers than in smokers, again suggesting that the biochemistry of secondhand smoke in passive smokers is different than in active smokers, with the passive smokers being more sensitive to the toxins in secondhand smoke.

MYOCARDIAL INFARCTION

There are also direct animal data to show that secondhand smoke promotes more tissue damage following myocardial infarction. Dogs exposed to secondhand smoke one hour daily for 10 days and then subjected to blockage of a coronary artery developed myocardial infarctions that were twice as large as those of controls who breathed clean air (112). This effect was not due to elevated circulating levels of nicotine or carboxyhemoglobin, since the infarcts were created the day after the last day of secondhand smoke exposure. Zhu et al. (39) conducted an experiment in rats, similar to the rabbit experiment discussed above, to investigate the effects of secondhand smoke exposure on infarct size. Rats were exposed to secondhand smoke six hours a day for three days, three weeks or six weeks, then subjected to a left coronary artery occlusion for 35 minutes, followed by reperfusion. There was a dose-dependent increase in infarct size, with the longest exposure (180 hours total secondhand smoke exposure) yielding infarcts that were nearly twice as large as those in the control group that breathed clean air (Fig. 4). It was also possible to block this effect by feeding the animals l-arginine, the amino acid which is a precursor for NO (113). This result suggests that the fact that secondhand smoke interferes with the vascular endothelium helps mediate the effects of secondhand smoke on myocardial infarction. There is no evidence of a threshold effect.

Although smokers seem to be less sensitive to effects of passive smoking than nonsmokers, it is important to recognize that even low doses of cigarette smoke can have important effects for smokers. For patients with coronary artery disease, smoking one cigarette significantly increases the coronary vascular resistance (114). Thus, at a time when demands for oxygen and blood supply to the heart are increasing (106,115), even a single cigarette can dramatically reduce the ability of smokers' coronaries to transmit blood. In addition, in habitual smokers, smoking a single cigarette causes an increase in the stiffness of

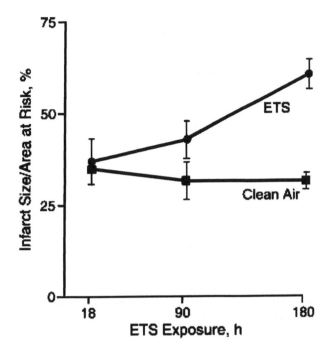

Figure 4 Passive smoking increases infarct size in rats subjected to a 35 minute occlusion of the left coronary artery, in a dose-dependent manner. There is no evidence of a threshold effect. *Source*: From Ref. 39.

coronary arterial walls, and this increased stiffness may be related to the rupturing of the atherosclerotic plaque, which can be an important step in the development of a myocardial infarction (116). It is likely that low doses of cigarette smoke will have similar effects in passive smokers.

NATURAL EXPERIMENTS: SHORT-TERM BENEFITS OF SMOKEFREE ENVIRONMENTS

Several of the effects of secondhand smoke, particularly the effects on platelets and endothelial function, occur quickly (within minutes) and are crucial elements in triggering and aggravating coronary events, particularly acute myocardial infarction (AMI). Given this fact, it was not all that surprising when Sargent et al. (117) reported a significant drop in hospital admissions for AMI (ICD-9 code 410), while a 100% smokefree law was in effect in Helena, Montana. In addition, when enforcement of the ordinance was suspended, AMI admissions inside Helena rebounded. Sargent et al. also examined admissions to the hospital from people living in the surrounding area (not covered by the ordinance) and found no change in AMI admissions from these people while the ordinance was in effect (Fig. 5).

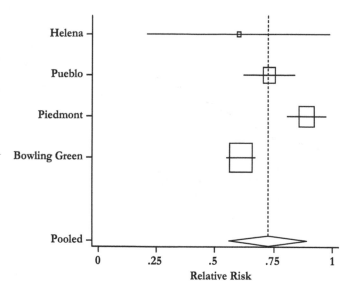

Figure 5 Reduction in hospital admissions in communities following implementation of smokefree workplace and public places laws. *Source*: From Ref. 121.

Just as the original epidemiological studies linking long-term exposure to secondhand smoke initially seemed too large, the Helena findings seemed too large and too fast to be plausible. Within two years of publication of the Helena study, three similar studies provided independent validation of the finding that eliminating secondhand smoke exposure was associated with significant drops in hospital admissions for AMI in Pueblo, Colorado (118) and the Piedmont region of Italy (119), and a third in Bowling Green, Ohio (120), for ischemic cardio-vascular disease and heart failure (Fig. 5). Overall, these four studies indicate that smokefree laws were associated with a 27% reduction (RR 0.73; CI 0.56, 0.89) in heart disease hospital admissions (121) (Fig. 5).

Like the Helena study (117), the Colorado (118) and Ohio (120) studies also examined hospital admission patterns in matched control community with no such law, and found no changes in admissions patterns during the time that the law was in effect. (The Italian law is national, so it was not possible to include a control community.) The fact that there were no changes in admission rates in the control communities is a major strength of all three studies that increases the confidence in the conclusion that the drop in admissions was actually due to a combination of reduced exposure to secondhand smoke associated with implementing a clean indoor air law and the fact that smokefree workplaces stimulate smokers to reduce cigarette consumption or stop smoking entirely (122). This reduction is also consistent with data demonstrating at least partial recovery of endothelial function after secondhand smoke exposure ends (65) and less systemic inflammation in bar workers after their workplaces were made smokefree (109).

CONCLUSION

The ability of the heart and vascular system to adapt to changing conditions is very important when considering the health effects of secondhand tobacco smoke, particularly when one compares the effects of secondhand smoke in nonsmokers with smokers. People who smoke cigarettes are chronically and continually adversely affecting their cardiovascular system (123), which adapts to compensate for all the deleterious effects of smoking. Nonsmokers, however, do not have the "benefit" of this adaptation, so the effects of passive smoking on nonsmokers are much greater than on smokers. This difference probably arises for two reasons: First, nonsmokers' hearts and vascular systems have not attempted to adapt to the chemicals in the secondhand smoke. Second, the cardiovascular system is extremely sensitive to many of the chemicals in secondhand smoke and that smokers may have achieved the maximum response possible to at least some of the toxins in the smoke, so the small additional exposures associated with passive smoking have little or no effect on habitual smokers because the additional dose of these toxins is so small compared with what the smoker normally receives.

As of January 2007, over half the U.S. population was covered by smokefree laws (124), and such laws were spreading around the world. Besides immediately improving indoor air quality and reducing long-term risk of cardiovascular diseases [and cancer and other diseases (2,4)], these laws immediately and substantially reduce the risk of AMI and other cardiovascular events. Using different methodologies, several investigators have estimated the population burden associated with passive smoking and heart disease, yielding estimates of 30,000 to 62,000 deaths annually in the United States (2,3,5,6,8,125,126), with about three times as many nonfatal cardiovascular events. Smokefree laws and policies have the additional advantage of creating an environment that makes it easier for smokers to reduce consumption or stop smoking (122). Indeed, smokefree workplaces are a more cost-effective smoking cessation intervention than directly delivered traditional cessation services (127). The large, consistent, and immediate effect of these laws and policies on health further strengthens the case for passing, fully implementing, and enforcing them.

REFERENCES

1. US Environmental Protection Agency. Respiratory Health Effects of Passive Smoking: Lung Cancer and Other Disorders: US Environmental Protection Agency; 1992. USEPA Document No. EPA/600/6-90/006F.
2. California Environmental Protection Agency. Proposed Identification of Environmental Tobacco Smoke as a Toxic Air Contaminant; 2005. Available at: www.arb.ca.gov/regact/ets2006/ets2006.htm.
3. California Environmental Protection Agency. Health Effects of Exposure to Environmental Tobacco Smoke. Final Report; 1997.
4. U.S. Department of Health and Human Services. The Health Consequences of Involuntary Exposure to Tobacco Smoke: A Report of the Surgeon General; 2006.

5. Wells AJ. Passive smoking as a cause of heart disease. J Am Coll Card 1994; 24: 546–554.
6. Wells AJ. Heart disease from passive smoking in the workplace. J Am Coll Cardiol 1998; 31(1):1–9.
7. Glantz S, Parmley W. Passive smoking and heart disease: mechanisms and risk. JAMA 1995; 273:1047–1053.
8. Glantz SA, Parmley WW. Passive smoking and heart disease: epidemiology, physiology, and biochemistry. Circulation 1991; 83:1–12.
9. Barnoya J, Glantz SA. Cardiovascular effects of secondhand smoke nearly as large as smoking. Circulation 2005; 111(20):2684–2698.
10. Taylor AE, Johnson DC, Kazemi H. Environmental tobacco smoke and cardiovascular disease: a position paper from the council on cardiopulmonary and critical care, American Heart Association. Circulation 1992; 86:1–4.
11. Gidding SS, Morgan W, Perry C, et al. Active and passive tobacco exposure: a serious pediatric health problem: a statement from the Committee on Atherosclerosis and Hypertension in Children, Council on Cardiovascular Disease in the Young, American Heart Association. Circulation 1994; 90:2582–2590.
12. Schick S, Glantz S. Philip Morris toxicological experiments with fresh sidestream smoke: more toxic than mainstream smoke. Tob Control 2005; 14(6):396–404.
13. Schick S, Glantz SA. Sidestream cigarette smoke toxicity increases with aging and exposure duration. Tob Control 2006; 15(6):424–429.
14. Pechacek TF, Babb S. How acute and reversible are the cardiovascular risks of secondhand smoke? BMJ 2004; 328(7446):980–983.
15. Raupach T, Schafer K, Konstantinides S, et al. Secondhand smoke as an acute threat for the cardiovascular system: a change in paradigm. Eur Heart J 2006; 27(4):386–392.
16. Law MR, Morris JK, Wald NJ. Environmental tobacco smoke exposure and ischaemic heart disease: an evaluation of the evidence. BMJ 1997; 315(7114):973–980.
17. He J, Vupputuri S, Allen K, et al. Passive smoking and the risk of coronary heart disease–a meta-analysis of epidemiologic studies. N Engl J Med 1999; 340(12): 920–926.
18. Thun M, Henley J, Apicella L. Epidemiologic studies of fatal and nonfatal cardiovascular disease and ETS exposure from spousal smoking. Environ Health Perspect 1999; 107(suppl 6):841–846.
19. Enstrom JE, Kabat GC. Environmental tobacco smoke and coronary heart disease mortality in the united states–a meta-analysis and critique. Inhal Toxicol 2006; 18(3): 199–210.
20. Enstrom JE, Kabat GC. Environmental tobacco smoke and tobacco related mortality in a prospective study of Californians, 1960-98. BMJ 2003; 326(7398):1057–1050.
21. Thun MJ. Passive smoking: tobacco industry publishes disinformation. BMJ 2003; 327(7413):502–503.
22. Whincup PH, Gilg JA, Emberson JR, et al. Passive smoking and risk of coronary heart disease and stroke: prospective study with cotinine measurement. BMJ 2004; 329(7459):200–205.
23. Benowitz NL. Cotinine as a biomarker of environmental tobacco smoke exposure. Epidemiol Rev 1996; 18(2):188–204.
24. Pittilo RM, Mackie IJ, Rowles PM, et al. Effects of cigarette smoking on the untrastructure of rat thoracic aorta and its ability to produce prostacyclin. Thromb Haemostas 1982; 48:173–176.

25. Davis J, Shelton L, Watanabe I, et al. Passive smoking affects endothelium and platelets. Arch Intern Med 1989; 149:386–389.
26. Sinzinger H, Kefalides A. Passive smoking severely decreases platelet sensitivity to antiaggregatory prostaglandines. Lancet 1982; 2:392–393.
27. Burghuber O, Punzengruber C, Sinzinger H, et al. Platelet sensitivity to prostacyclin in smokers and non-smokers. Chest 1986; 90:34–38.
28. Sinzinger H, Virgolini I. Are passive smokers at greater risk of thrombosis? Wien Klin Wochenschr 1989; 20:694–698.
29. Steinberg D, Parthasarathy S, Carew TE, et al. Beyond cholesterol: modifications of low-density lipoprotein that increase its atherogenicity. N Engl J Med 1989; 320: 915–924.
30. Elwood P, Renaud S, Sharp D, et al. Ischemic heart disease and platelet aggregation: the caerphilly collaborative heart disease study. Circulation 1991; 83:38–44.
31. Davis JW, Hartman CR, Lewis HD Jr., et al. Cigarette smoking-induced enhancement of platelet function: lack of prevention by aspirin in men with coronary artery disease. J Lab Clin Med 1985; 105:479–483.
32. Davis JW, Shelton L, Eigenberg DA, et al. Effects of tobacco and non-tobacco cigarette smoking on endothelium and platelets. Clin Pharmacol Ther 1985; 37: 529–533.
33. Davis J, Shelton L, Hartman C, et al. Smoking-induced changes in endothelium and platelets are not affected by hydroxyethlrutosides. Br J Exp Pathol 1986; 67: 765–771.
34. Davis JW, Shelton L, Eigenberg DA, et al. Lack of effect of aspirin on cigarette smoke-induced increase in circulating endothelial cells. Haemostasis 1987; 7:66–69.
35. Kato T, Inoue T, Morooka T, et al. Short-term passive smoking causes endothelial dysfunction via oxidative stress in nonsmokers. Can J Physiol Pharmacol 2006; 84(5): 523–529.
36. Rubenstein D, Jesty J, Bluestein D. Differences between mainstream and sidestream cigarette smoke extracts and nicotine in the activation of platelets under static and flow conditions. Circulation 2004; 109(1):78–83.
37. Zhu B-Q, Sun Y-P, Sievers R, et al. Passive smoking increases experimental atherosclerosis in cholesterol-fed rabbits. J Am Coll Cardiol 1993; 21:225–232.
38. Sun Y-p, Zhu b-q, SIevers RE, et al. Metoprolol does not attenuate atherosclerosis in lipid-fed rabbits exposed to environmentl tobacco smoke. Circulation 1994; 89:2260–2265.
39. Zhu B-Q, Sun Y-P, Sievers RE, et al. Exposure to environmental tobacco smoke increases myocardial infarct size in rats. Circulation 1994; 889:1282–1290.
40. Miyaura S, Eguchi H, Johnson JM. Effect of a cigarette smoke extract on the metabolism of the proinflammatory autacoid, platelet-activating factor. Circ Res 1992; 70:341–347.
41. Benowitz NL, Fitzgerald GA, Wilson M, et al. Nicotine effects on eicosanoid formation and hemostatic function: comparison of transdermal nicotine and cigarette smoking. J Am Coll Cardiol 1993; 22:1159–1167.
42. Bernhard D, Rossmann A, Henderson B, et al. Increased serum cadmium and strontium levels in young smokers: effects on arterial endothelial cell gene transcription. Arterioscler Thromb Vasc Biol 2006; 26(4):833–838.
43. Rader DJ. Lipid disorders. In: Topol EJ, ed. Textbook of Cardiovascular Medicine. 2nd ed. Philadelphia, PA: Lippincott Williams & Wilkins, 2002.

44. Iso H, Shimamoto T, Sato S, et al. Passive smoking and plasma fibrinogen concentrations. Am J Epidemiol 1996; 144(12):1151–1154.
45. Stavroulakis GA, Makris TK, Hatzizacharias AN, et al. Passive smoking adversely affects the haemostasis/fibrinolytic parameters in healthy non-smoker offspring of healthy smokers. Thromb Haemost 2000; 84(5):923–924.
46. Schmid P, Karanikas G, Kritz H, et al. Passive smoking and platelet thromboxane. Thrombosis Res 1996; 81:451–460.
47. Kroll MH, Resendiz JC. Mechanisms of platelet activation. In: Loscalzo J, Schafer AI, eds. Thrombosis and Hemorrhage. 3rd ed. Philadelphia, PA: Lippincott Williams & Wilkins, 2003:187–205.
48. Puranik R, Celermajer DS. Smoking and endothelial function. Prog Cardiovasc Dis 2003; 45(6):443–458.
49. Hutchison M, Stuart J, Sudhir M. Testosterone worsens endothelial dysfunction associated with hypercholesterolemia and environmental tobacco smoke exposure in male rabbit aorta. J Am Coll Cardiol 1997; 29(4):800–807.
50. Hutchison S, Sudhir K, Chou T, et al. Testosterone worsens endothelial dysfunction associated with hypercholesterolemia and environmental tobacco smoke exposure in male rabbit aorta. J Am Coll Cardiol 1997; 29:800–807.
51. Hutchison S, Glantz S, Zhu B-Q, et al. In-utero and neonatal exposure to secondhand smoke causes vascular dysfunction in newborn rats. JACC 1998; 32:1463–1467.
52. Zhu BQ, Parmley WW. Hemodynamic and vascular effects of active and passive smoking. Am Heart J 1995; 130(6):1270–1275.
53. Sumida H, Watanabe H, Kugiyama K, et al. Does passive smoking impair endothelium-dependent coronary artery dilation in women? J Am Coll Cardiol 1998; 31(4):811–815.
54. Widlansky ME, Gokce N, Keaney JF Jr., et al. The clinical implications of endothelial dysfunction. J Am Coll Cardiol 2003; 42(7):1149–1160.
55. Celermajer DS, Adams MR, Clarkson P, et al. Passive smoking and impaired endothelium-dependent arterial dilatation in healthy young adults. N Engl J Med 1996; 334(3):150–154.
56. Hutchison S, Ibarra M, Chou T, et al. L-arginine restores normal endothelium-medicated relaxation in hypercholesterolemic rabbits exposed to environmental tobacco smoke. J Am Coll Cardiol 1996; 27:(suppl 2):39A (abstr).
57. Hutchison S, Sudhir K, Sievers R, et al. Beneficial effects of chronic l-arginine supplementation on atherogenesis, endothelium-mediated relaxation, and nitric oxide production in hypersholesterolemic rabbits exposed to second hand smoke. Hypertension 1999; 34:44–50.
58. Hutchison S, Reitz M, Sudhir K, et al. Chronic dietary l-arginine prevents endothelial dysfunction secondary to environmental tobacco smoke in normocholesterolemic rabbits. Hypertension 1997; 29:1186–1191.
59. Otsuka R, Watanabe H, Hirata K, et al. Acute effects of passive smoking on the coronary circulation in healthy young adults. JAMA 2001; 286:436–441.
60. Glantz S, Parmley W. Even a little secondhand smoke is dangerous. JAMA 2001; 286:462–463.
61. Kato M, Roberts-Thomson P, Phillips BG, et al. The effects of short-term passive smoke exposure on endothelium-dependent and independent vasodilation. J Hypertens 1999; 17(10):1395–1401.

62. Barua RS, Ambrose JA, Eales-Reynolds LJ, et al. Dysfunctional endothelial nitric oxide biosynthesis in healthy smokers with impaired endothelium-dependent vasodilatation. Circulation 2001; 104(16):1905–1910.

63. Barua RS, Ambrose JA, Eales-Reynolds LJ, et al. Heavy and light cigarette smokers have similar dysfunction of endothelial vasoregulatory activity: an in vivo and in vitro correlation. J Am Coll Cardiol 2002; 39(11):1758–1763.

64. Mullick AE, McDonald JM, Melkonian G, et al. Reactive carbonyls from tobacco smoke increase arterial endothelial layer injury. Am J Physiol Heart Circ Physiol 2002; 283(2):H591–H597.

65. Raitakari OT, Adams MR, McCredie RJ, et al. Arterial endothelial dysfunction related to passive smoking is potentially reversible in healthy young adults. Ann Intern Med 1999; 130(7):578–581.

66. Cucina A, Sapienza P, Borrelli V, et al. Nicotine reorganizes cytoskeleton of vascular endothelial cell through platelet-derived growth factor Bb. J Surg Res 2000; 92(2):233–238.

67. Heiss C, Amabile N, Lee AC, et al. Second hand smoke causes acute vascular injury, and mobilization of dysfunctional endothelial progenitor cells. J Am Coll Cardiol 2008; 51(18):1760–1771.

68. Raij L, DeMaster EG, Jaimes EA. Cigarette smoke-induced endothelium dysfunction: role of superoxide anion. J Hypertens 2001; 19(5):891–897.

69. Jaimes EA, Demaster EG, Tian RX, et al. Stable compounds of cigarette smoke induce endothelial anion production via nadph oxidase activation. Arterioscler Thromb Vasc Biol 2004; 24:1031–1036.

70. Guthikonda S, Sinkey C, Barenz T, et al. Xanthine oxidase inhibition reverses endothelial dysfunction in heavy smokers. Circulation 2003; 107(3):416–421.

71. Ross R. The pathology of atherosclerosis: an update. N Engl J Med 1986; 314:488–500.

72. Ambrose JA, Barua RS. The pathophysiology of cigarette smoking and cardiovascular disease: an update. J Am Coll Cardiol 2004; 43(10):1731–1737.

73. Prerovsky I, Hladovec J. Suppression of the desquamating effect of smoking on the human endothelium by hydroxyethylrutosides. Blood Vessels 1979; 16:239–240.

74. Moskowitz W, Mosteller M, Schieken R, et al. Lipoprotein and oxygen transport alterations in passive smoking preadolescent children: the Mcv Irwin study. Circulation 1990; 81:586–592.

75. Feldman J, Shenker IR, Etzel RA, et al. Passive smoking alters lipid profiles in adolescents. Pediatrics 1991; 88:259–264.

76. White JR, Froeb HF. Serum lipoproteins in nonsmokers chonically exposed to tobacoo smoke in the workplace. Presented at: The 8th World Conference on Tobacco or Health (March 30–April 3, 1992); 1991; Buenos Aires, Argentina (abstr).

77. Valkonen M, Kuusi T. Passive Smoking Induces Atherogenic Changes in Low-Density Lipoprotein. Circulation 1998; 97(20):2012–2016.

78. Albert RE, Vanderlaan M, Burns FJ, et al. Effect of carcinogens on chicken atherosclerosis. Cancer Res 1977; 37:2232–2235.

79. Revis N, Bull R, Laurie D, et al. The Effectiveness of chemical carcinogens to induce atherosclerosis in the white carneau pigeon. Toxicology 1984; 32:215–227.

80. Penn A, Batastini G, Soloman J, et al. Dose-dependent size increases of aortic lesions following chronic exposure to 7.12-dimethybenz(a)anthracene. Cancer Res 1981; 41: 588–592.

81. Penn A, Garte S, Warren L, et al. Transforming gene is human atherosclerotic plaque DNA. Proc Natl Acad Sci U S A 1986; 83:7951–7955.

82. Penn A, Currie J, Snyder CA. Inhalation of carbon monoxide does not accelerate arteriosclerosis in cockerels. Eur J Pharmacol 1992; 228:155–164.
83. Penn A, Snyder CA. Inhalation of sidestream cigarette smoke accelerates development of artiosclerotic plaques. Circulation 1993; 88(pt 1):1820–1825.
84. Penn A, Snyder C. Sidestream cigarette smoke; Reply. Circulation 1994; 89: 2943–2944 (lettr).
85. Penn A, Chen LC, Snyder CA. Inhalation of steady-state sidestream smoke from one cigarette promotes atherosclerotic plaque development. Circulation 1994:1363–1367.
86. Penn A, Snyder C. 1,3 butadiene, a vapor phase component of environmental tobacco smoke, accelerates atheriosclerotic plaque development. Circulation 1996; 93:552–557.
87. Penn A, Keller K, Snyder C, et al. The tar fraction of cigarette smoke does not promote arterioschlerotic plaque development. Env Health Perspect 1996; 104: 1108–1113.
88. Penn A Snyder C. Butadiene inhalation accelerates arteriosclerotic plaque development in cockerels. Toxicology 1996; 113:351–354.
89. Majesky M, Yang H, Benditt E. Carcinogenesis and atherogenesis: differences in monoxygenase inducibility and bioactivation of benzo(a)pyrene in aortic and hepatic tissues of atherosclerosis-susceptible versus resistant pigeons. Carcinogenesis 1983; 4:647–652.
90. Howard D, Ota R, Briggs L, et al. Environmental tobacco smoke in the workplace induces oxidative stress in employees, including increased production of 8-hydroxy-2'-deoxyguanosine. Cancer Epidemiol Biomarkers Prev 1998; 7:141–146.
91. Ott W, Landan L, Switzer P. A time series model for cigarette smoking activity patterns: model validation for carbon monoxide and respirable particles in a chamber and an automobile. J Exposure Anal Environ Epidemiol 1992; 2(suppl 2): 175–200.
92. Howard G, Burke GL, Szklo M, et al. Active and passive smoking and are associated with increased carotid artery wall thickness: the atherosclerosis risk in communities study. Arch Int Med 1994; 154:1277–1282.
93. He Y, Lam T, LS L, et al. The number of stenotic coronary arteries is associated with the amount of passive smoking exposure. Atheroschlerosis 1996; 127:229–238.
94. Church DF, Pryor WA. Free-radical chemistry of cigarette smoke and its toxicological implications. Envirn Health Persp 1985; 64:111–126.
95. Ferrari R, Ceconi C, Curello S, et al. Oxygen free radicals and myocardial damage: protective role of thiol-containing agents. Am J Med 1991; 91 (suppl 3C):95S–105S.
96. Harrison D, Griendling KK, Landmesser U, et al. Role of oxidative stress in atherosclerosis. Am J Cardiol 2003; 91(3A):7A–11A.
97. Burke A, FitzGerald GA. Oxidative stress and smoking-induced vascular injury. Prog Cardiovasc Dis 2003; 46(1):79–90.
98. Tribble DL, Giuliano LJ, Fortmann SP. Reduced plasma ascorbic acid concentrations in nonsmokers regularly exposed to environmental tobacco smoke. Am J Clin Nutr 1993; 58(6):886–890.
99. Strauss RS. Environmental tobacco smoke and serum vitamin C levels in children. Pediatrics 2001; 107(3):540–542.
100. Preston AM, Rodriguez C, Rivera CE, et al. Influence of environmental tobacco smoke on vitamin C status in children. Am J Clin Nutr 2003; 77(1):167–172.

101. Alberg AJ, Chen JC, Zhao H, et al. Household exposure to passive cigarette smoking and serum micronutrient concentrations. Am J Clin Nutr 2000; 72(6): 1576–1582.
102. van der Vliet A. Cigarettes, cancer, and carotenoids: a continuing, unresolved antioxidant paradox. Am J Clin Nutr 2000; 72(6):1421–1423.
103. Dietrich M, Block G, Norkus EP, et al. Smoking and exposure to environmental tobacco smoke decrease some plasma antioxidants and increase {gamma}-tocopherol in vivo after adjustment for dietary antioxidant intakes. Am J Clin Nutr 2003; 77(1):160–166.
104. Hu FB, Willett WC. Optimal diets for prevention of coronary heart disease. JAMA 2002; 288(20):2569–2578.
105. Przyklenk K. Nicotine exacerbates postischemic contractile dysfunction of "stunned" myocardium in the canine model: possible role of free radicals. Circulation 1994; 89:1272–1281.
106. Benowitz NL. Nicotine and coronary heart disease. Trends Cardiovasc Med 1991; 1:315–321.
107. van Jaarsveld H, Kuyl JM, Alberts DW. Exposure of rats to low concentration of cigarette smoke increases myocardial sensitivity to ischaemia/reperfusion. Basic Res Cardiol. 1992; 87:393–399.
108. van Jaarsveld H, Kuyl JM, Alberts DW. Antioxidant vitamin supplementation of smoke-exposed rats partially protects against myocardial ischaemic/reperfusion injury. Free Rad Res Comms 1992; 17:263–269.
109. Knight-Lozano CA, Young CG, Burow DL, et al. Cigarette smoke exposure and hypercholesterolemia increase mitochondrial damage in cardiovascular tissues. Circulation 2002; 105(7):849–854.
110. McCusker K, Hoidal J. Selective increase of antioxidant enzyme activity in the alveolar macrophages from cigarette smokers and smoke-exposed hamsters. Am Rev Respir Dis 1990; 141:678–682.
111. Anderson R, Theron AJ, Richards GA, et al. Passive smoking by humans sensitizes circulating neutrophils. Am Rev Respir Dis 1991; 144:570–574.
112. Prentice RC, Carroll R, Scanlon PJ, et al. Recent exposure to cigarette smoke increases myocardial infarct size. J Am Coll Cardiol 1989; 13:124A (abstr).
113. Zhu B, Sun Y, Sievers RE, et al. L-arginine decreases infarct size in rats exposed to environmental tobacco smoke. Am Heart J 1996; 132(1 pt 1):91–100.
114. Quillen JE, Rossen JD, Oskarsson HJ, et al. Acute effect of cigarette smoking on the coronary circulation: constriction of epicardial and resistance vessels. J Am Coll Cardiol 1993; 22:642–647.
115. Fenton RA, Dobson JGJ. Nicotine increases heart adenosine release, oxygen consumption, and contractility. Am J Physiol (Heart) 1985; 249:H463–H469.
116. Kool MJF, Hoeks APG, Boudier HAJS, et al. Acute and chronic effects of smoking on arterial wall properties in habitual smokers. J Am Coll Cardiol 1993; 22: 1881–1886.
117. Sargent RP, Shepard RM, Glantz SA. Reduced incidence of admissions for myocardial infarction associated with public smoking ban: before and after study. BMJ 2004; 328(7446):977–980.
118. Bartecchi C, Alsever RN, Nevin-Woods C, et al. Reduction in the incidence of acute myocardial infarction associated with a citywide smoking ordinance. Circulation 2006; 114(14):1490–1496.

119. Barone-Adesi F, Vizzini L, Merletti F, et al. Short-term effects of italian smoking regulation on rates of hospital admission for acute myocardial infarction. Eur Heart J 2006; 27(20):2468.

120. Khuder SA, Milz S, Jordan T, et al. The impact of a smoking ban on hospital admissions for coronary heart disease. Prev Med 2007; 45(1):3–8.

121. Dinno A, Glantz SA. Clean indoor air laws immediately reduce heart attacks. Prev Med 2007; 45(1):9–11.

122. Fichtenberg CM, Glantz SA. Effect of smoke-free workplaces on smoking behaviour: systematic review. BMJ 2002; 325(7357):188.

123. US Centers for Disease Control and Prevention. The Health Consequences of Smoking: A Report of the Surgeon General. Washington, DC, 2004. Available at: http://www.cdc.gov/tobacco/sgr/sgr_2004/chapters.htm.

124. American Nonsmokers' Rights Foundation. Percent of U.S. State Populations Covered by Local or State 100% Smokefree Air Laws: American Nonsmokers' Rights foundation, 2007 January.

125. Wells AJ. An estimate of adult mortality in the united states from passive smoking. Environ Int 1988; 14:249–265.

126. Steenland K. Passive smoking and the risk of heart disease. JAMA 1992; 267:94–99.

127. Ong M, Glantz S. Cardiovascular health and economic effects of smoke-free workplaces. Am J Med 2004; 117:32–38.

128. Panagiotakos DB, Pitsavos C, Chrysohoou C, et al. Effect of exposure to secondhand smoke on markers of inflammation: the attica study*1. Am J Med 2004; 116(3): 145–150.

129. Stefanadis C, Tsiamis E, Vlachopoulos C, et al. Unfavorable effect of smoking on the elastic properties of the human aorta. Circulation 1997; 95(1):31–38.

130. Stefanadis C, Vlachopoulos C, Tsiamis E, et al. Unfavorable effects of passive smoking on aortic function in men. Ann Intern Med 1998; 128(6):426–434.

131. Moffatt RJ, Stamford BA, Biggerstaff KD. Influence of worksite environmental tobacco smoke on serum lipoprotein profiles of female nonsmokers. metabolism 1995; 44(12):1536–1539.

132. Howard G, Wagenknecht LE, Burke GL, et al. Cigarette smoking and progression of atherosclerosis: the atherosclerosis risk in communities (Aric) study. JAMA 1998; 279(2):119–124.

133. Ayaori M, Hisada T, Suzukawa M, et al. Plasma levels and redox status of ascorbic acid and levels of lipid peroxidation products in active and passive smokers. Environ Health Perspect 2000; 108(2):105–108.

134. Mannino DM, Mulinare J, Ford ES, et al. Tobacco smoke exposure and decreased serum and red blood cell folate levels: data from the Third National Health and Nutrition Examination Survey. Nicotine Tob Res 2003; 5(3):357–362.

14

Vascular Toxicology: A Cellular and Molecular Perspective

Kenneth S. Ramos

Department of Biochemistry and Molecular Biology, University of Louisville School of Medicine, Louisville, Kentucky, U.S.A.

E. Spencer Williams

Chemrisk, Inc., Houston, Texas, U.S.A.

INTRODUCTION

Epidemiologic and experimental evidence suggests that a direct correlation exists between occupational and environmental exposure to toxic chemicals and cardiovascular morbidity and mortality. This correlation is best exemplified by the recognition that exposure to tobacco smoke constituents is a major contributor to myocardial infarction, sudden cardiac death, arteriosclerotic peripheral vascular disease, and atherosclerotic aneurysm of the aorta. Similarly, recent studies have linked exposure to airborne environmental pollutants with increased risk for several cardiovascular diseases. Despite a wealth of new information on mechanisms of vascular injury, slow onset and long latency periods often obscure the relationship between toxic exposures and the development of cardiovascular pathology. Evidence implicating lipoproteins and oxidative stress as critical players in vascular pathogenesis continues to accumulate. A wide array of vascular toxins affect the vessels that serve as the circuitry for the transport and delivery of oxygen and nutrients to tissues throughout the body and for the removal of waste products of metabolism.

STRUCTURAL AND FUNCTIONAL CHARACTERISTICS
OF THE BLOOD VESSEL WALL

In view of the structural and cellular heterogeneity characteristic of the vascular tree, knowledge of blood vessel structure and function is essential to the elucidation of molecular mechanisms of chemical toxicity. Blood vessels are often classified as elastic or muscular vessels on the basis of their relative composition and abundance of extracellular matrix proteins. In primates, arteries vary in size from 300-μm internal diameter for large elastic vessels, such as the aorta and the carotid, to 30 μm for peripheral vessels, such as muscular arterioles. Veins are similar to their arterial counterparts but often are thinner and of larger diameter than arteries. Arterioles, capillaries, postcapillary venules, and venules constitute the microcirculation. In contrast to large blood vessels, which are distinct anatomical entities, microvessels are considered a part of the tissue in which they reside.

Mammalian blood vessels of large- and medium-size diameter are organized into three morphologically distinct layers (1,2). The innermost layer, referred to as the tunica intima, consists of a single layer of endothelial cells that rests on a loose layer of connective tissue formed by a thin basal lamina and a subendothelial layer. Luminal endothelial cells are flat and elongated, with their long axis parallel to the blood flow. These cells act as a semipermeable barrier between the blood and underlying components of the vessel wall. The subendothelial layer is formed by connective tissue bundles and elastic fibrils in which a few cells of smooth muscle origin may occasionally be oriented parallel to the long axis of the vessel. The subendothelial layer is only seen in large elastic arteries such as the human aorta.

Endothelial and vascular smooth muscle cells (vSMCs) are aligned around highly developed structures comprised of extracellular matrix proteins. Endothelial cells are anchored to a basal lamina, which includes fibrillar collagen and laminin. Fibrillar collagen types I and III are a major component of healthy vessels; these proteins, along with laminin, are thought to be quiescent in regard to vSMCs (3,4).

The medial layer, or tunica media, is composed of elastin and fibrillar collagen interwoven between multiple layers of smooth muscle cells. The media is separated from the outermost layer, the tunica adventitia, by a poorly defined external lamina. In the majority of vascular beds, smooth muscle cells dominate the media but may also be present in the intima of some vessels, as well as the adventitia of veins. The tunica adventitia consists of a loose layer of fibroblasts, collagen, elastin, and glycosaminoglycans. In larger vessels, this layer also includes the vasa vasorum, which supplies blood to the media and adventitia.

With the exception of capillaries, the walls of smaller vessels also have three distinct layers, which share many of the features described for larger vessels. However, in vessels of smaller diameter, the media is less elastic and consists of one to three layers of smooth muscle cells. An interesting feature of these vessels is the increased abundance of myoendothelial junctions. These features facilitate molecular transport and intercellular communication via Ca^{2+} and inositol 1,4,5-triphosphate signaling; they are particularly important in the regulation of vascular tone because they allow dissemination of endothelium-derived hyperpolarization factor (EDHF) and nitric oxide (NO$^-$) from endothelium into vascular smooth muscle (5,6). A recent review suggests that myoendothelial junctions are selective and communicate mainly in one direction, from endothelial cells to smooth muscle cells, to regulate cell-cell communication via secondary messengers (7).

As described for muscular arteries, venules are structurally similar to their arteriole counterparts. Because muscular venules are larger than arterioles, a large fraction of blood is contained in these capacitance vessels. Capillaries are endothelial tubes measuring 4 to 8 μm in diameter, which rest on a thin basal lamina to which pericytes are often attached. When one capillary converges with another, the vessel formed is referred to as a postcapillary venule. The capillary and the pericytic venule are the principal sites of exchange between the blood and tissues.

It has become increasingly apparent that the responses of smooth muscle cells are influenced by their relative location along the vascular tree. These distinctions are illustrated by phenotypic differences in growth characteristics and matrix-producing capabilities (8,9). This phenomenon may be explained by the contribution of multiple cell lineages to the vSMC population during embryonic development of the artery wall (10). Endothelial cells in different regions of the vasculature also differ in morphology and protein expression, stemming from genetic and epigenetic mechanisms (11,12).

VASCULAR CELL BIOLOGY

In humans, the development of the blood circulation (i.e., vasculogenesis) begins at four weeks of gestation, when simple diffusion of nutrients is no longer sufficient to support growth (13). Developing vessels are formed by cells of mesenchymal origin that become angioblasts and in turn differentiate into blood cells or endothelial cells. Endothelial cells form capillaries, which give rise to larger vessels by the apposition of pericytes and/or fibroblasts that ultimately differentiate into vSMCs. Cells that give rise to the development of vSMC layers appear to emanate from multiple sources in the developing embryo (14,15).

Endothelial cells play integral roles in the regulation of hemostasis, vascular tone, and angiogenesis. Endothelial cells are also involved in the regulation of macromolecular transport across the vessel wall, attachment and recruitment of inflammatory cells, trafficking of leukocytes, synthesis of connective tissue proteins, and generation of reactive oxygen species (ROS) (11,12,16–19). As part of their role in maintaining balance, endothelial cells can produce either molecules that promote or molecules that inhibit a variety of vascular processes, including vasoconstriction/vasodilation, coagulation, and inflammation (19).

Under normal conditions, medial smooth muscle cells are found primarily in a quiescent state of growth specialized for muscle contraction, though they are capable of cell cycle reentry (14,20,21). The hallmark of this state of specialization is an intricate and well-defined network of contractile machinery, characterized by the presence of smooth muscle myosin and actin isoforms, and anchoring proteins such as vinculin, metavinculin, α-actinin, and talin (22). Some components of this framework are useful as markers of vSMC identity, including SM22α, smooth muscle myosin heavy chains, smooth muscle α-actin, calponin, and β-tropomyosin to name a few (14,23). Mature vSMCs exhibit minimal proliferation or cell death, unless called upon for processes including regeneration or repair of vessel damage or myometrial development during pregnancy (24,25).

Physiologically, vSMCs of the media are responsible for maintenance of vascular tone; this function is mediated by an array of intracellular and extracellular signaling pathways, including the contribution of intimal endothelial cells. Smooth muscle cell responses to contractile agonists are mediated by receptors located on the plasma membrane. Activation of these receptors by endogenous transmitters, hormones, or xenobiotics is associated with changes in ionic conductance that ultimately activate the contractile apparatus. Membrane channels, sarcolemmal pumps, energy-dependent sequestration of calcium by intracellular organelles, and a number of calcium-binding proteins participate in the maintenance of ionic transport.

In addition to their central role in the regulation of vasomotor tone, smooth muscle cells participate in the synthesis of extracellular matrix proteins during arterial repair, the metabolism and/or secretion of bioactive substances, the regulation of monocyte function, and the generation of ROS (20,21,24). Fibroblasts within the adventitial layer secrete some of the collagen and glycosaminoglycans needed to lend structural support to the vessel wall (26).

MECHANISMS OF VASCULAR-SPECIFIC TOXICITY

Several types of chemicals including natural products, drugs, and anthropogenic chemicals have been recognized as potential vascular toxins. Angiotoxicity may be expressed at the mechanical, metabolic, epigenetic, or genetic level. As a general rule, vascular toxicity in vivo involves interactions of multiple cellular elements (Table 1). Alterations in the expression of cytoskeletal proteins, second-messenger molecules, or growth factors from any of these cell types may indicate vascular toxicity.

The most prevalent cellular mechanisms of vascular toxicity are listed in Table 2. These mechanisms include (*i*) selective alterations of vascular reactivity, (*ii*) vessel-specific bioactivation of protoxicants, (*iii*) erratic chemical detoxification, and (*iv*) preferential accumulation of the active toxin within vascular cells. As illustrated in Figure 1, multiple mechanisms may operate simultaneously for a given toxic agent. Vascular reactivity, defined as the intrinsic ability of blood vessels to respond to biologically active substances, can be regulated at multiple levels, including changes in signal transduction from the surface to the interior of the cell and/or modulation of contractile protein structure and function.

Table 1 Cell Types Implicated in the Vasculotoxic Response

Cell type	Function
Endothelial cells	First barrier to bloodborne toxins; synthesis and release of endothelium-derived relaxing factor; synthesis of pro- and antiaggregatory factors; attachment and recruitment of inflammatory cells; synthesis of connective tissue proteins; generation of oxygen-derived free radicals and other radical moieties.
Smooth muscle cells	Maintenance of vasomotor tone; synthesis of extracellular matrix proteins including collagen and elastin; synthesis of prostaglandins and other biologically active lipids; regulation of monocyte function; formation of free radicals.
Fibroblasts	Synthesis of extracellular matrix proteins, including collagens, structural support to the vessel wall.
Monocytes/ macrophages	Scavenger potential; synthesis of macrophage-derived growth factor; generation of reactive oxygen species; lymphocyte activation, progenitor of foam cells.
Platelets	Synthesis of proaggregatory substances and smooth muscle mitogens such as platelet-derived growth factor.
Lymphocytes	Release of activated oxygen species; cellular immunity; production of immunoglobulins.

Table 2 Putative Mechanisms of Vasculotoxic Insult

Mechanism	Prototype toxins
Alterations of vascular reactivity	Metals, catecholamines, carbon monoxide, nicotine, T-2 toxin
Vessel-specific bioactivation	Allylamine, polycyclic aromatic hydrocarbons, catecholamine, homocysteine, carbon disulfide
Erratic detoxification	Allylamine, dinitrotoluene, hydrazinobenzoic acid, metals
Preferential accumulation	Allylamine, polycyclic aromatic hydrocarbons, TCDD
Altered signal transduction	Allylamine, vitamin D, oxidized lipoproteins

Abbreviation: TCDD, tetrachlorodibenzo-p-dioxin.

Endothelial cells represent the first cellular barrier to the movement of bloodborne toxins from the lumen of the vessel to deeper regions of the wall. Constant exposure to luminal blood flow makes them particularly susceptible to toxic insult. Toxic chemicals that reach the subendothelial space as a protoxin or as substance metabolically activated by endothelial cells may cause injury to medial smooth muscle cells and/or adventitial fibroblasts. Adventitial and medial cells within large elastic arteries, such as the human aorta, may also be reached via the vasa vasorum. These exposures may result in adduction of the toxin to

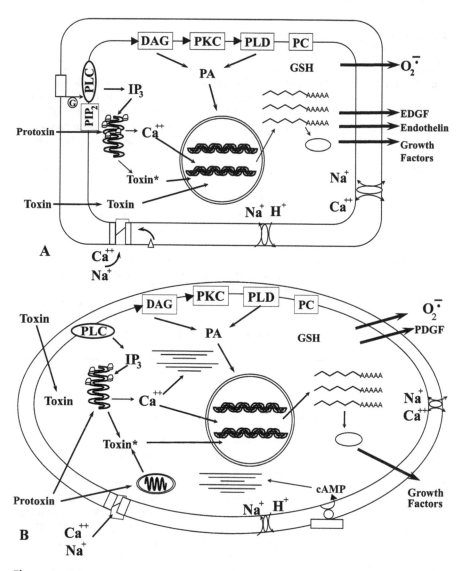

Figure 1 Selected cellular and molecular targets of vasculotoxic insult in (**A**) endothelial and (**B**) smooth muscle cells. Alterations of vascular reactivity are often mediated by changes in the distribution of ions across the membrane of vascular endothelial and/or smooth muscle cells. Alternatively, toxicant interference with signal transduction mechanisms at the receptor or second messenger level or structural/functional changes of contractile proteins may also interfere with vascular function. Enzyme systems capable of converting inactive chemicals to reactive forms that cause cell injury have also been identified. Deficient antioxidant capacity in vascular cells has also been suspected as a contributor to enhanced susceptibility to toxic injury. As in other organ systems, accumulation of toxicants within vascular cells has also been implicated in several vascular toxicities.

cellular macromolecules, such as protein and DNA. In addition, the vasculotoxic response may be dependent on the influence of (*i*) extracellular matrix proteins, which interact with vascular cells and initiate far-reaching signaling cascades; (*ii*) coagulation factors, which dictate the extent of hemostatic involvement; (*iii*) hormones and growth factors, which regulate proliferative/differentiation programs; (*iv*) plasma lipoproteins, some of which modulate cellular metabolism; (*v*) inflammation; and (*vi*) ROS in the intracellular and extracellular spaces.

As described for other organ systems, nontoxic chemicals can be converted by vascular enzymes to highly reactive species capable of causing injury to both intra- and extracellular targets. Enzyme systems present in vascular cells that have been implicated in the bioactivation of vascular toxins include amine oxidases, cytochrome P-450 monooxygenases, and prostaglandin synthetase. These enzymes play important roles in the regulation of vascular function under physiologic conditions. For instance, copper-containing amine oxidases are widespread enzymes that catalyze the oxidative removal of biogenic amines from blood plasma, the cross-linking of collagen and elastin in connective tissue, and the regulation of intracellular spermine and spermidine levels (27–29). Circulating levels of one of these enzymes, semicarbazide-sensitive amine oxidase (SSAO), is increased in diabetic patients as well as those with congestive heart failure (30). The existence of several cytochrome P-450 metabolites of arachidonic acid involved in the regulation of vascular tone, inflammation, cytokine production, and sodium pump activity has also been recognized (31,32). A complex of microsomal enzymes, collectively referred to as prostaglandin synthetase, catalyze the formation of biologically active lipid metabolites, including prostacyclin and thromboxane A_2. Prostacyclin, the major arachidonic acid metabolite in blood vessels, is a strong vasodilator and endogenous inhibitor of platelet aggregation, while thromboxane A_2, the major arachidonic acid metabolite in platelets, is a potent vasoconstrictor and promoter of platelet aggregation (32).

Evidence continues to accumulate, suggesting that vascular-specific activation of protoxins is a significant contributor to vasculotoxic insult. Cytochrome P-450 monooxygenases in both endothelial cells and vSMCs can activate protoxins to toxins, as shown recently for human cells (33). Similarly, vascular bioactivation of toxins has been demonstrated in several animal models (34–36). However, the bioactivation of vascular toxins need not be confined to vascular tissue. Angiotoxic chemicals may be bioactivated by other metabolically active organs such as the liver and lung. Lipophilic metabolites may be transported and delivered to the vessel wall by association with plasma lipoproteins (37).

Vascular toxicity may also be due to deficiencies in the capacity of target cells to detoxify the active toxin. Key components of the antioxidant defense system operative in vascular cells include the glutathione/glutathione reductase/glutathione peroxidase system, superoxide dismutase, and catalase. At low oxidant levels, glutathione is believed to be critical for cellular redox balance, while catalase is a major detoxifying enzyme at higher oxidant levels. It is well established that upregulation of glutathione synthesis machinery occurs in response to chemical and mechanical injury.

Significant differences in the antioxidant capacity of vascular cells relative to other cell types have been documented. For instance, vascular endothelial cells are more sensitive to oxidative stress than fibroblasts (38), while vSMCs appear to be fairly resistant to peroxide-induced injury relative to hepatocytes (39). Limited information is presently available regarding the cellular bases for the differential response of vascular and nonvascular cells, but the response is species-specific since rat cells are clearly more resistant to peroxide-induced injury than murine counterparts. The contractile properties of vSMCs and the role of ROS in intracellular signaling may account for the differential response to cellular oxidants. Ongoing production of ROS that occurs as a by-product of cellular bioenergetics may in effect prime detoxification of oxidant species in vSMCs. Interestingly, responses to oxidative stress may differ significantly even between populations of vSMCs from different regions of the vascular tree (40).

Finally, vascular toxicity may be due to selective accumulation of chemicals within the vascular wall. For example, benzo(a)pyrene (BaP), a prototypical polycyclic aromatic hydrocarbon (PAH), preferentially accumulates in the endoplasmic reticulum and the mitochondria of target cells (41). Although the mechanisms responsible for preferential accumulation of toxins within the vessel wall are not yet known, receptor-mediated internalization of low-density lipoproteins (LDLs) and chemical properties of the toxins in question may be critical in this process. It is evident that as the lesion progresses, oxidized low-density lipoprotein (oxLDL) and several types of extracellular matrix proteins accumulate in the vessel wall; these by-products may contribute to development of the lesion.

Ultimately, the consequences of vasculotoxic insult are dictated by the interplay between vascular and nonvascular cells, as well as intracellular signaling molecules and noncellular factors such as extracellular matrix proteins, coagulation factors, hormones, immune complexes, and plasma lipoproteins. This concept is exemplified by the lymphocytic and platelet involvement in various forms of toxic injury. Furthermore, the toxic response can be modulated by mechanical and hemodynamic factors such as arterial pressure, shear stress, and blood viscosity. An additional consideration is that kinetic and pharmacodynamic differences among different animal species, as well as age and sex, may also alter the toxicologic profile of a given chemical.

VASCULAR INJURY AND TOXICITY IN THE PATHOGENESIS OF VASCULAR DISEASE

Cardiovascular disease is still the leading cause of death in industrialized nations. The vast majority of these mortalities are associated with atherosclerosis. This common disease of the vasculature is characterized by the formation of a lesion in the wall of an artery, particularly those lesionsthat perfuse the heart (coronaries). Atherogenesis is initiated through several types of insults, including mechanical, chemical, and oxidative. An inflammatory-fibroproliferative response follows; macrophages, extracellular matrix components, and intra- and extracellular lipids accumulate as the lesion advances. Progression of athero-sclerosis involves hypertrophy, hyperproliferation, and migration of vSMCs into the intima, narrowing the available area for blood circulation (42,43). These lesions become more and more complex over time, including the formation of a fibrous cap, which protects a necrotic core, LDL-filled foam cells, and a body of extracellular matrix secreted by activated vSMCs. Rupture of the lesion can lead to thrombosis, the formation of a blood clot in the artery that occludes blood flow. Many risk factors for the development of atherosclerosis have been identified, including diabetes, hypercholesterolemia, obesity, smoking, and hypertension.

A popular theory of atherosclerosis as proposed originally by Russell Ross (44), and later modified (45,46), states that atherosclerotic lesions develop as a result of chronic cycles of vascular injury and repair. Consistent with this hypothesis, mechanical or toxic injury to the endothelium has been associated with initiation of atherogenesis (47–49). In fact, mechanical injury is commonly used as a model for atherosclerosis; balloon angioplasty in laboratory animals produces accelerated growth of lesions similar to those seen in atherosclerosis (50). As part of the repair process, smooth muscle cell mitogens and inflammatory cytokines are released from one or more of the cell types involved in the disease process, including endothelial cells, smooth muscle cells, macrophages, and fibroblasts.

However, the hypothesis that is generally accepted today is the monoclonal theory of atherogenesis as proposed by Benditt (51) and recently updated by Murry et al. (52). On the basis of the monotypism of glucose-6-phosphate dehydrogenase, these investigators proposed that smooth muscle cells within the atherosclerotic lesion are the progeny of a single smooth muscle cell. As such, development of atherosclerotic plaques would resemble benign neoplastic growth of smooth muscle tumors (leiomyomas). This theory was supported by genetic analysis of vSMCs arising from vascular lesions (10). Though the experiments of Schwartz and Murry appear to confirm the Benditt hypothesis of atherogenesis, inflammation and injury, central elements of the Ross theory, are certainly critical components of the disease process.

Following exposure to a toxic or infectious agent, smooth muscle cells may exist in a genetically altered state that gives rise to lesions upon exposure to chemotactic/growth-promoting factors. Alternatively, mutations could induce constitutive production of growth factors within smooth muscle cells themselves, resulting in autocrine stimulation of growth. DNA isolated from human athe-rosclerotic plaques is capable of transforming NIH3T3 cells and producing tumors in nude mice (53). Observations of DNA adducts found within human atherosclerotic lesions lend support to a genotoxic mechanism in vSMC dysre-gulation (54–56). Oxidative DNA damage may also contribute to genetic changes, which lead to atherosclerosis (57). Several genetic targets that may be altered in atherogenesis have been implicated, including myb, platelet-derived growth factor (PDGF), and ras (58–61).

One of the hallmarks of atherosclerosis is the so-called fatty streak, an accumulation of lipid material on the vessel wall. These deposits allow for concentration-dependent accumulation of LDL in the vessel wall (62). In recent years, the formation of oxLDL within the intima and the removal of oxLDL by macrophage scavenger receptors have been implicated in the development of atherosclerotic disease (63,64). A potent mediator of this oxidation may be the oxidant peroxynitrite ($ONOO^-$), which is the product of the reaction of superoxide (O_2^-) and NO^- (65,66). The presence of macrophages may also contribute to oxidation of LDL, as the presence of these lipids induces transcription of several inflammatory cytokines (62,67–69).

C-reactive protein (CRP) has been a subject of intense scrutiny in this context in recent years. This protein is expressed primarily by hepatocytes, yet has been confirmed as a marker for cardiovascular disease. CRP is present in atherosclerotic lesions, and levels of the protein correlate with the progression of atherosclerosis. It is unclear at this point if CRP is a marker or a contributor to the disease; however, it is worth noting that CRP can modulate the function of both endothelial cells and vSMCs as well as promote production of oxidant species and inflammatory pathways involved in atherosclerosis (70–73).

One of the critical events in initiation and progression of atherosclerotic lesions is the activation of vSMCs. Under the influence of various stimuli, smooth muscle cells lose their ability to contract and shift toward a phenotypic state characterized by enhanced synthetic and proliferative activity. This shift is accompanied by a decrease in expression of proteins associated with contractile activity (24,74). Cells in the synthetic state are distinguished from contractile counterparts by their ability to migrate, proliferate, and secrete extracellular matrix components. Phenotypic modulation of smooth muscle cells occurs during various physiologic processes, such as fetal and postnatal development, regeneration and repair of blood vessels, and myometrial development during pregnancy (25,75).

PDGF plays a central role in the modulation of this vSMC proliferation, migration, and contraction; epidermal growth factor (EGF) and insulin-like growth factor IGF are also thought to contribute to phenotypic modulation (46,76). Transcriptional activation of the growth-related proto-oncogene *c-Ha-ras* gene via redox mechanisms is associated with proliferation of vSMCs (77). The protein product of ras is a guanosine triphosphate (GTP)-binding protein, p21[ras]; this GTPase participates in multiple proliferation and injury response pathways. Downstream of ras, transcription factors AP-1 and NF-κB play important roles in proliferation and survival of vSMCs (78–80). A role for NF-κB in atherosclerosis is supported by several lines of evidence (81–84).

Aside from its role as a vasodilator, NO^- has been shown to inhibit proliferation and migration of vSMCs as a homeostatic function as well as during atherosclerotic lesion development. This effect involves activation of guanylate cyclase and cyclic guanosine mononucleotide (cGMP)-dependent protein kinase, concomitant with vasorelaxation pathways (85–87). In addition, vSMC mitogenesis can also be inhibited by estrogen and progesterone, in agreement with the suggestion that these hormones afford protective effects in the development of cardiovascular disease (88); however, evidence from recent clinical trials suggests that hormone replacement therapy does not have an effect on development or progression of atherosclerosis (89,90). The genetic basis for transition of vSMCs to proliferative phenotypes may involve activation of mobile genetic elements, retrotransposons, as described recently by this laboratory (91).

An important risk factor for atherosclerosis is hypertension. Increased vascular resistance has been associated with an overall increase in wall thickness and smooth muscle mass, which may be an early indicator of atherosclerosis (92,93). These changes appear to be due, at least in part, to hypertrophy of smooth muscle cells. Also, such increases of vascular resistance may involve increased levels of circulating vasoconstrictors, such as angiotensin II or catecholamines. However, local regulation by metabolic, myogenic, or angiogenic mechanisms may be involved in the pressor response (94). A sustained elevation in blood pressure has also been associated with destruction of capillaries at the tissue level.

SELECTED VASCULAR TOXINS

Allylamine

Allylamine (3-aminopropene) is an unsaturated aliphatic amine utilized as a precursor in the vulcanization of rubber and the synthesis of pharmaceuticals (95). In addition, several allylamine compounds have been developed as antifungal agents for human and veterinary use (96). Allylamine is more toxic than other unsaturated primary amines of higher molecular weight (97). Exposure to allylamine by a variety of routes in multiple animal species is associated with selective cardiovascular toxicity (98–101). The specificity of the toxic response may be related to its ability to accumulate in elastic and muscular arteries on administration in vivo (102). Gross lesions are evident in the myocardium, aorta, and coronary arteries of animals exposed to allylamine. Subacute and chronic administration is associated with the development of atherosclerotic-like lesions characterized by smooth muscle cell proliferation and fibrosis. Though human exposure to allylamine would be rare, use of this chemical in animal models have yielded many insights into mechanisms of vascular toxic injury.

Boor and colleagues first proposed that allylamine toxicity results from bioactivation of the parent compound to a toxic aldehyde, acrolein (103). Vascular-specific bioactivation of allylamine to acrolein and hydrogen peroxide (H_2O_2) by SSAO is considered a prerequisite for the manifestation of toxicity (103–105).

SSAO is a copper-containing amine oxidase found in cardiovascular tissue in higher concentrations than any other tissue (29,106). Elevated levels of this enzyme have been noted in diabetic patients as well as in those with congestive heart failure (30). Inhibition of this enzyme protects vascular cells from allyl-amine cytotoxicity (105). SSAO is most abundant in smooth muscle cells, both vascular and nonvascular, as well as adipocytes, chondrocytes, and odontoblasts. As a result of this, allylamine preferentially injures smooth muscle cells relative to other cell types within the vascular wall. Past work has shown that the enzymatic activity responsible for the metabolic conversion of allylamine to acrolein in aortic tissue is localized in the mitochondrial and microsomal fractions (107). These observations are in agreement with studies by others showing that allylamine, or its metabolites, are sequestered in close proximity to endoplasmic reticulum and mitochondria (108).

The selectivity of allylamine toxicity has been attributed to accumulation and preferential toxification, but other mechanisms including failure of detoxification systems may also contribute to the specificity of the toxic response. Glutathione-S-transferase 8-8 and γ-glutamylcysteine synthetase activity are upregulated in vSMCs exposed to allylamine (109).

Acrolein itself is a ubiquitous toxic chemical found in engine exhaust and cigarette smoke as well as cooked foods. Acrolein is an extremely reactive aldehyde, which disrupts the thiol balance of vascular cells (110). Acrolein is formed endogenously on oxidation of allylamine and as a by-product of lipid peroxidation and inflammation in biological systems (111,112). Although a large number of compounds react with acrolein under physiologic conditions, the main reaction products result from nucleophilic addition at the terminal ethylenic carbon. As such, toxicity most likely results from the reaction of acrolein with critical cellular sulfhydryls. This is reflected in depletion of glutathione. Acrolein can also be converted via nicotinamide adenosine dinucleotide phosphate (NADPH)-dependent microsomal enzymes to glycidaldehyde and acrylic acid (113).

Several studies have been conducted to examine the direct vascular toxicity of this aldehyde. Within the context of allylamine cytotoxicity, these studies are important since the toxicologic profile of acrolein may not replicate that of the parent compound. Exogenous acrolein results in extensive injury to the cell membrane before critical subcellular targets are compromised. In contrast, intracellular formation of acrolein allows simultaneous interaction of the aldehyde with multiple subcellular targets. In particular, acrolein can interfere with oxidative phosphorylation processes in the myocardium, resulting in loss of cellular adenosine triphosphate (ATP) (114). It is also clear that in vivo exposure to acrolein can cause changes in lipid proteins, regulation of vascular tone, activity of mitogen-activated protein kinase (MAPK) pathways, and expression of glutathione-S-transferases, all effects that may contribute to vascular disease (112,115–119). Studies by Kutzman et al. (120) also indicate that acrolein is more toxic to hypertension-sensitive animals than hypertension-resistant counterparts.

H_2O_2 and ammonia formed during the deamination process may contribute to allylamine-induced vascular injury. However, acute cytotoxicity studies have shown that vascular cells are relatively resistant to H_2O_2. The absence of overt cytotoxicity does not rule out the possibility that H_2O_2 enhances cellular proliferation, especially at low concentrations, and additional work to define its contribution to the overall cytotoxic injury is warranted (121). Further, the role of H_2O_2 in growth- and function-related signaling in vSMCs may further complicate this concept.

Because the expression of vasculotoxic insult is often a multifactorial phenomenon characterized by long latency periods, an in vivo/in vitro regimen has been used in our laboratory to evaluate the toxicity of allylamine (122,123). On completion of defined dosing regimens in vivo, aortic smooth muscle cells are isolated and established in primary or secondary culture. This culture system has been used to evaluate the impact of repeated cycles of injury and repair in vivo on smooth muscle cell phenotypes. Smooth muscle cells from rats exposed subchronically to allylamine grow more rapidly in primary culture than cells isolated from control animals (122). When seeded on a glass surface, control cells are elongated and spindle shaped, while allylamine cells are more broad and round. In contrast to cells from control animals, smooth muscle cells isolated from allylamine-treated animals do not respond to contractile challenge in vitro. Allylamine cells are characterized by numerous ribosomes and rough endoplasmic reticulum. These features are consistent with their enhanced ability to synthesize DNA and collagen relative to cells from control animals. Similar increases in collagenous proteins have been reported by Awasthi and Boor (124).

Subsequent studies showed that allylamine modulates both precursors and products of phosphoinositide metabolism in vSMCs (123). These actions appear to be mediated by enhanced phospholipase-C-mediated turnover of membrane phospholipids. Manipulation of phosphoinositide metabolism on exposure to dibutyryl cyclic adenosine monophosphate (cAMP) modulates the phenotypic expression of allylamine cells, as judged by changes in morphology, DNA synthesis, and inositol phosphate production (123). Although an intriguing association between cAMP levels and the phenotypic state of vSMCs has been established, the role of cAMP as a regulatory factor in phosphoinositide metabolism and phenotypic modulation is not yet clear.

It is likely that integrin-mediated signaling may regulate these intracellular processes through interactions with an allylamine-induced, thrombin-generated cleavage product of osteopontin in vSMCs, with α_v-coupled integrins (125). Along with changes in matrix protein production, modulation of the expression of integrin subunits and downstream signaling associated with focal adhesions has been described in allylamine-injured vSMCs (126). Microarray experiments have identified broad changes in expression of cytoskeletal, adhesion signaling, and signal transduction gene products (2).

Carbon Monoxide

Carbon monoxide (CO) induces vascular injury in laboratory animals at concentrations at which humans may be exposed from environmental sources such as automobile exhaust, tobacco smoke, and fossil fuels (127). Because most sources of CO represent a complex mixture of chemicals, attempts to distinguish the direct effects of CO from those of other chemicals such as sulfur oxides, nitrogen oxides, aldehydes, and hydrocarbons are problematic. CO is also produced in modest amounts as a result of physiologic processes (128). Short-term exposure to CO is associated with direct damage to vascular endothelial (129) and smooth muscle cells (130). Endothelial cells exposure increases intimal permeability and allows the interaction of blood constituents with underlying components of the vascular wall. This response may account, at least in part, for the ability of CO to induce atherosclerotic lesions in several animal species. Paradoxically, CO acts as a vasorelaxant, a function possibly related to its chemical similarity to NO^-.

Although CO enhances total arterial deposition of cholesterol in animals fed a lipid-rich diet (131), its vascular effects appear to be independent of serum cholesterol levels. CO potentiates cellular growth and suppresses collagen synthesis of cultured porcine endothelial cells, but inhibits cellular growth and causes no changes in the collagen synthesis of bovine endothelial cells (129). The mechanisms responsible for species differences have not been defined, but may account for conflicting reports in the literature. Consistent with phenotypic modulation seen in atherogenesis, smooth muscle cells exposed to CO in vitro exhibit partial loss of myofilaments and proliferation of intracellular organelles (130); however, CO inhibits proliferation of vSMCs.

A relative increase in the number of pinocytic vesicles at and below the cell surface and an increase in the number of lysosomes have also been observed. These alterations resemble those observed when smooth muscle cells are grown under hypoxic conditions (130). Hypoxia can also lead to increased expression of mitogens, such as PDGF-B, endothelin-1, and vascular endothelial growth factor in endothelial cells (132). Furthermore, hypoxia suppresses (NO^-) synthase, thereby decreasing cellular levels of (NO^-). VSMCs respond to hypoxia by increasing heme oxygenase, an enzyme that metabolizes heme to CO and biliverdin. CO in turn suppresses endothelin-1 and PDGF-B (133).

The observation that CO intoxication mimics hypoxia is not surprising, as the best-understood toxic effect of CO results from its reversible interaction with hemoglobin. The formation of carboxyhemoglobin in vivo is favored because binding of CO to hemoglobin is more cooperative than that of oxygen. As a result of this interaction, carboxyhemoglobin decreases the oxygen-carrying capacity of blood and shifts the oxyhemoglobin saturation curve to the left. These actions make it more difficult to unload oxygen and eventually cause functional anemia because of reduced oxygen availability. Evidence has also been presented that CO exerts toxic effects independent of those associated with carboxyhemoglobin formation (134). Elevated partial pressures of CO in the tissues may lead to the interaction of CO with cellular proteins such as myoglobin and cytochrome c oxidase (135,136). These metalloproteins contain iron and/or copper centers that form metal-ligand complexes with CO in competition with molecular oxygen.

CO elicits a direct vasodilatory response of the coronary circulation (137–139). This response is neither mediated by hypoxia nor by interference with adrenergic, adenosine, or prostaglandin receptors (137). Lin and McGrath (140) showed that CO directly relaxes the rat thoracic aorta. This relaxation is independent of the endothelium and does not appear to be agonist-specific. Because norepinephrine-induced contractions are inhibited to a greater extent than those induced by potassium, these investigators suggested that CO preferentially inhibits contractions initiated by calcium released from intracellular stores. In subsequent experiments, the relaxation of vascular smooth muscle induced by CO has been linked to activation of guanylate cyclase in a manner analogous to that of NO^- (141,142). CO produced in vSMCs under hypoxic conditions can modify guanylate cyclase levels in endothelial and smooth muscle cells (143). Furthermore, CO increases NO^- release from human platelets and bovine endothelial cells (144). This response is independent of NO^- synthase and appears to involve inhibition of NO^- sequestration in the tissue. These observations are consistent with studies showing that CO increases cGMP levels in cultured aortic smooth muscle cells (104). A role for hypoxia in CO-induced alterations of vascular tone should not be dismissed, given that cyanide, a well-known inhibitor of mitochondrial respiration and inducer of cytotoxic hypoxia, modulates aortic contractility (145). It has also been observed that CO can interfere with mitochondrial bioenergetics, potentially causing increased production of ROS.

The atherogenic potential of CO exposure is currently a topic of some controversy, as several studies have indicated that CO alone does not induce atherosclerotic lesions in animal models (134,146). As stated, CO is generally encountered as one component of a mixture of potential toxicants, including PAHs, formaldehyde, benzene, and dioxins.

Catecholamines

It has been noted that stress is a risk factor for development of cardiovascular disease. This may be explained by the fact that endogenous sympathomimetic amines including epinephrine, norepinephrine, and dopamine exert prominent physiologic effects mediated by receptors on the surface of target cells. Acute exposure to toxic concentrations of catecholamines is associated with cardiovascular and hemodynamic changes, some of which are mediated by alterations in peripheral vascular resistance. That catecholamines modulate progression of arterial disease is consistent with the observed enhancement of vascular reactivity to infused norepinephrine in essential hypertension (147).

Repeated exposure to catecholamines induces atherosclerotic lesions in several animal species (148–150). The atherosclerotic effect of catecholamines is related to their ability to induce endothelial cell injury and modulate the proliferation of vascular cells and the ability of these compounds to affect the expression of inflammatory mediators (151). The proliferative disturbances induced by catecholamines are partly mediated via α-receptors since prasozin, an α-receptor antagonist, effectively prevents the toxic response (152). Stimulation of α1-adrenergic receptors results in activation of protein kinase C and MAPK, leading to upregulation of c-fos, c-jun, and c-myc mRNAs (153), and stimulation of DNA synthesis in the vessel wall (154). Other studies have suggested that tyrosine kinase and phosphatidyl inositol-3-kinase mediate the gene induction response (155). Therefore, α1 stimulation may contribute to vascular remodeling in atherogenesis (154). However, Pettersson et al. (156) have shown that potentiation of the atherosclerotic process by sympathetic activation can be inhibited by β-adrenergic receptor blockade. Thus, the relative contribution of adrenergic receptor subtypes to changes in proliferation of vascular cells is not clear. The observation that both parent compounds and metabolites may be involved in the toxic response further complicates interpretation of these data (150). Sholley and coworkers (157) demonstrated that catecholamines inhibit endothelial migration and repopulation of small denuded areas in vitro. In this manner, catecholamines may interfere with repair of blood vessels in vivo. Smooth muscle cells exposed to atherosclerotic risk factors, such as diabetes, hypertension, and balloon injury are more susceptible to the effects of catecholamines (158,159). Hyperinsulinemia has also been linked to cardiovascular disease. For example, insulin and IGF-1 upregulate α1-D receptors, but not α1-B receptors, a pattern suggestive of differential α1-receptor functions (153). This suggestion is consistent with reports by Xin and coworkers (160) that norepinephrine-induced smooth muscle cell growth is mediated by α1-D receptors via an MAPK pathway. Thus, formation of arteriosclerotic lesions in certain forms of hypertension may be initiated and/or supported by high levels of circulating catecholamines. The atherogenic effect of catecholamines may also be related to their ability to induce contraction of vSMCs. A link may exist between vasoconstrictor and mitogenic mechanisms in vSMCs (161,162). The ability of vasoconstrictor agents to modulate the proliferation of smooth muscle cells may be related to modulation of oncogene expression. Angiotensin II, a powerful vasoconstrictor, increases the expression of various oncogenes, including c-fos and c-jun (163) as well as α1-D and α1-B receptors (164). Furthermore, angiotensin-converting enzyme inhibitors "reverse" remodeling of the vessel wall after injury (165).

Oxidative by-products of catecholamines have been implicated in their cardiac toxicity (166,167). The oxidation of catecholamines generates adrenochrome-like products that undergo spontaneous or enzyme-catalyzed oxidation to form oxygen-derived free radicals. Although a similar correlation has not been established for vascular cells, recent studies have demonstrated that 6-hydroxydopa, an oxidative by-product of catecholamines, is present at the active site of serum amine oxidase (27). These observations raise the possibility that oxidative by-products of catecholamines formed under physiologic conditions selectively modulate vascular function. In fact, O_2^- anions selectively attenuate the contractile responses to catecholamines (168). The vascular effects of oxygen-derived radicals have been reviewed by Rubanyi (169). Free radicals in vivo can be generated secondary to anoxic or reoxygenation injury (170), metabolism of xenobiotics (171), neutrophil/monocyte-mediated inflammation (172), and oxidative modification of LDLs (173). O_2^- anions inactivate endothelium-derived relaxing factor, while H_2O_2 and hydroxyl radicals cause direct vaso-dilation and stimulate the synthesis and release of relaxation factors. Oxygen radicals are considered important mediators of vascular damage in acute arterial hypertension and experimental brain injury (174–176). Hiebert and Liu (177) have suggested that toxic oxygen metabolites can damage endothelial cells and play an important role in the progression of atherosclerotic lesions. Free radicals generated from the xanthine/xanthine oxidase reaction increase the transfer of albumin across a barrier of endothelial cells in vitro (178). Rosenblum and Bryan (179) have presented evidence that hydroxyl radicals mediate the endothelium-dependent relaxation of brain microvessels. It has been suggested that calcium mobilization and activation of protein kinase C play significant roles in the generation and release of O_2^- by endothelial cells (180). This release of O_2^- may modulate vascular cell functions. Activated endothelial cells produce and secrete proteases in association with vessel penetration into surrounding con-nective tissue in response to angiogenic stimuli (181).

Dinitrotoluene

Dinitrotoluene is a nitroaromatic chemical used as a precursor in the synthesis of polyurethane foams, coatings, elastomers, and explosives. The manufacture of dinitrotoluene generates a technical grade mixture, which consists of 75.8% 2,4-dinitrotoluene, 19.5% 2,6-dinitrotoluene, and 4.7% other isomers. Several chronic toxicity studies in laboratory animals have shown that 2,4- and/or 2,6-dinitrotoluene causes cancers of the liver, gall bladder, and kidney as well as benign tumors of the connective tissues (182–184). In humans, however, retro-spective mortality studies in workers exposed daily to dinitrotoluene showed that dinitrotoluenes cause circulatory disorders of atherosclerotic etiology as well as ischemic heart disease (185–187). As in other instances of chronic occupational illness, increased mortality from cardiovascular disorders on exposure to dini-trotoluenes has been related to duration and intensity of exposure.

Studies in this laboratory established that repeated in vivo exposure of rats to 2,4- or 2,6-dinitrotoluene is associated with dysplasia and rearrangement of aortic smooth muscle cells (188). Marked inhibition of DNA synthesis occurred in medial smooth muscle cells isolated from dinitrotoluene-treated animals. The ability of dinitrotoluenes to modulate DNA synthesis in aortic smooth muscle cells was not due to direct genotoxic or cytotoxic effects (189). Dinitrotoluenes are metabolized in the liver to dinitrobenzylalcohol, which is then conjugated to form a glucoronide excreted in bile or urine. This conjugate is thought to be hydrolyzed by intestinal microflora and subsequently reduced to a toxic metabolite, or the precursor of a toxic metabolite (190,191). Dent et al. (192)

showed that rat cecal microflora convert dinitrotoluene to nitrosonitrotoluenes, aminonitrotoluenes, and diaminotoluenes. In vitro exposure of rat aortic smooth muscle cells to 2,4- or 2,6-diaminotoluene modulates DNA synthesis in a manner that resembles that observed on dinitrotoluene treatment in vivo (188). Interestingly, diaminotoluene retards the progression of smooth muscle cells through the G_1 phase of the cell cycle. This response resembles that observed on exposure of smooth muscle cells to other chemical carcinogens (193). However, diaminotoluene has not been detected in metabolism studies on in vivo exposure to dinitrotoluene (191). Because both dinitrotoluene and diaminotoluene must be activated to elicit toxic effects, metabolic intermediates common to both agents may actually be responsible for the vascular toxicity of dinitrotoluene.

The modulation of DNA synthesis in rat aortic smooth muscle cells by dinitrotoluene may be related to its ability to promote the atherosclerotic process in humans. Interestingly, in rats pretreated with aroclor 1254, a complex mixture of PAHs and chlorinated hydrocarbons, the genotoxicity of dinitrotoluene was potentiated possibly through alteration of nitroreductase activity, reduced pH, and/or changes in the microfloral population (194). However, additional studies are required to evaluate species differences in response to atherogenic insult, since the rat is relatively resistant to both spontaneously and chemically induced atherogenesis (195,196).

Homocysteine

An elevated plasma homocysteine level is an established risk factor for atherosclerotic coronary heart disease (CHD), cerebrovascular disease (CVD), and occlusive lower extremity disease (LED), and is associated with death in patients with CHD, CVD, and LED (197). Potential mechanisms by which levels of homocysteine might contribute to vascular injury and disease progression include impairment of endothelial function, stimulation of vSMC proliferation, increased monocyte adhesion, oxidation of LDL, and promotion of a prothrombotic environment (198). A polymorphism in methylene tetrahydrofolate reductase (MTHFR), an enzyme involved in clearance of homocysteine, may contribute to increased risk for cardiovascular disease (199).

Several investigators have established a correlation between homocysteine, an intermediate in cellular methionine metabolism and inducer of oxidative stress, and the formation of oxLDLs and H_2O_2 in the presence of cuprous and ferrous ions (200). Homocysteine has also been linked to myointimal cellular proliferation in baboons (201) and vSMC proliferation in vitro, following upregulation of cyclins D1 and A (202). Nishio and Watanabe (203) examined the effects of homocysteine on rat vSMC proliferation in vitro and found that homocysteine was only weakly mitogenic compared with PDGF-BB. When combined with PDGF-BB, however, homocysteine enhanced vSMC proliferation fourfold compared with controls (203). Interestingly, homocysteine decreased glutathione peroxidase activity, increased O_2^- dismutase activity, and had no effect on catalase activity (203). These results are consistent with the notion that mitogenic signaling in vSMCs involves alterations in cellular redox capacity.

During the initial stages of plaque formation, oxLDLs circulating in blood are engulfed by macrophages in the subendothelial space, giving rise to foam cells that eventually become "fatty streaks." OxLDLs also injure cells within the vessel wall (46) and modulate mitogenic signaling in vSMCs (204). Halvorsen and coworkers (205) observed that normal homocysteine plasma concentrations (6 μM) had no effect on LDL oxidation, while higher concentrations (25–500 μM) promoted lipid and protein modifications of LDL. Interestingly, in the presence of copper ions, homocysteine stimulated LDL oxidation; therefore, in the absence of circulating copper ions, homocysteine-induced atherosclerosis may be explained by mechanisms other than LDL oxidation (205). Treatment of elevated homocysteine levels by therapy with folate (197,206,207) and vitamins B6 and B12 has been suggested (197,207).

Multiple studies used methionine-rich diets to elevate blood levels of homocysteine in laboratory animals. These studies demonstrated that higher blood levels of homocysteine were correlated with increased rates of restenosis after balloon-mediated arterial injury, and that this response was attenuated by lowering of homocysteine levels by supplementing the diet with folic acid (208–210). Results from human clinical studies of this phenomenon are mixed; some studies appear to show benefit to lowering homocysteine with folic acid treatment while others show no such benefit (211,212).

Hydrazinobenzoic Acid

Hydrazinobenzoic acid is a nitrogen-nitrogen bonded chemical present in the cultivated mushroom *Agaricus bisporus*. McManus et al. (213) reported that this hydrazine derivative causes smooth muscle cell tumors of the aorta and large arteries of mice when administered over the life span of the animals. These tumors showed the characteristic appearance and immunocytochemical features of vascular leiomyomas and leiomyosarcomas. Smooth muscle cell lysis with vascular perforation apparently precedes malignant smooth muscle cell growth. The ability of hydrazinobenzoic acid to cause vSMC tumors is shared with other synthetic and naturally occurring hydrazines (214). Recently, a role for hydrazine-derived alkyl radicals in cytotoxicity and transformation of mouse fibroblasts was reported by Gamberini et al. (215). Although angiomyomas (or vascular leiomyomas) derived histogenetically from the media of blood and lymph vessels occur most commonly in the oral cavity and in the skin (216), evidence that primary leiomyosarcomas occur in the abdominal aorta has been presented (217,218). These observations are particularly significant when considering that primary leiomysarcomas in major arteries is an uncommon event, though several case reports are available for this tumor type in veins (219).

We have conducted in vitro studies to examine the direct cytotoxic effects of hydrazinobenzoic acid in cultured rat aortic smooth muscle cells. Exposure of smooth muscle cells to hydrazinobenzoic acid (0.1–100 μM) for various times was not lethal to the cells, as reflected by leakage of lactate dehydrogenase (Piron and Ramos, unpublished observations). However, significant fluctuations in cellular glutathione content on exposure to hydrazinobenzoic acid were observed.

Bioactivation of hydrazines to mutagenic products is accomplished by enzymes such as mushroom tyrosinase (220). Because free radicals can be generated from hydrazines by oxidizing systems, including metal-catalyzed autoxidation, prostaglandin synthetase, and cytochrome P-450/NADPH (221), the modulation of glutathione by hydrazinobenzoic acid may be mediated by free radical formation. This suggestion is consistent with previous reports showing that hydrazines bind covalently to macromolecules, promote lipid peroxidation, and induce DNA damage (222,223), as is the case with unsymmetrically alkylated hydrazines, which cause lethal DNA-lesions in repair-deficient strains (224).

Metals

Although epidemiologic and clinical reports regarding the vascular effects of metals have received some attention in past years (225–227), only a limited number of studies have been conducted to define the cellular and molecular mechanisms of metal-induced angiotoxicity. As in other systems, the vascular toxicity of food- and waterborne elements (selenium, chromium, copper, zinc, cadmium, lead, and mercury), as well as airborne elements (vanadium and lead), is thought to be due to nonspecific reactions of metals with sulfhydryl, carboxyl, or phosphate groups. In addition, the ability of metals such as cobalt, magnesium, manganese, nickel, cadmium, and lead to interact with and block calcium channels has been recognized for some time (228). Evidence that intracellular calcium-binding proteins are biologically relevant targets of heavy metal toxicity has also been presented. Calmodulin, a ubiquitous calcium-binding protein in eukaryotes, serves as a major intracellular calcium receptor in the regulation of multiple cellular processes. Certain heavy metals, including mercury and lead, effectively substitute for calcium within the calmodulin molecule (229). However, the contribution of this mechanism to the toxic effects of metals has been questioned on the basis of the inability of beryllium, barium, cobalt, zinc, and cadmium to bind readily to calmodulin in vitro (230).

Most vascular toxicity studies have focused on the effects of cadmium. Cadmium is not preferentially located in blood vessels relative to other tissues. However, when present, cadmium localizes to the elastic lamina of large arteries, with particularly high concentrations at arterial branching points (231). A large portion of cadmium accumulated in the body is tightly bound to hepatic and renal metallothionein, a detoxification mechanism (232,233). Thus, low metallothionein levels in vascular tissue may predispose to cadmium toxicity (231). Long-term exposure of laboratory animals to low levels of cadmium has been associated with the development of atherosclerosis and hypertension in the absence of other toxic effects (234). However, dietary cadmium has also been shown to reduce atherogenesis through suppression of free iron concentration (235).

In 1962, Schroeder and Vinton first reported that exposure of rats to 5-ppm cadmium in the drinking water causes hypertension (236). This observation has been corroborated by several independent laboratories (237–241). Perry et al. (231) suggested that cadmium-induced hypertension is only observed in a narrow concentration range of 0.1 to 5 ppm, above which toxicity without hypertensive effects is only observed. This observation may reflect dose-based biphasic induction of ERK1/2 signaling in vSMCs (241). Perry et al. (231) further proposed that failure to induce hypertension with chronic cadmium may be due to low levels of heavy metal contamination in the water or food supplies used in the course of experiments. This interpretation would be consistent with the observation that selenium and zinc inhibit (242), while lead potentiates the hypertensive effects of cadmium (243). Concentrations of cadmium, which increase blood pressure, fail to do so in the presence of calcium (234). In contrast, the protective effects of zinc and selenium may be related to their ability to increase the synthesis of cadmium-binding proteins and thus enhance cadmium detoxification.

Within the vasculature, the primary target for cadmium toxicity appears to be endothelium. As reviewed by Prozialeck et al. (244), several mechanisms have been proposed for cadmium toxicity, including induction of oxidative stress and associated changes to sulfhydryl groups, interference with homeostatic functions of other trace metals, and disruption of calcium-dependent signaling. Broadly, cadmium has been reported to increase sodium retention (245), induce vasoconstriction (246), increase cardiac output (247), and produce hyper-reninemia (248). Disruption of cadherin-dependent cell-cell junctions may be a critical effect of cadmium toxicity, an effect supported by the observations of Schlaepfer et al. (249). These investigators also noted vesiculation, vacuolization, and fragmentation of vascular endothelium. In vitro exposure to cadmium decreases prostacyclin formation in aortic rings and reduces adenosine diphosphate (ADP) clearance by arterial tissue (250). The responsiveness of rabbit platelets to nonaggregating concentrations of arachidonic acid or collagen can be potentiated by prior exposure to cadmium chloride (251).

Evidence continues to accumulate, which suggests that chronic exposure to lead is correlated with hypertension (252,253). Epidemiologic studies have shown that a large percentage of patients with essential hypertension have increased body stores of lead (254). The direct vasoconstrictor effect of lead may be related to the putative hypertensive response (255). This effect can be complemented by lead's ability to activate the rennin/angiotensin/aldosterone system (256). Lead also stimulates the proliferation of cultured vSMCs via a calcium-dependent pathway (257). The mechanism through which lead causes hypertension most likely involves oxidative stress and dysregulated expression of proteins involved in ROS handling (258–260).

A number of studies have focused on the toxic interactions of metals. For example, lead potentiates the vasopressor response to cadmium (242). In contrast to the protective effects of calcium in cadmium-induced hypertension, calcium is ineffective in reducing the toxic cardiovascular effects of lead (234). However, magnesium promotes the atherosclerotic and hypertensive effects of both lead and cadmium. Mercury and lead cause contraction of aortic smooth muscle in vitro, while cadmium is without effect (261). Mercury added to platelet-rich plasma causes a marked increase in platelet thromboxane B_2 production and increased platelet responsiveness to arachidonic acid (262). Although it is unlikely that mercury and lead compete with calcium for intracellular-binding sites, their accessibility to the intracellular compartment appears to be calcium dependent (261). Several investigators have proposed that acute lead-induced neuropathy is due to cerebral capillary dysfunction (263,264). This hypothesis is consistent with recent in vitro studies showing that lead causes dose- and time-dependent inhibition of cell division and glucose uptake in cerebral microvessel endothelium (265).

Nicotine

Nicotine, an alkaloid found in various plants, mimics the actions of acetylcholine at nicotinic receptors throughout the body. The cardiovascular effects of this toxin have been studied within the context of tobacco-associated toxicities as well as its use as a botanical insecticide. Epidemiologic and experimental studies have suggested that nicotine is a causative or aggravating factor in myocardial and cerebral infarction, gangrene, and aneurysm. Bull et al. (266) have shown that repeated subcutaneous infusion of nicotine for seven days is associated with reduced prostacyclin production in aortic segments. Reduced prostacyclin production has been observed in isolated rabbit hearts, rabbit aorta, human vein, rat aorta, and umbilical arteries when incubated with nicotine in vitro (267–270). It has been suggested that the effects of nicotine are due to competitive inhibition of cyclo-oxygenase, which precludes the formation of prostaglandin endoperoxides in vivo. Alterations in the structural integrity of the aortic endothelium following chronic oral administration of nicotine in vivo and on exposure of cultured aortic endothelial cells in vitro have also been noted (271,272). Because nicotine stimulates catecholamine release from sympathetic ganglia and nerve endings, as well as the adrenal medulla, its toxicologic profile may share features in common with those described for catecholamines. Stimulation of α-adrenergic receptors is thought to contribute to nicotine's hypertensive function, along with the generation of ROS and, possibly, inhibition of NO^- synthesis in the vascular endothelium (273).

At the cellular level, nicotine modulates the proliferation of vascular endothelial and smooth muscle cells. Nicotine increases the synthesis of DNA in luminal endothelial cells after in vivo administration (271). At concentrations lower than those present in blood after smoking, nicotine also increases the rate of DNA synthesis in growth-arrested subcultures of smooth muscle cells (274). This response appears to be independent of those of other mitogens present in the medium and additive to that of serum. Such changes in smooth muscle cell proliferation are consistent with the enhanced rate of phenotypic modulation from a contractile to a synthetic state induced by nicotine. Increased number of lysosomes with incompletely degraded inclusions and/or inhibition of intra-lysosomal proteolysis in macrophages on exposure to nicotine have been reported (275).

Recently, smokeless tobacco has been used as a vehicle to study nicotine intoxication. The use of this product removes the other potential contributors in smoked tobacco. It is worth noting that smokeless tobacco also contains licorice, which may also increase blood pressure (276). It is apparent that adverse cardiovascular outcomes are more highly associated with the use of cigarettes as opposed to smokeless tobacco, but the possibility that nicotine itself acts in concert with other toxins cannot be discounted. Ongoing study of effects associated with the use of nicotine gum, transdermal patches, and nasal sprays will continue to provide insight into nicotine's potential for cardiovascular effects.

Particulate Matter

Particles in the atmosphere originate from diverse sources, including emissions from motor vehicles, agricultural activity, wood combustion, power generation, industrial processes, and volcanic emissions to name a few. Environmental health scientists generally focus on particulate matter (PM) smaller than 10 μM in diameter (PM_{10}) as the size of these particles allows them to penetrate the respiratory tract. Often, particles are further described as coarse (between 2.5 and 10 μM, or $PM_{2.5-10}$), fine (less than 2.5 μM, or $PM_{2.5}$), or ultrafine (less than 0.1 μM, or $PM_{0.1}$).

Several lines of evidence indicate that elevation of PM levels cause increased hospital admissions and mortality related to cardiovascular issues (277). As with most environmental exposures, the contribution of other air pollutants (e.g., nitrogen oxides, sulfur dioxide) must be considered. However, PM alone can induce oxidative stress in cardiovascular systems (279,280). Increased levels of ROS caused by PM are concomitant with increases in markers of inflammation, including cytokine expression and activation of NF-κB and Nrf2 (281,282); expression of enzymes involved in vascular remodeling (matrix metalloproteinases or MMPs) is also increased (283,284). The presence of endotoxin in PM may be responsible for some of these effects (285,286).

Exposure to PM has also been associated with CRP expression (287,288), though epidemiologic evidence is mixed (289–291). Inflammation and oxidative stress subsequent to PM exposure appear to accelerate the development of atherosclerotic lesions in animal models (292,293). Inflammation and oxidative stress as central features of cardiovascular disease are likely major components of the mechanism causing atherosclerotic progression following PM exposure. Though the underlying mechanism remains unclear, the evidence indicates that air pollution as a mixture and PM specifically contribute to cardiovascular disease, including atherosclerosis.

Polycyclic Aromatic Hydrocarbons

Epidemiologic studies have demonstrated a convincing link between PAH-DNA adducts and atherosclerosis (55,56,294). Several lines of evidence suggest a link between PAH exposure and formation of atherosclerotic lesions, most likely through both genetic and epigenetic mechanisms (54).

Benditt and Benditt first proposed that atherosclerotic lesions, like benign smooth muscle tumors of the uterus, originate from the mutation of a single smooth muscle cell (295). Although this proposal was received with great skepticism, evidence implicating carcinogens (296) and radiation (297) in atherosclerosis has continued to accumulate over the years. Exposure of avian species to BaP and 7,12 dimethylbenz(a,h)anthracene causes atherosclerosis without alterations in serum cholesterol levels (296). Extensive work in my laboratory has supported the concept of AhR-independent mechanisms of atherogenesis, including DNA damage in vSMCs and subsequent inhibition of DNA repair by BaP and its metabolites (298). Parallel studies suggest a role for epigenetic regulation of dysregulated vSMC phenotypes through the antioxidant response element (ARE/EpRE) (91,299,300).

The atherogenic potential of BaP has been associated with cytochrome P-450-mediated conversion of the parent compound to toxic metabolic inter- mediates (301). Microsomal monooxygenases, including P-450 forms 2 and 6 and NADPH-cytochrome P-450 reductase, have been identified in rabbit aortic vascular tissue (302). The majority of the activity responsible for the bio- transformation of BaP is associated with the smooth muscle layers of the aorta (302). However, cytochrome P-450-dependent monooxygenase activity, which can potentially bioactivate carcinogens, is also present in the aortic endothelium (303,304). Interestingly, the activity of aortic aryl hydrocarbon hydroxylase (AHH) has been correlated with the degree of susceptibility to atherosclerosis in avian species (305).

AHH activity is primarily constituted by CYP1A1 and CYP1B1; these enzymes also act as mediators of PAH-dependent atherogenesis. BaP treatment induces AHH activity in vSMCs. It appears that CYP1B1 is largely responsible for this induction, as this enzyme is preferentially expressed in vSMCs (34,306,307). CYP1B1 is also expressed constitutively in vSMCs. Redox cycling of BaP quinone metabolites may contribute to the gene induction response. This response may be relevant to loss of coordinated cell cycle expression, leading to genomic instability and phenotypic modulation, as shown for fibroblasts by Stambrook and coworkers (308).

Concomitant with induction of phase I enzymes, PAHs also induce several phase II enzyme systems. The generation of phase II metabolites via sulfo- conjugation of 3-hydroxybenzo(a)pyrene has been demonstrated in aortic tissue (309). This reaction is important in the reduction of toxic phenolics. Sulfation takes place in cultured aortic smooth muscle cells and endothelial cells, in aortic whole organ explants, and in cytosolic fractions of cell-free preparations. The conjugation capacity of avian aortic tissues is 10% to 20% of the total avian hepatic capacity to sulfoconjugate 3-hydroxybenzo(a)pyrene. Avian aortic tissues also contain active uridine 5'-diphosphate (UDP)-glucuronosyltransferase activity, which catalyzes the glucuronidation of 3-hydroxybenzo(a)pyrene (310). In abdominal aortic segments, glucuronosyltransferase activity is eight- to ninefold higher than that of the thoracic aorta. Phenobarbital, but not 3-methylcholanthrene, increases the activity of microsomal fractions in both segments. Although glucuronidation of 3-hydroxybenzo(a)pyrene appears to be less active than sulfation in aortic tissues, the differential distribution of glucuronyltransferase activity may account for differences in the responses of abdominal versus thoracic regions of the aorta to BaP. This concept is supported by studies showing that glucuronidation decreases the mutagenic and carcinogenic effects of PAHs in the Ames test (311) but increases the generation of reactive intermediates in other preparations (312).

Albert et al. (296) and Penn and Synder (313) have reported that treatment with several polycyclic hydrocarbons increases the size but not the frequency of atherosclerotic lesions. These observations suggest that PAHs act as promoters of the atherosclerotic process, but do not initiate lesion formation. Majesky et al. (314) have shown that focal proliferation of intimal smooth muscle cells can be produced by an initiation/promotion sequence using 7,12 dimethylbenz[a]-anthracene and the α-1 selective adrenergic agonist, methoxamine. In contrast, Paigen et al. (315) have shown that 3-methylcholanthrene increases both the number and size of lipid-staining lesions in the aorta of animals fed an atherogenic diet for eight weeks. Further, in vivo exposure to BaP leads to the development of lesions in the aortic wall of Sprague-Dawley rats (316). The discrepancy between these studies may be accounted for by regional differences in the toxicologic response. Distal segments of aorta have been proposed as preferential sites for promotion, while initiation is thought to be confined to the thoracic region. The role of PAH-DNA adducts is not well understood in this context, but it has not been ruled out that these adducts contribute to development of atherosclerotic lesions in a process that mirrors carcinogenesis.

Because hydrocarbons associate readily with plasma lipoproteins, Revis et al. (317) have suggested that the atherogenic effect of PAHs is related to the mechanism by which these chemicals are transported in plasma. This proposal was based on the observation that carcinogens that do not associate with lipoproteins, such as 2,4,6-trichlorophenol, are not atherogenic.

The role of the aryl hydrocarbon receptor (AhR) in PAH-mediated atherogenesis has been the subject of recent study. Ah-responsive mice are more susceptible to 3-methylcholanthrene-induced atherosclerosis than Ah-resistant mice (318). We have recently found that epigenetic disturbances in vSMCs by BaP are absent in AhR nullizygous mice (319). Also, we have observed that AhR-null mice are more susceptible to methylcholanthrene (MC)-induced atherogenesis than their wild-type counterparts. Coupled with evidence that neither constitutive nor inducible expression of CYP1B1 rely solely on AhR function, these observations indicate that the AhR may not be a critical mediator of signaling and gene expression in atherogenic pathways (307).

More recently, we have shown that acute BaP exposure enhances expression of the *c-Ha-ras* oncogene in aortic smooth muscle cells (320). This induction is regulated at the transcriptional level and involves multiple protein-protein/DNA-protein interactions, including binding of antioxidant/electrophile response element (ARE/EpRE)-binding proteins to the ARE/EpRE (104,321,322) (Fig. 2). On the basis of our observations, it appears that induction of *c-Ha-ras* following BaP exposure is dependent on P-450-mediated metabolism; upregulation of this ras isoform contributes to development of atherosclerotic lesions in laboratory animals (91,299). On the basis of these observations, it is reasonable to suggest that metabolism of PAHs may cause redox cycling, which in turn could cause upregulation of *c-Ha-ras* through the ARE/EpRE.

Not surprisingly, many molecular targets downstream of ras are also altered following PAH exposure. In vivo exposure of quail to BaP modulates phosphorylation of medial aortic proteins. BaP enhances basal phosphorylation

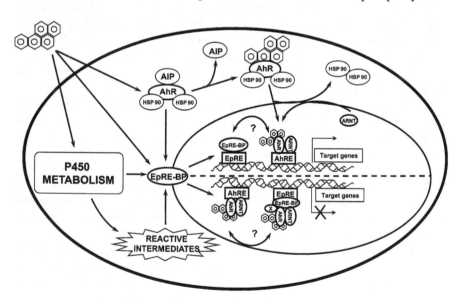

Figure 2 Proposed mechanisms of BaP-induced gene expression in vSMCs. BaP is metabolized by AhR-mediated P-450 monooxygenases to various hydroxylated and epoxidated intermediates. These intermediates induce activation of EpRE-BP, which interact with the EpRE of *c-Ha-ras*. Concomitantly, BaP interacts with the AhR, inducing translocation to the nucleus, interaction with Arnt, and association with the AhRE element of *c-Ha-ras*. Possible interactions between the activated AhR and EpRE-BP could lead to positive as well as negative regulation of target genes. *Abbreviations*: BaP, benzo(a)-pyrene; vSMC, vascular smooth muscle cell; AhR, aryl hydrocarbon receptor; EpRE-BP, electrophile response element–binding proteins; EpRE, electrophile responsive element; AhRE, AhR response element.

of several cytosolic proteins but inhibits C-kinase-mediated protein phosphorylation in the particulate fraction (323). This inhibition leads to disruption of mechanisms that regulate vSMC phenotypes (324). The profile of medial protein phosphorylation induced by BaP is altered when in vitro phosphorylation measurements are carried out in the presence of endothelial cells. Increased phosphorylation of cytosolic proteins is observed in aortic homogenates containing endothelial and smooth muscle cell proteins (323). Smooth muscle cells from BaP-treated rats are characterized by increased abundance of phosphatidylinositol metabolites, primarily products of phosphatidylinositol-3-kinase activity (299). These observations suggest that multiple cell interactions may be critical to the expression of the toxic response. Because phosphorylation mechanisms are intimately involved with the regulation of vSMC growth and differentiation, these results suggest that signal transduction pathways involved in the phosphorylation of proteins may be targeted by PAHs.

T-2 Toxin

Trichothecenes mycotoxins, commonly classified as tetracyclic sesquiterpenes, are naturally occurring cytotoxic metabolites of *Fusarium* species (325). These mycotoxins, including T-2 toxin [4β,15-diacetoxy-8α-(3-methylbutyryloxy)-3α-hydroxy-12,13-epoxytrichothec-9-ene], are major contaminants of foods and animal feeds and may cause illness in animals and humans. Although the carcinogenic effects of trichothecenes mycotoxins have been documented for many years, little is known about the vascular toxicity of these agents. Acute parenteral administration of T-2 toxin to laboratory animals induces shock, hypothermia, and death because of cardiovascular and respiratory failure (326). Wilson et al. (326) reported that intravenous infusion of T-2 toxin in rats causes an initial decrease in heart rate and blood pressure, followed by tachycardia and hypertension, and finally bradycardia and hypotension. These actions may be related to a central effect on blood pressure and catecholamine release (328). Siren and Feuerstein (328) also suggested that while T-2 toxin reduces blood flow and increases vascular resistance in skeletal muscle and mesenteric and renal vascular beds, no changes in mean arterial pressure and heart rate could be detected. Acute T-2 toxin exposure causes extensive destruction of myocardial capillaries, while repeated dosing promotes thickening of large coronary arteries (329). A more generalized atherosclerosis and hypertension are delayed consequences of repeated T-2 toxin exposure (330).

At the cellular level, T-2 toxin is a potent inhibitor of protein synthesis (331). T-2 toxin is thought to bind to the 60S subunit of the ribosome to interfere with peptidyl transferase activity. Inhibition of DNA synthesis is thought to be secondary to the interference with protein synthesis (332). A single large dose of 2-mg/kg, or four injections of 0.3 mg/kg, T-2 toxin causes necrosis of endothelial cells, accumulation of basement membrane-like material in the intima, and swelling and activation of smooth muscle cells in the media (333). Medial aortic smooth muscle cells decrease in number and increase in size on exposure to T-2 toxin. Marked inhibition of smooth muscle cell growth is observed in explant cultures of smooth muscle cells. This is followed by stimulation of the proliferative capacity of smooth muscle cells in vitro. The fragmentation and increase in basement membrane-like material in these cells suggest that long-term changes occur even after the endothelium has returned to normal.

Miscellaneous Toxins

Exposure of factory workers in rayon plants to carbon disulfide (CS_2) has been associated with a significant increase in mortality from CHD. A cohort epidemiologic study conducted in Poland showed a statistically significant excess in deaths due to circulatory system diseases in CS_2-exposed workers (334). A critical review of the epidemiologic literature was recently published by Sulsky et al. (335); the investigators indicate that the epidemiologic evidence is mixed with regard to CHD. This conclusion is bolstered by studies by Takebayashi et al. (336), which indicates an increased risk of abnormal electrocardiogram readings in workers exposed to CS_2, and Korinth et al. (337), which observed no alteration in heart chamber size or function due to exposure to CS_2. Similar conclusions about the epidemiologic data were reached through meta-analysis (338). Although the mechanism of toxicity is not known, alterations of glucose and/or lipid metabolism and blood coagulation have been suggested (339,340). It has also been suggested that CS_2 may create oxidative stress in exposed workers (341). Measurements of urinary 2-thiothiazotidine-4-carboxylic acid levels were shown to be a sensitive, precise, and selective marker to monitor CS_2 exposure in rats (342), and have also been monitored in humans (337).

Recent studies have shown that 1,3-butadiene, a chemical used in the production of styrene-butadiene, increases the incidence of cardiac hemangiosarcomas, rare tumors of endothelial origin (343,344). Occupational exposure to 1,3-butadiene has also been associated with significant increases in risk of arteriosclerotic heart disease, though it appears that African-Americans may be more susceptible than white counterparts (345,346). Penn and Snyder (347) have shown that 1,3-butadiene, a component of the vapor phase of cigarette smoke, accelerates plaque formation at environmentally relevant concentrations in cockerels; this response does not appear to rely on metabolism (348).

Tetrachlorodibenzo-p-dioxin (TCDD), a widely studied polychlorinated hydrocarbon, induces hyperlipoproteinemia in animals and humans (349,350). In guinea pigs, a single dose of TCDD induces a 19-fold increase in very low-density lipoproteins, and a fourfold increase in LDLs (351). The ability of TCDD to modulate lipid metabolism may be of serious consequences to the preservation of vascular function. Recent studies in our laboratory have shown that TCDD modulates protein phosphorylation in rat aortic smooth cells in vivo and in vitro (352). Specifically, TCDD selectively alters the phosphorylation status at the G_0/G_1 transition by decreasing the activity of several protein kinase C isoforms, α, β, and δ (353). Although the significance of these observations is presently unclear, the vascular responses to TCDD resemble some of those described for BaP. This parallelism raises the possibility that the vascular toxicity of these chemicals share common cellular and molecular pathways, most likely including oxidative stress (354). Recent studies by Puga and coworkers showed that TCDD increased urinary levels of vasoactive eicosanoids, mediators of ischemic heart disease, and partitioned lipoprotein particles, which may serve as a vehicle to deliver TCDD to atherosclerotic plaques (355,356). These effects may exacerbate the severity of ischemic heart disease. The vascular actions of TCDD may also involve deficits in vSMC function since cells isolated from TCDD-treated mice consistently exhibit atherogenic phenotypes (Ramos et al., unpublished observations). Investigations by the National Toxicology Program demonstrated that administration of TCDD to Sprague-Dawley rats causes development of degenerative cardiovascular lesions (357).

Vitamin D hypervitaminosis causes medial degeneration, calcification of the coronary arteries, and smooth muscle cell proliferation in laboratory animals (358–360). However, hypovitaminosis also may be associated with medial thickening (361). The toxic effects of vitamin D may be related to its structural similarity to 25-hydroxycholesterol, a potent vascular toxin (358). Koh et al. (357) have shown that 1,25-dihydroxyvitamin D binds specifically to surface receptors of rat vSMCs to stimulate proliferation in vitro. The toxicity of vitamin D may be related to alterations in cyclic nucleotide metabolism. This suggestion is consistent with studies showing that cyclic nucleotides play a critical role in the regulation of vSMC function (362). In this regard, phosphodiesterase inhibition has been associated with toxicity in medium-sized arteries of the mesentery, testis, and myocardium (363). Other reports showing that theophylline, an inhibitor of phosphodiesterase, causes cardiovascular lesions in mesenteric arterioles (364) and that isomazole and indolidan cause periarteritis of the media and adventitia of small- and medium-sized arteries have also been presented (365). More directly, 1α,25-dihydroxyvitamin D induces migration of vSMCs in culture via activation of phosphatidylinositol 3-kinase (366). This metabolite has also been shown to promote cell growth and calcification in SMCs (367,368).

From a toxicologic perspective, the recent demonstration that LDls are oxidized in vitro by oxygen-derived free radicals released by arterial cells is of particular interest (69). Modified LDLs attract macrophages and prevent their migration from the tissues (181). OxLDL may also promote osteoblastic differentiation of vascular cells, contributing to calcification (360,369,370). Oxidation derivatives of cholesterol, such as cholestane-3β,5α,6β-triol and 25-hydroxycholesterol are potent inhibitors of 3-hydroxy-3-methylglutaryl coenzyme A (HMG CoA) reductase, the rate-limiting enzyme in cholesterol biosynthesis (371). Interestingly, many of the oxidized products of cholesterol formed spontaneously are identical to those formed enzymatically by the microsomal and mitochondrial cytochrome P-450 systems (372). Inflammatory cytokines, including tissue necrosis factor (TNF)-α, IL-1, and macrophage colony–stimulating factor (M-CSF), promote binding of LDL to the epithelium (373). The presence of oxLDL in the vessel wall further amplifies the inflammatory response, inducing MCP-1 and M-CSF gene transcription, as well as alterations in the expression of VCAM-1 and ICAM-1 (62,67,68).

Studies conducted in recent years have focused on the causative role of infectious agents in cardiovascular disease, in particular atherosclerotic plaque formation (374–376). These studies are based on the suggestion that early life experience and exposure to pathogens may influence adult risk of CHD (377). Although numerous studies have identified the presence of viral and bacterial pathogens in atheromatous plaques, an etiologic mechanism has yet to be identified. A possible mechanism of injury involves direct infection of vascular cells, initiating a cascade of atherogenic inflammation (376). Researchers suggested that previous infection with *Chlamydia pneumoniae*, a common respiratory pathogen, is a major risk factor for stroke in young and middle-aged patients, possibly due to an enhanced hypercoagulable state that increases the risk of thrombosis (378). A recent survey of the available studies showed an association between antibodies to *C. pneumoniae* and cardiovascular disease (379). In clinical studies, seropositivity to *C. pneumoniae* has been independently associated with raised fibrinogen and malondialdehyde concentrations (380). A role for chlamydial lipopolysaccharide (cLPS), a gram-negative bacteria cell wall component, in the atherosclerotic process has been suggested by Kalayoglu and Byrne (381), in which *C. pneumoniae* induces macrophage foam cell formation in murine macrophage RAW-264.7 cells. Inhibition of cLPS prevented the uptake of cholesterol esters, suggesting that chronic exposure to cLPS may result in foam cell formation (381). Exposure of cultured macrophages to *C. pneumoniae* in combination with LDL resulted in foam cell formation that was not inhibited by the antioxidant-butylated hydroxytoluene, suggesting that scavenger receptors are not involved in chlamydia-induced LDL uptake (382). Furthermore, inhibition of LDL receptors blocked the uptake of LDL in macrophages, thus indicating that the mechanism of lipid accumulation was the result of unregulated LDL uptake and/or metabolism (382). It has also been suggested that chronic bacterial infection may aggravate preexisting plaques by enhancing T-cell activation as well as other inflammatory responses that may participate in the destabilization of the intimal cap, resulting in plaque rupture, progression to acute ischemic syndromes, and ultimate enlargement of the atherosclerotic plaque (383).

Human heat shock protein 60 (HSP 60) has previously been localized to atherosclerotic plaques, and a possible role for HSP 60 in atherogenesis has been proposed (384–386). The potential mechanism may include autocrine stimulation of vSMC proliferation (387). Kol and coworkers (388) found that chlamydial and human HSP 60 colocalized in human atherosclerotic plaques. *C. pneumoniae* can stimulate proliferation of vSMCs through the induction of HSP 60, which suggests a direct role for *C. pneumoniae* in the pathology of the vessel wall (389). Furthermore, chlamydial HSP 60 can induce proinflammatory cytokines, such as TNF-α and MMPs (388); a role for induction of EGR-1-dependent proteins, including PDFG-B, TGF-β, ICAM-1, and TNF-α, has also been postulated (375).

There are mixed reports in the literature regarding the role of *Helicobacter pylori*, a childhood-acquired bacterial infection, in cardiovascular disorders (377,390–393). Seropositivity to *H. pylori* has been independently associated with fibrinogen concentration and total leukocyte count (380). The Atherosclerosis Risk In Communities (ARIC) study found that *H. pylori* seropositivity was associated with other cardiovascular disease risk factors, such as higher homocysteine levels, lower plasma pyridoxal 5'-phosphate, decreased vitamin supplement use, and seropositivity for cytomegalovirus and herpes simplex type I (394). Therefore, these investigators concluded that *H. pylori* is probably not a factor in CHD. In contrast, Pasceri and colleagues (395) suggested that "low-grade" chronic exposure to *H pylori* may influence atherosclerotic plaque formation, while Markus and Mendall (393) suggested that *H. pylori* infection may be an independent risk factor for ischemic CVD. A proposed mechanism for *H. pylori*-induced cardiovascular disease involves decreases in folate bio availability, resulting in decreased methionine synthase activity and increased homocysteine levels (396). However, epidemiologic data have not been able to establish a correlation between *H. pylori* infection and cardiovascular disease (379,397).

CONCLUDING REMARKS

The proposed mechanisms of action for the vascular toxins surveyed in this chapter are summarized in Table 3. Although differences in cellular and subcellular targets are noted, many of these toxins share the ability to modulate growth and differentiation of vascular cells. Some of these chemicals require metabolic activation for the induction of toxicity, while others cause deleterious effects by virtue of their high chemical reactivity. Not discussed in this chapter were the vascular toxicities mediated by nonspecific alterations of membrane function on exposure to alcohols and solvents and the hypertensive episodes induced by a variety of autonomic agents. As highlighted throughout the chapter, vasculotoxic insult is potentially associated with injury to one or more of the cell types within the vessel wall. Toxicity often involves the interplay of multiple cellular and noncellular factors. The ultimate consequences of toxic challenge are influenced by the repair capacity of target cells and endocrine/paracrine influences on the tissue.

In recent years, the notion that toxic insult plays a significant role in the pathogenesis of vascular disorders, as well as various target-organ specific toxicities, has fueled interest in vascular toxicology. In attempting to unravel the cellular and molecular mechanisms of vasculotoxic insult, investigators must recognize the large degree of structural and functional heterogeneity that characterize the vascular system. Such differences add a level of complexity to the study of vascular toxicities, which is often disregarded.

Table 3 Selected Chemicals with Prominent Vascular Toxicity

Chemical	Source	Putative mechanism of action
Allylamine	Synthetic precursor/ antifungal analogs	Bioactivation of parent compound by amine oxidase to acrolein and hydrogen peroxide; smooth muscle cell lysis
Butadiene	Synthetic precursor	Endothelial injury
Carbon disulfide	Fumigant, solvent	Metabolic disturbances in glucose/lipid metabolism, protein cross-linking
Carbon monoxide	Environmental	Carboxyhemoglobin formation with resulting tissue hypoxia; modulation of second-messenger systems in vascular smooth muscle cells
Catecholamines	Endogenous amines	Adrenergic receptor-mediated alterations of contractile and proliferative behavior in vascular endothelial and/or smooth muscle cells
Dinitrotoluene	Synthetic precursor	Bioactivation-related changes of DNA synthesis in vascular smooth muscle cells
Hydrazinobenzoic acid	Constituent of *Agaricus bisporus*	Unknown; potential involvement of free radical–mediated genotoxicity
Metals	Environmental	Interference with cellular sulfhydryl, amino, and phosphate residues; interference with calcium-mediated cellular events
Nicotine	Tobacco smoke	Modulation of DNA synthesis in vascular endothelial and/or smooth muscle cells, altered signal transduction
Particulate matter	Tobacco smoke/ environmental	Stimulation of oxidative stress and inflammation, enhanced expression of CRP
Polycyclic aromatic hydrocarbons	Tobacco smoke/ environmental	Cytochrome P-450-mediated bioactivation of reactive metabolic intermediates, which bind to DNA in vascular smooth muscle cells
T-2 toxin	*Fusarium* mycotoxin	Endothelial and smooth muscle cell injury; modulation of smooth muscle cell proliferation
TCDD	Environmental	Modulation of lipid metabolism and hyperlipoproteinemia, altered signal transduction
Vitamin D	Dietary	Medial toxin, modulation of cyclic nucleotide metabolism

Abbreviation: CRP, C-reactive protein.

ACKNOWLEDGMENTS

The author's research cited in this chapter was supported in part by grants from the National Institute of Environmental Health Sciences (ES 04849, ES 09106). The contributions of present and past members of the laboratory are gratefully acknowledged.

REFERENCES

1. Rhodin, JAG. Architecture of the vessel wall. In: Bohr DF, Somlyo AP, Sparks HV, Geiger SR, eds. Handbook of Physiology: A critical comprehensive presentation of physiological knowledge and concepts, vol. II. Baltimore, Maryland: Waverly Press, 1980:1–31.
2. Partridge, CP, Williams, ES, Barmoui R, et al. Novel genomic targets in oxidant-induced vascular injury. J Mol Cell Cardiol 2005; 38(6):983–996.
3. Thyberg J, Blomgren K, Roy J, et al. Phenotypic modulation of smooth muscle cells after arterial injury is associated with changes in the distribution of laminin and fibronectin. J Histochem Cytochem 1997; 45(6):837–846.
4. Raines EW. The extraceullar matrix can regulate vascular cell migration, proliferation, and surivival: relationships to vascular disease. International J Exp Pathol 2000; 81(3):173–182.
5. Isakson BE, Rarmos SI, Duling BR. Ca2+ and inositol 1,4,5-triphosphate-mediated signaling across the myoendothelial junction. Circ Res 2007; 100(2):246–254.
6. de Wit C, Wolfle SE. EDHF and gap junctions: important regulators of vascular tone within the microcirculation. Curr Pharm Biotechnol 2007; 8(1):11–25.
7. Little TL, Xia J, Duling BR. Dye tracers define differential endothelial and smooth muscle coupling patterns within the arteriolar wall. Circ Res 1995; 76:498–504.
8. Frid MG, Dempsey EC, Durmowicz AG, et al. Smooth muscle cell heterogeneity in pulmonary and systemic vessels. Importance in vascular disease. Arterioscler Thromb Vasc Biol 1997; 17:1203–1209.
9. Yoshida T, Owens GK. Molecular determinants of vascular smooth muscle cell diversity. Circ Res 2005; 96(3):280–291.
10. Schwartz SM, Murry CE. Proliferation and the monoclonal origins of atherosclerotic lesions. Ann Rev Med 1998; 49:437–460.
11. Aird WC. Endothelial cell heterogeneity and atherosclerosis. Curr Atheroscler Rep 2006; 8(1):69–75.
12. Aird WC. Mechanisms of endothelial cell heterogeneity in health and disease. Circ Res 2006; 98(2):159–62.
13. Hudlicka O. Development of microcirculation: capillary growth and adaptation. In: Bohr Dr., Somlyo AP, Sparks HV, eds. Handbook of Physiology: A critical comprehensive presentation of physiological knowledge and concepts, vol. IV. Baltimore, Maryland: Waverly Press, 1980:165–216.
14. Katoh Y, Periasamy M. Growth and differentiation of smooth muscle cells during development. Trends Cardiovasc Med 1996; 6(3):100–106.
15. Gittenberger-de Groot AC, DeRuiter MC., Bergwerff M, et al. Smooth muscle cell origin and its relation to heterogeneity in development and disease. Atheroscler Thromb Vasc Biol 1999; 19(7):1589–1594.

16. King GL, Johnson SH. Receptor-mediated transport of insulin across endothelial cells. Science 1985; 227:1583–1586.
17. Jaffe EA. Physiologic functions of normal endothelial cells. Ann N Y Acad Sci 1985; 454:279–291.
18. Friedl HP, Till GO, Ryan US, et al. Mediator-induced activation of xanthine oxidase in endothelial cells. FASEB J 1989; 3:2512–2518.
19. Esper RJ, Nordabay RA, Vilarino JO, et al. Endothelial dysfunction: a comprehensive appraisal. Cardiovasc Diabetol 2006; 5:4.
20. Campbell GR, Campbell JH. Smooth muscle phenotypic changes in arterial wall homeostasis: implications for the pathogenesis of atherosclerosis. Expe Molr Pathol 1985; 42:139–162.
21. Gordon D, Schwartz SM. Arterial smooth muscle differentiation. In: Campbell JH, Campbell GR, eds. Vascular Smooth Muscle in Culture, vol. I. Boca Raton, Florida: CRC Press, 1987:1–14.
22. Hathaway DR., March KL, Lash LA, et al. Vascular smooth muscle. A review of the molecular basis of contractility. Circulation 1991; 83(2):382–390.
23. Small JV, Gimona M. The cytoskeleton of the vertebrate smooth muscle cell. Acta Physiol Scand 1998; 164(4):341–348.
24. Owens GK. Regulation of differentiation of vascular smooth muscle cells. Physiol Rev 1995; 75(3):487–517.
25. Cox LR, Ramos KS. Biochemical basis of allylamine-induced aortic smooth muscle cell proliferation. In: Chemically-Induced Cell Proliferation: Implications in Risk Assessment. Hoboken, NJ: John Wiley & Sons, 1991:429–438.
26. Sappino AP, Schurch W, Gabbiani G. Differentiation repertoire of fibroblastic cells: expression of cytoskeletal proteins as markers of phenotypic modulations. Lab Invest 1990; 63:144–161.
27. Janes SM, Mu D, Wemmer D, et al. A new redox cofactor in eukaryotic enzymes: 6-hydroxydopa at the active site of bovine serum amine oxidase. Science 1990; 248:981–987.
28. Langford SD, Trent MB, Balakumaran A, et al. Developmental vasculotoxicity associated with inhibition of semicarbazide-sensitive amine oxidase. Toxicol Appl Pharmacol 1999; 155(3):237–244.
29. Lyles GA. Mammalian plasma and tissue-bound semicarbazide-sensitive amine oxidases: biochemical, pharmacological and toxicological aspects. Int J Biochem Cell Biol 1996; 28:259–274.
30. Deng Y, Yu PH. Assessment of the deamination of aminoacetone, an endogenous substrate for semicarbazide-sensitive amine oxidase. Anal Biochem 1999; 270(1): 97–102.
31. Escalante B, Sessa WC, Falck JR, et al. Cytochrome P450-dependent arachidonic acid metabolites, 19- and 20-hydroxyeicosatetraenoic acids enhance sodium-potassium ATPase activity in vascular smooth muscle. J Cardiovasc Pharmacol 1990; 16: 438–443.
32. Das UN. Essential fatty acids: biochemistry, physiology, and pathology. Biotechnol J 2006; 1:420–439.
33. Zhao W, Parrish AR, Ramos KS. Constitutive and inducible expression of cytochrome P450IA1 and P450IB1 in human vascular endothelial and smooth muscle cells. In Vitro Cell Dev Biol Anim 1998; 34:671–673.

34. Moorthy B, Miller KP, Jiang W, et al. Role of cytochrome P4501B1 in benzo[a] pyrene bioactivation to DNA-binding metabolites in mouse vascular smooth muscle cells: evidence from 32P- postlabeling for formation of 3-hydroxybenzo[a]pyrene and benzo[a]pyrene -3,6-quinone as major proximate genotoxic intermediates. J Pharmacol Exp Ther 2003; 305(1):394–401.

35. Boor PJ, Nelson TJ. Biotransformation of the cardiovascular toxin, allylamine, by rat and human cardiovascular tissue. J Mol Cell Cardiol 1982; 14(11):679–682.

36. Bond JA, Hsueh-Ying LY, Majesky MW, et al. Metabolism of benzo(a)pyrene and 7,12-dimethylbenz(a)anthracene in chicken aortas: Monooxygenation, bioactivation to mutagens, and covalent binding to DNA *in vitro*. Toxicol Appl Pharmacol 1980; 52:323–335.

37. Ferrario JB, DeLeon IR, Tracy RE. Evidence for toxic anthropogenic chemicals in human thrombogenic coronary plaques. Arch Environ Contam Toxicol 1985; 14:529–534.

38. Bishop CT, Mirza Z, Crapo JD, et al. Free radical damage to cultured porcine aortic endothelial cells and lung fibroblasts: Modulation by culture conditions. In Vitro Cell Dev Biol 1985; 21:21–25.

39. Ramos KS, Thurlow CH. Comparative cytotoxic responses of cultured avian and rodent aortic smooth muscle cells to allylamine. J Toxicol Environ Health 1993; 40:61–76.

40. Wolin MS, Ahmad M, Gupte SA. Oxidant and redox signaling in vascular oxygen sensing mechanisms: basic concepts, current controversies, and potential importance of cytosolic NADPH. Am J Physiol Lung Cell Mol Physiol 2005; 289(2): L159–L173.

41. Barhoumi R, Mouneinme Y, Ramos KS, et al. Analysis of benzo(a)pyrene partinioning and cytotoxicity in rat liver cell line. Toxicol Sci 1999; 53:264–270.

42. McGill HC. The pathogenesis of atherosclerosis. Clin Chem 1988; 34:33–39.

43. Newby AC, Zaltsman AB. Molecular mechanisms in intimal hyperplasia. J Pathol 2000; 190(3):300–309.

44. Ross R, Glomset J. The pathogenesis of atherosclerosis. New Engl J Med 1976; 295:369–377.

45. Ross R. The pathogenesis of atherosclerosis-an update. New Engl J Med 1986; 314:488–500.

46. Ross R. The pathogenesis of atherosclerosis: a perspective for the 1990's. Nature 1993; 362:801–809.

47. Miano JM, Tota RR, Niksa V, et al. Early proto-oncogene expression in rat aortic smooth muscle cells following endothelial removal. Am J Pathol 1990; 137: 761–765.

48. Nishida K, Abiko T, Ishihara M, et al. Arterial injury-induced smooth muscle cell proliferation in rats is accompanied by increase in polyamine synthesis and level. Atherosclerosis 1990; 83:119–125.

49. Peng S-K, Taylor CB, Hill JC, et al. Cholesterol oxidation derivatives and arterial endothelial damage. Atherosclerosis 1985; 54:121–133.

50. Roller RE, Schnedl WJ, Korninger C. Predicting the risk of restenosis after angioplasty in patients with peripheral arterial disease. Clin Lab 2001; 47(11-12): 555–559.

51. Benditt EP. Evidence for a monoclonal origin of human atherosclerotic plaque and some implications. Circulation 1974; 50:650–652.

52. Murry CE, Gipaya TB, Benditt EP, et al. Monoclonality of smooth muscle cells in human atherosclerosis. Am J Pathol 1997; 151:697–706.

53. Penn A, Garte SJ, Warren L, et al. Transforming genes in human atherosclerotic plaque DNA. Proc the Natl Acad Sci U.S.A. 1986; 83:7951–7955.

54. Ramos KS, Moorthy B. Bioactivation of polycyclic aromatic hydrocarbon carcinogens within the vascular wall: implications for human atherogenesis. Drug Metab Rev 2005; 37(4):595–610.

55. Binkova B, Strejc P, Boubelik O, et al. DNA adducts and human atherosclerotic lesions. Int J Hyg and Environ Health 2001; 204(1):49–54.

56. De Flora S, Izzotti A, Randerath K, et al. DNA adducts and chronic degenerative disease. Pathogenic relevance and implications in preventative medicine. Mutat Res 1996; 366:197–238.

57. Andreassi MG. Coronary atherosclerosis and somatic mutations: an overview of the contributive factors for oxidative DNA damage. Mutat Res 2003; 543:67–86.

58. Barrett TB, Benditt EP. sis (platelet-derived growth factor B chain) gene transcript levels are elevated in human atherosclerotic lesions compared to normal artery. Proc Natl Acad Sci U.S.A. 1987; 84(4):1099–1103.

59. Simons M, Rosenberg RD. Antisense nonmuscle myosin heavy chain and c-myb oligonucleotides suppress smooth muscle cell proliferation in vitro. Circ Res 1992; 70(4):835–843.

60. Sadhu DN, Lundberg MS, Burghardt RC, et al. c-Ha-rasEJ transfection of rat aortic smooth muscle cells induces epidermal growth factor responsiveness and characteristics of a malignant phenotype. J Cell Physiol 1994; 161(3):490–500.

61. Matturri L, Cazzullo A, Turconi P, et al. Chromosomal alterations in atherosclerotic plaques. Atherosclerosis 2001; 154(3):755–761.

62. Berliner JA, Navab M, Fogelman AM, et al. Atherosclerosis: basic mechanisms. Oxidation, inflammation, and genetics. Circulation 1995; 91(9):2488–2496.

63. Kroon PA. Cholesterol and atherosclerosis. Aust N Z J Med 1997; 27:492–496.

64. Rader DJ, Pure E. Lipoproteins, macrophage function, and atherosclerosis: beyond the foam cell? Cell Metab 2005; 1(4):223–230.

65. Roger WC, Brock TA, Chang LY, et al. Superoxide and peroxynitrite in atherosclerosis. Proc Natl Acad Sci U.S.A. 1994; 91:1044–1048.

66. Rubbo H, Trostchansky A, Botti H, et al. Interactions of nitric oxide and peroxynitrite with low-density lipoprotein. Biol Chem 2002; 383(3–4):547–552.

67. Libby P, Ridker PM, Maseri A. Inflammation and atherosclerosis. Circulation 2002; 105(9):1135–1143.

68. Geng YJ, Libby P. Progression of atheroma: a struggle between death and procreation. Arterioscle Thromb Vasc Biol 2002; 22(9):1370–1380.

69. Navab M, Berliner JA, Watson AD, et al. The yin and yang of oxidation in the development of the fatty streak. A review based on the 1994 George Lyman Duff memorial lecture. Arterioscler Thromb Vasc Biol 1996; 16(7):831–842.

70. Paffen E, DeMaat MP. C-reactive protein in atherosclerosis: a causal factor? Cardiovasc Res 2006; 71(1):30–39.

71. Inoue N. Vascular c-reactive protein in the pathogenesis of coronary artery disease: role of vascular inflammation and oxidative stress. Cardiovasc Hematoll Disord Drug Targets 2006; 6(4):227–231.

72. Sun H, Koike T, Ichikawa T, et al. C-reactive protein in atherosclerotic lesions: its origins and pathological significance. Am J Pathol 2005; 167:1139–1148.

73. Torzewski J. C-reactive protein and atherogenesis: new insights from established animal models. Am J Pathol 2005; 167(4):923–925.
74. Worth NF, Rolfe BE, Song J, et al. Vascular smooth muscle cell phenotypic modulation in culture is associated with reorganization of contractile and cytoskeletal proteins. Cell Motil Cytoskeleton 2001; 49(3):130–145.
75. Campbell GR, Chamley-Campbell JH. The cellular pathobiology of atherosclerosis. Pathology 1981; 13:423–440.
76. Hughes AD, Clumm GF, Refson J, et al. Platelet-derived growth factor (PDGF): actions and mechanisms in vascular smooth muscle. Gen Pharmacol 1996; 27:1079–1089.
77. Gran CM, Sadhu DN, Ramos KS. Transcriptional activation of the c-Ha-Ras protooncogene in vascular smooth muscle cells by benzo(a)pyrene. In Vitro Cell Dev Biol 1996; 32:599–601.
78. Ahn JD, Morishita R, Kaneda Y, et al. Inhibitory effects of novel AP-1 oligonucleotides on vascular smooth muscle cell proliferation in vitro and neointimal formation in vivo. Circ Res 2002; 90(12):1325–1332.
79. Veidt C, Vogel J, Athanasiou T, et al. Monocyte chemoattractant protein-1 induces proliferation and interleukin-6 production in human smooth muscle cells by differential activation of nuclear factor kappa-B and activator protein-1. Arterioscler Thromb Vasc Biol 2002; 22(6):914–920.
80. Hoshi S, Goto M, Koyama N, et al. Regulation of vascular smooth muscle cell proliferation by nuclear factor-kappaB and its inhibitor, I-kappaB. J Biol Chem 2000; 275(2):883–889.
81. Brand K, Page S, Rogler G, et al. Activated transcription factor nuclear factor-kappaB is present in the atherosclerotic lesion. J Clin Invest 1996; 97:1715–1722.
82. Bourcier T, Sukhova G, Libby P. The nuclear factor-kappaB signaling pathway participates in dysregulation of vascular smooth muscle cells in vitro and in human atherosclerosis. J Biol Chem 1997; 272(25):15817–15824.
83. Breuss JM, Cejna M, Bergmeister H, et al. Activation of nuclear factor-kappaB significantly contributes to lumen loss in a rabbit iliac artery balloon angioplasty model. Circulation 2002; 105(5):633–638.
84. Squadrito F, Deodato B, Bova A, et al. Crucial role of nuclear factor-kappaB in neointimal hyperplasia of the mouse carotid artery after interruption of blood flow. Atherosclerosis 2003; 166(2):233–242
85. Sarkar R, Meinberg EG, Stanley JC, et al. Nitric oxide reversibly inhibits the migration of cultured vascular smooth muscle cells. Circ Res 1996; 78:225–230.
86. Boerth NJ, Dey NB, Cornwell TL, et al. Cyclic GMP-dependent protein kinase regulates vascular smooth muscle cell phenotype. J Vasc Res 1997; 34:245–259.
87. Tentolouris G, Tousoulis D, Goumas G, et al. L-arginine in coronary atherosclerosis. Int J Cardiol 2000; 75(2–3):123–128.
88. Morey AK, Pedram A, Razandi M, et al. Estrogen and progesterone inhibit vascular smooth muscle proliferation. Endocrinology 1997; 138:3330–3339.
89. Khan NS, Malhoutra S. Effect of hormone replacement therapy on cardiovascular disease: current opinion. Expert Opin Pharmacother 2003; 4(5):667–674.
90. Hodis HN, Mack WJ, Azen SP, et al. Hormone therapy and the progression of coronary-artery atherosclerosis in postmenopausal women. New Engl J Med 2003; 349(6):535–545.

91. Lu KP, Ramos KS. Identification of genes differentially expressed in vascular smooth muscle cells following benzo(a)pyrene challenge: Implications for chemical atherogenesis. Biochem Biophys Res Commun 1998; 253:828–833.

92. Owens GK, Schwartz SM. Alterations in vascular smooth muscle cells in the spontaneously hypertensive rat: Role of cellular hypertrophy, hyperploidy, and hyperplasia. Circ Res 1982; 9:264–277.

93. Van Bortel LM. What does intima-media thickness tell us? J Hypertens 2005; 23(1): 37–39.

94. Granger HJ, Schelling ME, Lewis RE, et al. Physiology and pathobiology of the microcirculation. Am J Otolaryngol 1988; 9:264–277.

95. Sutton WL. Aliphatic and alicyclic amines. In: Patty FA, Fassett DW, Irish DO, eds. Industrial Hygiene and Toxicology, vol. 2. Interscience, New York, New York: 1995:2038.

96. Ryder NS. Mechanism of action and biochemical selectivity of allylamine antimycotic agents. Ann N Y Acad Sci 1998; 544:208–220.

97. Beard RR, Noe JT. Aliphatic and alicyclic amines. In: Clayton GD, Clayton FE, eds. Patty's Industrial Hygiene and Toxicology, vol II. New York, NY: Wiley, 1981:3135–3173.

98. Hine CH, Kodama JK, Guzman RJ, et al. The toxicity of allylamines. Arch Environ Health 1960; 1:343–352.

99. Boor PJ, Moslen MJ, Reynolds ES. Allylamine cardiotoxicity: I. Sequence of pathologic events. Toxicol Appl Pharmacol 1979; 50:581–592.

100. Lalich JJ, Allen JR, Paik WCW. Myocardial fibrosis and smooth muscle cell hyperplasia in coronary arteries of allylamine-fed rats. Am J Pathol 1972; 66:225–233.

101. Guzman RJ, Loquvam GS, Kodama JK, et al. Myocarditis produced by allylamines. Arch Environ Health 1961; 2:62–73.

102. Boor PJ. Allylamine cardiovascular toxicity: V. Tissue distribution and toxicokinetics after oral administration. Toxicology 1985; 35:167–177.

103. Boor PJ, Hysmith RM, Sanduja R. A role for a new vascular enzyme in the metabolism of xenobiotic amines. Circ Res 1990; 66:249–252.

104. Ramos KS, Lin H, McGrath JJ. Modulation of cyclic guanosine monophosphate levels in cultured aortic smooth muscle cells by carbon monoxide. Biochem Pharmacol 1989; 38:1368–1370.

105. Conklin DJ, Trent MB, Boor PJ. The role of plasma semicarbazide-sensitive amine oxidase in allylamine and beta-aminopropionitrile cardiovascular toxicity: mechanisms of myocardial protection and aortic medial injury in rats. Toxicology 1999; 138(3):137–154.

106. Buffoni F. Biochemical pharmacology of amine oxidases. Trends Pharmacol Sci 1983; 4:313–315.

107. Grossman SL, Alipui C, Ramos K. Further characterization of the metabolic activation of allylamine to acrolein in rat vascular tissue. In Vitro Toxicol 1990; 3:303–307.

108. Hysmith RM, Boor PJ. Allylamine cardiovascular toxicity: VI. Subcellular distribution in rat aortas. Toxicology 1985; 35:179–187.

109. Misra P, Srivastava SK, Singhal SS, et al.. Glutathione S-transferase 8-8 is localized in smooth muscle cells of rat aorta and is induced in an experimental model of atherosclerosis. Toxicol Appl Pharmacol 1995; 133:27–33.

110. Ramos K, Cox LR. Primary cultures of rat aortic endothelial and smooth muscle cells. I. An *in vitro* model to study xenobiotic-induced vascular cytotoxicity. In Vitro Cell Dev Biol 1987; 21:495–504.

111. Uchida K, Kanematsu M, Morimitsu Y, et al. Acrolein is a product of lipid peroxidant reaction. Formation of free acrolein and its conjugate with lysine residues in oxidized low density lipoproteins. J Biol Chem 1998; 273:16058–16066.

112. Awe SO, Adeagbo AS, D'Souza SE, et al. Acrolein induces vasodilatation of rodent mesenteric bed via an EDHF-dependent mechanism. Toxicol Appl Pharmacol 2006; 217(3):266–276.

113. Patel JM, Gordon WP, Nelson SD, et al. Comparison of hepatic biotransformation and toxicity of allyl alcohol and [1,1-2H2] allyl alcohol in rats. Drug Metab Dispos 1983; 11:164–166.

114. Ghilarducci DP, Tjeerdema RS. Fate and effects of acrolein Rev Environ Contam Toxicol 1995; 144:95–146.

115. Ranganna K, Yousefipour Z, Nasif R, et al. Acrolein activates mitogen-activated protein kinase signal transduction pathways in rat vascular smooth muscle cells. Mol Cell Biochem 2002; 240(1–2):83–98.

116. Tsakadze NL, Srivastava S, Awe AO, et al. Acrolein-induced vasomotor responses of rat aorta. Am J Physiol Heart Circ Physiol 2003; 285(2):H727–H734.

117. Shao B, O'Brien KD, McDonald TO, et al. Acrolein modifies apolipoprotein A-1 in the human artery wall. Ann N Y Acad Sci 2005; 1043:396–403.

118. Yousefipour Z, Ranganna K, Newaz MA, et al. Mechanism of acrolein-induced vascular toxicity. J Physiol Pharmacol 2005; 56(3):337–353.

119. Conklin DJ, Bhatnagar A, Cowley HR, et al. Acrolein generation stimulates hypercontraction in isolated human blood vessels. Toxicol Appl Pharmacol 2006; 217(3):277–288.

120. Kutzman RS, Wehner RW, Haber SB. Selected responses of hypertension-sensitive and resistant rats to inhaled acrolein. Toxicology 1984; 31:53–65.

121. Ramos K, Grossman SL, Cox LR. Allylamine-induced vascular toxicity *in vitro*: prevention by semicarbizide-sensitive amine oxidase inhibitors. Toxicol Appl Pharmacol 1988; 96:61–71.

122. Cox LR, Ramos K. Allylamine-induced phenotypic modulation of aortic smooth muscle cells. J Exp Path 1990; 71:11–18.

123. Cox LR, Murphy SK, Ramos K. Modulation of phosphoinositide metabolism in aortic smooth muscle cells by allylamine. Exp Mol Pathol 1990; 53:52–63.

124. Awasthi S, Boor PJ. Allylamine and beta-aminopropionitrile-induced vascular injury: enhanced expression of high-molecular-weight protein. J Toxicol Environ Health 1998; 53:61–76.

125. Parrish AR, Ramos KS. Differential processing of osteopontin characterizes the proliferative vascular smooth muscle cell phenotype induced by allylamine. J Cell Biochem 1997; 65:267–275.

126. Wilson E, Parrish AR, Bral CM, et al. Collagen suppresses the proliferative phenotype of allylamine-injured vascular smooth muscle cells. Atherosclerosis 2002; 162(2):289–297.

127. Astrup P, Hellung-Larson P, Kjeldsen K, et al. The effect of tobacco smoking on the dissociation curve of oxyhemoglobin-investigations in patients with occlusive arterial diseases and in normal subjects. Scand J Clin Lab Invest 1966; 18:450–460.

128. Durante W, Johnson FK, Johnson RA. Role of carbon monoxide in cardiovascular function. J Cell Mol Med 2006; 10(3):672–686.

129. Levene CI, Barlet CP, Fornieri C, et al. Effect of hypoxia and carbon monoxide on collagen synthesis in cultured porcine and bovine aortic endothelium. Br J Exp Pathol 1985; 66:399–408.

130. Paule WJ, Zemplenyl TK, Rounds DE, et al. Light and Electron-Microscopic characteristics of arterial smooth muscle cell cultures subjected to hypoxia or carbon monoxide. Atherosclerosis 1976; 25:111–123.

131. Astrup P, Kjeldson K, Wanstrup J. Enhancing influence of carbon monoxide on the development of atheromatosis in cholesterol-fed rabbits. Journal of Atheroscler Res 1967; 7:343–354.

132. Morita T, Kourembanas S. Endothelial cell expression of vasoconstrictors and growth factors is regulated by smooth muscle cell-derived carbon monoxide. J Clin Invest 1995; 96:2676–2682.

133. Kourembanas S, Morita T, Liu Y, et al. Mechanisms by which oxygen regulates gene expression and cell-cell interaction in the vasculature. Kidney International 1997; 51:438–443.

134. Kao LW, Nanagas KA. Toxicity associated with carbon monoxide. Clin Lab Med 2006; 26:99–125.

135. Cobarn RF, Mayers LB. Myoglobin oxygen tension determined from measurements of carboxyhemoglobin in skeletal muscle. Am J Physiol 1971; 220:66–74.

136. Young LJ, Caughey WS. Pathobiochemistry of carbon monoxide poisoning. FEBS Letters 1990; 272:1–6.

137. McFaul SJ, McGrath JJ. Studies on the mechanism of carbon monoxide-induced vasodilation in the isolated perfused rat heart. Toxicol Appl Pharmacol 1987; 87:464–473.

138. Graser T, Vedernikov YP, Li DS. Study on the mechanism of carbon monoxide induced endothelium-independent relaxation in porcine coronary artery and vein. Biomed Biochim Acta 1990; 49:293–296.

139. Vedernikov YP, Graser T, Vanin AF. Similar endothelium-independent arterial relaxation by carbon monoxide and nitric oxide. Biomedica Biochimica Acta 1989; 48:601–603.

140. Lin H, McGrath JJ. Vasodilating effects of carbon monoxide. Drug Chem Toxicol 1988; 11(4):371–385.

141. Brune B, Ullrich V. Inhibition of platelet aggregation by carbon monoxide is mediated by activation of guanylate cyclase. Mol Pharmacol 1987; 32, 497–504.

142. Durante W, Kroll MH, Christodoulides N, et al. Nitric oxide induces heme oxygenase-1 gene expression and carbon monoxide production in vascular smooth muscle cells. Circ Res 1997; 80:557–564.

143. Morita T, Mitsialis SA, Koike H, et al. Carbon monoxide controls the proliferation of hypoxic vascular smooth muscle cells. J Biol Chem 1997; 272:32804–32809.

144. Thom SR, Ishirpoulos H. Mechanism of oxidative stress from low levels of carbon monoxide. Res Rep Health Eff Inst 1997; 80:1–9, (discussion 21-27).

145. Robinson CP, Baskin SI, Franz DR. The mechanisms of action of cyanide on the rabbit aorta. J Appl Toxicol 1985; 5:372–377.

146. Zevin S, Saunders S, Gourlay SG, et al. Cardiovascular effects of carbon monoxide and cigarette smoking. J Am Coll Cardiol 2001; 38(6):1633–1638.

147. Grimm M, Weidmann P, Keusch G, et al. Norepinephrine clearance and pressure effect in normal and hypertensive man. Klin Worhenschr 1980; 58:1175–1181.
148. Helin P, Lorenzen I, Garbarsch C, et al. Arteriosclerosis in rabbit aorta induced by noradrenaline. Atherosclerosis 1970; 12:125–132.
149. Kukreja RS, Datta BN, Chakravarti RN. Catecholamine-induced aggravation of aortic and coronary atherosclerosis in monkeys. Atherosclerosis 1981; 40:291–298.
150. Bauch HJ, Grunwald J, Vischer P, et al. A possible role of catecholamines in atherogenesis and subsequent complications of atherosclerosis. Expe Pathol 1987; 31:193–204.
151. Black PH. The inflammatory consequences of psychologic stress: Relationship to insulin resistance, obesity, atherosclerosis, and diabetes mellitus, type II. Medical Hypotheses 2006; 67(4):879–891.
152. Nakaki T, Nakayama M, Yamamoto S, et al. α_1-adrenergic stimulation and β_2-adrenergic inhibition of DNA synthesis in vascular smooth muscle cells. Mol Pharmacol 1989; 37:30–36.
153. Yu SM, Tsai SY, Guh JH, et al. Mechanism of catecholamine-induced proliferation of vascular smooth muscle cells. Circulation 1996; 94:547–554.
154. de Blois D, Schwartz SM, van Kleef EM, et al. Chronic alpha 1-adrenoreceptor stimulation increases DNA synthesis in rat arterial wall. Modulation of responsiveness after vascular injury. Arterioscler Thromb Vasc Biol 1996; 16: 1122–1129.
155. Hu ZW, Shi XY, Hoffman BB. Insulin and insulin-like growth factor I differentially induce alpha1-adrenergic receptor subtypes expression in rat vascular smooth muscle cells. J Clin Invest 1996; 98:1826–1834.
156. Pettersson K, Bejne B, Bjork H, et al. Experimental sympathetic activation causes endothelial injury in the rabbit thoracic aorta via β_1-adrenoceptor activation. Circ Res 1990; 67:1027–1034.
157. Sholley MM, Gimbrone MA, Cotran RS. Cellular migration and replication in endothelial regeneration. Lab Invest 1976; 36:18–25.
158. Grunwald J, Schaper W, Mey J, et al. Special characteristics of cultured smooth muscle cell subtypes of hypertensive and diabetic rats. Artery 1982; 11:1–14.
159. Grunwald J, Haudenschild CC. Intimal injury *in vivo* activates vascular smooth muscle cell migration and explant outgrowth *in vitro*. Arteriosclerosis 1984; 4:183–188.
160. Xin X, Yang N, Eckhart AD, et al. Alpha 1D-adrenergic receptors and mitogen-activated protein kinase mediate increased protein synthesis by arterial smooth muscle. Mol Pharmacol 1997; 51:764–75.
161. Berk BC, Alexander RW, Brock TA, et al. Vasoconstriction: A new activity for platelet-derived growth factors. Science 1986; 232:87–90.
162. Berk BC, Brock TA, Webb RC, et al. Epidermal growth factor, a vascular smooth muscle mitogen induces rat aortic contraction. J Clin Invest 1985; 75:1083–1086.
163. Naftilan AJ, Gilliland GK, Eldridge CS, et al. Induction of the protooncogene c-jun by angiotensin II. Mol Cell Biol 1990; 10:5536–5554.
164. Hu ZW, Shi XY, Okazaki M, et al. Angiotensin II induces transcription and expression of alpha 1-adrenergic receptors in vascular smooth muscle cells. Am J Physiol 1995; 268:H1006–H1014.
165. Chrysant SG. Vascular remodeling: the role of angiotensin-converting enzyme inhibitors. Am Heart J 1998; 135:S21–S30.

166. Dhalla NS, Yates JC, Lee SL, et al. Functional and subcellular changes in the isolated rat heart perfused with oxidized isoproterenol. J Mol Cell Cardiol 1978; 10:31–41.

167. Ramos K. Cellular and molecular basis of xenobiotic-induced cardiovascular toxicity: application of cell culture systems. In: Acosta D, ed. Cellular and Molecular Toxicology and In Vitro Toxicology. Boca Raton, Florida: CRC Press, 1990:139–155.

168. Wolin MS, Belloni FL. Superoxide anion selectivity attenuates catecholamine-induced contractile tension in isolated rabbit aorta. Am J Physiol 1985; 249:H1127–H1133.

169. Rubanyi GM. Vascular effects of oxygen-derived free radicals. Free Radic Biol Med 1988; 4:107–120.

170. McCord JM. Oxygen-derived free radicals in post ischemic tissue injury. New Engl J Med 1985; 312:159–163.

171. Machlin LJ, Bendich A. Free radical tissue damage: protective role of antioxidant nutrients. FASEB J 1987; 1:441–445.

172. Babior BM, Curnette JT, McMurick BJ. The particulate superoxide-forming system from human neutrophils: properties of the system and further evidence supporting its participation in the respiratory burst. J Clin Invest 1976; 58:989–996.

173. Heinecke JW. Free radical modification of low-density lipoprotein: mechanisms and biological consequences. Free Radic Biol Med 1987; 3:65–73.

174. Kontos HA, Wei EP, Dietrich WD, et al. Mechanism of cerebral arteriolar abnormalities after acute hypertension. Am J Physiol 1981; 240:H511–H527.

175. Wei EP, Kontos HA, Dietrich WD, et al. Inhibition by free radical scavengers and by cyclooxygenase inhibitors of pial arteriolar abnormalities from concussive brain injury in cats. Circ Res 1981; 48(1):95–103.

176. Wei EP, Kontos HA, Christman CW, et al. Superoxide generation and reversal of acetylcholine-induced cerebral arteriolar dilation after acute hypertension. Circ Res 1985; 57(5):781–787.

177. Hiebert LM, Liu JM. Heparin protects cultured arterial endothelial cells from damage by toxic oxygen metabolites. Atherosclerosis 1990; 83(1):47–51.

178. Shasby M, Lind SE, Shasby SS, et al. Reversible oxidant-induced increases in albumin transfer across cultured endothelium: alterations in cell shape and calcium homeostasis. Blood 1985; 65(3):605–614.

179. Rosenblum WI, Bryan D. Evidence that in vivo constriction of cerebral arterioles by local application of tert-butyl hydroperoxide is mediated by release of endogenous thromboxane. Stroke 1987; 18:195–199.

180. Matsubara T, Ziff M. Superoxide anion release by human endothelial cells: Synergism between a phorbol ester and a calcium ionophore. J Cell Physiol 1986; 127:207–210.

181. Gross JL, Moscatelli D, Rifkin DB. Increased capillary endothelial cell protease activity in response to angiogenic stimuli *in vitro*. Proc Natl Acad Sci U.S.A. 1983; 80:2623–2627.

182. Chemical Industry Institute of Toxicology. 104 week chronic toxicity study in rats. Dinitrotoluene. Final Report, vol. 1 and 2. Docket No. 12362. Research Triangle Park, North Carolina: CIIT, 1982.

183. Ellis HV, Hough CB, Dacre YC, et al. Chronic toxicity of 2,4-dinitrotoluene in the rat. Toxicol Appl Pharmacol 1978; 45:245.

184. Leonard TB, Graichen ME, Popp JA. Dinitrotoluene isomer-specific hepatocarcinogenesis in F344 rats. J Natl Cancer Inst 1987; 79:1313–1319.

185. Levine RJ. Dinitrotoluene: Human atherogen, carcinogen, neither or both? CIIT 1987; 7:2–5.

186. Levine RJ, Andjelkovich DA, Kersteter SL, et al. Heart disease in workers exposed to dinitrotoluene. J Occup Med 1986; 28:811–816.

187. Tchounwou PB, Newsome C, Glass K, et al. Environmental toxicology and health effects associated with dinitrotoluene exposure. Rev Environ Health 2003; 18(3): 203–229.

188. Ramos KS, McMahon KK, Alipui C, et al. Modulation of DNA synthesis in aortic smooth muscle cells by dinitrotoluene. Cell Biol Toxicol 1991; 7:111–128.

189. Ramos K, McMahon KK, Alipui C, et al. Modulation of smooth muscle cell pro-liferation by dinitrotoluene. In: Witmer CM, Snyder RR, Jollow DJ, eds. Biologic Reductive Intermediates, vol. V. New York, NY:Plenum Press, 1990:805–807.

190. Long RM, Rickert DE. Metabolism and excretion of 2,6-dinitro[14C]toluene *in vivo* and in isolated perfused rat livers. Drug Metab Dispos 1982; 10:455–458.

191. Mirsalis JC, Hamm TE, Sherrill JM, et al. Role of gut flora in the genotoxicity of dinitrotoluene. Nature 1982; 295:322–323.

192. Dent JG, Schnell SR, Guest D. Metabolism of 2,4-dinitrotoluene in rat hepatic microsomes and cecal flora. In: Proceedings of the Second International Sympo-sium on Biologically Reactive Intermediates. Chemical Mechanisms and Biologic Effects. New York, NY: Plenum Press, 1981:431–436.

193. Sadhu DN, Crum S, Ramos KS. Benzo(a)pyrene-induced alterations in [3H]-thymidine incorporation in cultured aortic smooth muscle cells. Toxicologist 1991; 11:339.

194. Chadwick RW, Elizabeth GE, Kohan MJ, et al. Potentiation of 2,6-dinitrotoluene genotoxicity in Fischer-344 rats by pretreatment with Aroclor 1254. Toxicology 1993; 80:153–171.

195. Vesselinovitch D. Animal models and the study of atherosclerosis. Arch Pathol Lab Med 1980; 112:1011–1017.

196. Jokinen MP, Clarkson TB, Prichard RW. Recent advances in molecular pathology. Animal models in atherosclerosis research. Exp Mol Pathol 1985; 42:1–28.

197. Taylor LM Jr., Moneta GL, Sexton GJ, et al. Prospective blinded study of the relationship between plasma homocysteine and progression of symptomatic peripheral arterial disease. J Vasc Surg 1999; 29: 8–21.

198. Kaul S, Zadeh AA, Shah PK. Homocysteine hypothesis for atherothrombotic car-diovascular disease: not validated. J Am Coll Cardiol 2006; 48(5):914–923.

199. Klerk M, Verhoef P, Clarke R, et al. JAMA 2002; 288(16):2023–2031.

200. McCully KS. Homocysteine and vascular disease. Nat Med 1996; 2:386–389

201. Harker LA, Harlan JM, Ross R. Effect of sulfinpyrazanone on homocysteine-induced endothelial injury and arteriosclerosis in baboons. Circ Res 1983; 53:731–739.

202. Tsai J-C, Perrella MA, Yoshizumi M, et al. Promotion of vascular smooth muscle cell growth by homocysteine: a link to atherosclerosis. Proc Natl Academy Sci U.S.A. 1994; 91:6369–6373.

203. Nishio E, Watanabe Y. Homocysteine as a modulator of platelet-derived growth factor action in vascular smooth muscle cells: a possible role for hydrogen peroxide. Br J Pharmacol 1997; 122:268–274.

204. Kusuhara M, Chait A, Cader A, et al. Oxidized LDL stimulates mitogen activated protein kinases in smooth muscle cells and macrophages. Arterioscler Thromb Vasc Biol 1997; 17:141–148.

205. Halvorsen B, Brude I, Drevon CA, et al. Effect of homocysteine on copper ion-catalyzed, azo compound-initiated, and mononuclear cell-mediated oxidative modification of low density lipoprotein. J Lipid Res 1996; 37:1591–1600.

206. Abby SL, Harris IM, Harris KM. Homocysteine and cardiovascular disease. J Am Board Fam Pract 1998; 11:391–398.

207. Hornstra G, Barth CA, Galli C, et al. Functional food science and the cardiovascular system. Br J Nutr 1998; 80(suppl 1):S113–S146.

208. Cook JW, Malinow MR, Moneta GL, et al. Neointimal hyperplasia in balloon-injured rat carotid arteries: the influence of hyperhomocysteinemia. J Vasc Surg 2002; 35(1):158–165.

209. Morita H, Kurihara H, Yoshida S, et al. Diet-induced hyperhomocysteinema exacerbates neointima formation in rat carotid arteries after balloon injury. Circulation 2001; 103(1):133–139.

210. Hofmann MA, Lalla E, Lu Y, et al. Hyperhomocysteinemia enhances vascular inflammation and accelerates atherosclerosis in a murine model. J Clin Invest 2001; 107(6):675–683.

211. Schnyder G, Roffi M, Pin R, et al. Decreased rate of coronary restenosis after lowering of plasma homocysteine levels. New Engl J Med 2001; 345(22):1593–1600.

212. Durga J, van Tits LJ, Schouten EG, et al. Effect of lowering of homocysteine levels on inflammatory markers: a randomized controlled trial. Arch Intern Med 2005; 165(12):1388–1394.

213. McManus BM, Toth B, Patil KD. Aortic rupture and aortic smooth muscle tumors in mice: Induction by p-hydrazinobenzoic acid hydrochloride of the cultivated mushroom Agaricusbisporus. Lab Invest 1987; 57(1):78–85.

214. Toth B, Nagel D, Patil K, et al. Tumor induction with N1-acetyl derivative of 4-hydroxy methyl phenyl hydrazine, a metabolite of agaritine of Agaricus bisporus. Cancer Res 1978; 38:177–180.

215. Gamberini M, Cidade MR, Valotta LA, et al. Contribution of hydrazine-derived alkyl radicals to cytotoxic and transformation induced in normal c-myc-over-expression mouse fibroblasts. Carcinogenesis 1998; 19:147–155.

216. Savage NW, Adkins KF, Young WG, et al. Oral vascular leiomyoma: review of the literature and report of 2 cases. Aust Dent J 1983; 28:346–349.

217. Hernandez FJ, Stanley JM, Ranganath KA, et al. Primary leiomyosarcoma of the aorta. Am J Surg Pathol 1979; 3:251–254.

218. Milili JJ, LaFlare RG, Nemir P. Leiomyosarcoma of the abdominal aorta: a case report. Surgery 1981; 89:631–634.

219. Blansfield JA, Chung H, Sullivan TR, et al. Leiomyosarcoma of the major peripheral arteries: case report and review of the literature. Ann Vasc Surg 2003; 17(5):565–570.

220. Walton K, Coombs MM, Walker R, et al. Bioactivation of mushroom hydrazines to mutagenic products mammalian and fungal enzymes. Mutat Res 1997; 381:131–139.

221. Kalyanaraman B, Sinha BK. Free radical-mediated activation of hydrazine derivatives. Environ Health Perspect 1985; 64:179–184.

222. Noda A, Ishizawa M, Ohino K, et al. Relationship between oxidative metabolites of hydrazine and hydrazine-induced mutagenicity. Toxicol Lett 1986; 31:131–137.

223. Whiting RF, Wei L, Stich HF. Enhancement by transition metals of unscheduled DNA synthesis induced by isoniazid and related hydrazines in cultured normal and xeroderma pegmentosum human cells. Mutat Res 1979; 62:505–510.

224. Poso A, Wright AV, Gynther J. An empirical and theoretical study on mechanisms of mutagenic activity of hydrazine compounds. Mutat Res 1995; 332:63–71.

225. Medeiros DM, Pellum LK. Blood pressure and hair cadmium, lead, copper, and zinc concentrations in Mississippi adolescents. Bull Environ Contam Toxicol 1985; 34:163–169.

226. Voors AW, Johnson WD, Shuman MS. Additive statistical effects of cadmium and lead on heart-related disease in a North Carolina autopsy series. Arch Environ Health 1982; 37:98–102.

227. Beevers DG, Campbell BC, Goldberts A, et al. Blood cadmium in hypertensives and normotensives. Lancet 1976; 2:12222–12224.

228. Carafoli E. How calcium crosses plasma membrane including the sarcolemma. In: Opie LH, ed. Calcium Antagonists and Cardiovascular Disease. New York, NY: Raven Press, 1984:29–41.

229. Cheung WY. Calmodulin: its potential role in cell proliferation and heavy metal toxicity. Fed Proc 1984; 43:2995–2999.

230. Habermann E, Richardt G. Intracellular calcium binding proteins as targets for heavy metal ions. Trends Pharmacol Sci 1986; 7:298–300.

231. Perry MH, Erlanger MW, Gustafsson TO, et al. Reversal of cadmium-induced hypertension by D-myo-inositol-1,2,6-triphosphate. J Toxicol Environ Health 1989; 28:151–159.

232. Georing PL, Klaassen CD. Zinc-induced tolerance to cadmium toxicity. Toxicol Appl Pharmacol 1984; 74:299–307.

233. Webb M. The metallothioneins. In: Webb M, ed. The Chemistry, Biochemistry and Biology of Cadmium. Amsterdam, the Netherlands: Elsevier/North Holland, 1979:195–266.

234. Revis NW, Zinsmeister AR, Bull R. Atherosclerosis and hypertension induction by lead and cadmium ions: an effect prevented by calcium ion. Proc Natl Acad Sci U.S.A. 1981; 78(10):6494–6498.

235. Meijer GW, Beems RB, Janssen GB, et al. Cadmium and atherosclerosis in rabbit: reduced atherogenesis by superseding of iron? Food Chem Toxicol 1996; 34: 611–621.

236. Schroeder HA, Vinton WH Jr. Hypertension in rats induced by small doses of cadmium. American Journal of Physiology 1962; 202:515–518.

237. Perry HM Jr., Erlanger MW, Perry EF. Elevated systolic pressure following chronic-level cadmium feeding. Am J Physiol 1977; 232:H114–H121.

238. Kopp SJ, Glonek T, Perry HM Jr., et al. Cardiovascular actions of cadmium at environmental exposure levels. Science 1982; 217:837–839.

239. Puri VN. Cadmium induced hypertension. Clin Exp Hypertens 1999; 21(1–2):79–84.

240. Varoni MV, Palomba D, Gianorso S, et al. Cadmium as an environmental factor of hypertension in animals: new perspectives on mechanisms. Vet Res Commun 2003; 27(suppl 1):807–810.

241. Washington B, Williams S, Armstrong P, et al. Cadmium toxicity on arterioles vascular smooth muscle cells of spontaneously hypertensive rats. Int J Environ Res Public Health 2006; 3(4):323–328.

242. Perry HM Jr., Perry EF, Erlanger MW. Possible influence of heavy metals in cardiovascular disease: an introduction and overview. J Environ Pathol Toxicol 1980; 3:195–203.

243. Perry HM Jr., Erlanger MW, Perry EF. Effect of a second metal on cadmium-induced hypertension. Arch Environ Health 1983; 8:80–85.

244. Prozialeck WC, Edwards JR, Woods JM. The vascular endothelium as a target of cadmium toxicity. Life Sci 2006; 79(16):1493–1506.

245. Doyle JJ, Bernhoft RA, Sandstead HH. The effects of a low level of dietary cadmium on blood pressure, ^{24} Na, ^{42} K and water retention in growing rats. J Lab Clin Med 1975; 86:57–83.

246. Perry HM Jr., Yunice A. Acute pressor effects of intra-arterial cadmium and mercuric ions in anesthetized rats. Proc Soc Expl Biol Med 1965; 120:805–808.

247. Perry HM Jr., Erlanger M, Yunice A, et al. Mechanism of the acute hypertensive effect of intra-arterial cadmium and mercury in anesthetized rats. J Lab Clin Med Lab 1967; 70:963–971.

248. Perry HM, Erlanger MW, Perry EF. Increase in the systolic pressure of rats chronically fed cadmium. Environ Health Perspect 1979; 28:251–260.

249. Schlaepfer WW. Sequential study of endothelial changes in acute cadmium intoxication. Lab Invest 1971; 25:556–564.

250. Togna G, Togna AR, Caprino L. Vascular endothelium and platelet preparations for the prediction of xenobiotic effects on the vascular system. Xenobiotica 1985; 15:661–664.

251. Caprino L, Togna G, Togna AR. Cadmium-induced platelet hypersensitivity to aggregating agents. Pharmacol Res Commun 1979; 11:731–737.

252. Vaziri ND. Pathogenesis of lead-induced hypertension: role of oxidative stress. J Hypertens Suppl 2002; 20(3):S15–S20.

253. Vaziri ND, Sica DA. Lead-induced hypertension: role of oxidative stress. Curr Hypertens Rep 2004; 6(4):314–320.

254. Batuman V, Landy E, Maesaka JK, et al. Contribution of lead to hypertension with renal impairment. New Engl J Med 1983; 309:17–21.

255. Chipino G, Constantine S, Cirla AM. Changes induced by cadmium, zinc, and lead on renal and peripheral vascular resistance in the anesthetized rabbit. Med Lav 1968; 59:522–533.

256. Fine BP, Vetrano T, Skurnick J, et al. Blood pressure elevation in young dogs during low level lead poisoning. Toxicol Appl Pharmacol 1988; 93:388–393.

257. Fujiwara Y, Kaji T, Yamamoto C, et al. Stimulatory effect of lead on the proliferation of cultured vascular smooth-muscle cells. Toxicology 1995; 98:105–110.

258. Farmand F, Ehdaie A, Roberts CK, et al. Lead-induced dysregulation of superoxide dismutases, catalase, glutathione peroxidase, and guanylate cyclase. Environ Res 2005; 98(1):33–39.

259. Ni Z, Hou S, Barton CH, et al. Lead exposure raises superoxide and hydrogen peroxide in human endothelial and vascular smooth muscle cells. Kidney Int 2004; 66(6):2329–2336.

260. Patrick L. Lead toxicity part II: the role of free radical damage and the use of antioxidants in the pathology and treatment of lead toxicity. Altern Med Rev 2006; 11(2):114–127.

261. Tomera JF, Harakal C. Mercury and lead-induced contraction of aortic smooth muscle in vitro. Arch Int de Pharmacodyn There 1986; 283:295–302.

262. Caprino L, Togna AR, Cebo B, et al. In vitro effects of mercury on platelet aggregation, thromboxane, and vascular prostacyclin production. Arch Toxicol Suppl 1983; 6:48–51.

263. Jhaveri R, Lavorgna L, Dube SK, et al. Relationship of blood pressure to blood lead concentrations in small children. Pediatrics 1979; 63:674–676.

264. Needleman HL, Schell AS, Bellinger D, et al. The long-term effects of exposure to low doses of lead in childhood: an 11 year follow-up report. New Engl J Med 1990; 322:83–88.

265. Maxwell K, Vinters HV, Berliner JA, et al. Effect of inorganic lead on some functions of the cerebral microvessel endothelium. Toxicol Appl Pharmacol 1986; 84:389–399.

266. Bull HA, Pittilo RM, Blow DJ, et al. The effects of nicotine on PGI$_2$ production by rat aortic endothelium. Thromb Haemost 1985; 54(2):472–474.

267. Wennmalm A. Nicotine inhibits the release of 6-keto-prostaglandin F1alpha from the isolated perfused rabbit heart. Acta Physiol Scand 1978; 103(1):107–109.

268. Sonnfield T, Wennmalm A. Inhibition by nicotine of the formation of prostacyclin-like activity in rabbit and human vascular tissue. Br J Pharmacol 1980; 71:609–613.

269. Stoel I, vd Giessen WJ, Zwolsman E, et al. Direct effect of nicotine on prostacyclin in human umbilical arteries. Acta Ther 1980; 6(4):32–34.

270. Alster P, Wennmalm A. Effect of nicotine on prostacyclin formation in rat aorta. Eur J Pharmacol 1983; 86:441–446.

271. Zimmerman M, McGeachie J. The effect of nicotine on aortic endothelial cell turnover: An autoradiographic study. Atherosclerosis 1985; 58:39–47.

272. Tulloss J, Booyse FM. Effect of various agents and physical damage in bovine endothelial cultures. Microvasc Res 1978; 16:51–58.

273. Hanna ST. Nicotine effect on cardiovascular system and ion channels. J Cardiovasc Pharmacol 2006; 47(3):348–358.

274. Thyberg J. Effects of nicotine on phenotypic modulation and initiation of DNA synthesis in cultured arterial smooth muscle cells. Virchows Arch 1986; 52:25–32.

275. Thyberg J, Nilsson J. Effects of nicotine on endocytosis and intracellular degradation of horseradish peroxidase in cultivated mouse peritoneal macrophages. Acta Pathol Microbiol Immunol Scand 1982; 90:305–310.

276. Gupta R, Gurm H, Bartholomew JR. Smokeless tobacco and cardiovascular risk. Arch Intern Med 2004; 164(17):1845–1849.

277. Brook RD, Franklin B, Cascio W, et al. Air pollution and cardiovascular disease. A statement for healthcare professionals from the expert panel on population and prevention science of the American Heart Association. Circulation 2004; 109:2655–2671.

278. Sorenson M, Daneshvar B, Hansen M, et al. Personal PM2.5 exposure and markers of oxidative stress in blood. Environ Health Perspect 2003; 111(2):161–166.

279. Gurgueira SA, Lawrence J, Coull B, et al. Rapid increases in the steady-state concentration of reactive oxygen species in the lungs and heart after particulate air pollution inhalation. Environ Health Perspect 2002; 110(8):749–755.

280. Li N, Sioutas C, Cho A, et al. Ultrafine particulate pollutants induce oxidative stress and mitochondrial damage. Environ Health Perspect 203; 111(4):455–460.

281. Shukla A, Timblin C, BeruBe K, et al. Inhaled particulate matter causes expression of nuclear factor (NF)-kappaB-related genes and oxidant-dependent NF-kappaB activation in vitro. Am J Respir Cell Mol Biol 2000; 23(2):182–187.

282. Xiao GG, Wang M, Li N, et al. Use of proteomics to demonstrate a hierarchical oxidative stress response to diesel exhaust particle chemicals in a macrophage cell line. J Biol Chem 2003; 278(50):50781–50790.
283. Thomson E, Kumarathasan P, Goegan P, et al. Differential regulation of the lung endothelin system by urban particulate matter and ozone. Toxicol Sci 2005; 88(1): 103–113.
284. Lund AK. Knuckles TL, Obot AC, et al. Gasoline exhaust emissions induce vascular remodeling pathways involved in atherosclerosis. Toxicol Sci 2007; 95(2): 485–494.
285. Soukup JM, Becker S. Human alveolar macrophage responses to air pollution particulates are associated with insoluble components of coarse material, including particulate endotoxin. Toxicol Appl Pharmacol 2001; 171(1):20–26
286. Monn C, Naef R, Koller T. Reactions of macrophages exposed to particles <10 micron. Environ Res 2003; 91(1):35–44.
287. Seaton A, Soutar A, Crawford V, et al. Particulate air pollution and the blood. Thorax 1999; 54(11):1027–1032.
288. Ridker PM. High-sensitivity C-reactive protein: potential adjunct for global risk assessment in the primary prevention of cardiovascular disease. Circulation 2001; 103(13):1813–1818.
289. Diez Roux AV, Auchincloss AH, Astor B, et al. Recent exposure to particulate matter and C-reactive protein concentration in the multi-ethnic study of atherosclerosis. Am J Epidemiol 2006; 164(5):437–448.
290. Venn A, Britton J. Exposure to secondhand smoke and biomarkers of cardiovascular disease risk in never-smoking adults. Circulation 2007; 115(8):990–995.
291. Pope CA, Hansen ML, Long RW, et al. Ambient particulate air pollution, heart rate variability, and blood markers of inflammation in a panel of elderly subjects. Environ Health Perspect 2004; 112(3):339–345.
292. Suwa T, Hogg JC, Quinlan KB, et al. Particulate air pollution induces progression of atherosclerosis. J Am Coll Cardiol 2002; 39(6):935–942.
293. Sun Q, Aixia W, Jin X, et al. Long-term air pollution exposure and acceleration of atherosclerosis and vascular inflammation in an animal model. JAMA 2005; 294(23):3003–3010.
294. Izzotti A, De Flora S, Petrilli GL, et al. Cancer biomarkers in human atherosclerotic lesions: detection of DNA adducts. Cancer Epidemiol Biomarkers Prev 1995; 4(2): 105–110.
295. Benditt EP, Benditt JM. Evidence for a monoclonal origin of human atherosclerotic plaques. Proc Natl Acad Sci U.S.A. 1973; 70:1753–1756.
296. Albert RE, Vanderlaan M, Burns FJ, et al. Effect of carcinogens on chicken atherosclerosis. Cancer Res 1977; 37:2232–2235.
297. Gold H. Production of arteriosclerosis in the rat: effect of x-ray and high-fat diet. Arch Pathol 1961; 71:268–273.
298. Lu KP, Hallberg LM, Tomlinson J, et al. Benzo(a)pyrene activates L1Md retrotransposon and inhibits DNA repair in vascular smooth muscle cells. Mutat Res 2000; 454(1–2):35–44.
299. Ramos KS, Zhang Y, Sadhu DN, et al. The induction of proliferative vascular smooth muscle cell phenotypes by benzo(a)pyrene is characterized by up-regulation of inositol phospholipid metabolism and *c-Ha-ras* gene expression. Arch Biochem Biophys 1996; 332:213–222.

300. Miller KP, Ramos KS. Impact of cellular metabolism on the biological effects of benzo(a)pyrene and related hydrocarbons. Drug Metab Rev 2001; 33(1):1–35.

301. Juchau MR, Bond JA, Benditt EP. Aryl 4-monooxygenase and cytochrome P-450 in the aorta: possible role in atherosclerosis. Proc Natl Acad Sci U.S.A. 1976; 73(10): 3723–3725.

302. Serabjit SCJ, Bend JR, Philpot RM. Cytochrome P-450 Monooxygenase system localization in smooth muscle of rabbit aorta. Mol Pharmacol 1985; 28:72–79.

303. Pinto A, Abraham NG, Mullane KM. Cytochrome P-450-dependent mono-oxygenase activity and endothelial-dependent relaxations induced by arachidonic acid. J Pharmacol Exp Ther 1986; 236:445–451.

304. Baird WM, Chemerys R, Grinspan JB, et al. Benzo(a)pyrene metabolism in bovine aortic endothelial and bovine lung fibroblast-like cell cultures. Cancer Res 1980; 40:1781–1786.

305. Majesky M, Yang HY, Benditt E, et al. Carcinogenesis and atherogenesis: differences in mono-oxygenase inducibility and bioactivation of benzo(a)pyrene in aortic and hepatic tissue of atherosclerosis-susceptible versus resistant pigeons. Carcinogenesis 1983; 4:647–652.

306. Moorthy B, Miller KP, Jiang W, et al. The atherogen 3-methylcholanthrene induces multiple DNA adducts in mouse aortic smooth muscle cells: role of cytochrome P4501B1. Cardiovasc Res 2002; 53(4):1002–1009.

307. Kerzee JK, Ramos KS. Constitutive and inducible expression of CYP1A1 and CYP1B1 in vascular smooth muscle cells: role of the AhR bHLH/PAS transcription factor. Circ Res 2001; 89(7):573–582.

308. Denko NC, Giaccia A, Stringer JR, et al. The human Ha-ras oncogene induces genomic instability in murine fibroblasts within one cell cycle. Proc Natl Acad Sci U.S.A. 1994; 91:5124–5128.

309. Yang HYL, Namkung MJ, Nelson WL, et al. Phase II Biotransformation of carcinogens/atherogens in cultured aortic tissues and cells: I. Sulfation of 3-Hydroxy-benzo(a)pyrene. Drug Metab Dispos 1986; 14:287–298.

310. Yang HYL, Majesky MW, Namkung MJ, et al. Phase II Biotransformation of carcinogens/atherogens in cultured aortic tissues and cells. II. Glucoronidation of 3-hydroxy-benzo(a)pyrene. Drug Metabolism and Disposition 1986; 14:293–298.

311. Owens IS, Koteen GM., Pelkonen O, et al. Activation of certain benzo(a)pyrene phenols and the effect of some conjugating enzyme activities. In: Aito A, ed. Conjugation Reactions in Biotransformation. Amsterdam, the Netherlands: Elsevier Biomedical, 1978:39.

312. Nemoto N, Kawana M, Tokoyama S. Effects of activation of UDP-glycuronyl transferase on metabolism of benzo(a)pyrene with rat liver microsomes. J Pharmacoio-yn 1983; 6:105–113.

313. Penn A, Snyder C. Arteriosclerotic plaque development is 'promoted' by poly-nuclear aromatic hydrocarbons. Carcinogenesis 1988; 9:2185–2189.

314. Majesky MW, Reidy MA, Benditt EP, et al. Focal smooth muscle proliferation in the aortic intima produced by an initiation-promotion sequence. Proc Natl Acad Sci U.S.A. 1985; 82:3450–3454.

315. Paigen B, Havens MB, Morrow A. Effect of 3-methylcholanthrene on the development of aortic lesions in mice. Cancer Res 1985; 45:3850–3855.

316. Zhang Y, Ramos KS. The induction of proliferative vascular smooth muscle cell phenotypes by benzo(a)pyrene does not involve mutational activation of ras genes. Mutat Res 1997; 373(2):285–292.

317. Revis NW, Bull R, Laurie D, et al. The effectiveness of chemical carcinogens to induce atherosclerosis in the white carneau pigeon. Toxicology 1984; 32: 215–227.

318. Paigen B, Holmes P, Morrow A, et al. Effects of 3-methylcholanthrene on atherosclerosis in two congenic strains of mice with different susceptibilities to methylcholanthrene-induced tumors. Cancer Res 1986; 46:3321–3324.

319. Kerzee JK, Ramos KS. Activation of c-Ha-ras by benzo(a)pyrene in vascular smooth muscle cells involves redox stress and aryl hydrocarbon receptor. Mol Pharmacol 2000; 58(1):152–158.

320. Sadhu DN, Ramos KS. Modulation by retinoic acid of spontaneous and benzo[a] pyrene-induced *c-Ha-ras* expression. Basic Life Sci 1993; 61:263–268.

321. Bral CM, Ramos KS. Identification of benzo(a)pyrene-inducible *cis*-acting elements within *c-Ha-ras* transcriptional regulatory sequences. Mol Pharmacol 1997; 52: 974–982.

322. Miller KP, Chen YH, Hastings VL, et al. Profiles of antioxidant/electrophile response element (ARE/EpRE) nuclear protein binding and c-Ha-ras transactivation in vascular smooth muscle cells treated with oxidative metabolites of benzo(a) pyrene. Biochem Pharmacol 2001; 60(9):1285–1296.

323. Ou X, Ramos KS. Modulation of aortic protein phosphorylation by benzo(a)pyrene: implications in PAH-induced atherogenesis. J Biochem Toxicoly 1992; 7:147–154.

324. Ou X, Weber TJ, Chapkin RS., et al. Interference with protein kinase C-related signal transduction in vascular smooth muscle cells by benzo(a)pyrene. Arch Biochem Biophys 1995; 318:122–130.

325. Schiefer HB, Rousseaux CG, Hancock DS, et al. Effects of low-level long-term oral exposure to T-2 toxin in CD-1 mice. Food Chemi Toxicol 1987; 25:593–601.

326. Feuerstein G, Goldstein DS, Ramwell RO, et al. Cardiorespiratory, sympathetic and biochemical responses to T-2 toxin in the guinea pig and rat. J Pharmacol Exp Ther 1985; 232:786–794.

327. Wilson CA, Everard DM, Schoental R. Blood pressure changes and cardiovascular lesions found in rats given T-2 toxin, a trichothecene secondary metabolite of certain Fusarium microfungi. Toxicol Lett 1982; 10:35–40.

328. Siren AL, Feuerstein G. Effect of T-2 toxin on regional blood flow and vascular resistance in the conscious rat. Toxicol Appl Pharmacol 1986; 83:438–444.

329. Yarom R, More R, Sherman Y, et al. T-2 toxin-induced pathology in the hearts of rats. Br J Exp Pathol 1983; 64:570–577.

330. Schoenthal R, Jaffe AZ, Yagen B. Cardiovascular lesions and various tumors found in rats given T-2 toxin, a trichothecene metabolite of Fusarium. Cancer Res 1979; 39:2179–2189.

331. Ueno Y. Trichothecenes: an overview. In: Rodrickes JV, Hesseltine CW, Mehlmann MA, eds. Mycotoxins in Human and Animal Health. Park forest, Illinois: Pathotox Pub, 1977; 189–207.

332. Cannon M, Smith KE, Carter CJ. Prevention, by ribosome-bound nascent polyphenylalanine chains, of the functional interaction of T-2 with its receptor site. Biochem J 1976; 156:289–294.

333. Yarom R, Sherman Y, Bergmann F, et al. T-2 toxin effect on rat aorta: cellular changes *in vivo* and growth of smooth muscle cells *in vitro*. Exp Mol Pathol 1987; 47:143–153.
334. Peplonska B, Szeszenia-Dabrowska N, Sobala W, et al. A mortality study of workers with reported chronic occupational carbon disulfide poisoning. Int J Occup Med Environ Health 1996; 9:291–299.
335. Sulsky SI, Hooven FH, Burch MT, et al. Critical review of the epidemiological literature on the potential cardiovascular effects of occupational carbon disulfide exposure. Int Arch Occup Environ Health 2002; 75(6):365–380.
336. Takebayashi T, Nishiwaki Y, Uemura T, et al. A six year follow up study of the subclinical effects of carbon disulfide exposure on the cardiovascular system. Occup Environ Med 2004; 61(2):127–134.
337. Korinth G, Goen T, Ulm K, et al. Cardiovascular function of workers exposed to carbon disulphide. Int Arch Occup Environ Health 2003; 76(1):81–85.
338. Tan X, Peng X, Wang F, et al. Cardiovascular effects of carbon disulfide: meta-analysis of cohort studies. Int J Hyg Environ Health 2002; 205(6):473–477.
339. Kurppa K, Hietanen E, Klockars M, et al. Chemical exposures at work and cardiovascular morbidity: Atherosclerosis, ischemic heart disease, hypertension, cardiomyopathy and arrhythmias. Scand J Work Environ Health 1984; 10:381–388.
340. Kotseva KP, De Bacquer D. Cardiovascular effects of occupational exposure to carbon disulfide. J Occup Med 2000; 50(1):43–47.
341. Wronska-Nofer T, Chojnowska-Jezierska J, Nofer JR, et al. Increased oxidative stress in subjects exposed to carbon disulfide (CS2)—an occupational coronary risk factor. Arch Toxicol 2002; 76(3):152–157.
342. Cox C, Que Hee SS, Lynch DW. Urinary 2-thiothiazolidine-4-carboxylic acid (TTCA) as the major urinary marker of carbon disulfide vapor exposure in rats. Toxicol Indust Health 1996; 12:81–92.
343. Huff JE, Melnick RL, Solleveld HA, et al. Multiple organ carcinogenicity of 1,3-butadiene in B6C3F$_1$ mice after 60 weeks of inhalation exposure. Science 1984; 227:548–549.
344. Miller RA, Boorman GA. Morphology of neoplastic lesions induced by 1,3-butadiene in B6C3F1 mice. Environ Health Perspect 1990; 86:37–48.
345. Matanoski GM, Santos-Burgoa C, Schwartz L. Mortality of a cohort of workers in the styreme-butadiene polymer manufacturing industry (1943–1982). Environ Health Perspect 1990; 86:107–117.
346. Divine BJ. An update on mortality among workers at a 1,3-butadiene facility—preliminary results. Environ Health Perspect 1990; 86:119–128.
347. Penn A, Snyder CA. 1,3 Butadiene, a vapor phase component of environmental tobacco smoke, accelerates arteriosclerotic plaque development. Circulation 1996; 93:552–557.
348. Penn A, Snyder CA. 1,3-Butadiene exposure and cardiovascular disease. Mutat Res, 2007; 621(1–2):42–49.
349. Lovati MR, Galbussera M, Franceschini G, et al. Increased plasma and aortic triglycerides in rabbits after acute administration of 2,3,7,8-tetrachlorodibenzo-p-dioxin. Toxicol Appl Pharmacol 1984; 75:91–97.
350. Walker AE, Martin JV. Lipid profiles in dioxin-exposed workers. Lancet 1979; 1:446–447.

351. Swift LL, Gasiewicz TA, Dunn GD, et al. Characterization of the hyperlipidemia in guinea pigs induced by 2,3,7,8-tetrachlorodi-benzo-p-dioxin. Toxicol Appl Pharmacol 1981; 59:489–499.

352. Weber TJ, Ou X, Narasimham T R, et al. Modulation of protein phosphorylation in rat aortic smooth muscle cells by 2,3,7,8 tetrachlorodibenzo-p-dioxin (TCDD). Toxicologist 1991; 11:340.

353. Weber TJ, Chapkin RS, Davidson LA, et al. Modulation of protein kinase C-related signal transduction by 2,3,7,8-tetrachlorodibenzo-p-dioxin exhibits cell cycle dependence. Arch Biochem Biophys 1996; 328:227–232.

354. Goldstone HM, Stegeman JJ. Molecular mechanisms of 2,3,7,8-tetrachlorodibenzo-p-dioxin cardiovascular embryotoxicity. Drug Metab Rev 2006; 38(1–2):261–289.

355. Dalton TP, Dieter MZ, Miller M, et al. TCDD increases the production of vasoactive eicosanoids and cofractionates with lipoprotein particles in hyperlipidemic mice. Toxicologist 1999; 48:219.

356. Dalton TP, Kerzee JK, Wang B, et al. Dioxin exposure is an environmental risk factor for ischemic heart disease. Cardiovasc Toxicol 1(4):285–298.

357. Jokinen MP, Walker NJ, Brix AE, et al. Increase in cardiovascular pathology in female Sprague-Dawley rats following chronic treatment with 2,3,7,8-tetrachlorodibenzo-p-dioxin and 3,3',4,4',5-pentachlorobiphenyl. Cardiovasc Toxicol 2003; 3(4):299–310.

358. Toda T, Ito M, Toda Y, et al. Angiotoxicity in swine of a moderate excess of dietary vitamin D3. Food Chem Toxicol 1985; 23(6):585–592.

359. Koh E, Morimoto S, Fukuo K, et al. 1,25-dihydroxyvitamin D_3 binds specifically to rat vascular smooth muscle cells and stimulates their proliferation *in vitro*. Life Sci 1988; 42:215–223.

360. Tang FT, Chen SR, Wu XQ, et al. Hypercholesterolemia accelerates vascular calcification induced by excessive vitamin D via oxidative stress. Calcif Tissue Int 2006; 79(5):326–339.

361. Targher G, Bertolini L, Padovani R, et al. Serum 25-hydroxyvitamin D_3 concentrations and carotid artery intima-media thickness among type 2 diabetic patients. Clin Endocrinol (Oxf) 2006; 65(5):593–597.

362. Murad F. Cyclic guanosine monophosphate as a mediator of vasodilation. J Clin Invest 1986; 78:1–5.

363. Westwood FR, Iswaran TJ, Greaves P. Pathologic changes in blood vessels following administration of an inotropic vasodilator (ICI 153,110) to the rat. Fundam Appl Toxicol 1990; 14(4):797–809.

364. Collins JJ, Elwell MR, Lamb JC, et al. Subchronic toxicity of orally administered (gavage and dosed-fed) theophylline in Fischer 344 rats and B6C3F$_1$ mice. Fundam Appl Toxicol 1988; 11:472–484.

365. Sandusky GE, Vodicnik MJ, Tamura RN. Cardiovascular and adrenal proliferative lesions in Fischer 344 rats induced by long-term treatment with type III phosphodiesterase inhibitors (Positive inotropic agents), isomazole and indolidan. Fundam Appl Toxicol 1991; 16:198–209.

366. Rebsamen MC, Sun J, Norman A, et al. 1alpha,25-hydroxyvitamin D_3 induces vascular smooth muscle cell migration via activation of phosphatidylinositol 3-kinase. Circ Res 2002; 91(1):17–24.

367. Inoue T, Kawashima H. 1,25-Dihydroxyvitamin D3 stimulates 45Ca2+ uptake by cultured vascular smooth muscle cells derived from rat aorta. Biochem Biophys Res Commun 1988; 152(3):1388–1394.
368. Mitsuhashi T, Morris RC, Ives HE. 1,25-dihydroxyvitamin D3 modulates growth of vascular smooth muscle cells. J Clin Invest 1991; 87(6):1889–1895.
369. Parhami F, Morrow AD, Balucan J, et al. Lipid oxidation products have opposite effects on calcifying vascular cell and bone cell differentiation. A possible explanation for the paradox of arterial calcification in osteoporotic patients. Arteriosclerosis, Thrombosis, and Vascular Biology 1997; 17(4):680–687.
370. Mody N, Parhami FSarafian TA, et al. Oxidative stress modulates osteoblastic differentiation of vascular and bone cells. Free Radic Biol Med 2001; 31(4): 509–519.
371. Naseem SM, Heald FP. Cytotoxicity of cholesterol oxides and their effects on cholesterol metabolism in cultured human aortic smooth muscle cells. Biochem Int 1987; 14(1):71–84.
372. Hayaishi O. Enzyme hydroxylation. Annu Rev Biochem 1969; 38:21–44.
373. Ross R. Atherosclerosis—an inflammatory disease. New Engl J Med 1999; 340(2): 115–126.
374. Belland RJ, Ouellette SP, Gieffers J, et al. Chlamydia pneumoniae and atherosclerosis. Cell Microbiol 2004; 6(2):117–127.
375. Campbell LA, Kuo CC. Chlamydia penumoniae—an infectious risk factor for atherosclerosis. Nat Rev Microbiol 2004; 2(1):23–32.
376. Fong IW. Infections and their role in atherosclerotic vascular disease. J Am Den Assoc 2002; 133:7S–13S.
377. Mendall MA, Goggin PM, Molineaux N, et al. Relation of Helicobacter pylori infection and coronary heart disease. Br Heart J 1994; 71:437–439.
378. Valtonen VV. Infection as a risk factor for infarction and atherosclerosis. Ann Med 1991; 23:539–543.
379. Fong IW. Emerging relations between infectious diseases and coronary artery disease and atherosclerosis. Can Med Assoc J 2000; 163(1):49–56.
380. Levy J, Blakeston C, Seymour CA, et al. Association of Helicobacter pylori and Chlamydia pneumoniae infections with coronary heart disease and cardiovascular risk factors. Br Med J 1995; 311:711–714.
381. Kalayoglu MV, Byrne GI. A Chlamydia pneumoniae component that induces macrophage foam cell formation is chlamydial lipopolysaccharide. Infect Immun 1998; 66:5067–5072.
382. Kalayoglu MV, Byrne GI. Induction of macrophage foam cell formation by Chlamydia pneumoniae. J Infect Dis 1998; 177:725–729.
383. Muhlestein JB. Bacterial infections and atherosclerosis. J Invest Med 1998; 46: 396–402.
384. Xu Q, Kleindienst R, Schett G, et al. Regression of arteriosclerotic lesions induced by immunization with heat shock protein 65-containing material in normocholesterolemic, but not hypercholesterolemic, rabbits. Atherosclerosis 1996; 123:145–155.
385. Birnie DH, Holme ERMcKay IC, et al. Association between antibodies to heat shock protein 65 and coronary atherosclerosis. Possible mechanism of action of Helicobacter pylori and other bacterial infections in increasing cardiovascular risk. Eur Heart J 1998; 19:387–394.

386. Xiao Q, Mandal K, Schett G, et al. Association of serum-soluble heat shock protein 60 with carotid atherosclerosis: clinical significance determined in a follow-up study. Stroke 2005; 36(12):2571–2576.
387. de Graaf R, Kloppenberg G, Kitslaar PJ, et al. Human heat shock protein 60 stimulates vascular smooth muscle cell proliferation through Toll-like receptors 2 and 4. Microbes Infect 2006; 8(7):1859–1865.
388. Kol A, Sukhova GK, Lichtman AH, et al. Chlamydial heat shock protein 60 localizes in human atheroma and regulates macrophage tumor necrosis factor-alpha and matrix metalloproteinase expression. Circulation 1998; 98:300–307.
389. Hirono S, Dibrov E, Hurtado C, et al. Chlamydia pneumoniae stimulates proliferation of vascular smooth muscle cells through induction of endogenous heat shock protein 60. Circ Res 2003; 93(8):710–716.
390. Murray LJ, Bamford KB, O'Reilly DP, et al. Helicobacter pylori infection: relation with cardiovascular risk factors, ischemic heart disease, and social class. Br Heart J 1995; 74:497–501.
391. Blasi F, Ranzi ML, Erba M, et al. No evidence for the presence of Helicobacter pylori in atherosclerotic plaques in abdominal aortic aneurysm specimens. Atherosclerosis 1996; 126(2):339–340.
392. Regnstrom J, Jovinge S, Bavenholm P, et al. Helicobacter pylori seropositivity is not associated with inflammatory parameters, lipid concentrations and degree of coronary artery disease. J Intern Med 1998; 243:109–113.
393. Markus HS, Mendall MA. Helicobacter pylori infection: a risk factor for ischemic cerebrovascular disease and carotid atheroma. J Neurol Neurosurg Psychiatr 1998; 64:104–107.
394. Folsom AR, Nieto FJ, Sorlie P, et al. Helicobacter pylori seropositivity and coronary heart disease incidence. Atherosclerosis Risk In Communities (ARIC) Study Investigators. Circulation 1998; 98:845–850.
395. Pasceri V, Cammarota G, Patti G, et al. Association of virulent Helicobacter pylori strains with ischemic heart disease. Circulation 1998; 97:1675–1679.
396. Markle HV. Coronary artery disease associated with Helicobacter pylori infection is at least partially due to inadequate folate status. Med Hypotheses 1997; 49:289–292.
397. Danesh J, Collins R, Peto R. Chronic infections and coronary heart disease: is there a link? Lancet 1997; 350(9075):430–436.

15

Pathobiology of the Vascular Response to Percutaneous Coronary Intervention and Drug-Eluting Stents

Brigitta C. Brott

Interventional Cardiology, University of Alabama at Birmingham, Birmingham, Alabama, U.S.A.

Zadok Ruben

Patoximed Consultants, Westfield, New Jersey, U.S.A.

Peter G. Anderson

Department of Pathology, University of Alabama at Birmingham, Birmingham, Alabama, U.S.A.

INTRODUCTION

In humans cardiovascular diseases, primarily atherosclerosis and hypertension, are the leading causes of morbidity and mortality in developed countries around the world, with estimates of almost 80 million American adults currently suffering from one or more types of cardiovascular disease (1). The response of the vasculature to lipids, inflammatory mediators, xenobiotics, infectious agents, and mechanical injury all importantly contribute to vascular function and dysfunction. The vulnerability of blood vessels to injury by numerous chemicals and drugs is well recognized and has previously been reviewed (2–5). The impact that these influences have on health and disease and on biomedical research aimed at investigating these health problems makes the understanding of the vascular response to injury of paramount clinical significance. Recent advances in vascular pathobiology have elucidated unique signaling and regulatory mechanisms that enable blood vessels to respond to and adapt to a variety of stresses and insults. The purpose of this chapter is to review the general mechanisms by which blood vessels respond to mechanical insults induced by percutaneous coronary interventions (PCI) and to explore the rationale behind stent engineering and the use of drug-eluting stents to impact the restenosis process.

REGULATION OF NORMAL VASCULAR STRUCTURE AND FUNCTION

The structural components that make up blood vessels vary according to the type and caliber of the vessel. Blood vessels are composed of an endothelial layer, a medial layer comprising primarily smooth muscle cells, and a fibrous connective tissue layer that makes up the adventitia. The endothelial cell layer serves as the interface between blood and tissues and plays a critical role in regulating blood flow, body fluids, and bidirectional traffic of humoral factors and cells. In the mid-19th century, Virchow referred to the vascular endothelium as "a membrane as simple as any that is ever met within the body" (6). Today, the endothelial cell is regarded as a complex, active regulator of vascular integrity. Endothelium regulates plasma-interstitial fluid exchange and intimal lipids, maintains a non-thrombogenic surface, produces mitogenic factors, and is a crucial element in the inflammatory response. The endothelial cell has also been shown to directly modulate the adjacent smooth muscle cells by secreting nitric oxide (NO$^{\bullet}$) (7–10).

In most blood vessels, the endothelial cells overlay an internal elastic lamina. This elastic lamina is produced by smooth muscle cells (11,12) and contains focal adhesion sites where filaments anchor endothelial cells to the subjacent elastic lamina (13). The elastic lamina is porous and contains ovoid fenestrations of varying diameters, which allow for vessel constriction and dilation and through which molecules can transit across the vessel barrier (14,15). The smooth muscle cells within the media function to maintain vascular tone. Smooth muscle cells normally have a "contractile phenotype" where the cells contain abundant myofilaments and are primarily suited for contraction. After vessel injury or when placed in culture, smooth muscle cells can modulate to a "synthetic phenotype" where the cells lose their myofilaments and contain abundant rough endoplasmic reticulum (16). This capacity to modulate from contractile to synthetic phenotype has a significant impact on how vessels respond to injury and is an important area of ongoing investigation (17,18).

The tunica adventitia has recently received considerable investigation because of its role in the remodeling that occurs after mechanical vascular intervention (19,20). The adventitia is also involved in vascular adaptation to pressure loads with significant thickening and fibrosis evident in models of increased intravascular pressure (21,22). The vasa vasorum, which enters the vessel via the adventitia and supplies circulation to the outer two-thirds of the vascular wall, is also known to play an important role in vascular structure and function. One primary example of vasa vasorum alterations leading to significant pathology is in the case of syphilitic aortitis. Syphilis can cause endarteritis obliterans of the vasa vasorum characterized by perivascular plasma cell and lymphocyte cuffing. This damage to the vasa vasorum leads to degeneration of the thoracic aorta and can result in ectasia and or rupture of that aorta (23). Additional studies have demonstrated the importance of the vasa vasorum in the pathogenesis of atherosclerosis and atherosclerotic plaque stability (24).

The discovery of NO• as the "endothelial-derived relaxing factor" greatly enhanced our understanding of the signaling pathways and the control mechanisms responsible for regulating cardiovascular function (25). The role of NO• in both the regulation of normal vascular function and as a major player in many pathologic states has generated extensive interest and investigation. The signaling pathways by which NO• affects cell function are protean, and these affects are due in part to the high affinity of NO• for heme-containing enzymes. Perhaps the most important intracellular signaling role for NO• is its capacity to activate guanylate cyclase, which leads to rapid and robust increases in cyclic GMP (cGMP) levels in target cells. The increased cGMP levels and subsequent cGMP-dependent phosphorylation of proteins appears to be involved in intracellular calcium sequestration or removal, which results in smooth muscle cell relaxation and reduction in vascular tone (18,26,27).

PATHOLOGY OF VASCULAR INTERVENTIONS

Direct mechanical injury to vessels elicits a wound-healing response similar to the response observed after any injury. The clinical importance of understanding this wound healing process is vital for patient care. The challenge for investigators interested in vascular biology is to identify the mechanisms involved in vascular repair and remodeling to impact the problem of restenosis.

PCI has become a frequently used clinically effective method for the revascularization of stenosed or occluded native arteries and vein grafts. However, the problem of restenosis continues to importantly impact the clinical utility of this procedure. Data from retrospective and prospective studies of angioplasty, atherectomy, laser ablation, and endovascular stenting demonstrate that with all of these interventional techniques the restenosis rate ranges from 25% to 40% (28–30). Even with the advent of drug-eluting stents, the restenosis rate varies from approximately 8% to 35% depending on patient and lesion characteristics (31). Thus, any revascularization technique that necessarily involves some degree of trauma to the vessel, may lead to restenosis in a certain cohort of patients. The specific factors that may lead to restenosis have not been well defined. The underlying basis for restenosis involves some form of vascular trauma with injury to endothelial and/or smooth muscle cells. Clinical and experimental studies have also shown that restenosis may result from other injurious procedures such as electrical stimulation, freezing, alcohol perfusion, crush injury, or physical injury produced by placement of a constricting band around the outside of the vessel (32–34). The trophic factors, either blood born or locally produced and/or released during these interventions, which result in active growth and phenotypic conversion of the smooth muscle cells with exuberant extracellular matrix production after vascular injury have been extensively studied with no clear consensus as to the specific factors responsible for restenosis (28,35–39). It is clear that restenosis is a complex pathophysiologic process, and the unraveling of the specific factors leading to restenosis will require precise experimental design and appropriate model systems. Various in vitro and in vivo model systems have been used to study restenosis and to investigate methods for preventing restenosis. Intravascular irradiation after vessel injury (brachytherapy) was initially thought to be an effective way to reduce the risk of repeated in-stent restenosis. However, concerns have been raised regarding a late catch-up in restenosis rates, reducing its long-term benefits compared with angioplasty for in-stent restenosis (40,41). More recent comparisons between radiation therapy and drug-eluting stents for the treatment of in-stent restenosis demonstrate that drug-eluting stents provide superior clinical outcomes (42,43). To date, the Food and Drug Administration (FDA) has approved three drug-eluting stents with somewhat different mechanisms of action. That both paclitaxel and sirolimus inhibit but do not prevent restenosis indicate that renarrowing after arterial injury is a complex process (37), the exact etiology of which continues to elude investigators. Results from these studies have elucidated many mechanisms involved in the restenosis process; however, there are some discrepancies in the efficacy of treatment protocols when comparative studies are performed on different animal species, including humans. Thus, there appear to be significant species differences in response to vascular injury that must be considered when performing and evaluating studies of restenosis (44–46).

MECHANICAL VASCULAR INJURY: EXPERIMENTAL MODELS AND STUDY PARADIGMS

The choice of model systems for studies of vascular biology and specifically studies of restenosis require clear identification of the experimental endpoint. It must be acknowledged from the outset that all model systems have limitations and that these experimental systems are just models of a process that occurs in humans. Thus, no experimental system can completely and accurately recapitulate the restenosis phenomena seen in an atherosclerotic coronary artery of human patients. However, it is possible, by careful experimental design, to answer specific questions related to the phenomena of restenosis using in vitro systems or animal models (47).

In vitro systems can be very precisely controlled, and specific factors or processes can be isolated and studied (48–52). If a specific hypothesis is to be tested, in vitro systems can be manipulated in such a way that only one variable is examined. These studies are useful in studies of the cell and molecular biology of endothelial cells or smooth muscle cells. Although beneficial in basic scientific investigation, in vitro studies cannot be used to mimic or recapitulate the restenosis process in vivo. The procedures used to isolate smooth muscle cells or endothelial cells and the techniques used to maintain them in culture are far removed from the milieu of an atherosclerotic coronary artery in a patient. Also, with in vitro techniques it is impossible to maintain the interaction that occurs between the various cell types and the blood-borne factors that impact the restenosis process in vivo. Studies of smooth muscle cells in culture demonstrate that after passage and after transition from the contractile to the secretary phenotype, key regulatory signaling pathways are altered or lost (53–55). These findings suggest that using cultured or passaged smooth muscle cells in studies of the vascular response to injury may be problematic. Thus, data from in vitro studies should be used to evaluate specific mechanisms of the cell and molecular biology of endothelial cell and smooth muscle cells, not to make definitive conclusions about the restenosis process in vivo.

Animal models are by far the most popular method for investigating restenosis. Investigators have used various animal species, different arteries or veins, and numerous types of interventions to induce restenosis. These model systems fall into three basic categories. In one group, models are designed to produce a very reproducible neointimal reaction that can be easily quantitated. Examples of this type of model system include the rat aortic or carotid artery balloon injury model and rabbit models of femoral or iliac artery injury. In these systems, the degree of restenosis is predictable and uniform. Thus, experiments designed to modify neointimal growth can be easily tested in these models. The second type of model system often uses coronary arteries in larger animals with artery sizes similar to humans. These model systems also endeavor to produce a consistent neointimal proliferative reaction; however, the reproducibility and ease of performing these experiments may be somewhat compromised to obtain the benefits of using a larger animal model. In these models, injury is produced in normal arteries, and the response to that injury is evaluated. Examples of models in this group include rabbit or pig coronary and carotid arteries. These models will be discussed in detail below. The third type of model system used to study restenosis attempts to recapitulate the conditions seen in human atherosclerotic coronary arteries. These systems use artery injury and atherosclerotic diets to induce atherosclerotic lesions in arteries. After development of atherosclerotic lesions, mechanical interventions are performed (e.g., angioplasty, stents, atherectomy), and the response of the diseased artery to this intervention is evaluated. These types of model systems are good for testing new equipment or new techniques. These models are also useful for evaluating the response of the diseased artery to these insults and the ability of therapeutic techniques to diminish the restenosis phenomena. Unfortunately, the complexity of these model systems makes it very difficult to obtain reproducible injury or reproducible restenosis; thus, statistical evaluation of the efficacy of therapeutic techniques is very difficult. In essence, trying to recapitulate human atherosclerosis makes these models so complex that these experiments have many of the same problems as human trials, i.e., large variability and large numbers of subjects needed to reach statistically significant endpoints. Examples of these types of animal models are femoral or iliac artery injury plus atherosclerotic diet in rabbits, injury plus atherosclerotic diet in minipigs, and atherosclerosis in nonhuman primates. These models have distinct advantages and disadvantages that will be discussed below.

The primary factor to be considered when choosing animal models of restenosis is the endpoint for the experiment. Each animal model has strengths and weaknesses that must be factored into the study plan. Each animal species has a slightly different anatomy and physiology, and these differences may or may not impact the experimental results when compared with humans. Thus, the model system should be carefully evaluated, and pilot studies should be performed prior to undertaking a large study.

Animal Models in the Study of Vascular Interventions

Numerous animal models are currently being used to investigate the pathogenesis of restenosis. This review will briefly discuss some of the more commonly used models and will describe the pros and cons of each model system.

Rodents

Rats are by far the most commonly used rodent model of restenosis; however, the use of transgenic mice has increased steadily. Transgenic mice have the benefit of allowing the investigator to modify specific genes and thus tailor-make the milieu of the restenosis process. Using these techniques, it is possible to directly investigate the role of specific factors in the restenosis process. Mouse models of atherosclerosis also increase the utility of this model system for studies of vascular response to mechanical injury, such as wire denudation of the femoral artery and more recently a model of balloon angioplasty and stenting (56–58). Use of specific mouse stains, transgenic or knockout mice, and special diets make it possible to induce the development of atherosclerotic lesions (Fig. 1) (59,60). The topographical locations of the lesions and the character of the atherosclerotic lesions in mice are quite variable depending on strain, diet, and which genes are knocked out. However, as seen in Figure 1, there are intimal cholesterol deposits and a fibrous cap overlying these lesions. These model systems have been used extensively to study pathogenic mechanisms of atherosclerosis and are powerful tools for studying this important disease process. Studies of restenosis in transgenic mice and knockout mice have been relatively few, and the procedures used to induce mechanical injury are technically demanding; but, the utility and power of this model system suggests that these model systems will evolve and become important additions to our experimental armamentarium.

Rats have the advantage that they are relatively inexpensive to procure and maintain. They are also amenable to a variety of experimental manipulations,

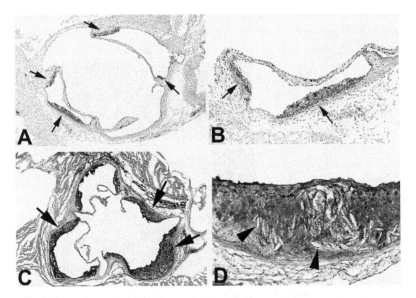

Figure 1 Atherosclerosis in mice. (**A** and **B**) Sections from the aortic root of an atherosclerosis-prone mouse strain fed a high-cholesterol diet. Note the lesions (*arrows*) are rather modest and are primarily restricted to the aortic root. (**C** and **D**) Similar sections from an ApoE knockout mouse demonstrating more sever lesions (*arrows*) with extensive cholesterol deposits within the lesions (*arrowheads*).

and large numbers of animals can be used for complex experimental protocols. One disadvantage of rodents as models of restenosis is the small size of the arteries that are used. Also, the most commonly used vessels, the aorta and carotid arteries, are elastic arteries as opposed to muscular arteries, and at least in the carotid artery, there is no vasa vasorum (61). In addition, rats are relatively resistant to atherosclerosis, and although atherosclerosis can be induced in certain strains of rats (62,63), there are no good models of atherosclerosis currently available in the rat. Despite these caveats, the rat is a very utilitarian model for studies of restenosis since they develop a very reproducible, rapid neointimal proliferative reaction.

Much of what we currently know about smooth muscle cell biology after vascular injury has been determined from studies using the rat carotid balloon injury model (64–68). In this model, a deflated Fogarty balloon or a small angioplasty balloon (39) is inserted into the carotid artery, the balloon is inflated and gently removed from the artery. This process results in dilation of the vessel wall and mechanical denudation of endothelial cells as the balloon is removed. The sequence of events after balloon injury, as initially described by Fishman et al. (64) and expounded by others (66–68), includes platelet adhesion and smooth muscle cell proliferation to form a neointima composed of almost 100% smooth muscle cells (Fig. 2). The initial sequences of platelet adhesion and degranulation result in thrombus formation and the release of numerous growth factors. If

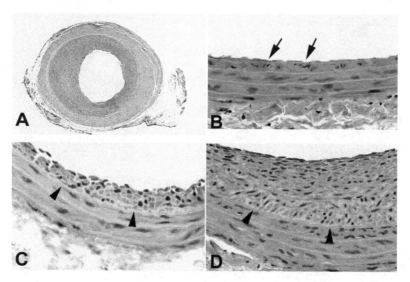

Figure 2 Balloon injury model in the rat carotid artery. (**A**) Low-power photomicrograph demonstrating the concentric neointimal response with preservation of the media in this rat carotid artery three weeks after balloon injury. (**B**) High-power view of carotid artery wall 24 hours after balloon injury. Note the absence of endothelial cells and the multiple breaks in the internal elastic membrane. There is also nuclear fragmentation in smooth muscle cells along the outermost layer of the vessel. (**C**) High-power view of carotid artery wall four days after balloon injury. Note the early formation of a neointima on the lumenal side of the internal elastic membrane (*arrowheads*). (**D**) At three weeks after balloon injury the neointima is well formed and has increased in thickness. Some of the smooth muscle cells have begun to develop a fusiform shape and line up circumferentially perpendicular to the direction of blood flow. Although difficult to appreciate at this magnification, the lumenal surface of the neointima is covered with endothelial cells. The arrowheads outline the internal elastic membrane.

rats are made thrombocytopenic by injection of antiplatelet antibodies, the neointimal response is abrogated (69). Medial injury by stretch and mechanical trauma also importantly impact on the neointimal proliferative response. Studies have demonstrated a significant loss of medial smooth muscle cells after balloon injury in this model. This has led many investigators to suggest that growth factors are released by the injured smooth muscle cells. In studies where the media was stretched by infusion of saline into the vessel lumen under pressure, resulting in little or no endothelial cell injury, the smooth muscle cell proliferation still occurred. These data support the contention that medial injury per se also induces the neointimal proliferative response. Additional studies have further characterized the pathogenesis of restenosis after balloon injury in the rat. At 24 to 72 hours after balloon injury, smooth muscle cells begin to divide and migrate from the media into the intima (70). Approximately 50% of the cells that migrate into the intima do not divide; rather they change to the secretory phenotype (loss of myofilaments) and increase rough endoplasmic reticulum (16,71,72) and begin to produce extracellular matrix material. The cell division in the neointima continued for up to eight weeks after injury in areas that were reendothelialized and cell division in the neointima continued up to 12 weeks in areas where endothelial cells did not regrow. In the balloon injury model, the central portion of the denuded artery segment may never reendothelialize (70), and the damage to the vessel wall limits pulsatile flow. It is evident that endothelial cell denudation plays a critical role in restenosis even without concurrent injury to the media. If a small region of the artery is denuded with a fine nylon thread that does not injure the underlying media, endothelial cells quickly grow over the denuded region and the proliferative process is greatly diminished (66,73). Addition studies have also demonstrated that adventitial myofibroblasts also play a role in the restenosis process in the rat (74–76). These findings are consistent with observations in other animal models and in humans, which suggest that cells other than medial smooth muscle cells are involved in the vessel injury/restenosis process.

With the rat carotid artery balloon injury model, the neointimal proliferation is very reproducible and accurate quantitation can be used to characterize the restenosis phenomenon. There are no breaks in the internal elastic membrane, thus the neointima is easily measured by morphometric techniques. This well-characterized model system, using animals that are relatively inexpensive and easy to handle, can be used to study specific pathogenic mechanisms in the restenosis process. This model system does have several caveats. First, the arteries are normal prior to the experimental manipulation. This is very different from what is seen in atherosclerotic human coronary arteries that undergo angioplasty or other interventions. A more disturbing finding has been that many of the treatments that have been successful in preventing restenosis in the rat model have not been successful in large animal species and in humans (77). Thus, there appear to be differences between rats and larger species that make it difficult to predict from rat studies the outcome of pharmacologic interventions on restenosis in humans.

Rabbits

Rabbits have been used extensively to study the pathogenic mechanisms of restenosis (16,72,78–82). Rabbits are relatively inexpensive to procure and maintain, and they lend themselves well to laboratory experiments. Most studies have used the femoral or iliac arteries; however, studies of the carotid arteries and aorta have also been performed. Of these vessels, only the femoral artery is a muscular artery. After vascular injury, rabbits develop a neointimal proliferative response that is uniform and reproducible and, as with rats, is composed primarily of smooth muscle cells. One advantage of the rabbit model over the rat is that the femoral and iliac arteries of an adult rabbit are similar in size to coronary arteries in humans (78). Rabbits on a normal diet do not develop naturally occurring atherosclerotic lesions; however, with a high-cholesterol diet, serum cholesterol levels of greater than 2,000 mg/dL can be achieved (63). In these hyperlipemic animals, lipid-laden macrophages (foam cells) are deposited in the media and intima of large arteries as well as in the parenchyma of the spleen, liver, and lymph nodes. This vascular foam cell deposition does not resemble the fibrocalcific atherosclerotic lesions seen in humans. Other model systems in rabbits use a moderately high-cholesterol diet and some form of vessel injury, e.g., air-drying or balloon injury (79,80). In these models, the arterial lesions consist of foam cells in the media and intima as well as a smooth muscle cell proliferative response similar to the type of response seen in human athero-sclerotic arteries that have undergone balloon injury. This model system does not usually have the well-developed atheromatous lesion with a fibrous cap or areas of calcification that is seen in human arteries; however, the major components of the atherosclerotic process are present in the rabbit atherosclerotic model. A third rabbit model that may be used in restenosis research is the Watanabe rabbit. This strain of rabbits has an inherited deficiency in low-density lipoprotein receptors, and the resultant hyperlipidemia predisposes the rabbits to atherosclerotic vas-cular disease (83). The pattern of atherosclerosis is similar to that found in patients with familial hyperlipidemia. Well-developed vascular lesions contain a cholesterol-filled necrotic core with areas of calcification and a fibrous cap. Some studies have used heterozygous Watanabe rabbits fed a high-cholesterol diet (81). This model may have advantages in that the morphology of the lesions more closely resembles human coronary artery disease as opposed to the foam cell lesions seen in normal rabbits fed high-cholesterol diets (Fig. 3).

Non-atherosclerotic rabbits have been used in studies of restenosis (84); however, most studies have involved some experimental manipulation to induce atherosclerosis. The major use of studies in atherosclerotic rabbits is that athe-rosclerosis is induced in the artery prior to the experimental intervention. In this way, the artery that is being investigated is already diseased, similar to the situation seen in patients who undergo vascular interventions. Even though the

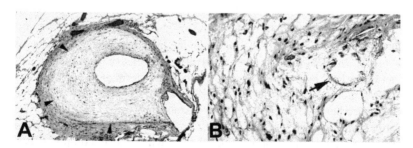

Figure 3   Atherosclerotic lesion in an F1 Watanabe-New Zealand White rabbit fed a high-fat diet. (**A**) Low-power view of the atherosclerotic lesion in a coronary artery. The arrowheads outline the internal elastic membrane. (**B**) High-power view of the atheroma demonstrating an area of calcification (*arrow*).

atherosclerotic lesion in rabbits is not identical to human atherosclerosis, there is intimal thickening, lipid accumulation (primarily foam cells), and fibrosis within the vessel wall and some atrophy or degeneration of the media with adventitial thickening by fibrosis. Thus, any additional intervention (angioplasty, stent placement, or atherectomy) is performed in a diseased artery, not a normal artery. This in itself may help to give credence to this model system as opposed to models where injurious interventions are performed on normal arteries. One negative aspect of the atherosclerotic rabbit model is that the degree of atherosclerosis and the underlying vascular injury is not uniform in all animals that are studied. Thus, the starting point for all the experiments and the morphologic characteristics of the vessels prior to the experimental intervention are not uniform. This lack of uniformity in the vessel prior to the intervention is not pronounced, but it does tend to increase the scatter in the data and make it more difficult to demonstrate statistically significant differences between experimental groups. The atherosclerotic rabbit model is very good for investigations of new angioplasty balloons, intravascular stents, and atherectomy devices. Evaluation of new devices and accurate quantitation of the degree of restenosis can be accurately evaluated in large numbers of animals. Thus, for a small animal model, the atherosclerotic rabbit and possibly the Watanabe rabbit have many benefits for studies of restenosis.

Nonhuman Primates

Several species of nonhuman primates develop spontaneous atherosclerosis and atherosclerosis can be induced by high-cholesterol diets (85–87). The location and morphology of these atherosclerotic lesions is very similar to lesions seen in humans. Both in spontaneously occurring atherosclerosis and in experimentally induced atherosclerosis, there is species variability in the susceptibility to lesion formation and the character of lesions. The cost of procuring and maintaining nonhuman primates makes this an unattractive model for many investigators. However, there are many regional primate centers around the country where large numbers of primates are housed and bred. Collaboration with investigators at these primate centers can provide an excellent opportunity to evaluate restenosis in animals that are very similar to humans.

Dogs

The size, the relatively easy vascular access, and the ease of working with dogs in the research laboratory make them amenable to many types of acute and chronic experimental protocols. Coronary arteries of dogs are similar in size and morphology to human coronary arteries (61,88). Dogs do not develop naturally occurring atherosclerosis, and even with high-cholesterol diets, there is little lipid accumulation within vessels. A model of atherosclerosis has been described in dogs, but this model required thyroidectomy and high-lipid diet, and this model is difficult to reproduce. Also, in this model the coronary arteries are not affected

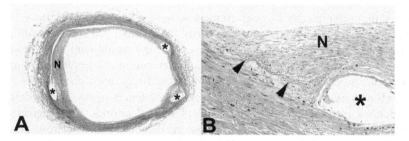

Figure 4 Dog coronary artery six months after stent placement. (**A**) Low-power view of the coronary artery after stent wires have been removed (*asterisk*). The neointima (N) is well formed but the thickness is variable. (**B**) High power of the vessel wall demonstrating the internal elastic membrane (*arrowheads*) that had been lacerated with the stent deployment. The neointima consists of primarily synthetic-type smooth muscle cells with a mild to moderate amount of extracellular matrix.

until late in the process, and the lesions consist mainly of lipid-laden macrophages (foam cells) in the media (89). This model is not generally considered as a viable model of atherosclerosis. Dogs also have a fibrinolytic system that is more active than in humans (90). Thus, studies of vascular devices and other interventions that may produce thrombosis may not receive adequate testing in the dog.

Despite these limitations, dog carotid, iliac, renal, and coronary arteries have been used in studies of restenosis and in trials to test interventional devices and intravascular stents (90–92). In studies of angioplasty and stent placement in normal dog arteries, the neointimal proliferative response appears to be minimal and seldom produces significant compromise of the vessel lumen. Studies from our laboratory show that at six months after stent placement there was neointima covering the stent wires, and this neointima was covered by endothelial cells (Fig. 4). The neointima ranged in thickness from 100 to 250 μm. The vessel lumen was patent, and the lumen contour was smooth. The neointima covering the stent wires was composed of smooth muscle cells with abundant eosinophilic cytoplasm and some small blood vessels (Fig. 4 **B**). These cells were primarily fusiform in shape along the lumenal surface, as would be expected for mature smooth muscle cells of the contractile phenotype. And, in deeper regions close to the stent wire, the smooth muscle cells were more irregular in appearance (secretory phenotype) and there was more extracellular matrix material. In the areas between the stent wires, the neointimal proliferative reaction was less pronounced and the smooth muscle cells were primarily of the contractile phenotype. In many areas, the extracellular material in the neointima after six months was fibrillar in nature and stained positively for collagen with the trichrome stain, with little elastic tissue present. Thus, in these specimens, the major portion of the extracellular matrix was composed of fibrous connective tissue. There was some rarefaction of the media underneath the stent wires, and there was a minimal inflammatory response. In some sections, particularly sections where the stent wire had lacerated the internal and the external elastic membrane, there was a mild accumulation of macrophages, lymphocytes, and plasma cells adjacent to the stent wire. Compared with humans, the dog appears to have a somewhat diminished response to vascular injury. This finding, along with the lack of a good atherosclerosis model in the dog, decreases the utility of this model system for studies of restenosis.

Swine

Swine models of vascular injury and restenosis are considered by most investigators to be the gold standard animal model for studies of vascular intervention. Pigs are relatively inexpensive to procure, are readily available, and are well suited for vascular research (93–95). Juvenile farm pigs can be used for acute and short-term experiments of vascular injury. However, farm pigs grow rapidly and can reach an adult weight of greater than 400 kg. Thus, all studies in farm pigs must necessarily be of short duration. This problem of extreme size in pig models can be overcome by the use of specially bred mini- or micropigs (96). These animals reach an adult weight of 30 to 40 kg. These animals are available commercially; however, the procurement costs are four to five times greater than farm pigs. This increased procurement cost is outweighed by the utility of these specially bred laboratory animals, the decreased cost of maintaining these animals, and the ability to perform long-term experiments with these animals. Adult farm pigs develop naturally occurring atherosclerotic lesions (63,97). Also, in both farm pigs and minipigs, high-cholesterol diets will produce an elevation in serum cholesterol and increased low-density lipoproteins. These serum lipid changes predispose to atherosclerosis. The lesions seen in the naturally occurring atherosclerosis closely resemble human atherosclerotic lesion, including lipid deposition, calcification, and development of a fibrous cap (96,98,99). Lesions from experimental models of atherosclerosis have some characteristics similar to humans; however, the overall character of the lesions demonstrates little similarity to those commonly seen in human autopsy cases (100,101).

Studies of balloon injury in pig coronary arteries involve overstretching and injury to the vessel wall (36,47,102). The type of injury and the restenotic process is quite dissimilar to the classic rat carotid balloon injury model. In the rat, the vessel is denuded of endothelium and there is little or mild medial injury. However, in the pig coronary artery model, there must be significant medial injury before you elicit a restenotic reaction. Since this model involves injury to a normal vessel, the type of lesion caused by the angioplasty balloon or the stent is somewhat different than what one sees after interventional procedures in human atherosclerotic vessels. In humans, it goes without saying that interventions are not usually performed unless there are underlying atherosclerotic lesions in the vessel. Work from our laboratory and others (103,104) have demonstrated that in atherosclerotic vessels, balloon injury usually causes laceration at the "shoulder region" of the atherosclerotic plaque with dissection between the plaque and media or the adventitia. In normal pig coronary arteries, there are no atherosclerotic plaques. Thus, as depicted in Figure 5, the

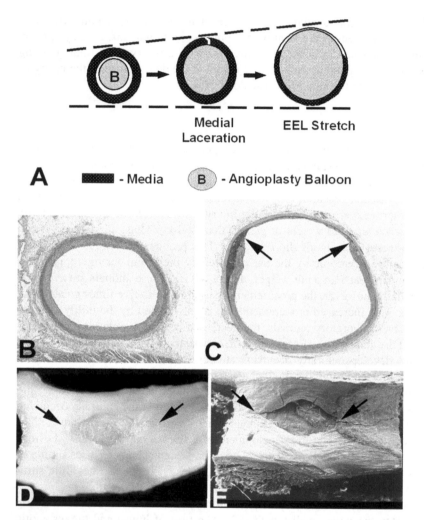

Figure 5 Overstretch balloon injury in the pig. (**A**) Diagrammatic representation of overstretch balloon injury in the pig coronary artery. As the balloon (**B**) is inflated, the vessel stretches until finally there is a focal area of laceration in the vessel wall (*center diagram*). As the balloon is inflated further, the adventitia is stretched. (**B**) Low-power view of a normal pig coronary artery just proximal to the site of balloon injury. (**C**) Low-power view of pig coronary artery at the site of balloon injury. Note that the media is lacerated (*arrows*), and there is an area of dissection between the media and the adventitia at both ends of the medial laceration. These focal areas of dissection are filled with thrombotic material. (**D**) Gross photographs of the lumenal surface of a pig coronary artery immediately after overstretch balloon injury. Note the area of medial laceration (*arrows*) that exposes the external elastic membrane and the adventitia. (**E**) Scanning electron micrograph of the same section seen in panel D. Again note the area of medial laceration (*arrows*) running longitudinally along the vessel lumen.

angioplasty balloon stretches the vessel until there is laceration of the media with stretching of the external elastic lamina and the adventitia. Immediately after the balloon injury, a layer of platelets and thrombus form on the exposed external elastic lamina (Fig. 5 **C**). Examination of vessel segments immediately after overstretch balloon injury demonstrates the laceration of the media and the exposed external elastic lamina (Figs. 5 **D,E**). Within four days after the injury, there is migration of smooth muscle cells into the thrombus that forms in the rent produced by the medial laceration (Figs. 6 **A,B**). Over time the space produced by the overstretch injury is filled in as neointima forms (Figs. 6 **C–F**). Studies from our laboratory have shown that most of the neointima forms by 14 days post injury with only a moderate increase in neointima between 14 and 28 days (102).

The response of pig coronary arteries to intravascular stenting in normal and atherosclerotic swine has been well characterized (45,47,105,106). In these studies, vascular injury is induced by placement of wire stents, which are deployed by an angioplasty balloon, thus producing endothelial denudation and stretch injury to the vessel wall. Stents and delivery balloons can be sized such that the size of the fully inflated balloon inside the vessel produces varying degrees of vessel wall stretch injury. In some studies, the balloons are purposely overstretched (50 to 100% over sizing, e.g., 3-mm diameter stent inside a 1.5–2.0-mm diameter vessel) to produce significant neointimal proliferative reaction. It is also possible to use balloons and stents that produce less vessel wall injury (10–20% oversizing), which produces less neointimal reaction (47,105).

In our studies of the severe overstretching model of stent placement in the pig (106,107), we have observed frequent laceration of the internal elastic membrane with stent wires being embedded into the media or adventitia. Despite this degree of vessel injury, only 1 of 45 pigs demonstrated very mild extravasation of blood that was clinically insignificant. In pigs that were sacrificed 28 days after stent implantation, there was a moderate thickening of the adventitia around the stented vessel segment, and the degree of neointimal and adventitial reaction is clearly visible (Fig. 7). The primary reaction within the vessel wall consisted of neointimal tissue, which was found overlying the stent wires where the vessel wall had been indented and, to a lesser extent, around the entire circumference of the vessel (Fig. 8). The neointimal tissue consisted of smooth muscle cells with varying amounts of eosinophilic extracellular material and occasional small blood vessels. Morphologically, the neointimal tissue is similar to human restenotic tissue seen after angioplasty or stenting (47,103). In vessels where the stent wires were embedded deep into the media or into the adventitia, there is often a chronic inflammatory reaction consisting of macrophages, lymphocytes, plasma cells, and occasional eosinophils.

A significant neointimal proliferative reaction is seen in the oversized stent coronary artery model in the pig (47,106,107). This neointimal reaction is morphologically similar to the reaction seen in humans after angioplasty; however, the degree of proliferation may be greater than what is usually seen in humans. This exuberant proliferative reaction may be so intense that

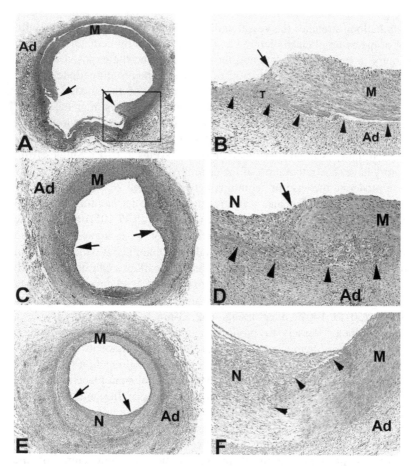

Figure 6 Time course of neointima formation after overstretch balloon injury in pig coronary arteries. (**A**) Low-power view of pig coronary artery four days after balloon injury. Note the laceration of the media with areas of dissection (*arrows*). (**B**) High-power view of an area of media (M) at the edge of the laceration (similar to the area outlined in panel **A**). The arrow points to the broken end of the internal elastic membrane. The arrowheads outline the external elastic membrane. Note that here is thrombotic material (T) adherent to the external elastic lamina. Near the surface of this thrombotic material, there are several smooth muscle cells beginning to form the neointima. Also note the abundance of inflammatory cells in the adventitia (Ad). (**C** and **D**) Similar sections of pig coronary artery seven days after balloon injury. Again note areas of medial laceration (*arrows*). The neointima (N) is much larger and more organized. Note that there is still some thrombotic material trapped in the neointima present along the external elastic lamina (*arrowheads*). (**E** and **F**) Similar sections of pig coronary artery 14 days after balloon injury. Again note areas of medial laceration (*arrows*). The neointima (N) is even larger and more organized and slightly impinges on the vessel lumen. Note at high power (panel F) that the media and the neointima blend together and broken end of the internal elastic membrane (*arrowheads*).

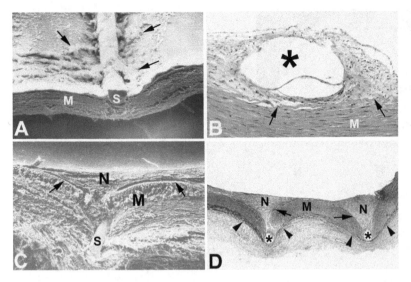

Figure 7 Balloon-expandable stents in pig coronary arteries. (**A**) Scanning electron micrograph of a pig coronary artery four hours after stent placement where the stents were carefully deployed to minimize vessel stretching. Note that the stent wires only slightly indent the vessel media and that there is an accumulation of platelet rich thrombotic material associated with the stent wires. (**B**) Three weeks after stent placement, there is a well-formed neointima that has surrounded the stent (*asterisk* where stent wire was removed). (**C**) Scanning electron micrograph of a pig coronary artery three weeks after stents were placed using an overstretch technique to purposely injure the vessel wall. The stent wire (S) is deeply embedded into the media (M), and the wire is adjacent to the external elastic membrane. There is a well-formed neointima (N) that has filled in the indentation produced by the stent wire and is much thinner along the area of media between the stent wires. (**D**) Histology of a longitudinal section from the artery seen in panel C. Note that the stent wires lacerated the internal elastic membrane (*arrows*) and completely lacerated the media (M). The stent wires (*asterisk* where wires were removed for processing) were contacting the external elastic lamina (*arrowheads*). Note that the contour of the vessel lumen is quite smooth. The neointima has "filled in" the indentations produced by the stent wires.

pharmacologic means of preventing restenosis would be unable to ameliorate the neointimal proliferative response. Thus, studies using compounds or techniques that may have promise in preventing restenosis in humans could give a negative result in the pig. Further studies must be undertaken to better characterize this model of restenosis.

Investigations of restenosis in conjunction with atherosclerosis in pigs have used minipigs for these long-term studies. In one study (108), minipigs were placed on an atherogenic diet consisting of 2% cholesterol, 15% fat, and 1.5% sodium cholate two weeks prior to balloon denudation of the coronary

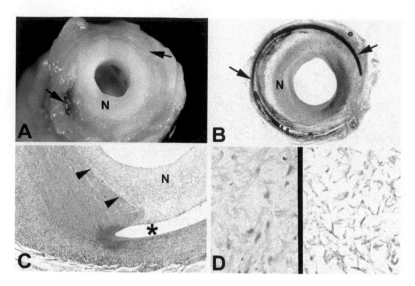

Figure 8 Neointima formation 28 days after stent placement in pig coronary arteries. (A) Gross photograph of stented pig coronary artery demonstrating the well-developed concentric neointimal formation indicative of in-stent restenosis. Also note the marked thickening of the adventitia. (B) Low-power view of plastic-embedded section of pig coronary artery showing the stent wire in the outer media and adventitial layer and the thick neointima. (C) Histologic section of vessel wall demonstrating the laceration of the internal elastic lamina (*arrowheads*) and the partial laceration of the media adjacent to the location of the stent wire (*asterisk*). Note the well-formed neointima (N). (D) High-power view of the neointima stained with hematoxylin and eosin (*left*) and immunostained for smooth muscle actin (*right*). Note the extensive extracellular matrix material that is especially evident in the section stained for smooth muscle actin (*right*). This morphology is virtually identical to that observed in human restenosis.

artery. Four to five months after the original vascular intervention, athero-sclerotic lesions had developed at the area of denudation. These lesions were then used as sites for stent implantation to evaluate the response of a diseased artery to stent implantation. At sacrifice, there was a significant neointimal proliferative reaction within the stented region of the vessel. The character of these lesions was similar to what was seen in the stented coronary arteries of pigs not on the atherogenic diet (described above), except that these arteries also contained foam cells and more fibrous connective tissue within the neointima. In additional studies with minipigs, stents were implanted in normal coronary arteries two weeks after the pigs had been started on an atherogenic diet (109). In these studies, the character of the neointimal proliferation was similar to the non-atherogenic stented arteries described above, and no mention was made of foam cells in these lesions.

It is apparent that swine models of vascular injury and restenosis are useful experimental tools for studies of the pathogenesis of restenosis. The neointimal proliferative response is very similar in character to that seen in humans; however, as mentioned above, the proliferative response is very intense and may be more severe than the proliferative response seen in humans. In addition, it is not apparent at this time what role the stent wire plays in producing the neointimal reaction seen in these animals. Further studies to characterize this restenosis reaction are needed to better determine the utility of these experimental systems as models for restenosis in humans.

MORPHOMETRIC TECHNIQUES IN STUDIES OF RESTENOSIS

The various model systems described above all have inherent strengths and weaknesses. In all the animal model systems, the production of a neointimal response to a vascular insult is the primary goal of each experimental model. In an ideal experimental model, the degree of neointimal proliferation should be reproducible and consistent from animal to animal. Accurate quantitation of the neointima requires correct use of morphometric techniques. Although simple in concept, valid morphometric evaluation of biologic tissues requires rigorous use of established morphometric techniques (110–112). The main tenant of morphometry is that the samples to be analyzed must be representative samples of the tissue reaction as a whole. This is especially germane to studies of restenosis in coronary arteries. In many of the models described above, focal areas of injury are produced in the vessel. A good example of this is the placement of stents in coronary arteries of pigs. In this instance, it is important to sample the entire region that is injured to properly evaluate the tissue response to injury. In many published studies of stent injury, tissue specimens are taken of the stented region and a single sample with the most severe stenosis is subjected to morphometric evaluation. Picking the region with the most severe stenosis is a valid technique in clinical cardiology since the maximum blood flow to the distal myocardium is dictated by the most severe stenotic lesion. However, in experiments designed to evaluate tissue response to injury, it is important to take representative samples from the entire region of the vessel that was injured. The degree of restenosis for a specific experimental procedure should be the mean or average restenosis for the entire injured area, not the degree of restenosis in the most severely affected area of the vessel. This basic requirement of adequate tissue sampling for valid morphometric evaluation of biologic tissues is especially important in studies designed to compare the degree of restenosis after specific experimental interventions or treatment regimens. Accurate and valid morphometric techniques are a prerequisite for scientific experiments of restenosis.

In models of endothelial denudation and angioplasty with little distortion of the vessel wall (e.g., rat carotid model), the degree of restenosis can be readily quantitated. In these cases, the tissue inside (lumenal to) the internal elastic membrane is easily identified as neointima. However, in experimental model systems where the internal elastic membrane is ruptured or lacerated (balloon overstretching, stents, or lasers), it becomes more difficult to accurately quantify the neointima. It is impossible to trace the internal elastic membrane for determinations of neointimal area in histologic sections if the internal elastic membrane is discontinuous. We developed protocols in our laboratory for evaluating restenosis in pig and dog arteries after angioplasty injury and stenting (36,47,102,106).

Plastic-embedded sections of stented vessels can be cut with special knives that can cut through the hard plastic and the metal stents. Alternatively, the plastic-embedded vessel segments can be cut with a saw and then sections ground to approximately 25 or 30 μm in thickness (46,113–115). In the former case, there tends to be significant artifacts in the histology specimens, while in the latter method, the thickness of the section preclude very precise visualization of histologic features at very high magnification. In both instances, the ability to visualize the stents, the vessel wall, and the neointima in situ provide a wealth of information to a trained observer.

INTRAVASCULAR STENTS: CLINICAL AND EXPERIMENTAL APPLICATIONS AND CHARACTERISTICS

In-stent restenosis is a complex process, involving vascular remodeling, elastic recoil, smooth muscle cell migration and proliferation, extracellular matrix production, and platelet activation. Although stent design and materials have significantly improved, nearly eliminating issues of vascular elastic recoil and contraction at the site of stent deployment, in-stent restenosis persists. Current efforts to improve stents have focused on stent designs to influence shear and wall stresses, thinner stent struts, materials with greater tissue compatibility, and methods to accelerate endothelial coverage after stent deployment.

STENT DESIGN

Stents deployed in coronary and peripheral arterial vessels are designed to be either balloon expandable or self-expanding. Those stents that are balloon expandable are primarily used in the coronary or renal arteries, whereas self-expanding stents more often are used in peripheral vessels. Self-expanding stents have shape memory and return to their expanded shape after undergoing compression or flexion. These stents are primarily placed in locations such as carotid and superficial femoral arteries, which undergo significant bending and compression. Balloon-expandable stents are used more in locations that require greater radial support, such as at the ostium of a vessel. Stent design itself significantly influences the rate of restenosis and thrombosis after deployment (116–119). Factors appear to include the number and method of connection of the stent struts (120,121), the degree of stent recoil after deployment (122,123), strut thickness and shape (124–126), and the degree of scaffolding of the artery by the strut distribution (127). There is general consensus that stents with less recoil and with thinner stent struts are associated with less restenosis.

Stent design and location of deployment significantly influences the stresses on the vessel wall itself, further influencing in-stent restenosis. Wall shear stress (WSS) is the "frictional" force exerted by the viscosity of the circulating blood on the intimal layer of a vessel (128). WSS is influenced by vessel geometry, such as curvature and branching, with regions of low WSS associated with accelerated atherosclerotic plaque development (129–132). Stent deployment creates regions of decreased WSS, which are associated with increased neointimal proliferation and greater intimal thickness (133–135). Regions of low WSS are influenced by strut thickness, number of stent struts, angle between struts, strut width, and arterial surface area covered by stent (136–138).

Another form of stress affecting the arterial wall is the perpendicular component of stress, associated with outward pressure such as from blood pressure. This is called wall normal stress. After a stent is deployed, this outward normal stress varies with stent design. Greater wall normal stress has been associated with increased atherosclerosis and neointimal proliferation (139,140). In addition, the stiffness of a stent placed in a curved vessel causes arterial straightening. There may be a threefold difference in stiffness between stent types (141). This straightening, and resultant greater curvature at the ends of the stents, appears to alter shear stress and influence restenosis (142,143).

STENT MATERIALS

When initially approved by the FDA, stents were created from 316L stainless steel. With the development of multiple stents, other metals have been used, most commonly Nitinol (nickel-titanium) and cobalt alloy (cobalt-chromium) (144). Although other materials continue to be used, balloon-expandable stents are made primarily of stainless steel and cobalt alloy; whereas self-expanding stents are primarily of Nitinol. Once a stent is deployed, the surface is rapidly covered with a monolayer of soluble proteins, binding based on surface affinity and plasma concentration. The proteins that bind, such as fibrinogen and albumin, play a key role in the cellular response to stent and platelet adhesion and activation (145–151). The stent materials used and their surface treatments significantly influence protein adhesion and cellular response (152–156).

CORROSION

All metals are subject to corrosion from their local environment, and blood is considered extremely corrosive to metallic materials (157). During production, stents undergo surface treatments, such as electropolishing, to create a uniform oxide layer and improve corrosion resistance (155,158,159). The durability and ability to repassivate or repair the surface layer varies on the basis of metal type and treatment used, and once there is a break in the coating, there is increased risk of corrosion (157). Release of ions from implanted metallic materials into local tissues has been associated with cytotoxicity in vitro and has been studied extensively in the orthopedic and dental literature (160–162). Corrosion products of Nitinol stent wire can cause smooth muscle cell necrosis, alter cell morphology, and decrease cell numbers (160). Likewise, stainless steel corrosion products, particularly nickel, may change smooth muscle cell morphology and induce cell necrosis (161). Low levels of metallic ions may be associated with proinflammatory activity (163), such as release of IL-6 (164). In addition, the presence of shear stress may influence a local inflammatory response (163). Limited in vivo and clinical trials data exist, evaluating the role of surface coatings and ion effects. Stainless steel stents coated with gold have increased restenosis rates compared with those without coating, suggesting the influence of local ion effects (165,166). In addition, improving electrochemical properties by the use of a titanium-nitride-oxide coating on a stainless steel stent has demonstrated decreased platelet adhesion, fibrinogen binding, and clinical in-stent restenosis (167,168). Diamond-like coatings have also been used, with some reduction in in vitro ion release. However, the use of diamond-like coating has not translated into a reduction in clinical restenosis (169–172). Analyses of stents obtained postmortem indicate that stent corrosion does occur, with measurable release of ions into surrounding tissues (173,174) (Figs. 9, 10). Studies are ongoing, evaluating their clinical significance.

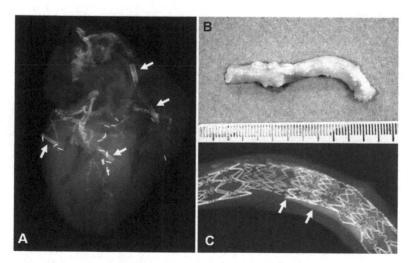

Figure 9 Overlapping stents in autopsy specimen. Image (**A**) is a postmortem radiograph of explanted heart from an autopsy patient. The radiograph demonstrates multiple stents (*arrows*) and marked calcification of the native coronary arteries and saphenous vein grafts. Image (**B**) shows a gross photograph of a section of coronary artery with implanted stents. Image (**C**) is a radiograph of the coronary artery section from (**B**) showing different types of overlapping stents. The overlapped portion is indicated by the arrows.

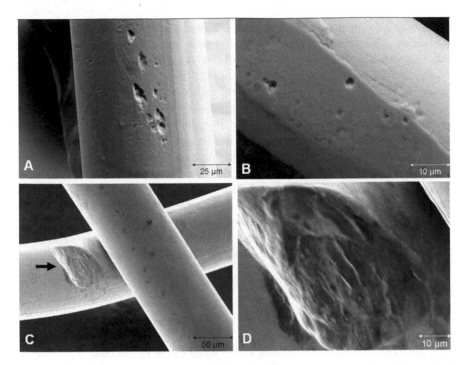

Figure 10 Scanning electron micrograph demonstrating stent corrosion in explanted stents from human patient. Stent with cobalt-chromium alloy surface. (**A** and **B**)—Region of overlap with a stainless steel stent. Cobalt-chromium surface stent struts have pitting corrosion. (**C**) Fretting wear (*arrow*) and pitting between struts of the cobalt-chromium surface stent. Image D is a high-power view of the area of stent wear demonstrated in image C.

DRUG-ELUTING STENTS

Drug-eluting stents have been developed, in an effort to inhibit neointimal proliferation and prevent in-stent restenosis. In general, medications are embedded in a polymer, which is coated on the metallic stents. The polymer controls drug release kinetics. The currently available systems have different medication/polymer combinations. Of the U.S. FDA-approved drug-eluting stents, there are two general groups of medications released: sirolimus and sirolimus derivatives and paclitaxel. The sirolimus-like drugs have similar mechanisms of action, although they may have different in vivo activities.

MEDICATIONS USED IN DRUG-ELUTING STENTS

Sirolimus (rapamycin) inhibits proliferation and migration of smooth muscle cells by interference with cell cycle regulation (175,176). It binds to the FK506-binding protein 12 (177–179). This drug-protein complex then binds to the regulatory protein mammalian target of rapamycin (mTOR) and inhibits its activation. This causes cell arrest. Everolimus and zotarolimus have similar mechanisms of action to sirolimus. Everolimus is a derivative of sirolimus that is orally active. Zotarolimus is more lipophilic than sirolimus, prolonging its retention in local tissues after its rapid release from the delivery polymer.

Paclitaxel is a lipophilic agent that binds to the β subunit of tubulin, promoting tubulin polymerization and cell cycle arrest (180,181). This causes apoptotic cell death by disrupting cell division and repair (182,183). Preclinical evaluation has been performed of paclitaxel release from biodegradable polymer coatings (different from the coating used in the Taxus stent). In a rabbit iliac artery model, there was incomplete healing of the vessel six months after stent deployment (184), with initial inhibition of growth but neointimal suppression no longer present at 90 days (185). Paclitaxel delivery from a different biodegradable polymer-coated stent resulted in medial necrosis and late neointimal thickening, suggesting that local paclitaxel release has a narrow therapeutic window (186).

POLYMERS

Sirolimus stent (Cypher)—The stainless steel stent is coated with three layers of polymer. The base layer is a coating of Parylene C. On to this base is attached a mixture of polyethylene-co-vinyl acetate (PEVA) and poly n-butylmethacrylate (PBMA)-containing sirolimus. The outer layer is a drug-free coating of PBMA, which is used to control drug release. The use of the outer drug-free layer allows the sirolimus to be released by diffusion control with the stent releasing 50% of its sirolimus content within the first week and 85% over 30 days (187).

Data regarding the local vascular response to the specific copolymer used in the Cypher stent in animal models is conflicting. In a porcine model, greater polymer thickness was associated with greater neointimal proliferation and a trend toward more arterial inflammation than bare-metal stents or thin polymer, although the arterial injury score also tended to be greater with the thicker polymer coating. In contrast, there was no relationship between the presence of polymer or polymer thickness with neointimal area or inflammation in a canine model (178). There is also no increase in neointimal area in a rabbit iliac model in the presence of polymer compared with bare-metal stents (188).

Paclitaxel Stent (Taxus)

The stent is coated with a nonbiodegradable polymer matrix that allows an initial burst of paclitaxel during the first 48 hours, followed by slow release over the next 10 days. No further drug is released after 30 days (187). Release of the drug into tissues is diffusion controlled. Vascular response to the polymer on the Taxus drug-eluting stent, poly(styrene-b-isobutylene-b-styrene) triblock copolymer (SIBS, Translute polymer) (189), is not publicly available. However, unpublished preclinical evaluation of the stent with Translute polymer suggests that the degree of neointimal proliferation is the same with or without polymer coating (190).

Zotarolimus Stent (Endeavor)

This stent is coated with phosphorylcholine and is loaded with zotarolimus. The phosphorylcholine coating is a methacrylate-based copolymer that includes a synthetic form of phosphorylcholine, the phospholipid found in the outer surface of red blood cell membranes (191,192). This coating appears to reduce the thrombogenicity of the metallic stent (193). The stent strut is coated with a thin phosphorylcholine base layer, covered by a layer of polymer that consists of 90% zotarolimus, which is then covered with a thin overlay of phosphorylcholine. The zotarolimus is completely released from the polymer coating within 15 days after implant, with 80% released within the first five days (4,194). However, some residual drug remains present in the arterial tissue up to 28 days, given its lipophilic properties (4).

Everolimus Stent (Xience V, Promus)

The polymer used to deliver everolimus is a thin layer of nonerodable copolymer of polyvinylidine fluoride and hexafluoropropylene. The dose of everolimus chosen was to achieve a similar quantity of released compound to that of the sirolimus-eluting stent. Eighty percent of the everolimus is released by 28 days, with 100% at 120 days (195). The polymer delivery system consists of two layers: a thin primer of PBMA and a drug matrix of a copolymer of vinylidene fluoride and hexafluoropropylene (PVDF-HFP) blended with everolimus. The low polymer thickness and stent strut thickness results in the thinnest stent strut of these drug-eluting stents.

DRUG RELEASE KINETICS

The rate and distribution of drug delivery from stents is dependent on stent design, strut distribution after deployment, polymer delivery system, drug characteristics, and the underlying vascular tissue. Ex vivo kinetics studies of drug release have been performed, modeling both paclitaxel and sirolimus drug delivery into the arterial wall. Both are hydrophobic compounds. Paclitaxel primarily travels through the arterial wall by binding to hydrophobic sites within the tissues. In addition, it moves by diffusion and by convection (196).

In studies comparing arterial distribution of hydrophilic and hydrophobic drugs released from stents, the hydrophobic drug concentration is greater, particularly near the intima (197). Stent design and inhomogeneous stent strut distribution in the artery wall causes greater maximal drug concentrations with hydrophobic than hydrophilic drugs (197). In addition to strut distribution, drug delivery is affected by the structure of the artery itself. There is greater distribution of drug in elastic arteries compared with muscular ones and greater distribution along the orientation of the elastic sheaths rather than into the thickness of the arterial wall (198).

The proteins to which the drugs bind within the vessel wall also determine their distribution. Rapamycin binds to the FKBP12-binding protein and distributes evenly throughout the vessel wall. Paclitaxel binds to microtubules and remains primarily in the subintimal space (199). The presence of thrombus adjacent to the stent struts affects local drug delivery. If thrombus is between the struts and vessel wall, it significantly decreases local drug delivery. However, if thrombus is in the lumen covering the stent, it may decrease local washout and increase drug delivery (200). Overlapping of stents and strut position also affect drug delivery and local response. Overlapping of rapamycin-eluting stents in a rabbit model leads to greater giant cell accumulation, whereas overlapping of paclitaxel-eluting stents is associated with more infiltration of eosinophils, fibrin deposition, and neointimal thickness at 90 days (201). In addition, there is delayed reendothelialization at the sites of overlap although there is greater coverage at the site of overlap with zotarolimus than with sirolimus or paclitaxel-eluting stents (114). Modeling of drug distribution shows significantly greater drug immediately downstream of overlapping struts. Histologic examination of explanted stents from a porcine model analyzed 30 days after stent implantation reveals greater fibrin deposition immediately distal to stent overlap zones, corresponding to the area of increased drug delivery in computational models (202).

PRECLINICAL DATA

Preclinical evaluation of drug-eluting stents has primarily been performed in the rabbit iliac and porcine coronary artery models (114). The time course for development of neointimal proliferation after bare-metal stent placement in humans peaks at six to nine months and then decrease up to three years (203). However, the neointimal growth in a porcine coronary artery model peaks at one month and then decreases for three to six months (113).

Sirolimus coating on stents significantly inhibits neointimal growth compared with bare-metal stents in both rabbit and porcine models at 28 days (178,188). However, at 90 and 180 days in a porcine model, there is no longer a reduction in neointimal area with sirolimus release compared with bare-metal stents, and there appears to be a greater inflammatory response in the coated stents at these later timepoints (204). Evaluation of paclitaxel coating in a porcine model revealed that at higher doses of paclitaxel there was significant fibrin deposition and at low doses, inadequate inhibition of neointimal proliferation (190). On the basis of these findings, clinical trials of the Taxus drug-eluting stent used a total dose of 1 $\mu g/mm^2$. Everolimus-eluting stents have been evaluated in an oversized stent porcine injury model. The degree of neointimal proliferation was equivalent for the everolimus- and sirolimus-eluting stents, and significantly less than bare-metal cobalt-chromium stents (195). Additional evaluation suggests that use of everolimus-eluting stents results in significantly greater reendothelization in rabbit arteries at 14 days than sirolimus, paclitaxel, or zotarolimus (205). Zotarolimus-eluting stents have been evaluated both in rabbit iliac and porcine coronary artery models. In the rabbit model, there was no significant reduction in neointimal proliferation with drug-elution compared with bare-metal stents at 28 days. However, in the porcine coronary artery, when compared with the sirolimus stent and bare-metal stent, there was lesser inflammation than with sirolimus release. In addition, although there was more neointima initially with zotarolimus release than sirolimus, by 180 days, there was significantly greater neointimal proliferation with sirolimus, whereas the neointimal size did not change over time with zotarolimus. There was also greater endothelialization with zotarolimus release than with sirolimus and paclitaxel in rabbit iliac arteries at 21 days (114).

CLINICAL DATA

Drug-eluting stents significantly decrease the risk of in-stent restenosis and overall major adverse cardiovascular events, compared with bare-metal stents (206–209). Prior to the advent of drug-eluting stents, restenosis accounted for approximately 300,000 repeat procedures a year worldwide, with an annual estimated economic burden of $1.2 billion in the United states (210). Of the drug-eluting stents, the Cypher and Taxus stents have the greatest clinical data (211), clearly demonstrating a significant reduction in in-stent restenosis rates compared with bare-metal stents (206,208,212–214).

The Cypher stent was the first drug-eluting stent approved in the United States, based on findings in the first-in-human study (215), the RAVEL trial (206), and the SIRIUS trial (208). The SIRIUS trial demonstrated 58% reduction in the combined endpoint of cardiac death, myocardial infarction, or target vessel revascularization at nine months compared with bare-metal stents. This significant reduction in need for target lesion revascularization persists to four years after the procedure (210). In a pooled analysis of three SIRIUS trials, target lesion revascularization was reduced from 22.6% with bare-metal stents to 5.7% with Cypher use (216).

The Taxus stent similarly has demonstrated a significant reduction in need for revascularization at nine months compared with bare-metal stents, as demonstrated in the TAXUS-I (207), TAXUS-II (212), and TAXUS-IV studies (209). In particular, the TAXUS-IV trial demonstrated a 73% reduction in target lesion revascularization with the Taxus stent at 12 months (217).

Several head-to-head comparisons between Cypher and Taxus have been performed. These studies demonstrated evidence of less neointimal proliferation (less late loss) with Cypher stent compared with Taxus, particularly when evaluated in patients at high risk for restenosis (168,218–220). However, the largest randomized multicenter trial (the REALITY trial) failed to show a clinical difference in restenosis rates (220). A subsequent meta-analysis combining randomized trials suggests an overall lower restenosis rate with the sirolimus-eluting stent, perhaps related to greater reduction in late lumen loss (221).

The Endeavor stent was initially compared to bare-metal stent in the ENDEAVOR-II trial, and demonstrated a 61% reduction in target lesion revascularization with the drug-eluting stent (222). Subsequent studies compared the Endeavor stent to the Cypher and Taxus stents. The ENDEAVOR-III study demonstrated a higher rate of restenosis but lower rate of in-hospital cardiac events with the Endeavor stent compared with the Cypher (223). Intravascular ultrasound evaluation also demonstrated significantly greater neointimal proliferation with zotarolimus release (224). Preliminary data from the ENDEAVOR-IV trial suggest no difference in restenosis rates between Endeavor and Taxus although there was evidence of greater neointimal proliferation with the Endeavor stent (225).

Everolimus-eluting stents have been evaluated in the series of SPIRIT and FUTURE trials. Combined analysis of the FUTURE I and II studies demonstrated a significant reduction in neointimal proliferation with everolimus-elution compared with bare-metal stents (226). Preliminary data from the SPIRIT III study demonstrated both a lesser degree of neointimal proliferation compared with the Taxus stent, and a 44% reduction in major adverse cardiac events (227).

DRUG-ELUTING STENT SAFETY

Stent Thrombosis

One of the main concerns regarding the use of drug-eluting stents is the risk of in-stent thrombosis, which appears to persist at least three years after deployment (228). Procedural factors appear to play a role, such as stent lumen dimension, stent length, stent malapposition to the arterial wall, the presence of dissections after deployment, and use in bifurcation lesions (229). Premature discontinuation of dual antiplatelet therapy is a particularly important risk factor for stent thrombosis (230,231). In addition, the polymer used may provoke an inflammatory response in a small percentage of patients (232,233). Both sirolimus and paclitaxel not only inhibit smooth muscle cell proliferation and migration but also suppress reendothelialization after stent implantation (176), thereby prolonging the time course for healing after stent placement (234). Although stent thrombosis remains a concern, clinical data indicate that there is no difference in myocardial infarction or death rates at four years with the use of drug-eluting stents compared with bare-metal stents (235).

Hypersensitivity, Inflammation, and Local Tissue Response

Reports of early and late hypersensitivity to components of drug-eluting stents have prompted FDA notification to physicians (236,237). The reactions described include pain, rash, respiratory alterations, hives, itching, fever, and blood pressure changes. However, some reactions have been severe, including ana-phylaxis. Additionally, Virmani et al. (238) describe a case of localized hyper-sensitivity vasculitis after Cypher stent placement, resulting in fatal stent thrombosis 18 months after stent implantation. This paper raises the possibility of long-term hypersensitivity to a stent, resulting in extensive inflammation, aneurysmal dilation, and stent thrombosis. These reports of clinically apparent inflammation, however, appear to be rare. Preclinical evaluation suggests that the newer drug-eluting stents (everolimus, zotarolimus stents) and their delivery polymers may provoke less of an inflammatory response (239).

Vasomotion and Collateral Flow Effects

Drug-eluting stent placement appears to also alter the vascular response of the vessel to the stent. This has been described after Cypher and Taxus stent placement. Asymptomatic vasoconstriction and abnormal vasomotion with exercise has been described six months after sirolimus-eluting stent deployment. Abnormal vasomotion was noted both proximal and distal to the drug-eluting stents. Paradoxical vasoconstriction was not seen in the bare-metal stent control group in this study (240). A second publication also demonstrates abnormal vasoconstriction in response to acetylcholine in patients receiving sirolimus-eluting stents compared with bare-metal stents (241). This is supported by an in vitro porcine coronary model, in which rapamycin caused significant impairment in vascular relaxation (242). A recent report describes abnormal vasoconstriction with acetylcholine after both sirolimus- and paclitaxel-eluting stents, particularly in the segments distal to the stents (243,244). Symptomatic spasm after drug-eluting stent placement has been described, and may be fatal (245,246). Similarly, anaphylaxis after paclitaxel-eluting stent placement has been reported, with severe diffuse coronary spasm (247). In addition to abnormal vasomotion, drug-eluting stent placement may also limit the development of coronary collateral vessels, thereby increasing the mortality associated with late stent thrombosis (248). Evaluation of coronary flow index and ST-segment elevation evaluated from an intracoronary guide wire revealed that coronary collateral function six months after drug-eluting stents placement was 30% to 40% less than after bare-metal stent placement.

Although adverse events have been reported after drug-eluting stent placement, overall their use has markedly benefited the care of patients with coronary artery disease, significantly reducing their rate of restenosis without affecting long-term rates of mortality or myocardial infarction.

CONCLUDING REMARKS

Cardiovascular disease is an increasingly important cause of morbidity and mortality in the developed world, and a thorough understanding of the response of blood vessels to injury is crucial for development of effective prevention and treatment approaches. Blood vessels are dynamic structures that respond in fairly predictable ways to chemical, infectious, and mechanical injury. Connective tissue cells and the extracellular matrix produced by synthetic smooth muscle cells also play a role in the response of blood vessels to injury. Blood constituents, particularly platelets and components of the coagulation cascade, are also primary participants in vascular injury and repair. The response to injury is somewhat limited, whereas the mechanisms of injury are numerous, complex, and often poorly understood. Thus, characterization of the morphologic changes often provides important directions for investigating the nature and mechanisms of injury. It is therefore essential that pathologists along with vascular biologists provide as accurate as possible an anatomic/morphologic description of the changes observed.

REFERENCES

1. Rosamond W, Flegal K, Furie K, et al. Heart disease and stroke statistics—2008 update: a report from the American Heart Association Statistics Committee and Stroke Statistics Subcommittee. Circulation 2008; 117:e25–e146.
2. Ruben Z, Arceo RJ, Wagner BM. Chemically induced injury of blood vessels. In: Acosta D, ed. Cardiovascular Toxicology. New York, NY: Raven Press, 1992:517–541.
3. Boor PJ, Gotlieb AI, Joseph EC, et al. Chemical-induced vasculature injury. Summary of the symposium presented at the 32nd annual meeting of the Society of Toxicology, New Orleans, Louisiana, March 1993. Toxicol Appl Pharmacol 1995; 132:177–195.
4. Burke A, Mullick FG, Virmani R. Characterization of toxic and drug-induced cardiovascular lesions in humans. In: Bishop SP, Kerns WD, eds. Comprehensive Toxicology. New York, NY: Pergamon, 1997:445–481.
5. Feuerstein GZ, Kerns WD. Molecular pharmacology of arterial endothelium and smooth muscles. In: Bishop SP, Kerns WD, eds. Molecular Pharmacology of Arterial Endothelium and Smooth Muscles. New York, NY: Pergamon, 1997:43–54.
6. Virchow RLK. Cellular Pathology as Based upon Physiological and Pathological Histology. London: John Churchill, 1860.
7. Furchgott RF. The 1996 Albert Lasker Medical Research Awards. The discovery of endothelium-derived relaxing factor and its importance in the identification of nitric oxide. JAMA 1996; 276:1186–1188.
8. Furchgott RF. Endothelium-derived relaxing factor: discovery, early studies, and identification as nitric oxide. Biosci Rep 1999; 19:235–251.
9. Ignarro LJ, Cirino G, Casini A, et al. Nitric oxide as a signaling molecule in the vascular system: an overview. J Cardiovasc Pharmacol 1999; 34:879–886.
10. Murad F. Discovery of some of the biological effects of nitric oxide and its role in cell signaling. Biosci Rep 1999; 19:133–154.
11. Noishiki Y, Yamane Y, Tomizawa Y, et al. Rapid neointima formation with elastic laminae similar to the natural arterial wall on an adipose tissue fragmented vascular prosthesis. ASAIO J 1994; 40:M267–M272.
12. Davis EC. Elastic lamina growth in the developing mouse aorta. J Histochem Cytochem 1995; 43:1115–1123.

13. Plump AS, Smith JD, Hayek T, et al. Severe hypercholesterolemia and atherosclerosis in apolipoprotein E-deficient mice created by homologous recombination in ES cells. Cell 1992; 71:343–353.
14. Clark JM, Glagov S. Luminal surface of distended arteries by scanning electron microscopy: eliminating configurational and technical artefacts. Br J Exp Pathol 1976; 57:129–135.
15. Crissman RS. SEM observations of the elastic networks in canine femoral artery. Am J Anat 1986; 175:481–492.
16. Campbell GR, Campbell JH, Manderson JA, et al. Arterial smooth muscle. A multifunctional mesenchymal cell. Arch Pathol Lab Med 1988; 112:977–986.
17. Boerth NJ, Dey NB, Cornwell TL, et al. Cyclic GMP-dependent protein kinase regulates vascular smooth muscle cell phenotype. J Vasc Res 1997; 34:245–259.
18. Anderson PG, Boerth NJ, Liu M, et al. Cyclic GMP-dependent protein kinase expression in coronary arterial smooth muscle in response to balloon catheter injury. Arterioscler Thromb Vasc Biol 2000; 20:2192–2197.
19. Gibbons GH, Dzau VJ. The emerging concept of vascular remodeling. N Engl J Med 1994; 330:1431–1438.
20. Shi Y, O'Brien JE, Fard A, et al. Adventitial myofibroblasts contribute to neointimal formation in injured porcine coronary arteries. Circulation 1996; 94: 1655–1664.
21. Regan CP, Anderson PG, Bishop SP, et al. Captopril prevents vascular and fibrotic changes but not cardiac hypertrophy in aortic-banded rats. Am J Physiol 1996; 271: H906–H913.
22. Regan CP, Anderson PG, Bishop SP, et al. Pressure-independent effects of AT1-receptor antagonism on cardiovascular remodeling in aortic-banded rats. Am J Physiol 1997; 272:H2131–H2138.
23. Heggtveit HA. Nonatherosclerotic diseases of the aorta. In: Silver MD, ed. Cardiovascular Pathology. Philadelphia, PA: Churchill Livingstone, 1983:707–737.
24. Kwon HM, Sangiorgi G, Ritman EL, et al. Enhanced coronary vasa vasorum neovascularization in experimental hypercholesterolemia. J Clin Invest 1998; 101:1551–1556.
25. Ignarro LJ, Buga GM, Wood KS, et al. Endothelium-derived relaxing factor produced and released from artery and vein is nitric oxide. Proc Natl Acad Sci U S A 1987; 84:9265–9269.
26. Johnson RM, Lincoln TM. Effects of nitroprusside, glyceryl trinitrate, and 8-bromo cyclic GMP on phosphorylase a formation and myosin light chain phosphorylation in rat aorta. Mol Pharmacol 1985; 27:333–342.
27. Lincoln TM, Komalavilas P, Boerth NJ, et al. cGMP signaling through cAMP- and cGMP-dependent protein kinases. Adv Pharmacol 1995; 34:305–322.
28. Liu MW, Roubin GS, King SB III. Restenosis after coronary angioplasty. Potential biologic determinants and role of intimal hyperplasia. Circulation 1989; 79: 1374–1387.
29. Windecker S, Meier B. Intervention in coronary artery disease. Heart 2000; 83: 481–490.
30. Ellis SG, Popma JJ, Stone GW, et al. Restenosis, statistics, and reasonable inferences. J Am Coll Cardiol 2006; 47:470–471; author reply 471.
31. Moussa I, Leon MB, Baim DS, et al. Impact of sirolimus-eluting stents on outcome in diabetic patients: a SIRIUS (SIRolImUS-coated Bx Velocity balloon-expandable

stent in the treatment of patients with de novo coronary artery lesions) substudy. Circulation 2004; 109:2273–2278.

32. Banai S, Shou M, Correa R, et al. Rabbit ear model of injury-induced arterial smooth muscle cell proliferation. Kinetics, reproducibility, and implications. Circ Res 1991; 69:748–756.

33. Stanley WC, Connett RJ. Regulation of muscle carbohydrate metabolism during exercise. FASEB J 1991; 5:2155–2159.

34. Willerson JT, Eidt JF, McNatt J, et al. Role of thromboxane and serotonin as mediators in the development of spontaneous alterations in coronary blood flow and neointimal proliferation in canine models with chronic coronary artery stenoses and endothelial injury. J Am Coll Cardiol 1991; 17:101B–110B.

35. Forrester JS, Fishbein M, Helfant R, et al. A paradigm for restenosis based on cell biology: clues for the development of new preventive therapies. J Am Coll Cardiol 1991; 17:758–769.

36. Liu MW, Hearn JA, Luo JF, et al. Reduction of thrombus formation without inhibiting coagulation factors does not inhibit intimal hyperplasia after balloon injury in pig coronary arteries. Coron Artery Dis 1996; 7:667–671.

37. Bennett MR. In-stent stenosis: pathology and implications for the development of drug eluting stents. Heart 2003; 89:218–224.

38. Kolodgie FD, Nakazawa G, Sangiorgi G, et al. Pathology of atherosclerosis and stenting. Neuroimaging Clin N Am 2007; 17:285–301.

39. Sun ZS, Zhou SH, Guan X. Impact of blood circulation on reendothelialization, restenosis and atrovastatin's restenosis prevention effects. Int J Cardiol 2007. doi:10.1016/j.icard.2007.05.116.

40. Grise MA, Massullo V, Jani S, et al. Five-year clinical follow-up after intracoronary radiation: results of a randomized clinical trial. Circulation 2002; 105:2737–2740.

41. Baierl V, Baumgartner S, Pollinger B, et al. Three-year clinical follow-up after strontium-90/yttrium-90 beta-irradiation for the treatment of in-stent coronary restenosis. Am J Cardiol 2005; 96:1399–1403.

42. Holmes DR Jr., Teirstein P, Satler L, et al. Sirolimus-eluting stents vs vascular brachytherapy for in-stent restenosis within bare-metal stents: the SISR randomized trial. JAMA 2006; 295:1264–1273.

43. Stone GW, Ellis SG, O'Shaughnessy CD, et al. Paclitaxel-eluting stents vs vascular brachytherapy for in-stent restenosis within bare-metal stents: the TAXUS V ISR randomized trial. JAMA 2006; 295:1253–1263.

44. Ferrell M, Fuster V, Gold HK, et al. A dilemma for the 1990s. Choosing appropriate experimental animal model for the prevention of restenosis. Circulation 1992; 85:1630–1631.

45. Schwartz RS, Edelman ER, Carter A, et al. Drug-eluting stents in preclinical studies: recommended evaluation from a consensus group. Circulation 2002; 106:1867–1873.

46. Schwartz RS, Chronos NA, Virmani R. Preclinical restenosis models and drug-eluting stents: still important, still much to learn. J Am Coll Cardiol 2004; 44:1373–1385.

47. Anderson PG. Restenosis: animal models and morphometric techniques in studies of the vasuclar response to injury. Cardiovasc Pathol 1992; 1:263–278.

48. Blank RS, Owens GK. Platelet-derived growth factor regulates actin isoform expression and growth state in cultured rat aortic smooth muscle cells. J Cell Physiol 1990; 142:635–642.

49. Dartsch PC, Voisard R, Bauriedel G, et al. Growth characteristics and cytoskeletal organization of cultured smooth muscle cells from human primary stenosing and restenosing lesions. Arteriosclerosis 1990; 10:62–75.

50. Pukac LA, Hirsch GM, Lormeau JC, et al. Antiproliferative effects of novel, nonanticoagulant heparin derivatives on vascular smooth muscle cells in vitro and in vivo. Am J Pathol 1991; 139:1501–1509.

51. Carere RG, Koo EWY, Liu PP, et al. Porcine coronary artery organ culture: a model for study of angioplasty injury. Cardiovasc Pathol 1992; 1:107–115.

52. Wang XJ, Maier KG, Fuse S, et al. Thrombospondin-1-induced migration is functionally dependent upon focal adhesion kinase. Vasc Endovascular Surg 2008. PMID:18319354.

53. Cornwell TL, Soff GA, Traynor AE, et al. Regulation of the expression of cyclic GMP-dependent protein kinase by cell density in vascular smooth muscle cells. J Vasc Res 1994; 31:330–337.

54. Lincoln TM, Komalavilas P, Cornwell TL. Pleiotropic regulation of vascular smooth muscle tone by cyclic GMP-dependent protein kinase. Hypertension 1994; 23:1141–1147.

55. Lincoln TM, Dey NB, Boerth NJ, et al. Nitric oxide–cyclic GMP pathway regulates vascular smooth muscle cell phenotypic modulation: implications in vascular diseases. Acta Physiol Scand 1998; 164:507–515.

56. Sata M, Maejima Y, Adachi F, et al. A mouse model of vascular injury that induces rapid onset of medial cell apoptosis followed by reproducible neointimal hyperplasia. J Mol Cell Cardiol 2000; 32:2097–3104.

57. Ali ZA, Alp NJ, Lupton H, et al. Increased in-stent stenosis in ApoE knockout mice: insights from a novel mouse model of balloon angioplasty and stenting. Arterioscler Thromb Vasc Biol 2007; 27:833–840.

58. Zou Y, Qi Y, Roztocil E, et al. Patterns of kinase activation induced by injury in the murine femoral artery. J Surg Res 2007; 142:332–340.

59. Paigen B, Morrow A, Holmes PA, et al. Quantitative assessment of atherosclerotic lesions in mice. Atherosclerosis 1987; 68:231–240.

60. Breslow JL. Mouse models of atherosclerosis. Science 1996; 272:685–688.

61. Sims FH. A comparison of structural features of the walls of coronary arteries from 10 different species. Pathology 1989; 21:115–124.

62. Wilgram GF, Ingle DJ. "Spontaneous" cardiovascular lesions in rats. In: Roberts JC Jr., Straus R, eds. Comparative Atherosclerosis: The Morphology of Spontaneous and Induced Atherosclerotic Lesions in Animals and Its Relation to Human Disease. New York, NY: Harber & Row, 1965:87–91.

63. Gross DR. Animal Models in Cardiovascular Research. Boston, MA: Martinus Nijhoff, 1985.

64. Fishman JA, Ryan GB, Karnovsky MJ. Endothelial regeneration in the rat carotid artery and the significance of endothelial denudation in the pathogenesis of myointimal thickening. Lab Invest 1975; 32:339–351.

65. Clowes AW, Clowes MM, Au YP, et al. Smooth muscle cells express urokinase during mitogenesis and tissue-type plasminogen activator during migration in injured rat carotid artery. Circ Res 1990; 67:61–67.

66. Fingerle J, Au YP, Clowes AW, et al. Intimal lesion formation in rat carotid arteries after endothelial denudation in absence of medial injury. Arteriosclerosis 1990; 10:1082–1087.

67. Prescott MF, Webb RL, Reidy MA. Angiotensin-converting enzyme inhibitor versus angiotensin II, AT1 receptor antagonist. Effects on smooth muscle cell migration and proliferation after balloon catheter injury. Am J Pathol 1991; 139:1291–1296.

68. Majesky MW, Giachelli CM, Reidy MA, et al. Rat carotid neointimal smooth muscle cells reexpress a developmentally regulated mRNA phenotype during repair of arterial injury. Circ Res 1992; 71:759–768.

69. Fingerle J, Johnson R, Clowes AW, et al. Role of platelets in smooth muscle cell proliferation and migration after vascular injury in rat carotid artery. Proc Natl Acad Sci U S A 1989; 86:8412–8416.

70. Clowes AW, Reidy MA, Clowes MM. Mechanisms of stenosis after arterial injury. Lab Invest 1983; 49:208–215.

71. Schwartz SM, Campbell GR, Campbell JH. Replication of smooth muscle cells in vascular disease. Circ Res 1986; 58:427–444.

72. Manderson JA, Mosse PR, Safstrom JA, et al. Balloon catheter injury to rabbit carotid artery. I. Changes in smooth muscle phenotype. Arteriosclerosis 1989; 9:289–298.

73. Clowes AW, Clowes MM, Fingerle J, et al. Kinetics of cellular proliferation after arterial injury. V. Role of acute distension in the induction of smooth muscle proliferation. Lab Invest 1989; 60:360–364.

74. Li G, Chen SJ, Oparil S, et al. Direct in vivo evidence demonstrating neointimal migration of adventitial fibroblasts after balloon injury of rat carotid arteries. Circulation 2000; 101:1362–1365.

75. Frosen J, Calderon-Ramirez L, Hayry P, et al. Quantitation of cell migration in a rat carotid artery balloon injury model. Indications for a perivascular origin of the neointimal cells. Cardiovasc Drugs Ther 2001; 15:437–444.

76. Siow RC, Mallawaarachchi CM, Weissberg PL. Migration of adventitial myofibroblasts following vascular balloon injury: insights from in vivo gene transfer to rat carotid arteries. Cardiovasc Res 2003; 59:212–221.

77. Lafont A, Faxon D. Why do animal models of post-angioplasty restenosis sometimes poorly predict the outcome of clinical trials? Cardiovasc Res 1998; 39:50–59.

78. Block PC, Baughman KL, Pasternak RC, et al. Transluminal angioplasty: correlation of morphologic and angiographic findings in an experimental model. Circulation 1980; 61:778–785.

79. Faxon DP, Weber VJ, Haudenschild C, et al. Acute effects of transluminal angioplasty in three experimental models of atherosclerosis. Arteriosclerosis 1982; 2: 125–133.

80. Faxon DP, Sanborn TA, Weber VJ, et al. Restenosis following transluminal angioplasty in experimental atherosclerosis. Arteriosclerosis 1984; 4:189–195.

81. Atkinson JB, Swift LL, Virmani R. Watanabe heritable hyperlipidemic rabbits. Familial hypercholesterolemia. Am J Pathol 1992; 140:749–753.

82. Carter AJ, Farb A, Gould KE, et al. The degree of neointimal formation after stent placement in atherosclerotic rabbit iliac arteries is dependent on the underlying plaque. Cardiovasc Pathol 1999; 8:73–80.

83. Oshima R, Ikeda T, Watanabe K, et al. Probucol treatment attenuates the aortic atherosclerosis in Watanabe heritable hyperlipidemic rabbits. Atherosclerosis 1998; 137:13–22.

84. Consigny PM, Tulenko TN, Nicosia RF. Immediate and long-term effects of angioplasty-balloon dilation on normal rabbit iliac artery. Arteriosclerosis 1986; 6:265–276.

85. Coats WD Jr., Currier JW, Faxon DP. Remodelling and restenosis: insights from animal studies. Semin Interv Cardiol 1997; 2:153–158.

86. Clarkson TB. Nonhuman primate models of atherosclerosis. Lab Anim Sci 1998; 8:569–572.

87. Giese NA, Marijianowski MM, McCook O, et al. The role of alpha and beta platelet-derived growth factor receptor in the vascular response to injury in non-human primates. Arterioscler Thromb Vasc Biol 1999; 19:900–909.

88. Sims FH, Gavin JB, Vanderwee MA. The intima of human coronary arteries. Am Heart J 1989; 118:32–38.

89. Geer JC, Guidry MA. Experimental canine atherosclerosis. In: Roberts JC Jr., Straus R, eds. Comparative Atherosclerosis: the Morphology of Spontaneous and Induced Atherosclerotic Lesions in Animals and Its Relation to Human Disease. New York, NY: Harper & Row, 1962:170–185.

90. Bates ER, McGillem MJ, Mickelson JK, et al. A monoclonal antibody against the platelet glycoprotein IIb/IIIa receptor complex prevents platelet aggregation and thrombosis in a canine model of coronary angioplasty. Circulation 1991; 84:2463–2469.

91. Roubin GS, Robinson KA, King SB III, et al. Early and late results of intracoronary arterial stenting after coronary angioplasty in dogs. Circulation 1987; 76:891–897.

92. Schatz RA, Palmaz JC, Tio FO, et al. Balloon-expandable intracoronary stents in the adult dog. Circulation 1987; 76:450–457.

93. Michel G. Swine in Biomedical Research. Seattle, WA: Frayn Printing Co., 1966.

94. Hughes HC. Swine in cardiovascular research. Lab Anim Sci 1986; 36:348–350.

95. Swindle MM, Horneffer PJ, Gardner TJ, et al. Anatomic and anesthetic considerations in experimental cardiopulmonary surgery in swine. Lab Anim Sci 1986; 36: 357–361.

96. Gal D, Rondione AJ, Slovekai GA, et al. Atherosclerotic Yucatan microswine: an animal model with high-grade fibrocalcific, nonfatty lesions suitable for testing catheter-based interventions. Am Heart J 1990; 119:291–300.

97. Vesselinovitch D. Animal models and the study of atherosclerosis. Arch Pathol Lab Med 1988; 112:1011–1017.

98. Reitman JS, Mahley RW, Fry DL. Yucatan miniature swine as a model for diet-induced atherosclerosis. Atherosclerosis 1982; 43:119–132.

99. Weiner BH, Ockene IS, Jarmolych J, et al. Comparison of pathologic and angiographic findings in a porcine preparation of coronary atherosclerosis. Circulation 1985; 72:1081–1086.

100. Carter AJ, Laird JR, Kufs WM, et al. Coronary stenting with a novel stainless steel balloon-expandable stent: determinants of neointimal formation and changes in arterial geometry after placement in an atherosclerotic model. J Am Coll Cardiol 1996; 27:1270–1277.

101. Post MJ, de Smet BJ, van der Helm Y, et al. Arterial remodeling after balloon angioplasty or stenting in an atherosclerotic experimental model. Circulation 1997; 96:996–1003.

102. Liu MW, Anderson PG, Luo JF, et al. Local delivery of ethanol inhibits intimal hyperplasia in pig coronary arteries after balloon injury. Circulation 1997; 96: 2295–2301.

103. Farb A, Virmani R, Atkinson JB, et al. Long-term histologic patency after percutaneous transluminal coronary angioplasty is predicted by the creation of a greater lumen area. J Am Coll Cardiol 1994; 24:1229–1235.

104. Anderson PG, Atkinson J. Atherosclerosis. In: McManus BMB, ed. Atlas of Cardiovascular Pathology. Philadelphia, PA: Current Medicine, 2001:60–78.

105. Schwartz RS, Murphy JG, Edwards WD, et al. Restenosis after balloon angioplasty. A practical proliferative model in porcine coronary arteries. Circulation 1990; 82:2190–2200.

106. Cox DA, Anderson PG, Roubin GS, et al. Effect of local delivery of heparin and methotrexate on neointimal proliferation in stented porcine coronary arteries. Coron Artery Dis 1992; 3:237–248.

107. Waller BF, Anderson PG. The pathology of interventional coronary artery techniques and devices. In: Topol EJ, ed. Textbook of Interventional Cardiology. Philadelphia, PA: W.B. Saunders Co., 1999.

108. Rodgers GP, Minor ST, Robinson K, et al. Adjuvant therapy for intracoronary stents. Investigations in atherosclerotic swine. Circulation 1990; 82:560–569.

109. Santoian EC, King SB III. Intravascular stents, intimal proliferation and restenosis. J Am Coll Cardiol 1992; 19:877–879.

110. Elias H, Hyde DM. An elementary introduction to stereology (quantitative microscopy). Am J Anat 1980; 159:412–446.

111. Reid IM. Morphometric methods in veterinary pathology: a review. Vet Pathol 1980; 17:522–543.

112. Weibel ER. Stereological Methods. Theoretical Foundations. London: Academic Press, 1980.

113. Virmani R, Kolodgie FD, Farb A, et al. Drug eluting stents: are human and animal studies comparable? Heart 2003; 89:133–138.

114. Nakazawa G, Finn AV, John MC, et al. The significance of preclinical evaluation of sirolimus-, paclitaxel-, and zotarolimus-eluting stents. Am J Cardiol 2007; 100:36M–44M.

115. Waksman R, Pakala R, Baffour R, et al. Efficacy and safety of pimecrolimus-eluting stents in porcine coronary arteries. Cardiovasc Revasc Med 2007; 8:259–274.

116. Rogers C, Edelman ER. Endovascular stent design dictates experimental restenosis and thrombosis. Circulation 1995; 91:2995–3001.

117. Barth KH, Virmani R, Froelich J, et al. Paired comparison of vascular wall reactions to Palmaz stents, Strecker tantalum stents, and Wallstents in canine iliac and femoral arteries. Circulation 1996; 93:2161–2169.

118. Sheth S, Litvack F, Dev V, et al. Subacute thrombosis and vascular injury resulting from slotted-tube nitinol and stainless steel stents in a rabbit carotid artery model. Circulation 1996; 94:1733–1740.

119. Escaned J, Goicolea J, Alfonso F, et al. Propensity and mechanisms of restenosis in different coronary stent designs: complementary value of the analysis of the luminal gain-loss relationship. J Am Coll Cardiol 1999; 34:1490–1497.

120. Garasic JM, Edelman ER, Squire JC, et al. Stent and artery geometry determine intimal thickening independent of arterial injury. Circulation 2000; 101:812–818.

121. Baim DS, Cutlip DE, Midei M, et al. Final results of a randomized trial comparing the MULTI-LINK stent with the Palmaz-Schatz stent for narrowings in native coronary arteries. Am J Cardiol 2001; 87:157–162.

122. Okabe T, Asakura Y, Ishikawa S, et al. Evaluation of scaffolding effects of five different types of stents by intravascular ultrasound analysis. Am J Cardiol 1999; 84:981–986.
123. Lansky AJ, Roubin GS, O'Shaughnessy CD, et al. Randomized comparison of GR-II stent and Palmaz-Schatz stent for elective treatment of coronary stenoses. Circulation 2000; 102:1364–1368.
124. Kastrati A, Mehilli J, Dirschinger J, et al. Intracoronary stenting and angiographic results: strut thickness effect on restenosis outcome (ISAR-STEREO) trial. Circulation 2001; 103:2816–2821.
125. Briguori C, Sarais C, Pagnotta P, et al. In-stent restenosis in small coronary arteries: impact of strut thickness. J Am Coll Cardiol 2002; 40:403–409.
126. Pache J, Kastrati A, Mehilli J, et al. Intracoronary stenting and angiographic results: strut thickness effect on restenosis outcome (ISAR-STEREO-2) trial. J Am Coll Cardiol 2003; 41:1283–1288.
127. Gurbel PA, Callahan KP, Malinin AI, et al. Could stent design affect platelet activation? Results of the Platelet Activation in STenting (PAST) Study. J Invasive Cardiol 2002; 14:584–589.
128. Reneman RS, Arts T, Hoeks AP. Wall shear stress—an important determinant of endothelial cell function and structure—in the arterial system in vivo. Discrepancies with theory. J Vasc Res 2006; 43:251–269.
129. Stone PH, Coskun AU, Kinlay S, et al. Effect of endothelial shear stress on the progression of coronary artery disease, vascular remodeling, and in-stent restenosis in humans: in vivo 6-month follow-up study. Circulation 2003; 108:438–444.
130. Chatzizisis YS, Coskun AU, Jonas M, et al. Role of endothelial shear stress in the natural history of coronary atherosclerosis and vascular remodeling: molecular, cellular, and vascular behavior. J Am Coll Cardiol 2007; 49:2379–2393.
131. Chatzizisis YS, Coskun AU, Jonas M, et al. Risk stratification of individual coronary lesions using local endothelial shear stress: a new paradigm for managing coronary artery disease. Curr Opin Cardiol 2007; 22:552–564.
132. Chatzizisis YS, Jonas M, Coskun AU, et al. Prediction of the localization of high-risk coronary atherosclerotic plaques on the basis of low endothelial shear stress: an intravascular ultrasound and histopathology natural history study. Circulation 2008; 117:993–1002.
133. Benard N, Coisne D, Donal E, et al. Experimental study of laminar blood flow through an artery treated by a stent implantation: characterisation of intra-stent wall shear stress. J Biomech 2003; 36:991–998.
134. LaDisa JF Jr., Guler I, Olson LE, et al. Three-dimensional computational fluid dynamics modeling of alterations in coronary wall shear stress produced by stent implantation. Ann Biomed Eng 2003; 31:972–980.
135. LaDisa JF Jr., Olson LE, Hettrick DA, et al. Axial stent strut angle influences wall shear stress after stent implantation: analysis using 3D computational fluid dynamics models of stent foreshortening. Biomed Eng Online 2005; 4:59.
136. LaDisa JF Jr., Olson LE, Guler I, et al. Stent design properties and deployment ratio influence indexes of wall shear stress: a three-dimensional computational fluid dynamics investigation within a normal artery. J Appl Physiol 2004; 97:424–430.
137. LaDisa JF Jr., Olson LE, Molthen RC, et al. Alterations in wall shear stress predict sites of neointimal hyperplasia after stent implantation in rabbit iliac arteries. Am J Physiol Heart Circ Physiol 2005; 288:H2465–H2475.

138. Seo T, Schachter LG, Barakat AI. Computational study of fluid mechanical disturbance induced by endovascular stents. Ann Biomed Eng 2005; 33:444–456.
139. Thubrikar MJ, Robicsek F. Pressure-induced arterial wall stress and atherosclerosis. Ann Thorac Surg 1995; 59:1594–1603.
140. Lally C, Dolan F, Prendergast PJ. Cardiovascular stent design and vessel stresses: a finite element analysis. J Biomech 2005; 38:1574–1581.
141. Ormiston JA, Dixon SR, Webster MW, et al. Stent longitudinal flexibility: a comparison of 13 stent designs before and after balloon expansion. Catheter Cardiovasc Interv 2000; 50:120–124.
142. Wentzel JJ, Whelan DM, van der Giessen WJ, et al. Coronary stent implantation changes 3-D vessel geometry and 3-D shear stress distribution. J Biomech 2000; 33:1287–1295.
143. LaDisa JF Jr., Olson LE, Douglas HA, et al. Alterations in regional vascular geometry produced by theoretical stent implantation influence distributions of wall shear stress: analysis of a curved coronary artery using 3D computational fluid dynamics modeling. Biomed Eng Online 2006; 5:40.
144. Taylor A. Metals. In: Sigwart U, ed. Endoluminal Stenting. London: WB Saunders, 1996:28–33.
145. Dion I, Baquey C, Candelon B, et al. Hemocompatibility of titanium nitride. Int J Artif Organs 1992; 15:617–621.
146. Dion I, Roques X, Baquey C, et al. Hemocompatibility of diamond-like carbon coating. Biomed Mater Eng 1993; 3:51–55.
147. Niimi Y, Yamane S, Yamaji K, et al. Protein adsorption and platelet adhesion on the surface of an oxygenator membrane. ASAIO J 1997; 43:M706–M710.
148. Werthen M, Sellborn A, Kalltorp M, et al. In vitro study of monocyte viability during the initial adhesion to albumin- and fibrinogen-coated surfaces. Biomaterials 2001; 22:827–832.
149. Thierry B, Merhi Y, Bilodeau L, et al. Nitinol versus stainless steel stents: acute thrombogenicity study in an ex vivo porcine model. Biomaterials 2002; 23: 2997–3005.
150. Botnar RM, Buecker A, Wiethoff AJ, et al. In vivo magnetic resonance imaging of coronary thrombosis using a fibrin-binding molecular magnetic resonance contrast agent. Circulation 2004; 110:1463–1466.
151. Santin M, Mikhalovska L, Lloyd AW, et al. In vitro host response assessment of biomaterials for cardiovascular stent manufacture. J Mater Sci Mater Med 2004; 15:473–477.
152. Simon C, Palmaz JC, Sprague EA. Protein interactions with endovascular prosthetic surfaces. J Long Term Eff Med Implants 2000; 10:127–141.
153. Sprague EA, Palmaz JC, Simon C, et al. Electrostatic forces on the surface of metals as measured by atomic force microscopy. J Long Term Eff Med Implants 2000;10:111–125.
154. Tepe G, Wendel HP, Khorchidi S, et al. Thrombogenicity of various endovascular stent types: an in vitro evaluation. J Vasc Interv Radiol 2002;13:1029–1035.
155. Shih CC, Shih CM, Su YY, et al. Impact on the thrombogenicity of surface oxide properties of 316l stainless steel for biomedical applications. J Biomed Mater Res A 2003; 67:1320–1328.
156. Clarke B, Kingshott P, Hou X, et al. Effect of nitinol wire surface properties on albumin adsorption. Acta Biomater 2007; 3:103–111.

157. Singh R, Dahotre NB. Corrosion degradation and prevention by surface modification of biometallic materials. J Mater Sci Mater Med 2007; 18:725–751.
158. ASTM-F86. Standard Practice for Surface Preparation and Marking of Metallic Surgical Implants. Annual Book of ASTM Standards: Medical Devices and Services. Philadelphia: American Society for Testing and Materials, 1995:6–8.
159. Shih CC, Shih CM, Chou KY, et al. Stability of passivated 316L stainless steel oxide films for cardiovascular stents. J Biomed Mater Res A 2007; 80:861–873.
160. Shih CC, Lin SJ, Chen YL, et al. The cytotoxicity of corrosion products of nitinol stent wire on cultured smooth muscle cells. J Biomed Mater Res 2000; 52:395–403.
161. Shih CC, Shih CM, Chen YL, et al. Growth inhibition of cultured smooth muscle cells by corrosion products of 316 L stainless steel wire. J Biomed Mater Res 2001; 57:200–207.
162. Eliades T, Pratsinis H, Kletsas D, et al. Characterization and cytotoxicity of ions released from stainless steel and nickel-titanium orthodontic alloys. Am J Orthod Dentofacial Orthop 2004; 125:24–29.
163. Messer RL, Mickalonis J, Lewis JB, et al. Interactions between stainless steel, shear stress, and monocytes. J Biomed Mater Res A 2007. doi:10.1002/jbm.a.31730.
164. Schmalz G, Schuster U, Schweikl H. Influence of metals on IL-6 release in vitro. Biomaterials 1998; 19:1689–1694.
165. Kastrati A, Schomig A, Dirschinger J, et al. Increased risk of restenosis after placement of gold-coated stents: results of a randomized trial comparing gold-coated with uncoated steel stents in patients with coronary artery disease. Circulation 2000; 101:2478–2483.
166. Nolan BW, Schermerhorn ML, Powell RJ, et al. Restenosis in gold-coated renal artery stents. J Vasc Surg 2005; 42:40–46.
167. Windecker S, Mayer I, De Pasquale G, et al. Stent coating with titanium-nitride-oxide for reduction of neointimal hyperplasia. Circulation 2001; 104:928–933.
168. Windecker S, Remondino A, Eberli FR, et al. Sirolimus-eluting and paclitaxel-eluting stents for coronary revascularization. N Engl J Med 2005; 353:653–662.
169. Gutensohn K, Beythien C, Bau J, et al. In vitro analyses of diamond-like carbon coated stents. Reduction of metal ion release, platelet activation, and thrombogenicity. Thromb Res 2000; 99:577–585.
170. Airoldi F, Colombo A, Tavano D, et al. Comparison of diamond-like carbon-coated stents versus uncoated stainless steel stents in coronary artery disease. Am J Cardiol 2004; 93:474–477.
171. Jung JH, Min PK, Kim JY, et al. Does a carbon ion-implanted surface reduce the restenosis rate of coronary stents? Cardiology 2005; 104:72–75.
172. Sick PB, Brosteanu O, Ulrich M, et al. Prospective randomized comparison of early and late results of a carbonized stent versus a high-grade stainless steel stent of identical design: the PREVENT Trial [corrected]. Am Heart J 2005; 149:681–688.
173. Brott BC, Halwani D, Anderson PG, et al. Scanning electron microscopy analysis of corrosion of stainless steel and nitinol stents from autopsy retrievals. J Am Coll Cardiol SCAI-ACCi2 Summit 2008; 51(10), Suppl 2:2900–305.
174. Halwani D, Brott BC, Anderson PG, et al. Local release of metallic ions from stents into vascular tissue. J Am Coll Cardiol SCAI-ACCi2 Summit 2008; 51(10), Suppl 2:2900–310.
175. Poon M, Marx SO, Gallo R, et al. Rapamycin inhibits vascular smooth muscle cell migration. J Clin Invest 1996; 98:2277–2283.

176. Matter CM, Rozenberg I, Jaschko A, et al. Effects of tacrolimus or sirolimus on proliferation of vascular smooth muscle and endothelial cells. J Cardiovasc Pharmacol 2006; 48:286–292.

177. Gallo R, Padurean A, Jayaraman T, et al. Inhibition of intimal thickening after balloon angioplasty in porcine coronary arteries by targeting regulators of the cell cycle. Circulation 1999; 99:2164–2170.

178. Suzuki T, Kopia G, Hayashi S, et al. Stent-based delivery of sirolimus reduces neointimal formation in a porcine coronary model. Circulation 2001; 104: 1188–1193.

179. Indolfi C, Mongiardo A, Curcio A, et al. Molecular mechanisms of in-stent restenosis and approach to therapy with eluting stents. Trends Cardiovasc Med 2003; 13:142–148.

180. Sollott SJ, Cheng L, Pauly RR, et al. Taxol inhibits neointimal smooth muscle cell accumulation after angioplasty in the rat. J Clin Invest 1995; 95:1869–1876.

181. Crown J, O'Leary M. The taxanes: an update. Lancet 2000; 355:1176–1178.

182. Rowinsky EK, Donehower RC. Paclitaxel (taxol). N Engl J Med 1995; 332: 1004–1014.

183. Parry TJ, Brosius R, Thyagarajan R, et al. Drug-eluting stents: sirolimus and paclitaxel differentially affect cultured cells and injured arteries. Eur J Pharmacol 2005; 524:19–29.

184. Drachman DE, Edelman ER, Seifert P, et al. Neointimal thickening after stent delivery of paclitaxel: change in composition and arrest of growth over six months. J Am Coll Cardiol 2000; 36:2325–2332.

185. Farb A, Heller PF, Shroff S, et al. Pathological analysis of local delivery of paclitaxel via a polymer-coated stent. Circulation 2001; 104:473–479.

186. Jabara R, Chronos N, Tondato F, et al. Toxic vessel reaction to an absorbable polymer-based paclitaxel-eluting stent in pig coronary arteries. J Invasive Cardiol 2006; 18:383–390.

187. Acharya G, Park K. Mechanisms of controlled drug release from drug-eluting stents. Adv Drug Deliv Rev 2006; 58:387–401.

188. Klugherz BD, Llanos G, Lieuallen W, et al. Twenty-eight-day efficacy and pharmacokinetics of the sirolimus-eluting stent. Coron Artery Dis 2002; 13:183–188.

189. Ranade SV, Miller KM, Richard RE, et al. Physical characterization of controlled release of paclitaxel from the TAXUS Express2 drug-eluting stent. J Biomed Mater Res A 2004; 71:625–634.

190. Kamath KR, Barry JJ, Miller KM. The Taxus (TM) drug-eluting stent: a new paradigm in controlled drug delivery. Adv Drug Deliv Rev 2006; 58:412–436.

191. Lewis AL, Tolhurst LA, Stratford PW. Analysis of a phosphorylcholine-based polymer coating on a coronary stent pre- and post-implantation. Biomaterials 2002; 23:1697–1706.

192. Burke SE, Kuntz RE, Schwartz LB. Zotarolimus (ABT-578) eluting stents. Adv Drug Deliv Rev 2006; 58:437–446.

193. Lewis AL. Phosphorylcholine-based polymers and their use in the prevention of biofouling. Colloids Surf B Biointerfaces 2000; 18:261–275.

194. Chen YW, Smith ML, Sheets M, et al. Zotarolimus, a novel sirolimus analogue with potent anti-proliferative activity on coronary smooth muscle cells and reduced potential for systemic immunosuppression. J Cardiovasc Pharmacol 2007; 49:228–235.

195. Carter AJ, Brodeur A, Collingwood R, et al. Experimental efficacy of an everolimus eluting cobalt chromium stent. Catheter Cardiovasc Interv 2006; 68:97–103.

196. Creel CJ, Lovich MA, Edelman ER. Arterial paclitaxel distribution and deposition. Circ Res 2000; 86:879–884.

197. Hwang CW, Wu D, Edelman ER. Physiological transport forces govern drug distribution for stent-based delivery. Circulation 2001; 104:600–605.

198. Hwang CW, Edelman ER. Arterial ultrastructure influences transport of locally delivered drugs. Circ Res 2002; 90:826–832.

199. Levin AD, Vukmirovic N, Hwang CW, et al. Specific binding to intracellular proteins determines arterial transport properties for rapamycin and paclitaxel. Proc Natl Acad Sci U S A 2004; 101:9463–9467.

200. Hwang CW, Levin AD, Jonas M, et al. Thrombosis modulates arterial drug distribution for drug-eluting stents. Circulation 2005; 111:1619–1626.

201. Finn AV, Kolodgie FD, Harnek J, et al. Differential response of delayed healing and persistent inflammation at sites of overlapping sirolimus- or paclitaxel-eluting stents. Circulation 2005; 112:270–278.

202. Balakrishnan B, Tzafriri AR, Seifert P, et al. Strut position, blood flow, and drug deposition: implications for single and overlapping drug-eluting stents. Circulation 2005; 111:2958–2965.

203. Kimura T, Yokoi H, Nakagawa Y, et al. Three-year follow-up after implantation of metallic coronary-artery stents. N Engl J Med 1996; 334:561–566.

204. Carter AJ, Aggarwal M, Kopia GA, et al. Long-term effects of polymer-based, slow-release, sirolimus-eluting stents in a porcine coronary model. Cardiovasc Res 2004; 63:617–624.

205. Sudhir K. US FDA: Abbott Vascular Drug Eluting Stent Program. Available at: http://www.fda.gov/ohrms/dockets/ac/06/slides/2006–4253oph2_18_Sudhir.pdf, 2006.

206. Morice MC, Serruys PW, Sousa JE, et al. A randomized comparison of a sirolimus-eluting stent with a standard stent for coronary revascularization. N Engl J Med 2002; 346:1773–1780.

207. Grube E, Silber S, Hauptmann KE, et al. TAXUS I: six- and twelve-month results from a randomized, double-blind trial on a slow-release paclitaxel-eluting stent for de novo coronary lesions. Circulation 2003; 107:38–42.

208. Moses JW, Leon MB, Popma JJ, et al. Sirolimus-eluting stents versus standard stents in patients with stenosis in a native coronary artery. N Engl J Med 2003; 349:1315–1323.

209. Stone GW, Ellis SG, Cox DA, et al. One-year clinical results with the slow-release, polymer-based, paclitaxel-eluting TAXUS stent: the TAXUS-IV trial. Circulation 2004; 109:1942–1947.

210. Moses JW. Clinician's Perspective on Drug-Eluting Stents: Balancing Safety and Efficacy. US FDA, 2008.

211. Popma JJ, Weiner B, Cowley MJ, et al. FDA advisory panel on the safety and efficacy of drug-eluting stents: summary of findings and recommendations. J Interv Cardiol 2007; 20:425–446.

212. Colombo A, Drzewiecki J, Banning A, et al. Randomized study to assess the effectiveness of slow- and moderate-release polymer-based paclitaxel-eluting stents for coronary artery lesions. Circulation 2003; 108:788–794.

213. Stone GW, Ellis SG, Cannon L, et al. Comparison of a polymer-based paclitaxel-eluting stent with a bare metal stent in patients with complex coronary artery disease: a randomized controlled trial. JAMA 2005; 294:1215–1223.

214. Morice MC, Serruys PW, Barragan P, et al. Long-term clinical outcomes with sirolimus-eluting coronary stents: five-year results of the RAVEL trial. J Am Coll Cardiol 2007; 50:1299–1304.

215. Sousa JE, Costa MA, Abizaid A, et al. Four-year angiographic and intravascular ultrasound follow-up of patients treated with sirolimus-eluting stents. Circulation 2005; 111:2326–2329.

216. Schampaert E, Moses JW, Schofer J, et al. Sirolimus-eluting stents at two years: a pooled analysis of SIRIUS, E-SIRIUS, and C-SIRIUS with emphasis on late revascularizations and stent thromboses. Am J Cardiol 2006; 98:36–41.

217. Stone GW, Ellis SG, Cox DA, et al. A polymer-based, paclitaxel-eluting stent in patients with coronary artery disease. N Engl J Med 2004; 350:221–231.

218. Dibra A, Kastrati A, Mehilli J, et al. Paclitaxel-eluting or sirolimus-eluting stents to prevent restenosis in diabetic patients. N Engl J Med 2005; 353:663–670.

219. Mehilli J, Dibra A, Kastrati A, et al. Randomized trial of paclitaxel- and sirolimus-eluting stents in small coronary vessels. Eur Heart J 2006; 27:260–266.

220. Morice MC, Colombo A, Meier B, et al. Sirolimus- vs paclitaxel-eluting stents in de novo coronary artery lesions: the REALITY trial: a randomized controlled trial. JAMA 2006; 295:895–904.

221. Kastrati A, Dibra A, Eberle S, et al. Sirolimus-eluting stents vs paclitaxel-eluting stents in patients with coronary artery disease: meta-analysis of randomized trials. JAMA 2005; 294:819–825.

222. Fajadet J, Wijns W, Laarman GJ, et al. Randomized, double-blind, multicenter study of the Endeavor zotarolimus-eluting phosphorylcholine-encapsulated stent for treatment of native coronary artery lesions: clinical and angiographic results of the ENDEAVOR II trial. Circulation 2006; 114:798–806.

223. Kandzari DE, Leon MB, Popma JJ, et al. Comparison of zotarolimus-eluting and sirolimus-eluting stents in patients with native coronary artery disease: a randomized controlled trial. J Am Coll Cardiol 2006; 48:2440–2447.

224. Miyazawa A, Ako J, Hongo Y, et al. Comparison of vascular response to zotarolimus-eluting stent versus sirolimus-eluting stent: intravascular ultrasound results from ENDEAVOR III. Am Heart J 2008; 155:108–113.

225. NIH. The ENDEAVOR IV Clinical Trial. Available at: http://ClinicalTrials.gov/ National Library of Medicine, 2008.

226. Tsuchiya Y, Lansky AJ, Costa RA, et al. Effect of everolimus-eluting stents in different vessel sizes (from the pooled FUTURE I and II trials). Am J Cardiol 2006; 98:464–469.

227. NIH. SPIRIT III Clinical Trial of the XIENCET V Everolimus Eluting Coronary Stent System (EECSS). Available at: http://ClinicalTrials.gov/National Library of Medicine, 2008.

228. Daemen J, Wenaweser P, Tsuchida K, et al. Early and late coronary stent thrombosis of sirolimus-eluting and paclitaxel-eluting stents in routine clinical practice: data from a large two-institutional cohort study. Lancet 2007; 369:667–678.

229. Kuchulakanti PK, Chu WW, Torguson R, et al. Correlates and long-term outcomes of angiographically proven stent thrombosis with sirolimus- and paclitaxel-eluting stents. Circulation 2006; 113:1108–1113.

230. Iakovou I, Schmidt T, Bonizzoni E, et al. Incidence, predictors, and outcome of thrombosis after successful implantation of drug-eluting stents. JAMA 2005; 293:2126–2130.

231. Mauri L, Hsieh WH, Massaro JM, et al. Stent thrombosis in randomized clinical trials of drug-eluting stents. N Engl J Med 2007; 356:1020–1029.

232. Joner M, Finn AV, Farb A, et al. Pathology of drug-eluting stents in humans: delayed healing and late thrombotic risk. J Am Coll Cardiol 2006; 48:193–202.

233. Nebeker JR, Virmani R, Bennett CL, et al. Hypersensitivity cases associated with drug-eluting coronary stents: a review of available cases from the Research on Adverse Drug Events and Reports (RADAR) project. J Am Coll Cardiol 2006; 47:175–181.

234. Luscher TF, Steffel J, Eberli FR, et al. Drug-eluting stent and coronary thrombosis: biological mechanisms and clinical implications. Circulation 2007; 115:1051–1058.

235. Stone GW, Moses JW, Ellis SG, et al. Safety and efficacy of sirolimus- and paclitaxel-eluting coronary stents. N Engl J Med 2007; 356:998–1008.

236. FDA. FDA advises physicians of adverse events associated with Cordis Cypher coronary stents. U.S. Food and Drug Administration Public Health Web Notification. T03-71 ed., 2003.

237. FDA. FDA updates information for physicians on Cordis Cypher Stent. U.S. Food and Drug Administration Public Health Web Notification. T03-81 ed., 2003.

238. Virmani R, Guagliumi G, Farb A, et al. Localized hypersensitivity and late coronary thrombosis secondary to a sirolimus-eluting stent: should we be cautious? Circulation 2004; 109:701–705.

239. Togni M, Windecker S, Cocchia R, et al. Sirolimus-eluting stents associated with paradoxic coronary vasoconstriction. J Am Coll Cardiol 2005; 46:231–236.

240. Hofma SH, van der Giessen WJ, van Dalen BM, et al. Indication of long-term endothelial dysfunction after sirolimus-eluting stent implantation. Eur Heart J 2006; 27:166–170.

241. Jeanmart H, Malo O, Carrier M, et al. Comparative study of cyclosporine and tacrolimus vs newer immunosuppressants mycophenolate mofetil and rapamycin on coronary endothelial function. J Heart Lung Transplant 2002; 21:990–998.

242. Shin DI, Kim PJ, Seung KB, et al. Drug-eluting stent implantation could be associated with long-term coronary endothelial dysfunction. Int Heart J 2007; 48: 553–567.

243. Kim JW, Suh SY, Choi CU, et al. Six-month comparison of coronary endothelial dysfunction associated with sirolimus-eluting stent versus Paclitaxel-eluting stent. J Am Coll Cardiol 2008; 1:65–71.

244. Brott BC, Anayiotos AS, Chapman GD, et al. Severe, diffuse coronary artery spasm after drug-eluting stent placement. J Invasive Cardiol 2006; 18:584–592.

245. Wheatcroft S, Byrne J, Thomas M, et al. Life-threatening coronary artery spasm following sirolimus-eluting stent deployment. J Am Coll Cardiol 2006; 47: 1911–1912; author reply 1912–1913.

246. Turkoglu S, Simsek V, Abaci A. Possible anaphylactic reaction to taxus stent: a case report. Catheter Cardiovasc Interv 2005; 66:554–556.

247. Meier P, Zbinden R, Togni M, et al. Coronary collateral function long after drug-eluting stent implantation. J Am Coll Cardiol 2007; 49:15–20.

16

The Arterial Media as a Target of Structural and Functional Injury by Chemicals

Paul J. Boor

*Department of Pathology, University of Texas Medical Branch,
Galveston, Texas, U.S.A.*

Daniel J. Conklin

*Department of Medicine, Division of Cardiology, University of Louisville,
Louisville, Kentucky, U.S.A.*

INTRODUCTION

The vasculature, which is a complex and highly integrated system of conduits, is deceptively simple from the standpoint of the cellular composition of each individual blood vessel. All vessels of the entire vasculature are composed, at most, of only two cell types, the endothelial cell and the vascular smooth muscle cell. Vessels of all sizes are also surrounded by the specialized supporting cells and structures known as the adventitia. The space around capillaries, which varies greatly from tissue to tissue, also contains an additional cell, the pericyte, which is not contractile and about which relatively little is known. Large muscular arteries, elastic arteries, and veins are surrounded by adventitial fibroblastic cells and a great number of other specialized structures, including nervous tissue and, in the case of large elastic arteries, vasa vasorum. Thus, while the basic cellular components of blood vessels per se are simple, the characteristics of these elements vary greatly from vessel to vessel and the integration of varying types of blood vessel with adjacent structures is quite complex.

The endothelial cells lining the vasculature vary greatly in the basic "barrier" function they serve between blood and tissue through their highly specialized cell-cell junctions. The tightest barrier regulation is achieved by brain capillaries (which are responsible for the well-known blood-brain barrier). Much looser control of transvascular movement is exerted by the endothelial linings of specialized sinusoids that are found in liver, spleen, bone marrow, adrenal glands, and hypophysis. The endothelial cells that line the large capillaries of the liver, known as hepatic sinusoids, form the only truly discontinuous endothelium. These specialized endothelial cells, or Kupffer cells, are highly phagocytic and frequently overlap without tight junctions at their borders, as do lymphatic endothelial cells (1).

The structures and consequently the functions of the media of blood vessels also differ from vessel to vessel, perhaps to an even greater degree than endothelium. The vascular media is composed of vascular smooth muscle cells and an intercellular matrix that varies dramatically in composition from the largest to the smallest arteries and between arteries and veins. In the large elastic arteries and muscular arteries, which are the focus of this chapter, the muscle layers and medial composition lend these vessels their unique physical and physiologic properties. The large elastic arteries, i.e., the aorta and vessels of the aortic arch, are rich in elastin (ELN) aligned in heavy concentric bands, or lamellae. The vascular smooth muscle cells in these larger vessels function primarily in the production and maintenance of interstitial molecules, especially the complex proteins ELN and collagen that give tensile strength and elasticity to the arterial wall. The medium-sized muscular arteries have a relative paucity of elastic lamellae, which is more suited to the more pronounced contractile function that these vessels serve. As the arterial vasculature tapers further, the contractile function of arterioles exquisitely controls blood flow to the tissues. This control is also affected and modified by neural mechanisms and numerous circulating paracrine influences.

This chapter addresses medial injury. Thus, the vascular smooth muscle cell is the prime cell of interest for these discussions. Specific emphasis will be placed on environmental chemicals or drugs as etiologic agents of both structural and functional effects on the media. Examples of both the pathologic lesions that are caused by chemicals and the aberrations of normal vascular function that may result will be discussed. Emphasis will be placed on human diseases with great clinical importance and also on potential human exposure to chemicals or drugs that may be injurious to the vascular media and medial function. Because the blood vessel is a well-integrated functional and structural unit, it is often difficult to sort out the role of endothelium versus that of vascular smooth muscle cells. Wherever possible, an attempt will be made to clarify the contribution of different cell types to the pathobiology that is reflected in the arterial media. Furthermore, the hugely important topic of atherosclerosis will not be addressed in any great depth, since this topic is discussed elsewhere in this volume.

MEDIAL INJURY—STRUCTURAL

The major structural alteration that follows medial injury is the arterial aneurysm. On the basis of the structural pathology that characterizes them, both human and experimental arterial aneurysms may be divided conveniently into two types, dilated aneurysms and dissecting aneurysms. Dilatation, or an increase in vascular diameter, is the hallmark of dilated types of aneurysms. The increase in vascular diameter may occur concentrically, or along one side of the vessel only, forming a prominent outpouching, or irregular dilated area described as a saccular aneurysm. Whether dilatation is concentric or saccular, an increase in vascular diameter is almost universally accompanied by thinning of the vascular wall, primarily of the media, at the site of the aneurysm. The human abdominal aortic aneurysm (AAA) will be reviewed briefly in this section, but it should be mentioned that localized dilated aneurysms can form in virtually any large to midsized artery secondary to localized trauma or infection.

The other type of aneurysm, the dissecting aneurysm, is actually somewhat of a misnomer, because "dissecting" or "dissection" refers to tearing or splitting of the vascular wall, or media, of a medium-sized to large artery, frequently resulting in rupture of the vessel and death. Hence, the true medial diameter of a dissecting aneurysm may or may not be increased, but rather the media is torn, or dissected, by blood under systemic arterial pressure. Often, it should be mentioned, the definitive type of aneurysm resulting from experimental chemical-induced arterial damage is not clear, or the structural damage may actually result in both dissection and dilation.

Abdominal Aortic Aneurysm

By far the most frequent of dilated types of aneurysms is the AAA. AAA is a deadly disease of humans characterized by the dilatation, weakening, and sudden rupture of the lower, abdominal, or infrarenal portion of the largest elastic artery—the aorta. Recent clinical and basic science studies support the idea that the progressive dilatation of aorta that is characteristic of AAA is caused by structural weakening of the aortic wall's connective tissues, especially of ELN. AAA is a common disorder and a frequent cause of rapid or sudden death, especially prevalent in men older than 60 years. In the United States, AAA is the 13th leading cause of death, and its incidence appears to be rising, most likely due to increased diagnosis and an aging population (2,3). AAA causes fatalities by acutely rupturing into the abdominal cavity or by hemorrhaging into adjacent structures such as retroperitoneum, duodenum, or colon. Slower, or recurrent, hemorrhage leads to a host of symptoms that prove extremely difficult to diagnose, although these clinical scenarios may lead to death within a matter of days or weeks.

Autopsy studies estimate the incidence of AAA at 1% to 6% (3). However, sensitive clinical methods of detecting aneurysmal dilatation of the aorta show a fairly high prevalence of asymptomatic aneurysms. For instance, the ultrasound screening study of Collin et al. (4) found an incidence of 5.4% in men between the ages of 65 and 74; nearly half of these were 4 cm or greater in diameter—a size that is associated with more rapid widening and clinically significant symptoms that indicate the need for surgical aneurysm repair. Improved diagnosis and treatment have raised serious cost-efficiency issues about screening programs and surgical intervention (5). Although AAA is a known, common cause of morbidity and mortality in the elderly, it has received much less experimental interest than other aging-associated vascular diseases.

Since the original report in 1977 of a family with a high incidence of AAA (6), a wealth of clinical studies have supported the idea that AAA is a familial disorder. Large studies have found that the relative risk of AAA for siblings of a proband case is from 10% to 20% (3). The study of Bengtsson et al. (7), which used clinically sensitive prospective screening methods, confirmed that male relatives of patients stricken with AAA have a remarkably high incidence (29%) of asymptomatic AAA themselves. While the familial aggregation of AAA appears indisputable, very few studies have addressed its genetic mode of inheritance. Some authors have proposed an X-chromosome-linked dominant form as well as a less frequent autosomal dominant form. Verloes et al. suggest that in AAA—a common disorder with late onset—irregular familial expression may be due to partial or age-dependent penetrance, polygenic inheritance, the effect of environmental factors, or possibly a combination of factors (3). Although several genes have been proposed as candidates that play a role in the vascular weakening that leads to AAA, none have been definitely implicated experimentally. Candidate genes include those associated with collagen or ELN metabolism and the matrix metalloproteinases (MMPs) (8–11).

Although the etiology of AAA is not completely understood, much suggests that chemical exposure, especially cigarette smoking, may be a factor. Historically, AAA had been viewed as a complication of atherosclerosis; however, in recent years, AAA has been clearly *disassociated* from the ubiquitous pathologic process of atherosclerosis. The current thought is that atherosclerosis is at least in part a *secondary* event in AAA, occurring because of flow abnormalities in the dilated aorta. Many of the human risk factors for atherosclerosis do not appear to correlate well with AAA. For instance, hypertension and smoking are the only atherosclerotic risk factors epidemiologically associated with AAA, but smoking is thought by many to represent an environmental factor only in genetically susceptible individuals (2,3). An additional risk factor for rupture of AAA is chronic obstructive lung disease, which is not a risk factor for atherosclerosis (12). Overall, observations on the familial incidence of AAA, as well as most other studies, suggest that AAA results from an age-related process of ELN loss, with consequent weakening in normal elastic properties, most marked in the distal aorta, where AAA occurs. This process is likely hastened by alterations in collagen and ELN metabolism, and the role of metalloproteinases (8,9) in this process may also be enhanced by chemical exposures such as cigarette smoking and air pollution. The specific toxins involved, however, have not been adequately defined.

No completely satisfactory experimental model of AAA exists. Toxin-induced models of medial vascular injury, which have been a long-term focus of this laboratory, have been thought for years to be due to inhibition of the well-characterized connective tissue enzyme, lysyl oxidase (13). These intoxications, however, are also associated with systemic bone, connective tissue, and even central nervous system abnormalities, and the vascular lesions affect aorta diffusely, rather than localizing to the distal aorta, as does AAA. Spontaneous aneurysms in the turkey, as well as those produced by copper deficiency, have also been linked to alterations in lysyl oxidase. The *blotchy* (*Blo*), or "mottled," mouse may represent the experimental model most close to the human disease. This X-linked mutation results in aortic aneurysms at all sites of aorta, including the ascending thoracic portion (14). The genetic phenotype is also characterized by coat and skin changes, skeletal and neurologic abnormalities, abnormal copper metabolism, and defects in collagen metabolism. Recent evidence indicates that the mottled gene is homologous to the gene identified in human Menkes disease, a rare disease with a wide constellation of findings, including the development of thoracic aortic aneurysms (14). Finally, surgical manipulations in rats, designed to physically weaken the abdominal aorta by local digestion with elastase or other means, have been used to simulate aneurysm development (15). In summary, no animal model appears to mimic the particular anatomic distribution or structural changes of the human disease exactly.

Dissecting Aortic Aneurysm

Dissection is the tearing or splitting of the vascular wall, or media, of a medium-sized to large artery, frequently resulting in sudden death. The largest elastic artery—the aorta—is by far the most common site for dissection to begin, and dissecting aortic aneurysm (DAA) almost universally involves the thoracic aorta, with splitting extending into abdominal aorta, or virtually any branching vessel (16). The true incidence of DAA in the United States (as distinct from the more common, dilated AAA) is difficult to know. A large international registry suggests an incidence of 5 to 30 per million person-years (17), corresponding to as many as 10,000 DAA in the United States annually. In a large Japanese study of over 10,000 medicolegal deaths (18), ruptured DAA accounted for 170 sudden deaths, which was more than three times the number dying from acute myocarditis and far greater than the deaths due to Takayasu's arteritis. For unknown reasons, a dramatic seasonal variation in DAA deaths occurs in Japan, with the peak in the winter months (18). In the United States, there is growing recognition of DAA as a deadly and frequently undiagnosed disorder in young adults (19).

Clinically, DAAs are classified according to extent of aortic involvement—from ascending aorta alone (DeBakey classification type II) to ascending and descending aorta (DeBakey classification type I) (20). The vast majority of

DAAs, therefore, involve the ascending aorta and aortic arch, where the great vessels of the upper body (carotids, etc.) arise. This is distinctly different from AAA, which occurs in the lower aorta (see above). Clinical diagnosis of DAA is difficult, but if diagnosed quickly, appropriate surgical therapy is well described and carries a 25% to 31% in-hospital mortality (21,22). Recently, percutaneous stent placement has been employed successfully (17). Isolated dissection of smaller vessels also occurs in the absence of aortic involvement. For instance, isolated dissection of coronary arteries has recently been recognized as a cause of sudden death in women in the peripartum period (23). Similarly, Murai et al. reported that 40% of fatal, spontaneous intracranial subarachnoid hemorrhages are due to isolated vertebral arterial dissection of unknown cause (24).

DAA is two- to threefold more frequent in men. In younger patients (ages 20s–30s), it may be associated with Marfan syndrome or other connective tissue disorders. However, a familial occurrence of isolated DAA has also been established with autosomal dominant inheritance in the absence of stigmata of Marfan or other connective tissue syndrome (25). Surprisingly, the majority of DAA occurs without known association to connective tissue disorders (26), and are considered "sporadic." DAA is associated with hypertension in patients older than 60 years. A high incidence of DAA is found in the third trimester of pregnancy. DAA is also a known complication of aortic defects such as inflammatory aortitis (Takayasu's arteritis), coarctation of the aorta, bicuspid aortic valve, and rare congenital aortic valve abnormalities linked to mutations in the ELN gene (discussed below).

DAAs are usually characterized as having an entrance point (Fig. 1) and often an exit point, establishing large tracts or "false lumens" that dissect through the media (Fig. 2). These tracts may completely encircle the aorta or may break out, causing massive hemorrhage into pleural cavities or pericardium, which are common causes of the rapid, sudden death associated with human DAA. Microscopically, the tears typically run along the heavy, parallel layers of ELN, or elastic lamellae, of the great thoracic vessels (Fig. 2). Historically, DAAs have been ascribed to a medial lesion known as "Erdheim's cystic medial necrosis," or "degeneration," which is characterized by medial areas devoid of ELN that accumulate mucopolysaccharides (27). This pathologic lesion is not universally found in DAA, even in genetically well-characterized cases of Marfan syndrome.

Etiology of DAA as a "Connective Tissue" Disorder

It is generally accepted that changes in the structural components of the vascular wall are the precursor to dissection, but the details of these structural changes are not completely understood. Although hypertension may play a role in precipitating arterial dissection, hypertension by itself should not rupture a normal adult aorta, since it was shown over 50 years ago that a normal aorta will not tear until an intravascular pressure many times greater than physiologic pressure is reached (16,28). The pathologic changes in the media that predispose to DAA

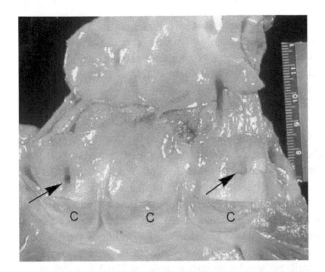

Figure 1 DAA in a 28-year-old male with Marfan syndrome. Opened ascending aorta, aortic valve cusps (c), and coronary artery ostia (*arrows*) indicated massive tear begins in first part of ascending aorta. Tear extended ("dissected") into the cartoid arteries and into the pericardial sac, causing sudden death. *Abbreviation*: DAA, dissecting aortic aneurysm.

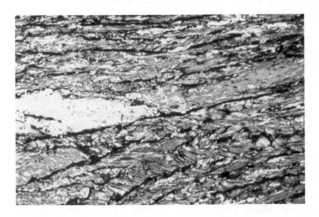

Figure 2 Microscopic view of edge of human dissection (*space*) splitting aortic media; elastin layers, or "lamellae," are black. (Movat's stain; patient with Marfan syndrome as in Fig. 1).

are thought to involve the complex, layered matrix proteins that give this largest of vessels its strength and elasticity—*collagen* and *elastin*. The collagens give tensile strength to the vascular wall, while the elastic layers or "lamellae" provide elasticity. The intricately interconnected elastic lamellae are a complex mix of the large, complex protein, ELN, laid down on a substrate of the microfibrillar protein, fibrillin (FBN), and tethered together by collagen. This structural complex—ELN plus collagens I and III—makes up greater than 95% of the extracellular matrix. Another 3% is a mixture of proteoglycans, of which more than 30 have been identified. Many other, less abundant proteins are thought to contribute to the extracellular matrix. Recent interest has also focused on the family of matrix MMPs that includes a great number of enzymes capable of degrading matrix proteins including collagen, ELN, laminin, fibronectin, and the proteoglycans (8–11).

Three-dimensional structural changes have been defined in the aortic ELN of patients with DAA; these consist of marked thinning of lamellae with less interconnection, fraying of ELN fibers, and gross disruption or "cystic" areas, as described above (29). Biochemically, a decrease in total ELN has been documented, with decreased cross-linked, or mature ELN, and increased type I collagen. These structural and biochemical changes are also known to occur with aging (30,31), accompanied by alterations in MMPs, remodeling of the vascular wall, and aortic stiffening and dilatation. Although many of these factors may be operative in the vascular wall, no single initiating cause of DAA is evident.

Genetic Aspects of DAA—ELN Gene

Human mutations in the ELN gene result in a wide variety of abnormalities. It is a reflection of the complexity of the aortic interstitium; however, none of the known human or experimentally-induced ELN gene defects results in DAA. For example, the disorder "supravalvular aortic stenosis" is an autosomal dominant disorder associated with point mutations of ELN, with a predominance of premature termination mutations the majority being nonsense and frameshift mutations (25,32). Supravalvular aortic stenosis is characterized by diffuse or localized *narrowing* of the ascending aorta accompanied by marked *thickening* of the vascular media. Elastic lamellae are irregular and disrupted, and vascular smooth muscle cells are hypertrophic. Other ELN mutations result in the skin disease known as cutix laxa, a disorder characterized by redundant, loose, sagging, and inelastic skin (33). Hence, none of the known human ELN defects show vascular changes at all similar to DAA.

Experimental deletion of the ELN gene in mice ($ELN^{-/-}$) results in a total lack of ELN in the aorta and other large elastic arteries (34). Surprisingly, however, all arteries examined in these animals (including aorta) undergo striking *obliterative* lesions, which are due to proliferating medial vascular smooth muscle cells occurring in the late gestational and early postnatal period. Mice presumably die from the occlusive vascular lesions by day 5 of life. On the basis of these findings, a major regulatory function for ELN in embryonic morphogenesis of blood vessels has been suggested, expanding the role of ELN from a simple structural component to an essential determinant of normal vascular development. A regulatory role for ELN has also been suggested in the remodeling that follows vascular injury. It has recently been proposed that integrins and a variety of matrix molecules contribute to vascular repair, remodeling, and response to mechanical stress through the exposure of specific intra-molecular sites that regulate cell adhesion, migration, and proliferation (35–42).

Genetic Aspects of DAA—FBN Genes (FBN1, FBN2)

Marfan syndrome is an autosomal dominant disorder with ocular and skeletal pathology, and a high incidence of DAA, which is a frequent cause of sudden death. It has long been established that classic Marfan syndrome is associated with mutations in the gene for FBN1, which codes for a 350 kDa glycoprotein that is widely distributed in the body as a major component of the microfibrillar system and is largely responsible for the mechanical properties of elastic fibers (25,43). Well over a hundred FBN1 mutations have been catalogued; the majority of mutations causing Marfan are missense mutations, occurring in one of the 47 tandemly repeated EGF-like domains (25). The cellular metabolism of FBN has been well studied; it results from a series of posttranslational modifications, including proteolytic processing of a proprotein, profibrillin-1. Marfan patients exhibit markedly depressed biochemical levels of FBN, and structural studies of Marfan microfibrils show a lack of identifiable fibrils, deranged assembly, and abnormalities in morphology.

The wide spectrum of FBN1-related syndromes exhibits a continuum of phenotypes. For instance, a large family of patients with isolated DAA (without other Marfan phenotype) was found to have a mutation in exon 26; a similar family was described with mutations in the region of exon 27. Other defects in FBN1 result in a wide variety of skin and visceral effects (as in systemic sclerosis, or scleroderma) or severe skeletal abnormalities (congenital contractural arachnodactyly, or Beals syndrome). Thus, a wide range of human mutations and phenotypic aberrations have been ascribed to the FBN1 gene. Experimental manipulation of the FBN1 gene in animals, however, has not been achieved. Similarly, the lack of experimental cell strains that synthesize FBN2 has slowed progress in its understanding. Although 90% of Marfan patients studied have been found to exhibit genetic defects in FBN1, recent defects in transforming growth factor beta (TGFβ), specifically in TGFβ type 2 receptor (TGFβR2), a putative tumor suppressor gene associated with known connective tissue disorders have been described (44,45). These patients exhibit prominent cardiovascular-skeletal phenotypes, including DAA, but are negative in FBN1 genetic screening.

Genetic Aspects of DAA—Collagen Knockouts

A great deal has been learned about collagen metabolism through targeted mutations. Specifically, genetic manipulations of the genes-encoding collagens I, II, V, and IX have added to the understanding of these collagens' localization and function (46–49). Most relevant to DAA, however, is the recent inactivation of the gene-encoding collagen type III (Col3A1) in mutant mice created by Liu et al. (50). In their study, homozygous Col3A1$^{-/-}$ mice had a survival of 5% at weaning and a phenotype that includes DAA morphologically identical to the developmental DAA recently described by our laboratory (51). Col3A1$^{-/-}$mice die from ruptured DAA and also show intestinal enlargement and rupture and defective wound healing. Liu et al. suggest that lack of type III collagen disrupts normal collagen fibrillogenesis and results in defective mature collagen type I fibrils in the media and adventitia of aorta as well as in collagen of skin, lung, and heart. Collagen type III acts as a "procollagen" critically involved in fibrillogenesis and maturation of collagen type I, the main structural collagen in the adult. Interestingly, collagen type III is most abundant in vascular, and other, highly elastic tissues such as bowel, lung, and skin. Further support for a role of Col3A1 in defective aortic connective tissue is the demonstration of frameshift mutations in the Col3A1 gene in patients with Ehlers-Danlos syndrome type IV, the dominantly inherited form of the disease characterized by large-joint hypermobility, thin and fragile skin, classic DAA, and bowel rupture (52).

Environmental Exposures and DAA

Few examples of arterial dissection related to environmental exposures are known. Copper deficiency induces vascular lesions with similarities to DAA in several species (13). Toxin-induced models of medial vascular injury characterized by vascular smooth muscle cell degeneration and defective collagen and ELN cross-linking have been known for years as "lathyrism" or "angiolathyrism." The classic lathyrogenic intoxicant is ß-aminopropionitrile, the toxic component of the toxic sweet pea *Lathyrus odoratus*. ß-aminopropionitrile intoxication results in systemic bone, connective tissue, and central nervous system abnormalities. Vascular lesions include overt medial necrosis and degeneration of matrix proteins with ELN fragmentation and dissolution (13). It is generally agreed that lathyrism is due to inhibition of the collagen cross-linking enzyme, lysyl oxidase, by ß-aminopropionitrile. The degenerative changes in aortas, however, are not localized to the thoracic aorta as in DAA and include bizarre chondroid and osseous metaplasia of the media (13). These changes, while potentially leading to aortic rupture, differ from the more subtle changes found in DAA.

Other Environmental Concerns

The recent discovery of trace amounts of semicarbazide in bottled baby foods (as a contaminant from Press On-Twist Off® cap technology) has raised serious concern in the food industry and prompted a review of semicarbazide toxicity (53). Semicarbazide is deemed a weak carcinogen, causing lung and vascular tumors in mice at high doses (54,55). A single fetal exposure study (51) found that high doses of semicarbazide cause embryonic or fetal death and cleft palate in surviving fetuses in rats, although no mention of vascular malformations was made (56). On the basis of estimates of human exposure to infants consuming bottled baby foods, recent risk-benefit analysis has concluded that trace levels of semicarbazide pose little threat to human health (53). The potential for human exposure to other environmental compounds or drugs that are semicarbazide-sensitive amine oxidase–inhibitors, or SSAO-inhibitors, is not known. Whether semicarbazide induces DAA following fetal exposure due to SSAO inhibition or some other molecular effect is not clear. Nevertheless, human exposure to common monoamine oxidase inhibitors, or MAO inhibitors, either as drugs or environmental chemicals, has long been known to cause a wide range of serious detrimental toxic effects (57), suggesting that the potential for adverse effects by SSAO inhibitors is real.

Recent Studies of a New Model of DAA

In earlier studies from this laboratory, we sought to uncover the physiologic role of SSAO by treating weanling (21-day-old) rats with a series of SSAO-inhibitors for one to three weeks (58). (The weanling period in rats is a time of rapid growth and production of connective tissues akin to human adolescence.) Treatment consisted of daily i.p. injections of the classic SSAO inhibitor, semicarbazide ($H_2NCONHNH_2$), or halo-substituted allylamines (AAs) originally developed by Merrill-Dow-Lynch, Inc. as specific SSAO inhibitors: MDL-72274 and MDL-72145 (kindly supplied by Dr. Lawrence Sayre). In the absence of systemic toxicity, we found striking pathology isolated to aorta. Aortic histology showed thinned, discontinuous, and frayed ELN fibers and increased fibrosis (Fig. 3). These alterations are well-described lesions of aging in the human aorta (31,59,60). Inhibition of aorta and lung SSAO activity was confirmed. The activity of the collagen and ELN cross-linking enzyme, lysyl oxidase, was unaltered in vascular tissue. Subsequent physiologic length-tension measurements in isolated aortic rings demonstrated dysfunctional elasticity of the aortic wall of weanling rats treated with SSAO inhibitors; this finding is also well described in aging aorta of several species (Fig. 4).

Biochemically, insoluble (mature) ELN was decreased, while total collagen was increased by SSAO inhibition during the weanling period. Abnormal collagen metabolism was confirmed in fetal aortic vascular smooth muscle cells

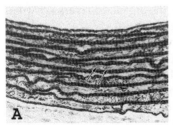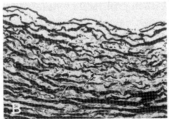

Figure 3 Weanling rat, SSAO inhibitor–treated; elastic tissue stain of thoracic aorta of control (**A**) versus treated (**B**) shows fragmented elastic lamellae. *Abbreviation*: SSAO, semicarbazide-sensitive amine oxidase.

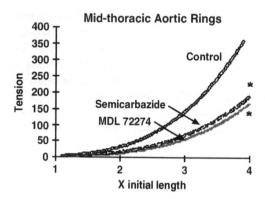

Figure 4 SSAO inhibition causes dysfunctional elasticity of aortic wall. Length-tension relationship is shown for aortic rings from conrol weanling rats vs. those from rats treated with SSAO inhibitors semicarbazide or MDL 72274 (arrows) for 21 days. An incremental increase in length (stretching) resulted in lower final resting tension in rings from inhibitor-treated rats, indicative of dysfunctional elasticity, i.e., inability to maintain tension after stretching. This finding is consistent with increased collagen and proportionally decreased elastin, and is a known aging-related change in connective tissues of several species. *Abbreviation*: SSAO, semicarbazide-sensitive amine oxidase.

grown in vitro (61). In these experiments, primary vascular smooth muscle cells, isolated from fetal or newborn aortas, as originally described by Jones et al. (62,63), served as a model for the study of interstitial protein production by isolated vascular smooth muscle cells. When kept in continuous culture for four weeks, these cells lay down a complex matrix of collagen, ELN, and other matriceal structural proteins.

We next explored the effects of SSAO inhibition on pregnant rats (dams) during the last trimester of fetal development. Gestational days 14 to 21 (GD, 14–21) were chosen for exposure to the environmental insult because this represents the most significant period of development of large elastic arteries. Specifically, the embryology and early development of the aorta in the rat indicate that mesenchymal myoblasts migrate into the vascular media from GD 14 to 17, with subsequent development of elastic fibers and collagen. Vascular smooth muscle cells then proliferate and lay down the organized layers known as elastic lamellae through extensive elastogenesis (33,64–66).

When newborn pups in these experiments were killed for histopathologic examination, a striking gross lesion was noted—a massive dissection of blood in the thoracic aorta that extended to the carotids and other vessels of the aortic arch (Fig. 5). At some doses, virtually 100% of pups showed the lesion (51). No other systemic lesions were found. Hemorrhage was contained by adventitia in all vessels examined. Fragments of ELN and vascular smooth muscle cells were seen mixed with the dissecting blood at points of juncture of dissection to normal media. Small tears of media, or "entry points" from the false lumen created by the dissection, were identified in a minority of cases and only in thoracic aorta.

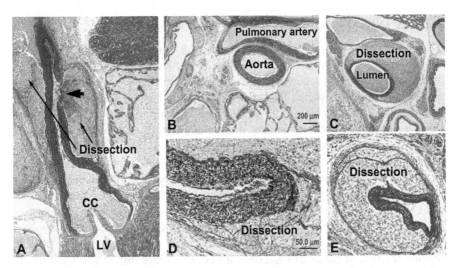

Figure 5 Histopathology of DAA in newborn rat. Transverse section through aortic root (**A**) shows left ventricular outflow tract (*LV*) and aortic valve cusps (*C*); Dissection of ascending aorta; note focal tear through media ("entry point") at arrowhead (Compare to human DAA, Fig. 1). Panel **B** shows cross section of intact control aorta; (**C**) newborn of treated dam. Higher power (**D**) shows fragmented elastin and shearing at outer third of media with few residual layers of smooth muscle and adventitia containing dissected blood. A high power view of carotid artery dissection is shown in (**E**). A and **E**: Verhoff von Giesen elastic tissue stains; **B–D**: Movat pentachrome. *Abbreviation*: DAA, dissecting aortic aneurysm.

Inflammatory cells were not seen. Dissection extended in a high percentage to the brachiocephalic arteries or abdominal aorta. These similarities to the human event of DAA were most remarkable.

In all arteries without dissection, the vascular wall, including elastic lamellae, showed no observable morphologic difference from control. Compared with control pups, experimental animals showed no differences in maternal weight, stillbirths, pup numbers/litter, or pup weights. Most interesting, however, was the fact that when we examined fetuses the day before birth (GD, 20) after the full range of doses used, DAAs were not found. This indicates that dissection occurred at birth or in the immediate postnatal period, perhaps associated with the sudden rise in systemic blood pressure and alterations in cardiac and vascular flow that accompany birth.

In summary, this recently described, acute animal model of DAA affords a unique opportunity to examine the underlying molecular flaws that result in aortic dissection in the absence of factors that confound most existing models of aneurysm (e.g., mechanical trauma, direct chemical injury, complex genetic manipulations, aging, or other degenerative changes). It is hoped that through studies of such in vivo phenomena, a better understanding of how injurious environmental exposures weaken the vascular wall will be forthcoming.

MEDIAL INJURY—FUNCTIONAL (PATHOPHYSIOLOGY)

Because the role of endothelial dysfunction [i.e., diminished bioavailability of endothelium-derived nitric oxide (NO)] is a well-recognized risk factor of cardiovascular disease of atherosclerosis, diabetes, and hypertension, its contribution to chemically-mediated medial dysfunction and injury will not be covered herein. Altered vascular reactivity in standard agonist tests is commonly observed in blood vessels of humans in vivo and experimental models ex vivo in response to disease or chemical exposure. The majority of these altered function tests involve hypercontractility or diminished relaxation (or both simultaneously) as a result of a decreased endothelium-derived release of NO. Relaxation of a precontracted blood vessel with a NO donor (e.g., sodium nitroprusside) indicates the presence of a competent soluble guanylyl cyclase-cGMP-PKG system in the vascular smooth muscle. However, when there is a deficit in blood vessel relaxation to a NO donor, as in murine coronary arteries exposed to volatile organic fraction of diesel exhaust (67), it becomes more difficult to functionally evaluate the status of endothelium-derived NO. Moreover, intimal injury involves a coordinated repair response that predictably alters endothelium and vascular smooth muscle cell structure and function, and thus, responses to chemically or surgically induced intimal injury is not covered herein.

Two basic dysfunctions prevail in the vasculature: too much vaso-relaxation, leading to decreased peripheral resistance and a drop in blood pressure (hypotension) or too much vasoconstriction, possibly leading to tissue ischemia and hypoxia (e.g., vasospasm). Targets of smooth muscle cells for chemical modification include surface membrane proteins such as G-protein-coupled receptors (GPCR), voltage- and stretch-dependent ion channels (Ca^{++}, K^{+}), junctional and adhesion molecules (connexin 43), and numerous enzymes (Na^{+}/K^{+} ATPase) to name but a few. Additional intracellular targets of modification regulate release and uptake of calcium (Ca^{++}-ATPase), cyclic nucleotide metabolism (e.g., phosphodiesterases, PDE), mitochondrial electron transport/ATP synthesis (cytochrome c oxidase), and myofilament function. Whatever the specific chemical and target, typically foreign compounds undergo bioactivation mediated by specific enzymes located where they presumably function with endogenous substrates. By studying specific cases of chemically induced medial injury, we can learn both the mechanism of action of a compound but also, and importantly, the endogenous function of a specific enzyme. In any case, xenobiotic bioactivation is often accompanied by free radical and reactive oxygen species (ROS) production, which may be a common denominator in subsequent vascular injury and dysfunction.

Role of Oxidative Stress and Aldehyde Generation in Vascular Wall Injury

Oxidation of unsaturated fatty acids of lipoproteins and lipids forms alkoxyl and peroxyl radicals that decompose into several metastable carbonyl end products including the α,β-unsaturated aldehydes acrolein and 4-hydroxy-*trans*-2-nonenal (4HNE) (68,69). Additional sources of tissue acrolein include glucose oxidation of fatty acids (70) and the oxidation of polyamines by amine oxidase (71). Generation of acrolein by amine oxidase has been linked to the ability of polyamines to induce phase 2 enzymes (72) and produce cytotoxicity (73). Several disease states associated with oxidative stress and lipid peroxidation lead to the generation and accumulation of acrolein and 4HNE and their protein and DNA adducts. Increased levels of acrolein and 4HNE have been measured in plasma of patients with renal failure (74), in Alzheimer's patients' brain tissues (75), and human and experimental models of heart failure. Moreover, increased acrolein-protein adducts have been detected in vascular tissues of patients with diabetes (76–78), Alzheimer's disease (79,80), and atherosclerosis (81,82). Additionally, inflammation can also generate acrolein. Acrolein is generated upon oxidation of L-threonine by myeloperoxidase, and its production by neutrophils could contribute to vascular damage at sites of inflammation (83). Finally, acrolein is specifically derived from oxidative deamination of AA by primarily smooth muscle-localized SSAO enzyme (*vide supra*). Thus, unsaturated aldehydes generated from a variety of sources, including oxidative stress, could act as final common denominators in chemical toxicity of the vascular wall and, as demonstrated for the specific case of AA and ß-aminopropionitrile cotreatment, medial injury and aortic dysfunction (84,85).

Aldehydes and Vasorelaxation

To understand the role of unsaturated aldehydes, in general, and acrolein, specifically, in functional medial injury, blood vessel responses to acrolein in vitro have been studied. In precontracted isolated human and rodent arteries and perfused mesenteric beds, invariably, acrolein (or 4HNE) stimulates vasorelaxation at sub-µM to mM concentrations (86–89). These aldehyde-induced relaxations appear species and blood vessel independent and endothelium dependent, although the specific relaxing factors and mechanisms are not fully defined. For example, in rat aorta LNAME (NOS inhibitor) or indomethacin (COX inhibitor) pretreatment inhibits acrolein-induced relaxation (87), while LNAME or indomethacin pretreatment has no effect on acrolein-induced dilatation in rat mesenteric bed, thus, implicating release of an endothelium-derived relaxing factor (EDRF) that is neither NO nor a prostanoid but perhaps an endothelium-derived hyperpolarizing factor (EDHF) in this vascular bed (86). However, the toxicologic significance of these exposures is not clear, as most studies do not report subsequent effects of acrolein or 4HNE exposure on blood vessel ex vivo viability. In perfused rat mesenteric bed preparations, acrolein-induced relaxations were repeatable and did not alter subsequent agonist-induced precontractions or relaxations, indicating little toxicity under these conditions (86).

Acrolein Generation and Vasospasm—A Medial Injury Model

By comparison, the effects of the acrolein generator, AA, are more varied and dramatic with definitive toxicity to both endothelium and smooth muscle. For example, AA addition to precontracted isolated blood vessels induces a biphasic

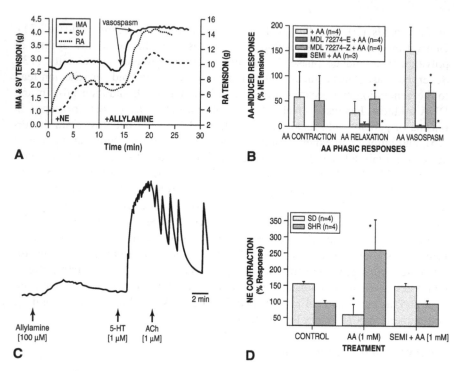

Figure 6 AA induces vasospasm (hypercontraction) in human coronary artery bypass graft blood vessels (internal mammary artery, IMA; radial artery, RA; saphenous vein, SV; **A,B**), naïve Sprague-Dawley (SD) rat left coronary artery (**C**) and spontaneously hypertensive rat (SHR; **D**) aorta in a SSAO-dependent manner (**B,D**). *Abbreviations:* Allylamine, AA; NE, norepinephrine; SEMI, semicarbazide; 5-HT, serotonin; ACh, acetylcholine; SSAO, semicarbazide-sensitive amine oxidase.

response where rapid relaxation is abruptly reversed to a powerful contraction (vasospasm) by 1 mM AA (Fig. 6 **A**). This AA-induced contraction (or spasm) is SSAO dependent in rodent and human blood vessels, as it is inhibited by pretreatment with semicarbazide or with a more specific SSAO inhibitor, MDL 72274-*E* (Fig. 6 **B**) (90,91). It is well established that all observed forms of AA-induced cardiovascular toxicity in vivo and in vitro are inhibited by semicarbazide pretreatment (92–95). Similarly, in uncontracted rat aorta and rat coronary artery blood vessels, AA induces concentration-dependent, although modest, contractions (Fig. 6 **C**) (90,96).

Increased Susceptibility to Acrolein-Induced Vasospasm

What is particularly striking about AA-induced vasoaction is that preexposure to AA or oxidative stress in vivo enhances blood vessel responses to subsequent AA exposure in vitro. This increased susceptibility, likely due to acrolein-induced medial injury, is best illustrated by the observed increases in AA-induced contractile behavior in isolated aorta of rats treated for 10 days with AA (96) or from spontaneously hypertensive rats (SHR) (Fig. 6 **D**)—both models sharing an increased oxidative stress in the vessel wall (97–100). Moreover, AA-induced effects are largely independent of endothelium function indicating that smooth muscle localization of the SSAO enzyme likely provides both the site of acrolein generation and proximity to the target of acrolein toxicity. Acrolein exposure in isolated tracheal smooth muscle also increases contractility and eicosanoid release by increasing cytoplasmic free calcium (101–103)—a mechanism that easily accommodates both increased release of EDRFs/EDHFs and smooth muscle hypercontractility but for which there is limited experimental data in blood vessels (86,91). Thus, sensitivity to AA- (or acrolein)-induced injury could be enhanced by prior oxidative stress, and this likely contributes to the dramatic vasospasm observed in human coronary artery bypass graft (CABG) blood vessels, which are obtained from patients with many risk factors, including hypertension, hypercholesterolemia, diabetes, and smoking (91).

Medial Metabolism of Other Vasoactive and Potentially Toxic Amines

Exogenous and endogenous amines represent a pool of compounds that can be metabolized by SSAO [or related amine oxidases, such as VAP-1 (104–106)] in and around the vascular wall and potentially damage the adventitia, endothelium, and media. However, excepting AA, the majority of metabolized exogenous amines have limited toxicity in isolated blood vessels, perfused vascular beds, and cultured smooth muscle cells (107–110). For example, benzylamine (BZA) and methylamine (MA), both very good substrates of vascular SSAO (111–113), stimulate relaxation in precontracted isolated human CABG blood vessels without injury or vasospasm (91,114). In fact, MA-induced relaxation in human CABG vessels is SSAO dependent but produced no toxicity even at 1-mM concentration for greater than 40-minute exposure (114). Similarly, BZA induces a robust and sensitive relaxation in human CABG blood vessels without toxicity. Published data also support the weak toxicity of these amines in cultured smooth muscle cells (109,110), although a variety of studies implicate MA metabolism to formaldehyde in endothelium toxicity, including from nicotine exposure (115–118). Moreover and importantly, these data indicate that acrolein, and not H_2O_2 or NH_3, is the primary injurious molecule generated from SSAO-mediated metabolism of AA, hence use of the term "acrolein generator." Thus, it appears that acrolein generation in the vascular wall is mechanistically linked with increased contractility independent of changes in endothelium function, which indicates that the medial layer (like the endothelium) is sensitive to the effects of aldehyde exposure—a susceptibility that is exacerbated by pre-existing oxidative stress. It is critical to better understand the role of metabolism of ROS and ROS-induced aldehydes in the blood vessel wall to identify the mechanisms and targets of aldehyde action in the blood vessel wall (99,119).

CONCLUSION

This chapter has addressed medial injury from both a structural and physiologic point of view, with emphasis on environmental influences as etiologic agents of vascular injury. The examples of structural injury given, along with descriptions of the importance of these lesions to common human diseases, illustrate the many areas in which further research is needed. For example, it is important to more fully understand how cigarette smoke causes injury to the blood vessel wall or how prenatal exposures might result in subtle vascular injury that becomes manifest only later during life.

From a functional standpoint, cardiovascular diseases, including atherosclerosis and heart failure, are associated with increased ROS and aldehyde formation and protein-aldehyde adducts of acrolein and 4HNE indicating a potential causal role for aldehyde-related injury to the arterial media during the progression of cardiovascular diseases. While endothelium dysfunction likely contributes to decreased physiologic vasorelaxation, increased thrombosis, and propensity for plaque rupture, the direct effects of aldehydes on medial function and pathophysiology, including vasospasm, have been less well studied.

In our examples, amine metabolism by the medially located SSAO leads to robust vascular effects and in the specific case of the acrolein generator, AA, vasospasm (hypercontraction) in human CABG blood vessels. Susceptibility to acrolein-induced hypercontraction appears to be increased in vasculature under oxidative stress, and thus, these data indicate that medial injury could contribute to overall vascular pathophysiology in addition (or independently) to the well-established role of endothelial dysfunction. Future studies should be designed to identify those factors that increase susceptibility for medial oxidative stress and injury (e.g., polymorphisms in aldehyde-metabolizing enzymes), and thus, potentially contribute to vascular structural and functional defects in distinct human populations.

ACKNOWLEDGMENT

We acknowledge funding for work presented in this chapter from NIH HL-26145 (PJB), NIEHS ES-013038 (PJB), 1R15 ES-011141-01 (DJC), 1P01 ES-11860 (DJC), ES-12062 (DJC), and the University of Louisville E0566 (DJC). Research described in this article was supported in part by Philip Morris USA, Inc. and Philip Morris International (DJC).

REFERENCES

1. Kofoed KF, Czernin J, Johnson J, et al. Effects of cardiac allograft vasculopathy on myocardial blood flow, vasodilatory capacity, and coronary vasomotion. Circulation 1997; 95:600–606.

2. Reilly JM, Tilson MD. Incidence and etiology of abdominal aortic aneurysms. Surg Clin North Am 1989; 69:705–711.
3. Verloes A, Sakalihasan N, Limet R, et al. Genetic aspects of abdominal aortic aneurysm. In: Tilson MD, Boyd CD, eds. The Abdominal Aortic Aneurysm: Genetics, Pathophysiology, and Molecular Biology. New York, NY: The New York Academy of Science, 1996:44–55.
4. Collin J, Araujo L, Walton J, et al. Oxford screening programme for abdominal aortic aneurysm in men aged 65 to 74 years. Lancet 1988; 2:613–615.
5. Ascer E, DePippo PS, Hanson J, et al. A modern series of ruptured infrarenal aortic aneurysms. Improved survival at a cost. Ann N Y Acad Sci 1996; 800:231–233.
6. Clifton MA. Familial abdominal aortic aneurysms. Br J Surg 1977; 64:765–766.
7. Bengtsson H, Norrgard O, Angquist KA, et al. Ultrasonographic screening of the abdominal aorta among siblings of patients with abdominal aortic aneurysms. Br J Surg 1989; 76:589–591.
8. Yu AE, Hewitt RE, Connor EW, et al. Matrix metalloproteinases-novel targets for directed cancer therapy. Drugs and Aging 1997; 11:229–244.
9. Stetler-Stevenson WG. Matrix metalloproteinases in angiogenesis: a moving target for therapeutic intervention. J Clin Invest 1999; 103:1237–1241.
10. Westermarck J, Kahari V-M. Regulation of matrix metalloproteinase expression in tumor invasion. FASEB J 1999; 13:781–792.
11. Lemaire SA, Wang X, Wilks JA, et al. Matrix metalloproteinases in ascending aortic aneurysms: bicuspid versus trileaflet aortic valves. J Surg Res 2005; 123:40–48.
12. Cronenwett JL. Variables that affect the expansion rate and rupture of abdominal aortic aneurysms. Ann N Y Acad Sci 1996; 800:56–67.
13. Boor PJ, Langford SA. Pathogenesis of chemically induced arterial lesions. In: Sipes IG, McQueen CA, Gandolfi AG, eds. Comprehensive Toxicology. New York, NY: Elsevier Science, 1997:309–332.
14. Levinson B, Vulpe C, Elder B, et al. The mottled gene is the mouse homologue of the Menkes disease gene. Nature Genet 1994; 6:369–373.
15. Nackman GB, Karkowski FJ, Halpern VJ, et al. Elastin degradation products induce adventitial angiogenesis in the Anidjar/Dobrin rat aneurysm model. Surgery 1997; 122:39–44.
16. Stehbens WE. Aneurysm. In: Stehbens WE, Lie JT, eds. Vascular Pathology. New York, NY: Chapman and Hall Medical, 1995:353–414.
17. Hagan PG, Nienaber CA, Isselbacher EM, et al. The International Registry of Acute Aortic Dissection (IRAD): new insights into an old disease3. JAMA 2000; 283:897–903.
18. Murai T, Baba M, Ro A, et al. Sudden death due to cardiovascular disorders: a review of the studies on the medico-legal cases in Tokyo. Keio J Med 2001; 50: 175–181.
19. Hayward C, Brock DJ. Medical ignorance contributes to toll from aortic illness. Wall Street Journal, New York, NY: 2003:A12–A13.
20. Dzau V, Creager MA. Diseases of the aorta. In: Braunwald E, Fauci AS, Kasper DL, et al, eds. Harrison's Principles of Internal Medicine. New York, NY: McGraw-Hill, 2001:1430–1434.
21. Mehta RH, Suzuki T, Hagan PG, et al. Predicting death in patients with acute type a aortic dissection. Circulation 2002; 105:200–206.

22. Trimarchi S, Nienaber CA, Rampoldi V, et al. Contemporary results of surgery in acute type A aortic dissection: The International Registry of Acute Aortic Dissection experience. J Thorac Cardiovasc Surg 2005; 129:112–122.

23. Basso C, Morgagni GL, Thiene G. Spontaneous coronary artery dissection: a neglected cause of acute myocardial ischaemia and sudden death. Br Heart J 1996; 75:451–454.

24. Murai T, Saito K, Takada A, et al. Subarachnoid hemorrhage from ruptured dissecting aneurysm of the vertebral artery: a clinico-pathological study. Res Pract Forens Med 1993; 36:175–183.

25. Milewicz DM, Urban Z, Boyd C. Genetic disorders of the elastic fiber system. Matrix Biol 2000; 19:471–480.

26. Albornoz G, Coady MA, Roberts M, et al. Familial thoracic aortic aneurysms and dissections—incidence, modes of inheritance, and phenotypic patterns. Ann Thorac Surg 2006; 82:1400–1405.

27. Isselbacher EM. Diseases of the aorta. In: Zipes DP, Libby P, Bonow RO, et al., eds. Braunwald's Heart Disease. Philadephia, PA: Elsevier Saunders, 2005:1403–1435.

28. Sailer S. Dissecting aneurysms of the aorta in persons under forty years of age. Arch Pathol 1942; 33:704–730.

29. Nakashima Y, Shiokawa Y, Sueshi K. Alterations of elastic architecture in human aortic dissecting aneurysm. Lab Invest 1992; 62:751–760.

30. Dobrin PB, Schwarcz TH, Baker WH. Mechanisms of arterial and aneurysmal tortuosity. Surgery 1988; 104:568–571.

31. Tilson MD, Elefteriades JBCM. Tensile strength and collagen in abdominal aortic aneurysm disease. In: Greenhalgh RM, Mannick JA, Powell JT, eds. The Cause and Management of Aneurysms. London, UK: W.B. Saunders, 1990:97–103.

32. Curran M, Atkinson DL, Ewart AK, et al. The elastin gene is disrupted by a translocation associated with supravalvular aortic stenosis. Cell 1993; 73:159–168.

33. Prockop DJ, Kuivaniemi H, Tromp G, et al. Inherited disorders of connective tissue. In: Braunwald E, Fauci AS, Kasper DL, et al., eds. Harrison's Principles of Internal Medicine. New York, NY: McGraw-Hill, 2001:2290–2300.

34. Li DY, Brooke B, Davis EC, et al. Elastin is an essential determinant of arterial morphogenesis. Nature 1998; 393:276–280.

35. Davis GE, Bayless KJ, Davis MJ, et al. Regulation of tissue injury responses by the exposure of matricryptic sites within extracellular matrix molecules. Am J Path 2000; 156:1489–1498.

36. Chao JT, Martinez-Lemus LA, Kaufman SJ, et al. Modulation of alpha7-integrin-mediated adhesion and expression by platelet-derived growth factor in vascular smooth muscle cells. Am J Physiol Cell Physiol 2006; 290:C972–C980.

37. Sun Z, Martinez-Lemus LA, Trache A, et al. Mechanical properties of the interaction between fibronectin and alpha5beta1-integrin on vascular smooth muscle cells studied using atomic force microscopy. Am J Physiol Heart Circ Physiol 2005; 289:H2526–H2535.

38. Partridge CR, Williams ES, Barhoumi R, et al. Novel genomic targets in oxidant-induced vascular injury. J Mol Cell Cardiol 2005; 38:983–996.

39. Jones M, Sabatini PJ, Lee FS, et al. N-cadherin upregulation and function in response of smooth muscle cells to arterial injury. Arterioscler Thromb Vasc Biol 2002; 22:1972–1977.

40. Nili N, Zhang M, Strauss BH, et al. Biochemical analysis of collagen and elastin synthesis in the balloon injured rat carotid artery. Cardiovasc Pathol 2002; 11:272–276.

41. Franco CD, Hou G, Bendeck MP. Collagens, integrins, and the discoidin domain receptors in arterial occlusive disease. Trends Cardiovasc Med 2002; 12:143–148.
42. Orr AW, Helmke BP, Blackman BR, et al. Mechanisms of mechanotransduction. Dev Cell 2006; 10:11–20.
43. Behan WMH, Longman C, Petty RKH, et al. Muscle fibrillin deficiency in Marfan's syndrome myopathy. J Neurol Neurosurg Psychiatry 2003; 74:633–639.
44. Mizuguchi T, Collod-Beroud G, Akiyama T, et al. Heterozygous TGFBR2 mutations in Marfan syndrome. Nat Genet 2004; 36:855–860.
45. Loeys BL, Chen J, Neptune ER, et al. A syndrome of altered cardiovascular, craniofacial, neurocognitive and skeletal development caused by mutations in TGFBR1 or TGFBR2. Nat Genet 2005; 37:275–281.
46. Li S-W, Prockop DJ, Helminen H, et al. Transgenic mice with targeted inactivation of the Col2a1 gene for collagen II develop a skeleton with membranous and periosteal bone but no endochondral bone. Genes Dev 1995; 9:2821–2830.
47. Fassler R, Schnegelsberg PNJ, Dausman J, et al. Mice lacking alpha1 (IX) collagen develop noninflammatory degenerative joint disease. Proc Natl Acad Sci 1994; 91: 5070–5074.
48. Andrikopoulos K, Liu X, Keene DR, et al. Targeted mutation in the col5a2 gene reveals a regulatory role for type V collagen during matrix assembly. Nature Genetics 1995; 9:31–36.
49. Liu X, Hong W, Byrne M, et al. A targeted mutation at the known collagenase cleavage site in mouse Type I collagen impairs tissue remodeling. J Cell Biol 1995; 130:227–237.
50. Liu X, Hong W, Byrne M, et al. Type III collagen is crucial for collagen I fibrillogenesis and for normal cardiovascular development. Proc Natl Acad Sci 1997; 94:1852–1856.
51. Gong B, Trent MB, Srivastava D, et al. Chemical-induced, nonlethal, developmental model of dissecting aortic aneurysm. Birth Defects Res 2006; 76:29–38.
52. Schwarze U, Schievink WI, Petty E, et al. Haploinsufficiency for one COL3A1 allele of type III procollagen results in a phenotype similar to the vascular form of Ehlers-Danlos syndrome, Ehlers-Danlos syndrome type IV. Am J Hum Genet 2001; 69:989–1001.
53. Nestmann ER, Lynch BS, Musa-Veloso K, et al. Safety assessment and risk-benefit analysis of the use of azodicarbonamide in baby food jar closure technology: putting trace levels of semicarbazide exposure into perspective—a review. Food Addit Contam 2005; 22:875–891.
54. Toth B, Shimizu H. Tumorigenic effects of chronic administration of benzylhydrazine dihydrochloride and phenylhydrazine hydrochloride in Swiss mice. Z Krebsforsch Klin Onkol Cancer Res Clin Oncol 1976; 87:267–273.
55. Toth B, Shimizu H. 1-Carbamyl-2-phenylhydrazine tumorigenesis in Swiss mice. Morphology of lung adenomas. J Natl Cancer Inst 1974; 52:241–251.
56. Steffek AJ, Verrusio AC, Watkins CA. Cleft palate in rodents after maternal treatment with various lathyrogenic agents. Teratology 1972; 5:33–38.
57. Gong B, Boor PJ. The role of amine oxidases in xenobiotic metabolism. Expert Opin Drug Metab Toxicol 2006; 2:559–571.
58. Langford SA, Trent MB, Balakumaran A, et al. Developmental vasculotoxicity associated with inhibition of semicarbazide-sensitive amine oxidase. Toxicol Appl Pharmacol 1999; 155:237–244.

59. Cox RH, Kikta DC. Age related changes in thoracic aorta of obese Zucker rats. Am J Physiol 1992; 262:H1548–H1556.

60. Cox RH, Detweiler DK. Comparison of arterial wall properties in young and old racing greyhounds. Mech of Aging and Devel 1988; 44:51–67.

61. Langford SA, Trent MB, Boor PJ. Semicarbazide-sensitive amine oxidase and extracellular matrix deposition by smooth muscle cells. Cardiovas Toxicol 2002; 2: 141–150.

62. DeClerk YA, Jones PA. The effects of ascorbic acid on the nature and production of collagen and elastin by rat smooth muscle cells. In: 1980:217–225.

63. Jones PA, Scott-Burden T, Gevers W. Glycoprotein, elastin, and collagen secretion by rat smooth muscle cells. Proc Natl Acad Sci 1979; 76:353–357.

64. Berry CL, Looker T, Germain J. The growth and development of the rat aorta. I. Morphological aspects. J Anat 1972; 113:1–16.

65. Looker T, Berry CL. The growth and development of the aorta. II. Changes in nucleic acid and scleroprotein content. J Anat 1972; 113:17–34.

66. Iredale RB, Eccleston-Joyner CA, Rucker RB, et al. Ontogenic development of the elastic component of the aortic wall in spontaneously hypertensive rats. Clin Exp Hypertens A 1989; A11:173–187.

67. Campen MJ, Babu NS, Helms GA, et al. Nonparticulate components of diesel exhaust promote constriction in coronary arteries from ApoE-/- mice. Toxicol Sci 2005; 88:95–102.

68. Grosch W. Reactions of hydroperoxides-products of low molecular weights. In: Chan HWS, ed. Autoxidation of Unsaturated Lipids. London, UK: Academic Press, 1987:95–139.

69. Porter NA, Caldwell SE, Mills KA. Mechanisms of free radical oxidation of unsaturated lipids. Lipids 1995; 30:277–290.

70. Medina-Navarro R, Duran-Reyes G, Diaz-Flores M, et al. Glucose-stimulated acrolein production from unsaturated fatty acids. Hum Exp Toxicol 2004; 23:101–105.

71. Gahl WA, Pitot HC. Polyamine degradation in foetal and adult bovine serum. Biochem J 1982; 202:603–611.

72. Kwak MK, Kensler TW, Casero RA Jr. Induction of phase 2 enzymes by serum oxidized polyamines through activation of Nrf2: effect of the polyamine metabolite acrolein. Biochem Biophys Res Commun 2003; 305:662–670.

73. Sharmin S, Sakata K, Kashiwagi K, et al. Polyamine cytotoxicity in the presence of bovine serum amine oxidase. Biochem Biophys Res Commun 2001; 282:228–235.

74. Sakata K, Kashiwagi K, Sharmin S, et al. Increase in putrescine, amine oxidase, and acrolein in plasma of renal failure patients. Biochem Biophys Res Commun 2003; 305:143–149.

75. Lovell MA, Xie C, Markesbery WR. Acrolein is increased in Alzheimer's disease brain and is toxic to primary hippocampal cultures. Neurobiol Aging 2001; 22:187–194.

76. Daimon M, Sugiyama K, Kameda W, et al. Increased urinary levels of pentosidine, pyrraline and acrolein adduct in type 2 diabetes. Endocr J 2003; 50:61–67.

77. Suzuki D, Miyata T. Carbonyl stress in the pathogenesis of diabetic nephropathy. Intern Med 1999; 38:309–314.

78. Uesugi N, Sakata N, Nangaku M, et al. Possible mechanism for medial smooth muscle cell injury in diabetic nephropathy: glycoxidation-mediated local complement activation. Am J Kidney Dis 2004; 44:224–238.

79. Calingasan NY, Uchida K, Gibson GE. Protein-bound acrolein: a novel marker of oxidative stress in Alzheimer's disease. J Neurochem 1999; 72:751–756.

80. Lovell MA, Xie C, Markesbery WR. Acrolein is increased in Alzheimer's disease brain and is toxic to primary hippocampal cultures. Neurobiol Aging 2001; 22:187–194.

81. Uchida K, Kanematsu M, Sakai K, et al. Protein-bound acrolein: potential markers for oxidative stress. Proc Natl Acad Sci U S A 1998; 95:4882–4887.

82. Uchida K, Kanematsu M, Morimitsu Y, et al. Acrolein is a product of lipid peroxidation reaction. Formation of free acrolein and its conjugate with lysine residues in oxidized low density lipoproteins. J Biol Chem 1998; 273:16058–16066.

83. Anderson MM, Hazen SL, Hsu FF, et al. Human neutrophils employ the myeloperoxidase-hydrogen peroxide-chloride system to convert hydroxy-amino acids into glycolaldehyde, 2-hydroxypropanal, and acrolein. A mechanism for the generation of highly reactive alpha-hydroxy and alpha, beta-unsaturated aldehydes by phagocytes at sites of inflammation. J Clin Invest 1997; 99:424–432.

84. Kumar D, Hysmith RM, Boor PJ. Allylamine and b-aminopropionitrile induced vascular injury: an in vivo and in vitro study. Toxicol Appl Pharmacol 1990; 103:288–302.

85. Conklin DJ, Trent MB, Boor PJ. The role of plasma semicarbazide-sensitive amine oxidase in allylamine and beta-aminopropionitrile cardiovascular toxicity: mechanisms of myocardial protection and aortic medial injury in rats. Toxicology 1999; 138:137–154.

86. Awe SO, Adeagbo AS, D'Souza SE, et al. Acrolein induces vasodilatation of rodent mesenteric bed via an EDHF-dependent mechanism. Toxicol Appl Pharmacol. 2006; 217:266–276.

87. Tsakadze NL, Srivastava S, Awe SO, et al. Acrolein-induced vasomotor responses of rat aorta. Am J Physiol Heart Circ Physiol 2003; 285:H727–H734.

88. Martinez MC, Bosch-Morell F, Raya A, et al. 4-hydroxynonenal, a lipid peroxidation product, induces relaxation of human cerebral arteries. J Cereb Blood Flow Metab 1994; 14:693–696.

89. Romero FJ, Romero MJ, Bosch-Morell F, et al. 4-hydroxynonenal-induced relaxation of human mesenteric arteries. Free Rad Biol Med 1997; 23:521–523.

90. Conklin DJ, Boyce CL, Trent MB, et al. Amine metabolism: a novel path to coronary artery vasospasm. Toxicol Appl Pharmacol 2001; 175:149–159.

91. Conklin DJ, Bhatnagar A, Cowley HR, et al. Acrolein generation stimulates hypercontraction in isolated human blood vessels. Toxicol Appl Pharmacol 2006; 217:277–288.

92. Awasthi S, Boor PJ. Semicarbazide protection from in vivo oxidant injury of vascular tissue by allylamine. Tox Letters 1993; 66:157–163.

93. Boor PJ, Nelson TJ. Allylamine cardiotoxicity: III. Protection by semicarbazide and in vivo derangement of monoamine oxidase. Toxicology 1980; 18:87–102.

94. Awasthi S, Boor PJ. Lipid peroxidation and oxidative stress during acute allylamine-induced cardiovascular toxicity. J Vasc Res 1994; 31:33–41.

95. Ramos K, Grossman SL, Cox LR. Allylamine-induced vascular toxicity in vitro: prevention by semicarbazide-sensitive amine oxidase inhibitors. Toxicol. Appl. Pharmacol. 1988; 95(1):61–71.

96. Conklin DJ, Boor PJ. Allylamine cardiovascular toxicity: evidence for aberrant vasoreactivity in rats. Toxicol Appl Pharmacol 1998; 148:245–251.

97. Chu Y, Alwahdani A, Iida S, et al. Vascular effects of the human extracellular superoxide dismutase R213G variant. Circulation 2005; 112:1047–1053.

98. Misra P, Srivastava SK, Singhal SS, et al. Glutathione S-transferase 8-8 is localized in smooth muscle cells of rat aorta and is induced in an experimental model of atherosclerosis. Toxicol Appl Pharmacol 1995; 133:27–33.

99. McBride MW, Brosnan MJ, Mathers J, et al. Reduction of Gstm1 expression in the stroke-prone spontaneously hypertension rat contributes to increased oxidative stress. Hypertension 2005; 45:786–792.

100. Nabha L, Garbern JC, Buller CL, et al. Vascular oxidative stress precedes high blood pressure in spontaneously hypertensive rats. Clin Exp Hypertens 2005; 27:71–82.

101. Hyvelin JM, Roux E, Prevost MC, et al. Cellular mechanisms of acrolein-induced alteration in calcium signaling in airway smooth muscle. Toxicol Appl Pharmacol 2000; 164:176–183.

102. Roux E, Hyvelin JM, Savineau JP, et al. Calcium signaling in airway smooth muscle cells is altered by in vitro exposure to the aldehyde acrolein. Am J Respir Cell Mol Biol 1998; 19:437–444.

103. Ben-Jebria A, Crozet Y, Eskew ML, et al. Acrolein-induced smooth muscle hyperresponsiveness and eicosanoid release in excised ferret tracheae. Toxicol Appl Pharmacol 1995; 135:35–44.

104. Bono P, Salmi M, Smith DJ, et al. Isolation, structural characterization, and chromosomal mapping of the mouse vascular adhesion protein-1 gene and promoter. J Immunol 1998; 161:2953–2960.

105. Jaakkola K, Kaunismaki K, Tohka S, et al. Human vascular adhesion protein-1 in smooth muscle cells. Am J Path 1999; 155:1953–1965.

106. Salmi M, Jalkanen S. VAP-1: an adhesin and an enzyme. Trends Immunol 2001; 22:211–216.

107. Elliott J, Callingham BA. Effect of benzylamine and its metabolites on the responses of the isolated perfused mesenteric arterial bed of the rat. J Auton Pharmacol 1991; 11:323–335.

108. Elliott J, Callingham BA, Sharman DF. The influence of amine metabolizing enzymes on the pharmacology of tyramine in the isolated perfused mesenteric arterial bed of the rat. Br J Pharmacol 1989; 98:515–522.

109. Conklin DJ, Langford SD, Boor PJ. Contribution of serum and cellular semicarbazide-sensitive amine oxidase to amine metabolism and cardiovascular toxicity. Toxicol Sci 1998; 46:386–392.

110. Langford SD, Trent MB, Boor PJ. Cultured rat vascular smooth muscle cells are resistant to methylamine toxicity: no correlation to semicarbazide-sensitive amine oxidase. Cardiovasc Toxicol 2001; 1:51–60.

111. Boor PJ, Trent MB, Lyles GA, et al. Methylamine metabolism to formaldehyde by a vascular enzyme. Toxicology 1992; 73:251–258.

112. Yu PH. Oxidative deamination of aliphatic amines by rat aorta semicarbazide-sensitive amine oxidase. J Pharm Pharmacol 1990; 42:882–884.

113. Precious E, Gunn CE, Lyles GA. Deamination of methylamine by semicarbazide-sensitive amine oxidase in human umbilical artery and rat aorta. Biochem Pharmacol 1988; 37:707–713.

114. Conklin DJ, Cowley HR, Wiechmann RJ, et al. Vasoactive effects of methylamine in isolated human blood vessels: role of semicarbazide-sensitive amine oxidase,

formaldehyde, and hydrogen peroxide. Am J Physiol Heart Circ Physiol 2004; 286:667–676.

115. Deng Y, Boomsma F, Yu PH. Deamination of methylamine and aminoacetone increases aldehydes and oxidative stress in rats. Life Sci 1998; 63:2049–2058.

116. Gubisne-Haberle D, Hill W, Kazachkov M, et al. Protein cross-linkage induced by formaldehyde derived from semicarbazide-sensitive amine oxidase-mediated deamination of methylamine. J Pharmacol Exp Ther 2004; 310:1125–1132.

117. Yu PH, Zuo DM. Formaldehyde produced endogenously via deamination of methylamine. A potential risk factor for initiation of endothelial injury. Atherosclerosis 1996; 120:189–197.

118. Yu PH. Increase of formation of methylamine and formaldehyde in vivo after administration of nicotine and the potential cytotoxicity. Neurochem Res 1998; 23:1205–1210.

119. Conklin D, Prough R, Bhatnagar A. Aldehyde metabolism in the cardiovascular system. Mol BioSyst 2007; 3:136–150.

Index

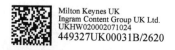